AN OUTLINE OF ORAL SURGERY

An Outline of Oral Surgery

Part One

Gordon R. Seward MDS(Lond), FDS RCS(Eng), FRCS, FRCS(Edin), MBBS(Lond)
Emeritus Professor of Oral and Maxillo-Facial Surgery in the University of London at the London Hospital Medical College; Consulting Oral and Maxillo-Facial Surgeon to the Royal London Hospital

Malcolm Harris MD(Lond), FDS RCS(Eng), FFDRCSI
Professor of Oral and Maxillo-Facial Surgery, University of London; Head of the Departments of Oral and Maxillo-Facial Surgery, The Eastman Dental Hospital and University College Hospital; Honorary Consultant at the Eastman Dental Hospital and University College Hospital

David A. McGowan MDS(QU Belfast), PhD(Lond), FDS RCS(Eng), FFDRCSI, FDSRCPS(Glas)
Professor of Oral Surgery and Head of the Department of Oral Surgery, University of Glasgow; Honorary Consultant Oral Surgeon to Greater Glasgow Health Board (Glasgow Dental Hospital and Glasgow Royal Infirmary)

Part Two

H.C. Killey FDS RCS(Eng), FDS, HDD RCS(Edin), LRCP(Lond), MRCS(Eng)
Professor of Oral Surgery, London University; Head of Department of Oral Surgery, Eastman Dental Hospital and Westminster Hospital Teaching Group

G.R. Seward MDS(Lond), MBBS(Lond), FDS RCS(Eng)
Professor of Oral Surgery, London University; Head of Department of Oral Surgery, The London Hospital Medical College; Hon. Consultant, The London Hospital Group

L.W. Kay MDS, FDS RCS(Eng), LRCP(Lond), MRCS(Eng)
Reader in Oral Surgery, London University; Honorary Consultant, Eastman Dental Hospital

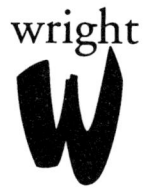

Wright
An imprint of Butterworth-Heinemann
Linacre House, Jordan Hill, Oxford OX2 8DP
A division of Reed Educational and Professional Publishing Ltd

℞ A member of the Reed Elsevier plc group

OXFORD   BOSTON   JOHANNESBURG
MELBOURNE   NEW DELHI   SINGAPORE

Part One
First published by IOP Publishing Ltd 1971
Reprinted 1975, 1979, 1981, 1982, 1983
Second edition 1987
Revised reprint 1992
Reprinted 1996

Part Two
First published by John Wright 1971
Revised reprint 1975
Reprinted 1979, 1983, 1984, 1987, 1989, 1993

Single volume edition 1998

© Reed Educational and Professional Publishing Ltd 1998

All rights reserved. No part of this publication may be reproduced in
any material form (including photocopying or storing in any medium by
electronic means and whether or not transiently or incidentally to some
other use of this publication) without the written permission of the
copyright holder except in accordance with the provisions of the Copyright,
Designs and Patents Act 1988 or under the terms of a licence issued by the
Copyright Licensing Agency Ltd, 90 Tottenham Court Road, London,
England W1P 9HE. Applications for the copyright holder's written
permission to reproduce any part of this publication should be addressed
to the publishers

British Library Cataloguing in Publication Data
A catalogue record for this book is available from the British Library

ISBN 0 7236 1061 4

Printed and bound in Great Britain by
Hartnolls Limited, Bodmin, Cornwall

Part One

PREFACE TO THE SECOND EDITION

The sad demise of both Professor Killey and Mr Kay left a serious gap in the field of academic oral surgery. Both were skilled and popular teachers whose books had a deserved popularity. Two new authors have joined me to write this second edition: Professor Malcolm Harris, who succeeded Professor Killey at the Postgraduate Institute of Dental Surgery, and Professor David McGowan from Glasgow Dental School. In revising the text we hope we have preserved the tradition established by the former authors.

It has again been our intention that Part I should embrace those aspects of oral surgery which are essential in the undergraduate course and for daily general dental practice. Part II deals with aspects of oral surgery seen more often in hospital, but the division is arbitrary and senior undergraduates will find that the topics in Part II are also covered during the latter part of their course. We hope also that general dental practitioners will find Part II useful for reference.

In Part I sufficient detail of practical technique is covered to ensure that the beginner develops sound habits, but obviously coverage in depth for all procedures is impossible in a book of this size and indeed practical surgery is often best taught by example and by close supervision by a senior oral surgeon.

Young trainees need to revise what was taught during the undergraduate course, to round out their knowledge to match their greater clinical responsibilities and to prepare for higher examinations. We hope this book will continue to serve them also.

Once again we have omitted consideration of traumatic injuries to the mandible and maxilla which are covered in other books in the Dental Practitioner Handbook series.

G. R. S.
M. H.
D. A. M.

PREFACE TO THE FIRST EDITION

This *Outline of Oral Surgery* is written as a guide for postgraduate and senior undergraduate students and for practitioners with a special interest in oral surgery. It is not intended as a textbook for the established consultant in the specialty, for in a book of this size it is impossible to consider the subject in the necessary detail.

The field of oral surgery covers a wide range of topics and in a work of this nature it is impossible to discuss the entire specialty. Space has therefore been devoted to the more important aspects of oral surgery, but even so it has been necessary to divide the work into two volumes. Although these two books are complementary, each volume is more or less complete in itself. Part I is mainly devoted to the practical aspects of minor oral surgery and should be of value to all dental practitioners who perform surgery, while Part II deals with the needs of the dental surgeon working in a hospital.

At the request of the publisher, fractures of the mandible and middle third of the facial skeleton have not been discussed as these subjects have been dealt with elsewhere in the Dental Practitioner Handbook series, and illustrations have been cut to a minimum in order to reduce costs.

It is the authors' sincere hope that this *Outline of Oral Surgery* will be of help to students preparing for undergraduate final examinations and for higher examinations in dentistry.

H. C. K.
G. R. S.
L. W. K.

CONTENTS

1. Patient Management, Preoperative Planning, Instruments and Sterilization 1
2. Intraoral Incisions and Suturing 28
3. The Removal of Roots 43
4. Unerupted and Impacted Teeth 52
5. Surgical Preparation of the Mouth for Dentures 92
6. Pyogenic Infections of the Soft Tissues 121
7. Inflammatory Diseases of Bone 174
8. The Control of Infections 208
9. Sinusitis, Oroantral Fistula and Removal of a Tooth or Root from the Maxillary Sinus 235
10. Surgical Endodontics 254
11. Cysts of the Jaws 263
12. Soft Tissue Swellings of the Oral Mucosa 297
13. The Diagnosis and Management of Orofacial Pain 313
14. Drugs and Oral Surgery 341

Index 367

CHAPTER 1

PATIENT MANAGEMENT, PREOPERATIVE PLANNING, INSTRUMENTS AND STERILIZATION

INTRODUCTION TO PATIENT MANAGEMENT

The practice of any branch of surgery requires diagnostic ability, technical skill, judgement and compassion. Diagnostic ability is founded upon a knowledge of the natural history of diseases and of the varied way in which they are manifest in patients. It depends upon the ability to listen patiently to the history while establishing a rapport with the patient so as to develop a level of confidence and trust. The consultation is likely to be accompanied by an undercurrent of varying emotions for the patient, though often they are successfully suppressed. If the clinician fails to recognize their presence and respond appropriately, but in a controlled fashion, the patient will think him or her unsympathetic. On the other hand, the clinician must preserve a degree of detachment to ensure that judgement is not impaired. Some patients will be frankly fearful and indeed if their disease is serious may have just cause for being so. They may express their fear by a show of aggression and it is particularly important that the clinician should not respond to this by irritation or anger. Others may put on a light hearted air or become garrulous in order to conceal their fear.

The history of the present condition (HPC) is taken first because this is what the patient has come about and is anxious to relate to you. Initially the patient is encouraged to tell his or her story with the minimum of interference or prompting. Then the detail is filled out by more direct questioning and the order and relationship of events is established. With tact, facts are gently separated from opinions, including those of the patient, friends and relatives. A pattern of events will be established which may be recognized and one or more possible diagnoses can be tested by other questions designed either to confirm or exclude a particular condition. The nature of the principle complaint or complaints can now be expressed briefly as a title to the history and placed before the start of the account under the heading 'complaining of' (C/O).

It is necessary to review the patient's general health (GH). This may involve no more than an enquiry if he or she is generally fit and well, supplemented perhaps by questions about breathlessness, cough, pain in the chest, ankle swelling and whether the weight is steady. Alternatively, if the case so demands, a detailed system by system enquiry may be undertaken seeking evidence of any other bodily malfunctions.

The past history (PH) is usually enquired into next, often briefly by asking if the patient has had any serious illnesses in the past, any prolonged periods at home and particularly in bed, or any admissions to hospital. Problems with the heart or chest and rheumatic fever and chorea in particular may be specially mentioned.

During a hospital admission and before an operation it may be relevant to enquire systematically into the patient's past illnesses from childhood to the present time. The past history should of course include an account of dental problems and experiences of dental treatment.

The family history (FH) can be unexpectedly useful, leading the patient to tell you about the children, of elderly dependent relatives or the ill health of a husband or wife, all of which may enhance the understanding of the patient's own illness or warn of possible problems with postoperative care.

Similarly the social history (SH) is important as this too may reveal social and work pressures which may be relevant to the diagnosis or difficulties to be surmounted as a result of the illness or which might arise from an admission to hospital. (Who will look after a young widow's small child if mother and father live abroad?). Details of medicines, injections or tablets which are taken regularly must not be overlooked, nor an enquiry into allergies to drugs, dressings or other substances.

The patient will expect you to examine the site of the complaint first and will be puzzled, possibly disturbed if your routine of examination doesn't permit this. The examination of the lesion should be systematic and methodical, actively relating what is found to the details of the history. Do not forget to look for physical signs that are appropriate to the differential diagnosis which should have formed already in your mind, even if negative observations have to be recorded as these are as valuable as the positive ones. Next examine the structures which are functionally related to the part complained of, such as the regional lymph nodes. Finally, take a look at the rest of the head and neck and oral cavity. A more general examination of the patient is always appropriate and normally sufficient information can be gleaned by simple observation during the consultation. The patient may have mentioned palpitations and breathlessness. Think back: was he or she breathless while entering the room or giving the history? Is the patient using the sternomastoid muscles now when taking a breath? Feel the pulse: is it in fact fast, and regular or irregular? What about finger clubbing while you are holding the hand. Is the patient pale and were the mucous membranes pale when you examined them? Is the thyroid enlarged or is there ankle oedema, and so on.

However, where in-patient surgery is required and in the case of the physically ill out-patient, a full general physical examination is indicated. For a patient attending a general dental practice, the patient's general medical practitioner will usually provide the necessary information or will examine the patient afresh if this is appropriate.

PATIENT MANAGEMENT

Radiographic and other imaging investigations, clinical laboratory tests and the question of a biopsy come next. Special investigation should be requested thoughtfully and sparingly, selecting those which will answer specific questions, or provide information essential for diagnosis and treatment planning. Automation of laboratory investigations has made various tests cheaper to process, provides the results more rapidly, and often with greater accuracy than when they were all done individually by hand, but the batch ordering of liver function tests, 'bone profiles' and haematological 'print-outs' has worked against precision of thought. It is too easy to tick all the boxes on the computer form and forget the cost and resources involved. The results of modern imaging methods have considerable visual appeal, but their cost can be very high and an investigation should not be ordered unless it confers a real benefit for the patient's management.

A differential diagnosis involves the consideration and comparison initially of groups of diseases but ultimately of perhaps two or three individual conditions all of which share various clinical and pathological features in common. First, whole groups of conditions and then individual diseases are eliminated because certain of their features are unlike those of the particular patient's illness. Ultimately a single condition is chosen on a 'best-fit' basis.

A diagnosis therefore involves the recognition of a specific pattern in the available data. Even with straightforward cases alternative possibilities should be considered even if they are rapidly dismissed in favour of the obvious. This way any item of data which may be inconsistent with the obvious solution and which suggests the possibility of some alternative explanation will not be disregarded. Dealing successfully with the variability of the disease and of the patient in which it is manifest is part of the intellectual pleasure to be gained from surgical practice. Herein lies the value of a large clinical experience. No clinician has seen it all, but the more he or she has seen the more valued the opinion.

From time to time all clinicians find themselves unable to make a diagnosis or reach a conclusion about the best management for a difficult case and must seek the aid of a colleague. This may be done by a straight referral or by consultation. The advantage of the latter approach is that one is able to watch the other practitioner at work and learn directly from him or her. Sometimes one's failure is seen to result from not properly following the basic techniques of clinical and diagnostic methodology. Often one requires the knowledge and skills of a more experienced dental practitioner, frequently a consultant or specialist with in-depth knowledge and ability in a particular field. At other times expert advice from a practitioner in some quite different discipline appears appropriate. Where this other discipline is a speciality of medicine rather than dentistry it is usual for the general dental practitioner to contact the patient's general medical practitioner who, if he agrees, will arrange the referral. Indeed, often the medical GP is the appropriate person to whom the patient should be directed, with of course a letter or telephone call (or both) from the referring dentist. In hospital practice it is usually more convenient to refer the patient to another department directly.

Increasingly during practising life the dentist will be able to make the correct diagnosis even when the condition is unusual in its presentation or is uncommon. However, it may still be necessary to refer the patient to a colleague who has the requisite treatment skills or relevant special facilities. Wise general dental practitioners will develop their own special interests as a source of professional satisfaction and as a means of increasing the interests of professional life. Discussion of cases and problems either with or without the patient being present is always fruitful. Where a decision is difficult, discussion even with a more junior and less experienced colleague will help to clarify one's own viewpoint, and of course enlist the advice and moral support of one's fellow practitioner. Simply a different way of thinking about the matter may be what is required. Without falling into the trap of always 'talking shop', general chat about professional matters at the practice and at meetings and conferences is an important part of continuing professional education.

The skills required for successful oral surgery are no less demanding than those of surgery in other regions of the body and the same basic principles apply. Dentists trained and experienced mainly in the disciplines of restorative dentistry bring to oral surgery skills in the handling of patients and in manual technique but these need to be applied thoughtfully to bone and soft tissues which respond to cutting in a way which is quite different to that of the dental hard tissues. Above all the tissues must be handled gently because rough retraction and unnecessarily vigorous instrumentation bruises the soft tissues and leads to excessive oedema and delayed wound healing. Bone which has been overheated by burs or crushed by elevators will die and must be resorbed or sequestrated before healing occurs and such damage creates unnecessary postoperative pain. The rigorous avoidance of bacterial contamination will maximize the healing potential and ensure that postoperative recovery is as rapid and comfortable as possible.

Successful surgery depends on thorough preparation which anticipates the requirements of the operation and avoids the necessity for compromise, or risk of failure, during the procedure. The preparation involves not only physical preparation, such as having available all the equipment and instruments which may be needed from the beginning, but mental preparation. As much information as possible about the task to be undertaken and the circumstances and problems to be encountered is obtained by examining the patient, relevant radiographs and models, etc. Each stage in the proposed operation is reviewed in the mind and for the more complicated procedures the order in which the various stages are to be tackled is determined. Time spent in preparation and planning reduces

PATIENT MANAGEMENT

operating time and the increased efficiency decreases the level of stress for both the operator and the patient.

Students are always closely supervised and experienced help is never far away from the postgraduate trainee so that if unexpected difficulties arise advice can be given quickly or the teacher or senior practitioner can take over and bring the operation to a successful conclusion. But what does the experienced surgeon him or herself do under such circumstances? The first lesson is to keep calm. Apprehension and uncertainty reduce rational thinking and excited or loud behaviour transmits itself to others, preventing the effective teamwork which is necessary to meet the challenge.

Most often the answer lies in improved vision and better access. Difficulties develop at the bottom of deep, dark oozing holes: increase exposure by extending soft tissue wounds and by removing unimportant obscuring bone, control ooze—usually by simple pressure with a pack for a measured period of time—adjust the light and retraction, position the sucker to remove any blood and get a good look at the problem. If to continue the operation at one site is difficult, turn your attention to where progress can be made more easily. This way the area of difficulty will be reduced until all that is required finally is a limited procedure demanding the maximum of concentration. If, on rare occasions you have genuine thoughts about the need to abandon an operation, and this can be done without immediate hazard to the patient, you should. To proceed under these circumstances invites disaster. The patient needs to live to be operated upon another day!

Only three emergencies spell real danger for the patient and you and your team must know what to do should the occasion arise, and must be prepared to act promptly and efficiently to give effective treatment. You must know how to clear an obstructed airway, how to inflate the chest if there is respiratory failure and, if the form of the obstruction warrants it, how to perform a tracheostomy. Cardiac arrest requires immediate, effective, external cardiac massage in addition to ventilation of the lungs. Serious haemorrhage is the third life-threatening emergency. During surgery pressure on the bleeding site will always control haemorrhage. Mostly a general ooze will be stopped by sustained pressure and it will reduce bleeding from vessels to a level where the source can be seen and dealt with. Postoperative bleeding manifests itself by a rapidly increasing swelling, blood seeping through the suture line, or a sudden flow of blood along a drain. With small wounds a local anaesthetic with a vasoconstrictor is injected and the wound re-opened to stop the bleeding. With bleeding from a large operation site the patient is promptly re-anaesthetized with a general anaesthetic while an intravenous infusion of blood is set up. Usually the wound is not reopened before anaesthesia is achieved as this releases the pressure in the wound and increases the bleeding before it can be controlled. Only where the swelling threatens the airway is the wound opened at once. Once the bleeding can be controlled by direct pressure haste is no longer appropriate. Then deliberate action can be taken to remove clot, improve visibility and to search for the bleeding vessel, so achieving precise control without damage to nerves and other adjacent important structures.

Most textbooks give the impression that the prescription of treatment follows automatically once a diagnosis is reached. In practice things are rarely quite that straightforward. There may be several choices of treatment, or even a decision not to treat at all. The patient's age, general health, family and work responsibilities and the distance to the surgery can all affect the particular mode of treatment to be proposed. Also the broader concept of patient management embraces not only advice but patient participation in the selection of appropriate therapy. Possible complications, the degree of temporary disability and discomfort, and the chances of a successful or satisfactory outcome must all be weighed where the proposed treatment involves an operation. Sound advice is difficult to give if the condition is not currently causing trouble and where it is difficult to predict when or whether—or if ever—it will do so. The patient may be pleased now if you decide that nothing needs to be done, but sorry if in years to come an operation becomes essential, and is by then more difficult and more hazardous because the patient is no longer fit and well. Conversely, to persuade an unwilling patient to have elective surgery can lead to considerable trouble, particularly if through a mischance, it results in some permanent deficit, say a numb lip. The patient may make the decision for you if the reasons for and against the procedure are carefully explained, but often the final choice is thrown back to you. This informed approach enables the patient to give what is termed 'informed consent' to the surgical procedure.

For minor procedures on conscious, unsedated patients operated upon under local anaesthesia, a reasonable explanation with agreement by the patient in front of the staff is sufficient. Where sedation or a general anaesthetic is involved the more formal signing of a consent form by the patient, or a parent or guardian in the case of a child, is necessary with a counter signature by the clinician. Most operations carry some risks of complications or unwanted sequelae. Patients are usually warned about these and a formal note should be made to record what has been said. The list of rare and occasional complications can be long and quite frightening. It is not usual to add unreasonably to the patient's natural preoperative anxiety by recounting them unless a particular hazard is recognised. Where the surgeon foresees serious, possibly untreatable problems for the patient if nothing is done, it is right for him to urge an unwilling patient to have the surgery, but if after sensible discussion the patient declines, clearly he or she has the right to do so. Under the circumstances the clinician should continue to see the patient and offer what help will be accepted. If decisions are made thoughtfully and compassionately, in conjunction with the patient, on the basis of the data currently available, there should be no personal recriminations if in the light of future events the decision proves to be faulty. Any lessons that might be learnt should be added to one's experience.

Oral surgery operations are generally performed either under local anaesthesia in the general practitioner's own surgery or in a hospital outpatient clinic, or under general anaesthesia in the operating theatre either as an in-patient or on a day-stay basis. As the demands of these two situations are different, they will be discussed separately.

OPERATIONS UNDER LOCAL ANAESTHESIA IN THE DENTAL SURGERY OR CLINIC

Preparations

A preoperative check-list should include the following points.

1. *Preparation of the Patient*

The need for accurate preoperative diagnosis and careful assessment of the patient is obvious, but the need for their psychological preparation is sometimes neglected. A routine minor procedure for the operator may be a major traumatic episode for his patient, and every effort must be made to gain willing co-operation and to reduce mental stress. Time spent at the preoperative consultation in explanation of the planned procedure, perhaps with the help of radiographs, and relating it to the patient's previous experience of dental treatment, will help to reduce apprehension. At the same time the need for sedation as an adjunct to local analgesia, or even the desirability of general anaesthesia, can be discussed.

Immediately prior to the operation, the patient should be received in a courteous and unhurried fashion and seated comfortably in the dental chair. Unnecessary outer clothing should be removed since surgical drapes will be applied, and the heat from the operating light can lead to discomfort which may enhance the common tendency to fainting. The proposed procedure should be confirmed with the patient and a few words of reassurance and encouragement given. The appropriate local anaesthetic injections are given and the patient positioned so as to allow the operator a comfortable working posture and adequate vision. A backwards tilt of the patient of about 50° usually permits the dentist to see the operation site without bending. A more horizontal posture may be appropriate for some procedures, but blood and irrigation solutions must not be allowed to gravitate backwards into the throat as this produces a sensation of choking.

2. *Patient Information*

The patient's notes, and especially the radiographs, should be to hand and so mounted that there is no temptation to handle them once the surgeon has scrubbed. Radiographs must be of adequate quality, show the whole operative field clearly, and should be displayed on a viewing screen adjacent to the surgery chair. Avoid doing surgical procedures 'blind' without radiographs.

3. *Light*
Standard dental operating lights provide sufficient illumination for minor oral surgery but a means of adjustment without contamination of the operator's hands should be available. This may be either by the use of sterilizable handles or by the use of a dry swab, later discarded, which acts as a barrier between the fingers and the handle.

4. *Suction*
High vacuum, low velocity suction is most suitable for surgery and will be available in hospital, but the high flow low vacuum aspirators used in practice for restorative dentistry will suffice, provided a sterile tip of a suitable size and shape is used.

5. *Instruments*
The operating kit will be discussed in detail in the next section. Sets rather than individual instruments should be prepared and assembled in trays which can be sterilized and stored dry in sterile paper bags or cloth wrappings. It may, however, be convenient to prepare separately in individual bags special instruments which are only used occasionally.

6. *Assistance*
Skilled assistance is essential to efficient surgery, and no operation should be attempted without it. Staff have to be trained not only in the anticipation of the operator's needs, but also in the discipline of aseptic technique so that correct reactions are instinctive and the sterile chain is not broken. Even simple manoeuvres, such as suture removal, require assistance for their speedy and comfortable achievement. Good team work creates an atmosphere of efficiency which sustains the patient's morale.

7. *The Operator*
The surgeon must be mentally prepared, comfortably positioned and confident that the preoperative planning has been comprehensive and complete. The time available while awaiting the onset of local anaesthesia may be used conveniently for a final check on the instrument set and for setting up the suction and drill. During this time also the patient should be engaged in general conversation to prevent him or her dwelling unnecessarily upon the forthcoming procedure, a task which is often shared by the surgeon and the surgery assistant.

Sterilization
Scrupulous sterilization of all instruments and material is essential in oral surgery. Used instruments must be thoroughly cleaned before sterilization

and all deposits of blood and debris removed. Though contamination of oral wounds by the patient's resident bacterial flora is unavoidable, cross-infection from one patient to another or from operator to patient must be avoided.

1. *Disposable Items*
Many materials are supplied in sterile form by manufacturers, who can apply methods such as gamma irradiation which are not feasible for the treatment of small batches. Provided the source is a reputable manufacturer and the wrappings have not been damaged in transit, the sterility of such products can be relied upon. The use of manufacturer sterilized, single use scalpel blades and suture needles is particularly recommended, since adequate sterilization of such items in the surgery without damage to their cutting efficiency is difficult to achieve.

2. *Autoclaving*
Small autoclaves have virtually replaced water boilers, because of the abundant evidence that exposure to boiling water alone is insufficient to kill bacterial spores and destroy viruses. A satisfactory autoclave for oral surgical instruments should reach a temperature of 134° at 32 psi pressure and maintain it for 3½ minutes. If instrument packs are to be stored and not used shortly after sterilization, the autoclave cycle should end with a drying phase. Not all small surgery autoclaves have a drying phase and surgical instruments put away damp to store will tarnish, corrode or rust.

3. *Dry Heat Sterilization*
Instruments with a sharp cutting edge, such as chisels, are preferably sterilized by exposure to dry heat at 160 °C for one hour since autoclaving may reduce their sharpness and promote rusting.

Sterilization of handpieces is a particular problem and for some dry heat is preferable, but it must be preceded by careful cleaning and lubrication with special heat resistant oils. Others with sealed bearings or handpieces which have been pressure lubricated with appropriate oils can be autoclaved.

Knowledgeable manufacturers will offer advice about their equipment and the way in which it may be cleaned, lubricated and sterilized.

4. *Chemical Disinfection*
Unfortunately, no chemical solution is available which will sterilize instruments immersed in it without the risk of producing tissue damage if drops of the material are carried over into the wound at the time of use. The formerly common practice of storing cleaned and sterilized instruments in chemical solutions is unnecessary since both trays of instruments and individual items can be wrapped in paper or cloth packs for sterilizing. Then individual items can be unwrapped without contaminating the rest.

5. Hand Disinfection

Proprietary preparations are now available for preoperative washing of the hands of surgeon and assistant, which have an effective bactericidal effect that is cumulative with repeated use and which do not cause excessive drying of the skin. Three suitable preparations are 'Hibiscrub' and 'Phisomed', which contain 4 per cent chlorhexidine gluconate, and 'Betadine', which contains 7·5 per cent povidone-iodine. If these are not available, then a soap containing a disinfectant like hexachlorophane should be used and washing must be continued for 5 minutes in running water. Following drying of the hands and forearms, 70 per cent alcohol or 'Hibisol' (2·5 per cent chlorhexidine in 70 per cent alcohol) lotion may be applied as an extra precaution.

Whatever agent is used, nails should be cut short and all jewellery removed before washing, and the nails should be scrubbed first thoroughly with a brush. Provided this cleansing routine is conscientiously followed, the wearing of surgical gloves during the performance of minor procedures is not essential for the avoidance of wound infection. However, gloves do help to protect the operator from infection by bacteria and more importantly from viruses in the patient's blood, and when worn for this purpose may be washed and worn for more than one operation, provided that they have not been punctured or damaged. Dentists are strongly advised to wear gloves when treating patients and even when merely examining patients.

In dental practice and outpatient clinic conditions a clean, freshly laundered gown is perfectly adequate and more readily available than packed sterile operating gowns. A surgical mask in certain circumstances is a sensible measure, but recent work on wound infection suggest that there is probably little benefit from its use during out-patient minor oral surgery. However, some operators prefer to follow the full operating theatre procedure and set up the appropriate facilities to permit this.

Where the operator has good eyesight and does not normally wear glasses a pair with plain lenses will protect the eyes from sprayed debris when rotary cutting instruments are used and from splashes of blood or pus.

6. Preparation and Isolation of the Operation Site

The circumoral skin should be cleaned with either the same preparation used for the operator's hands or aqueous or alcoholic solutions of the same agents. Disinfection of the oral mucosal surface is more difficult to achieve effectively, but a rinse with aqueous 0·5 per cent chlorhexidine can be used if desired. It is much more important that plaque and debris should be removed from the gingival margin and interdental embrasures before surgery, and when the oral hygiene has been poor, a preoperative scaling is desirable. Following this the patient should be instructed in oral hygiene techniques. Several days of tooth cleaning preoperatively will materially

PATIENT MANAGEMENT

reduce the local bacterial population even where patients have neglected the mouth for some time.

Needle puncture sites in the oral mucosa should be dried and an antiseptic, such as alcoholic chlorhexidine 0·5 per cent in 70 per cent alcohol or povidone-iodine solution may be applied, if desired. It is probable, however, that the main benefit is achieved by drying the surface of the mucosa and excluding saliva from the area. Sterile towels may be draped round the patient's head to cover the hair, leaving only the mouth and eyes exposed. A towel covering the chest and shoulders is essential since this is the area most likely to be touched by the operator's or assistant's hands or the dangling end of a suture. The suction tubing may be conveniently clipped to this towel so that its weight is supported and so that loops of tubing close to the end do not trail on dirty surfaces.

Instruments and Equipment

The selection of instruments for oral surgery is obviously a matter of personal choice but the basic set which will be described is typical of those which are currently in general use for out-patient oral surgery in the United Kingdom (*Fig.* 1.1). They will be discussed in the usual order of use, which

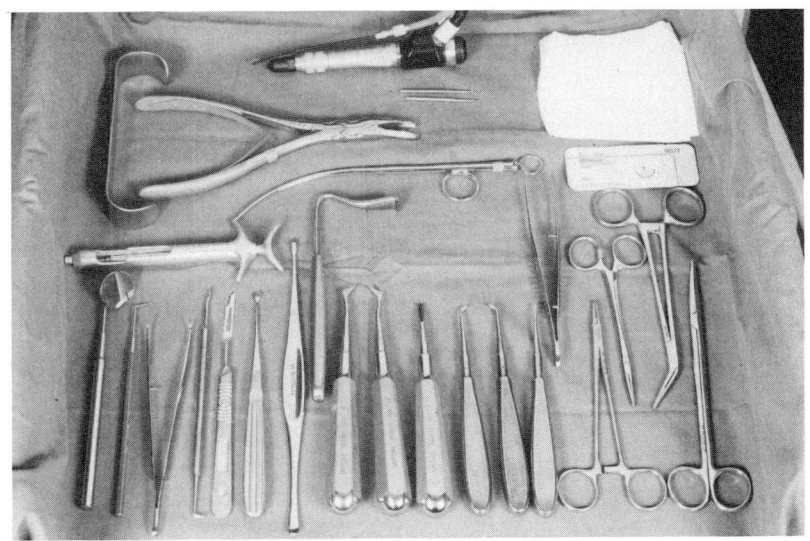

Fig. 1.1. Instruments for minor oral surgery. *Front row, left to right:* dental mirror, probe, college tweezers, cumine scaler, scalpel, Ward's periosteal elevator, Howarth's rougine, Bowdler-Henry rake retractor, Cryer's elevators right and left, Coupland's chisel, Warwick James' elevators right, left and straight, toothed dissecting forceps, needle holders, mosquito artery forceps, toothed Fickling's forceps, MacIndoe's scissors. *Across the back, left to right:* Astra self-aspirating syringe, Kilner retractor, bone nibblers, sucker tip, Svedia handpiece and tungsten carbide burs, black silk suture pack and swabs.

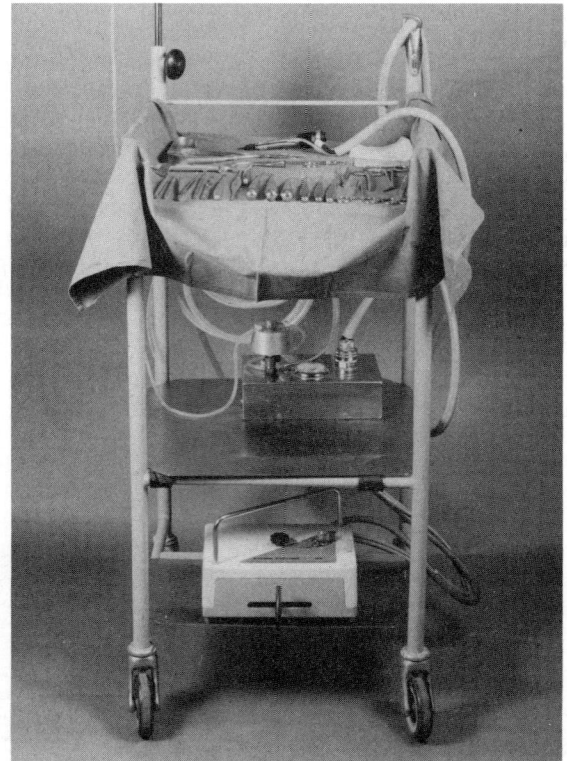

Fig. 1.2. A small surgical trolley, suitable for out-patient or practice minor oral surgery with a built-in Svedia surgical airmotor unit. The rod (*left, rear*) forms a drip stand and supports the irrigation water bag. An electrical Kavo Oral Surgery Unit can be installed in a similar way.

is also the order in which they are most conveniently laid out on the instrument trolley (*Fig.* 1.2). Many of the instruments described come originally from a variety of other surgical specialties, but all have been chosen because of their proven suitability for oral operations.

1. *Local Anaesthetic Syringe*

There have been major advances in the last two decades in the development, not only of local anaesthetic preparations, but of syringe systems for their delivery. Many and varied patterns are available to suit the circumstances of different practices and clinics, and no single type is paramount.

A syringe system for administration of local anaesthetic for oral surgery should be autoclavable, robust and mechanically efficient, convenient and comfortable to use and should have an aspirating facility. The requirement for sterility is met also by the use of disposable plastic syringes, which are pre-packed and sterilized by the manufacturer. Local anaesthetic solutions prepared in glass cartridges are in general use and those with specially designed rubber plungers, as in the 'Astra' system which allow easy repeated aspiration prior to injection, are to be preferred.

Disposable single use needles are sharper and therefore more comfortable for the patient, and of course avoid difficulties with cleaning and sterilization after use, which used to be the case with the re-usable type.

Most operators prefer proprietary solutions of 2 per cent lignocaine with 1 : 80000 adrenaline for general use, or prilocaine 3 per cent with felypressin 0·03 i.u. per ml for procedures which can be completed within 45–50 minutes and for patients for whom adrenaline is contraindicated. A clot forms in the socket more promptly and there is a less frequent occurrence of reactionary haemorrhage if prilocaine and felypressin can be used. The shorter acting mepivacaine, 3 per cent without added vasoconstrictor, is a useful alternative when these two solutions are unsuitable, and a 5 per cent solution of lignocaine may be valuable when analgesia is incomplete and a further injection is needed, but should be used only in small quantities and with particular care to avoid intravenous injection. Six 2 ml cartridges of the 2 per cent solution should normally be regarded as a maximum dose on a single occasion.

2. *Retractors*

There are many suitable instruments for retraction of the lips and cheeks, but a small and large version of the double-ended Kilner cheek retractor is the most versatile, and when properly held at an angle to the cheek pouches out the cheek most effectively (i.e. Kilner's double-ended retractors, small with 25 mm (1 in) and 19 mm (¾ in) wide ends and large with 35 mm (1⅜ in) and 29 mm (1⅛ in) wide ends).

Retraction of the mucoperiosteal flap is more difficult to achieve and again there are many suitable instruments available, but the Howarth's periosteal elevator and the specially designed Bowdler–Henry retractor are commonly used. A Lack's retractor is suitable for retracting the tongue or a palatal flap. Retractors also serve to guard the soft tissue from accidental damage, especially by burs. The shanks of retractors or other instruments which may rub against the angles of the mouth should be smeared with petroleum jelly to prevent frictional sores.

3. *Scalpel*

The majority of oral surgical incisions can be made conveniently with a No. 3 Bard–Parker type of scalpel handle and a No. 15 (BP) detachable blade. A No. 10 (BP) blade may be preferred for skin incisions and the pointed triangular No. 11 (BP) blade is used for the incision of intraoral abscesses by stabbing it into the swelling and cutting upwards through the mucoperiosteum.

4. *Periosteal Elevators*

The Howarth's nasal rugine (curved on flat) is widely used for periosteal elevation, the flat, round blade end for insertion into the incision beneath the cut edge of the periosteum to strip it off the bone, and the rugine end for the detachment of muscle insertions. Some find the smaller and shorter Fickling type more convenient to use, and a Ward's fan shaped periosteal elevator or a Mitchell's trimmer is also helpful in separating tough fibrous tissues from around the crowns of unerupted teeth. Retraction of the tissues with a Howarth's rugine in one hand while the flap is elevated from the bone with another periosteal elevator in the other, ensures precise movements with good visibility.

5. *Bone-cutting Instruments*

The choice lies between the use of bone-cutting burs in a suitable handpiece and the use of chisels, but each method has its own advantages and disadvantages and the most appropriate tool should be selected for the work in hand. Bone rongeurs are a useful adjunct to remove accessible sheets of bone and sharp points and edges.

Ideally, burs used for oral surgery should be those specially designed for the purpose. As compared with those intended for cutting enamel and dentine, the number of blades is less so as to reduce clogging with debris and consequent loss of cutting efficiency. Ordinary dental steel burs are acceptable, but tungsten carbide burs cut more efficiently because they have a wider clearance between the blades and because they retain their sharpness during lengthy or repeated use. Specially designed burs are produced for major bone-cutting procedures and these will be referred to in the sections concerned with such operations. They are often substantially more expensive than dental burs.

Either round or 'fissure' burs or both can be used according to the operator's preference and the demands of particular circumstances. Very large diameter bone burs may be used for removal of wide areas of bone or for smoothing the margin of bony defects prior to wound closure. In most cases, however, the use of either size 6 or 8 dental burs will enable the production of deep narrow slots in the bone, which are less destructive of bony tissue, and the edge of the slot provides a fulcrum during elevation of teeth or roots. Individual burs can be hot-air sterilized in small, paper packets for convenient storage. A range of burs should always be available.

Chisels 3 mm wide and 5 mm wide are used to split bone in a controlled fashion taking advantage of its anatomical grain and the relative thinness of the alveolar plates around most of the teeth. Bone in young individuals has a marked grain and a predictable direction of split. As a person gets older the bone becomes harder and more brittle and pieces of an unpredictable size split off when it is cut with a chisel. Oral surgery chisels should be long enough to grasp with a fist grip with the hand outside the mouth where it will not obstruct the field of view. The Eastman pattern chisels which are 191 mm (7½ in) long are suitable. The use of an 8½ oz, all-metal mallet to strike the chisel is mainly applicable to operations under general anaesthesia since conscious patients may be somewhat alarmed by this approach and upset by the noise which is conducted through the bones of the face and ears. However, a great deal of bone removal can be achieved rapidly and atraumatically with a chisel held in the palm of the hand. The Read's pattern and Coupland's chisel are specially designed for this purpose. Chisels are bevelled on one side and, when driven into a surface, the bone on the bevel side of the edge is wedged away, creating a split. It is also crushed by the bevel as it is separated from the undisturbed bone on the unbevelled side. The direction of split with a chisel lies mid-way between the plane of the flat side and the bevel and this must be taken into account or unexpectedly large pieces will be removed.

Gouges, which are chisels with a curved cross-section, are used by some operators because they can create a trough around a tooth like that cut with a bur, or cut a round hole in the cortex, but they need to be struck with a mallet because they cut, not only along, but also across the grain of the bone.

Osteotomes differ from chisels in that they are bi-bevelled to form a narrow wedge-shaped end, and cut in a direction in line with the blade. Therefore they are used to split apart two segments of bone. They may be used also for splitting teeth. Where part of the crown is to be split off the tooth should not be loosened in its socket. Indeed a loose tooth requires a considerably greater force to achieve the split and this may result in the tooth being driven through the lingual plate. Where it is intended that the split should pass on between the roots the tooth should be eased a little in the socket. Care should be taken that the edge of the oesteotome does not strike the bone during the tooth splitting process or a fracture may be created through the jaw.

Tungsten carbide tipped or tungsten steel osteotomes and chisels may be needed to cut hard bone and split teeth (Ward's tungsten steel osteotomes 3 mm and 5 mm wide and 178 mm (7 in) long). All these instruments require special care in sharpening after use and dry heat sterilization to preserve the quality of the metal of the cutting edge.

Bone-cutting rongeurs (bone 'nibblers') such as the Ward's pattern with multiple action joints 178 mm (7 in) long and slightly curved on the flat are extremely useful for cutting off sharp spikes of bone or biting off thin curved plates of bone and even the tough accompanying soft tissue of the gubernaculum which overlies unerupted teeth. They can be used safely only when the blades can be applied to both sides of the piece of bone without soft tissue intervening, and this is a limitation. Glasgow pattern contouring forceps are a simpler but also suitable pattern. Special rongeurs with narrow blades are available to remove interdental bone and the wall of sockets.

A variety of drills are available for oral surgery and all have their advantages and disadvantages. The ultra high speed (250000 r.p.m.) air-rotor drills, so convenient for restorative dentistry, are unsuitable for surgery since the shape and size of the heads and burs are wrong for this purpose and many exhaust air and finely dispersed lubricants close to the cutting area, risking contamination and surgical emphysema. If this type of rotary cutting instrument is needed, a purpose designed surgical air-rotor must be used which takes special long shank burs and exhausts air away from the wound. The relative lack of torque of these tools destroys the discrimination of touch between bone and tooth substance during the process of cutting, which is often essential in oral surgery, and they and their coolant are not easily sterilized to surgical standards. Medium speed drills (12 000–20 000 r.p.m.) are therefore preferred for dento-alveolar surgery and they may be driven by air motors (*Fig.* 1.2) or miniature electric motors, according to convenience. The relatively old-fashioned electric bench type motor, with a flexible drive shaft, is perhaps the simplest and most robust available, and its reliability and ease of maintenance is a great advantage. Unfortunately the spark hazard rules out its use alongside gaseous anaesthetics. Furthermore the torque in the flexible drive strains the hand and reduces accuracy of work. Either sealed bearing handpieces or surgical handpieces with extra ball bearings must be used as ordinary handpieces overheat after prolonged cutting with lateral pressure such as is common in minor oral surgery, particularly when teeth are divided. Overheated handpieces burn the lip or cheek and the bearings seize up.

Irrigation of the bur with sterile saline during bone cutting is essential both for lubrication and cleaning of the bur blades, to improve vision and in order to avoid bone damage due to overheating. This may be arranged in a variety of ways, ranging from syringing by the assistant to automatic systems which switch on and off with the drill. A suitably modified infusion set is the simplest arrangement. Narrow bore spray tubes on handpieces may become obstructed by salt crystals if saline is passed through them so sterile water should be used instead. Some form of sterile syringe is also needed to wash away debris during and after the operation. The simplest is a 20 ml disposable syringe fitted with a sterile anaesthetic drawing up quill.

6. *Dental Forceps and Elevators*

A limited range of extraction forceps is useful during minor oral surgery as opposed to routine exodontia to loosen teeth and finally deliver roots or impacted teeth. Fig. 76N, 74N, 110 (or 111) and 73S form a suitable selection. For most surgical cases elevators are required. Many types are available but a set comprising a right, left and straight Warwick James' elevators and right and left Cryer's elevators will meet most requirements. Coupland's chisels should be keep sharp for bone cutting by regular sharpening between cases and should not be blunted by use as a heavy straight elevator, for which purpose anyway they are too thick. However, they will conveniently wedge out teeth with conical roots or turn out already loosened curved roots when pushed into the periodontal membrane.

7. *Curettes*

One of the most versatile instruments for use in oral surgery is the Mitchell's trimmer. Designed originally for carving wax patterns in restorative dentistry, it has been employed for a whole variety of purposes. The spike end can be used as a probe to pierce thin bone plates or to separate soft tissues from teeth or as a fine pointed elevator. The round spoon end is useful as a small periosteal elevator and as a curette, and additional instruments for this purpose alone are seldom needed. Occasionally, access may be difficult and a double ended and bi-angled curette such as Exner's is required. Large spoon bi-angled excavators are also useful as miniature curettes to separate the lining of small cysts or to reach into difficult corners of bone cavities.

8. *Artery Forceps*

An incision should not be made unless suitable artery forceps are available to control haemorrhage from cut vessels. The curved Halsted's mosquito type (125 mm; 5 in) are most useful in minor oral surgery and a minimum of two should be available. The blades and hinges of these fine forceps can be damaged if they are used to grasp fragments of hard tissue so that a longer and more robust pair such as Spencer Wells (152 mm; 6 in) should also be available and kept solely for this purpose. Fickling's angled forceps are invaluable for the removal of small fragments from deep wounds or sockets, the toothed version being used for soft tissue and the non-toothed for hard tissue.

9. *Suturing Instruments*

The essential instruments for suturing are needle holders and toothed dissecting forceps. Needle holders are either ratchet or non-ratchet in type, and many variations of each are available. The instrument kit should contain one of each type since, though most operators prefer one or other for general use, occasions arise in which a change to the alternative type may greatly simplify suturing. With a ratchet type of needle holder (e.g. Mayo or Crile Wood pattern with tungsten carbide jaw inserts) the needle is held rigidly in the blades by springing closed the ratchet between the handles, whereas the non-ratchet type, e.g. Gillies' or Ward's, the needle is held firmly in the blades by finger pressure alone. The Gillies' needle holder with tungsten carbide jaw inserts 165 mm (6½ in) are combined with suture scissors, which facilitate the cutting of thread while working with only one assistant. Mobile soft tissues must be held firmly by dissecting forceps, such as Gillies' toothed dissecting forceps, or with skin hooks, while the flap is positioned and pierced by the suture needle (Gillies' dissecting forceps, light model with 1 × 2 teeth, 152 mm (6 in) long and either Gillies' fine skin hooks 165 (6½ in) or McIndoe's skin hooks 191 mm (7½ in), two of each).

10. *Scissors*
A pair of sharp pointed scissors such as Kilner's straight fine sharp pointed 115 mm (6½ in) scissors, is required for cutting and removing sutures and occasionally for sharp dissection of soft tissues. It is wise to reserve the suture cutting scissors exclusively for this purpose as the hard thread blunts the blades, and to have available another pair of scissors for cutting tissues. McIndoe's light blunt tipped 191 mm (7½ in) long curved on flat scissors are also needed for soft tissue dissection.

11. *Suture Materials*
A traditional material for routine suturing of intraoral wounds is 3/0 (metric size 2) black silk. It is easy to handle and knot, sufficiently strong without being too bulky, and the cut ends are soft and comfortable for the patient. However, the braided, coated, synthetic polyglactin suture, Vicryl (Ethicon) is becoming increasingly popular, particularly as it slowly resorbs and therefore may be left in inaccessible parts of the mouth.

Catgut is also popular to close intraoral wounds, especially when suture removal is likely to be difficult or impossible. Conventional gut is more difficult to handle and knot than silk, and the knots tend to absorb moisture and unravel in the oral fluids. The cut ends of chromic gut are sufficiently stiff to be irritating to the patient and as the catgut is a foreign protein an intense polymorphonuclear leucocyte tissue reaction surrounds the suture material. The synthetic, resorbable materials do not induce this reaction, but may persist for 3 weeks or longer when used to close the oral mucosa. However, the new 'soft gut' (Davis and Geck) has overcome many of these disadvantages, knots well and can be left to slough off the healed wound margin.

The cut ends of many of the non-absorbable synthetic materials are also sharp and uncomfortable and they seem to offer little advantage over the traditional black silk.

For intraoral suturing a 21 or 22 mm half-circle or a 25 mm, ⅝ circle cutting needle is commonly used, although individual oral surgeons may have a preference for other sizes and patterns for particular purposes. Individually packed sutures, which are supplied attached to the needle and sterilized by the manufacturer, are the most convenient. Examples are Ethicon 577 which is 2 metric (3/0) black silk on a 22 mm half-circle cutting needle. Ethicon 576 is the 25 mm Denis Browne ⅝ circle cutting needle with 2 metric (3/0) black silk, and Ethicon W9730 is the same needle with 2 metric (3/0) Vicryl. Plain or chromic 3/0 and 2/0 softgut are also supplied by Davis and Geck on oral surgery needles, i.e. the 21 mm ½ circle cutting or the 25 mm ⅝ circle cutting. Where supplies are difficult or economy is necessary, sutures can be prepared on eyed needles from a roll of suture silk or thread and then sterilized. The best method of attachment is to insert the end of the suture thread through the eye and pass the short end round and back through the same side of the eye. This procedure will attach the thread firmly to the needle without the necessity for a knot, which would drag in its passage through the tissues.*

12. *Suction Tips and Tubing*

A fine metal suction tip is required to keep the operation field clear of blood. Fraziers' (8FG or 9FG) suction tips have a small side hole in the finger plate which, when uncovered, reduces the strength of suction at the end of the tube which might damage delicate tissues. Hu–Friedy's self-clearing suction tubes (2 mm and 3 mm diameter) have a built in stylet with which a blockage in the tube can be cleared. It is also wise to have either a metal or disposable plastic pharyngeal sucker which is useful if there is gross bleeding or vomiting or other emergency situation.

Suitable autoclavable plastic suction tubing is also necessary to connect the tip to the vacuum outlet via, of course, a water trap bottle and filter to prevent aspirated liquids entering the vacuum pipe.

13. *Swabs and Dressings*

Ten cm square sterile gauze swabs with radiopaque markers (BP) should be available in sufficient quantity. A pre-packaged bundle of 5 will serve for most simple procedures but more should be immediately to hand if needed. Most oral wounds are repaired by suturing but, in some circumstances, a material is required to cover or pack a tissue defect. One cm wide sterile ribbon gauze impregnated with iodoform paint (BP) (Whitehead's varnish) or Bismuth in iodoform-paraffin paste BIPP (BP) is widely used for this purpose and is usually retained by suitably placed sutures. An alternative approach is to use a packing material designed for periodontal surgery (e.g. Coe-Pak) which can be ligated to or packed round neighbouring teeth or which can be held in position by a plate or denture.

OPERATIONS UNDER GENERAL ANAESTHESIA IN THE OPERATING THEATRE

Every hospital has its own particular customs and practice so that the description which follows can only be a general guide to procedure and will

---

*The correspondence between metric and gauge size for catgut differs from that of other suture materials.

be modified by local circumstances. The oral surgeon has to fit in with general surgical practice while ensuring that his own special needs are met.

1. *Preparation of the Patient*

Patients are usually admitted to hospital for major oral surgery at least 24 hours before the operation so that their general health and fitness may be assessed prior to the anaesthetic and so that any necessary preoperative investigations can be arranged. These will include a haemoglobin estimation, urinalysis and, where appropriate, a chest radiograph and electrocardiogram. The surgeon has a further opportunity to discuss the operation and its effects with the patient and to obtain informed consent in writing. The history is reviewed and the adequacy of available radiographs is checked. Every effort is made to allay anxiety and ensure that the patient has a comfortable and restful night, using sedative drugs if necessary. Food and drink are withheld for at least 4 hours before the anaesthetic (nil after midnight for a morning list and nil by mouth after 8 a.m. for an afternoon one). On the morning of the operation, the patient should have a bath using an antiseptic preparation such as Savlon (cetrimide and chlorhexidine gluconate) which is added to the water or Phisomed or Hibiscrub which are used instead of soap. They should clean the teeth carefully with brush and paste even though they haven't eaten and male patients should have a close shave. Premedication is administered as prescribed by the anaesthetist. The patient is robed in a loose gown and transported to the anaesthetic room.

2. *Preparations in the Operating Theatre*

Theatre staff have to be notified in advance of the operations which are scheduled and warned of any special equipment or instruments which will be required. In the case of a long or complex procedure the order of the various phases should be given to the theatre sister. In a properly equipped operating theatre all the instruments etc. listed in the preceding section will be readily available.

3. *Instruments*

The basic operating list described above is suitable for most dento-alveolar operations under general anaesthetic, with the addition of a suitable set of mouth props (e.g. set of Mackintosh rubber props and a set of 4 Mushin's metal props) and spoon shaped 'cold light' or plastic concave and convex tongue retractors. These control a tongue made bulky by a throat pack and are particularly appropriate if coagulation diathermy has to be used to control bleeding.

Electric laboratory type motors to drive a slip joint handpiece are no longer permitted as they are not spark proof and the handpieces tend to overheat. Surgical air motors may be run off the compressed air supply or compressed air bottles. Some orthopaedic air tools include a straight handpiece. Alternatively, sealed miniature electric motors specially designed for surgery may be required.

For skin incisions a No. 10 blade on a No. 3 handle is mostly sufficient but larger scalpels are required for some procedures. Where the soft tissues are to be dissected additional artery forceps will be required. Ten curved mosquito artery forceps and ten Dunhill's artery forceps are sufficient for many procedures. Coagulation diathermy and specially insulated diathermy forceps are normally available. Additional retractors such as two small Langenbeck's and two large Langenbeck's with a set of Seward's double-ended retractors will be needed.

A pair of strong scissors, such as Aufricht heavy model straight dissecting scissors 140 mm (5½ in), are needed to cut tough tissues and a Farabeuf's periosteal elevator to raise obstinate tendons from bone.

Not infrequently bones have to be cut and joined and on rare occasions jaw fractures occur as an unexpected complication, so a suitable wiring kit is required. It may be necessary also to apply eyelet wires or arch bars to the teeth or attach plastic splints such as Gunning's splints, and the necessary forceps and awls to do this should be assembled as a basic wiring kit. Artery forceps used for this work should be specially marked and those used for haemostasis should not be misused. Neither should the theatre wire cutters be sent with the patient to recovery and to the wards. Additional wire cutters should be available for this purpose.

Complex fractures, operations for facial deformity, bone and skin grafting and other special procedures all require additional sets of instruments which the operator will order to meet his own particular techniques and preferences. These should be assembled as add on sets which do not duplicate the basic instruments.

4. *Scrub Technique and Theatre Dress*

Access to the operating theatre, anaesthetic rooms, theatre corridor and immediate recovery area is usually restricted to staff who have changed into special clean clothing and footwear. Caps to cover the hair and masks are also worn in theatres, but may be put on outside the anaesthetic or scrub room rather than in the changing room. In this and other details practice varies between hospitals.

The correct methods of gowning and gloving can be learned effectively only by demonstration and practice and those unsure of the procedure current in a particular theatre suite should seek the guidance of the theatre staff. Nails should be kept short and either the hair worn in a relatively short style, or arranged so that it can be completely enclosed in the theatre cap or hood. Surgeons view beards which cannot be completely contained within a face mask with concern.

In the scrub room the hands are washed under running hot water and the nails scrubbed with a brush. The hands themselves are not usually scrubbed

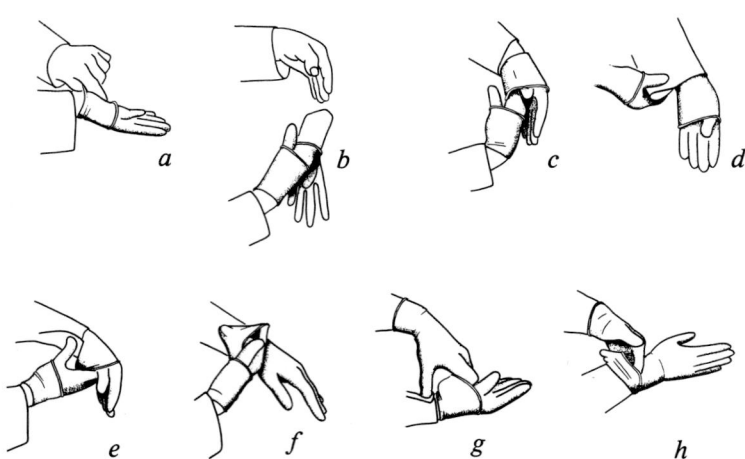

Fig. 1.3. Gloving with gown without cuffs (it is a matter for personal preference whether the right or the left glove is put on first). *a*, Pull on the right glove by grasping the turned back cuff. *b*, Pick up the left glove by inserting gloved fingers of the right hand under cuff. *c*, Insert left hand. *d*, Grasp outside of sleeve and fold tightly across the wrist. To prevent the cuff rolling, keep the left thumb across the palm of the hand. *e*, Hold sleeve with right thumb and insert right fingers under the left cuff. *f*, Pull left cuff over gown at the wrist by spreading right fingers and rotating left wrist. *g* and *h*, Repeat as in diagrams *e* and *f* with the opposite hand.

as this abrades the skin and spreads organisms out of the pores. The hands and arms, up to the elbows, are washed and rinsed repeatedly with scrub solution, for between 3 and 5 minutes, keeping the elbows down so that the water runs away from the hands. Each hand and arm is dried separately from the hands down to the elbows, after which a sterile gown may be picked up. The gowns are folded inside out so that only the inside is touched. As it is unfolded the hands are inserted into and through the sleeves. A 'circulating nurse' ties the gown at the back and any covering back flap and waist ties are drawn around by a gowned and gloved colleague. Gloves may be put on by holding the turned back cuff with the opposite hand and the palm side of the folded cuff with the opposite gloved hand. Alternatively, gloves are handled with the ends of long sleeves to the gown which are drawn back onto the wrist under the cuffs as the gloves are pulled on (*Figs.* 1.3 and 1.4).

Once gowned and gloved self-discipline is essential as any sterile item of clothing or equipment which becomes contaminated as a result of accidental or thoughtless contact with an unsterile area must be removed and replaced immediately. Gloved hands are best held above waist height in front of the chest so that such accidental contacts are avoided. Common errors by students which can attract censure by the theatre sister are to hand

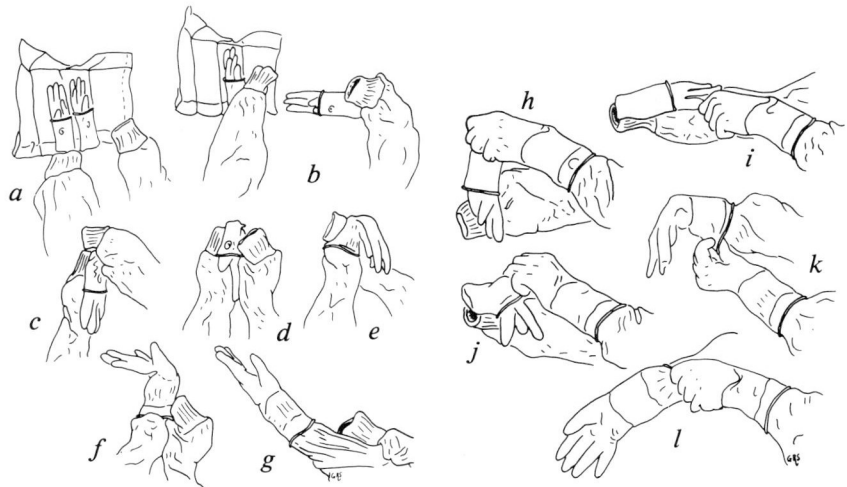

Fig. 1.4. Gloving with a cuffed gown. *a* and *b*, The left glove is picked up by its cuff with the right hand. *c*, The glove is placed against the left hand, thumb towards the hand and fingers lying up the arm. *d*, The rim of the cuff is gripped by thumb and fingers, by both hands. *e*, The part of the cuff held in the right hand is flicked over the gown cuff of left gown sleeve, inside of which are the tips of the fingers of the left hand. *f*, The glove cuff is gripped by the right hand through the gown sleeve and both glove and the left arm sleeve are pulled together over the left hand, until the hand is fully in the glove. *g*, The sleeve of the gown is pulled down until the gown cuff sits on the wrist inside the glove cuff. *h*, The right-hand glove is picked up by the already gloved left hand. *i*, It is placed over the right hand which is still within the gown sleeve, thumb of the glove towards the hand and fingers up the arm. *j*, The glove cuff is gripped with the fingers and thumbs of both hands. *k*, And flicked over the gown cuff. *l*, Glove cuff and gown are pulled together down over the right hand until it is fully within the glove. By pulling on the sleeve the gown cuff is settled around the wrist.

instruments across behind operators backs, to touch the gowned back of another assistant, to move a light other than by the sterile handle or to retrieve an instrument which has slipped down the side of the drapes.

5. *Preparation and Isolation of Operation Area*

The patient is laid on the operating table with the head firmly supported by a suitable rest, such as the horseshoe-shaped Whitlock pattern which will prevent it from rotating from side to side. Special care should be taken to protect the patient's eyes (*Fig.* 1.5). Petroleum jelly gauze is placed over the closed lids with thick protective pads taped into place on top. A throat pack is placed by the anaesthetist to protect the airway, even if a cuffed tube is used. The skin of the lower part of the face, the mandibular angle and

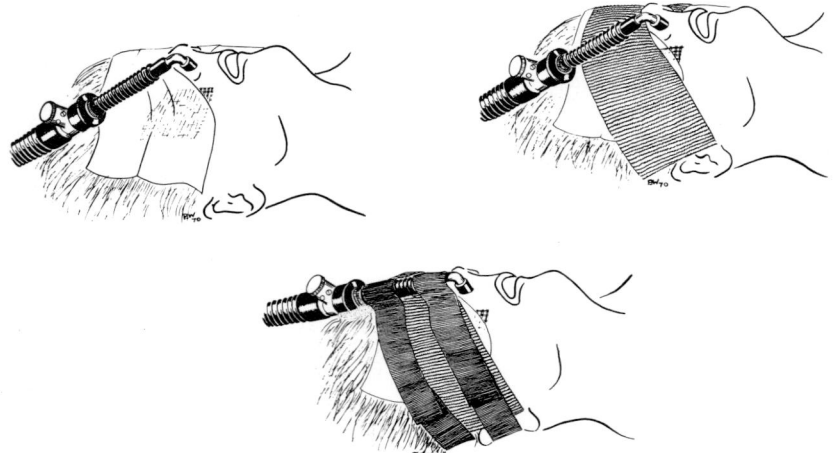

Fig. 1.5. Protection of the patient's eyes during anaesthesia. Each eye is covered with a 5 cm square of tulle gras and this is in turn covered with a sheet of cellophane and then a sheet of polythene sponge. These protection layers are secured by the anaesthetic harness.

mastoid region and the upper part of the neck are thoroughly washed with an antiseptic solution such as 0·5 per cent Hibitane or Savlon. The mouth may be irrigated with a similar lotion. During all these procedures the surgeon or assistant must avoid contact with unsterile areas and the swabs used in the washing process are held in a pair of sponge holders which are discarded after use.

When operative procedures more extensive than dento-alveolar surgery are to be performed more elaborate procedures may be necessary to control contamination of the operation site. Not only does the patient have a preoperative bath but the hair is washed with an antiseptic scrub solution.

Bone graft donor sites are shaved and a preliminary skin preparation may be made before the patient is given the premedication. Hibitane pastels or a chlorhexidine mouth wash can be used for two hours preoperatively, provided the mouth is checked free of pastille fragments before the premedication is given. Skin graft sites are not shaved in case hair bearing skin is transferred to the mouth.

The operation site is washed, prior to draping, with lotion, then dried and an alcoholic povidone-iodine 10 per cent preparation applied. Adhesive skin drapes may be applied and the incisions made through them, but if they are in place for any considerable period of time the patient may sweat beneath them, bringing organisms to the surface. Extra towels sewn to the wound edge (wound towels) may be preferred for this reason.

PATIENT MANAGEMENT

In normal circumstances the face and the endotracheal tube end and anaesthetic tubing are covered by surgical towels. Two towels and a waterproof sheet are placed under the patient's head and the top towel is folded across the face with the lower edges beneath the nose. It is secured at the edge by towel clips, taking care to avoid piercing the ears or placing the clips near the eyes. A sterile sheet covers the patient's torso and legs and is drawn up under the chin to be clipped to the head towels at either side. Two side towels are placed, one on either side of the head, to cover the side of the table. Sterile petroleum jelly or 18 per cent hydrocortisone cream is applied to the lips to avoid drying and to lubricate them and prevent friction sores.

If other operative fields are required as well the arrangement of the drapes is adjusted accordingly. Prepared areas which are not needed until later in the operation are covered by a sterile towel after the drapes have been placed and clipped in position. This towel is removed just before the site is operated upon. A further wipe with alcoholic povidone-iodine can be applied before the procedure is commenced.

The Operation Record

Details of the operation are usually written up on a special sheet. The date, the theatre number or name, the time at which the operation began and ended, who performed it and who assisted, and the names of the anaesthetist, scrub nurse and circulating nurses are usually entered at the top. While a lengthy 'blow by blow'account is unnecessary the type of operation performed, the surgeon's findings and in particular any unusual findings or problems and how they were dealt with are recorded. Where it is usual to safeguard any important structure at risk the fact that this was done should be mentioned. For lengthy and complex procedures a summary of what took place and how the operation was performed in this instance is necessary. The mode of closing the wound and the use of drains, packs and dressings should be noted. Finally the account should be signed. Some intra-operative happenings, such as unusual or unexpected haemorrhage, can be of importance during the postoperative period and these may be highlighted.

Postoperative Care

The initial recovery and in some cases the patient's management during the first twenty-four or forty-eight hours may be controlled by the staff of the recovery ward or intensive care unit. Routine cases are usually returned to the general ward once the patient is conscious and orientated. Postoperative care involves two facets, the general care of the patient and local care of the operation site. Even with relatively minor procedures, incorrect general management of the patient postoperatively can lead to life threatening incidents. Few complications are directly related to inadequate post-operative care of dento-alveolar wounds, but a carefully conducted major procedure can be ruined by inept handling in the postoperative period. Resident staff must be assiduous in monitoring the progress of patients under their care and must be certain of the way in which the consultant would wish the operative sites to be cared for. Ward sisters can be a valuable source of information upon the correct procedures and upon individual consultant's personal likes and dislikes.

The nursing staff will always provide the patients with mouth washes on a regular basis but it is up to the resident dental staff to see that the patients are encouraged to clean the teeth with brush and paste as far as is practical. Where splints or other forms of intermaxillary fixation have been applied a dental hygienist can provide a valuable service in maintaining oral cleanliness while the patient is in the ward and teaching the patient appropriate oral hygiene methods for use at home.

One aspect of drug therapy which may be given inadequate attention is the question of postoperative pain control and sedation. Too little, too infrequently will permit the patient to suffer unnecessarily. Too frequent administration of potent drugs will produce an over-sedated and drowsy patient. Even after quite major procedures, pain often gives way to soreness and discomfort after 24–48 hours. Severe pain after this time may signify complications. Sometimes there is a simple mechanical cause of the pain such as an appliance which is pressing into the soft tissues. Be certain you know why a patient is in pain. Do not ignore any complaints from patients which suggest that something is wrong even when a particular patient seems to make a habit of complaining for trivial reasons.

The Discharge from Hospital

Ask well ahead of the time where the patient will go when discharged and who will look after them. This is a matter which can be enquired into with the admission procedure, but may be more relevant as the day approaches and relatives or friends can see for themselves what home care is likely to be needed. Preferably patients should be accompanied on the way home even if the stay in hospital has been short. They may well feel tired or even unwell after travelling for a while. They should be discouraged from driving themselves in a car until fit to do so and in any case not for the first 24 hours after leaving hospital for the same reason. Find out how far the journey will be. This may influence the date of discharge. Patients should take with them any medical certificates which they may need and it is helpful to give the patient a brief note to be delivered as soon as practical to their general medical practitioner. This should outline what has been done, give details of any drugs or prescriptions given to the patient and record the name, address and telephone number of the surgeon.

A more detailed report is usually sent to the GP by post and if the patient has been referred by a dental colleague it is usual to write to the referring practitioner also, giving a summary of the operation, what was found and events in hospital. All patients must be given clear instructions as to whom

PATIENT MANAGEMENT

to contact in the event of problems. The first postoperative out-patient appointment is best fixed before the patient leaves the ward, rather than sending it by post. While the removal of any sutures may loom large in the patient's mind, at this appointment the opportunity should be taken to assess thoroughly the patient's general progress and the healing of the wounds. Any symptoms must be recorded and evaluated and all operative sites carefully examined. If appropriate, postoperative X-rays or other follow-up investigations are arranged. Once healing is complete or at least progressing normally such that uneventful further progress is likely the patient can be discharged with advice to contact the surgeon and return if necessary. It is as well to remember the aphorism that the operation is not complete until the patient stops complaining. In discharging the patient see that they understand that they are being returned to their dental practitioner for routine care, and where the surgery forms part of some overall treatment plan, such as a course of orthodontic treatment, make sure that a further appointment is booked with the appropriate practitioner so that the remainder of the treatment may be completed.

SUGGESTED READING

Editorial (22 November 1980) The risk of assessing risk. *Br. Med. J.* **281**, 1374.
Listening and talking to patients:
1. The problem: *Br. Med. J.* **281**, 845–846 (1980).
2. The clinical interview: *Br. Med. J.* **281**, 931–933 (1980).
3. The exposition: *Br. Med. J.* **281**, 994–996 (1980).
4. Some special problems: *Br. Med. J.* **281**, 1056–1058 (1980).

Hoy A. M. (1985) Breaking bad news to patients. *Br. J. Hosp. Med.* **34**, 2, 96–99.
Kirk R. M. (1978) *Basic Surgical Technique,* 2nd ed. Edinburgh, London & New York, Churchill Livingstone.
Shovelton D. S. (1982) The prevention of cross infection in dentistry. *Br. Dent. J.* **153**, 260–264.
Simpson H. E. (1960) Experimental investigation into the healing of extraction wounds in Macacus rhesus monkeys. *J. Oral Surg. Anaesth. & Hosp. D. Serv.* **18**, 391–399.
Simpson H. E. (1961) Healing of surgical extraction wounds in Macacus rhesus monkeys: I. The effect of burs. *J. Oral Surg. Anaesth. & Hosp. D. Serv.* **19**, 3–9.
II. The effects of chisels. *J. Oral Surg. Anaesth. & Hosp. D. Serv.* **19**, 126–129.
III. Effect of removal of alveolar crests after extraction of teeth by means of forceps. *J. Oral Surg. Anaesth. & Hosp. D. Serv.* **19**, 228–231.
Simpson H. E. (1960) Effects of suturing extraction wounds in Macacus rhesus monkeys. *J. Oral Surg. Anaesth. & Hosp. D. Serv.* **18**, 11–464.
Trieger N. and Goldblatt L. (1978) The art of history taking. *J. Oral Surg.* **36**, 118–124.

CHAPTER 2

INTRAORAL INCISIONS AND SUTURING

INCISIONS

A gingival margin incision which divides the mandibular interdental papillae will permit the insertion of a periosteal elevator and the reflection of either the buccal or lingual mucoperiosteum or both. If necessary, the papillae can be divided from one third molar around to the other without the operator encountering any sizeable vessel. Similarly, an incision along the crest of the mandibular edentulous ridge will also permit buccal and lingual mucoperiosteal flaps to be raised. Such flaps are described as envelope flaps.

If required the incision can be extended backwards into the retromolar region and then distobuccally up the external oblique ridge and anterior border of the coronoid process. No vessel of a size requiring formal ligation will be encountered until this upwards extension of the incision reaches a point just below the level of the occlusal surface of the upper 3rd molar. Here, the buccal artery and long buccal nerve lie side by side and cross the anterior border of the coronoid from medial to lateral on the superficial aspect of the buccinator muscle. The deep facial vein runs either with the artery and nerve or a little higher up.

By dividing the interdental papillae or by incising along the edentulous ridge, depending upon whether teeth are present or not, and then raising flaps, the outer and palatal aspects of the maxillary alveolar process can be exposed in a similar fashion. Again no sizeable vessel will be cut while making these incisions.

A second incision can be added which starts at one end of the crestal incision and is carried towards the buccal sulcus. The second incision can be a straight one which leaves the first at an obtuse angle, or with the edentulous ridge the crestal incision can be continued in a curve onto the buccal aspect of the alveolar process. In the dentulous patient the oblique relieving incision should include an interdental papilla at the corner to locate the flap on replacement. This two-sided, or triangular, flap is easy to retract and allows sufficient access for many small dento-alveolar procedures to be carried out, and is easy to suture. The addition of a second buccal incision at the other end of the crestal incision so creating a three-sided rhomboidal flap increases still further the degree of surgical access. By curving the sulcus ends of the incisions along the bottom of the sulcus in a direction away from the centre of the flap the length of these relaxing incisions can be increased. This permits the reflection of the tissues to a higher level in the case of the maxilla or a lower one in the case of the mandible.

It is a basic principle of flap design that the base of the flap should be as wide as is practical to ensure a good blood supply. However, where teeth are standing, the angle at the gingival margin should be no more than around 100 ° or a narrow V-shaped strip will be left which will have an inadequate blood supply at its tip.

In order to raise the flap along the gingival margin of the teeth the papillae needs to be divided interdentally. A No. 15 scalpel blade on a No. 3 handle is held parallel to the long axis of the teeth with the back of the blade interproximally and the cutting tip used to incise vertically downwards, first the distal attachment of the papilla then the mesial attachment so dividing it like a wedge of cake (*see Fig.* 3.1). The blade may then be passed along the gingival crevice to divide the next papilla, but if this is done it should not cut the periodontal fibres below the alveolar crest. Often as the flap is reflected it will separate readily from the alveolar bone and the neck of the tooth so that the connecting incisions are not essential. In the edentulous jaw, however, the attachment of the mucoperiosteum to the crest of the ridge is particularly strong and not only must the crestal incision be made firmly down to bone but reflection of the flap may need the assistance of the knife to cut the tough fibrous connections and to free it from the adjacent bone. The use of excessive force with a periosteal elevator may tear the flap, either at this narrow zone of strong attachment, or at the sulcus end of a two limbed incision.

It is important to design the incision so that a complete interdental papilla is present at each end of a three-sided flap, because this facilitates suturing through each interdental space. Bringing together the buccal and lingual papillae in this way produces excellent healing without clinically detectable increase in the depth of the gingival crevices. If such an incision is made in the experimental animal and the healing studied, a small downgrowth of epithelium will be found at the depth of the gingival crevice. The extent is microscopic, however, and not detectable clinically.

Recommendations have been made from time to time that the marginal gingiva should be avoided when outlining a flap, in order to prevent injury to the epithelial attachment. Those who follow this advice make a horizontal incision 2–3 millimetres away from, and parallel to, the gingival margin. Unfortunately the strip of gingiva which is left covers the margin of the alveolar bone. Should the excision of bone be carried too close to the concealed socket margin while, for example, removing an unerupted upper canine, the crestal alveolar bone may be damaged. Loss of the marginal bone will not be repaired and permanent damage to the tooth attachment will result. Retention of such a strip of gum also reduces surgical access with the result that it becomes traumatised both during the operation and when suturing, so producing necrosis with breakdown of the suture line. In addition, at the end of the operation, a bone cavity, such as the socket of a tooth or a cyst cavity, may lie close to the line of closure so that the wound edges are not adequately supported. Again the suture line will tend to break down and the flap fall into the underlying bony defect.

In general incision lines should be planned so that at the end of the operative procedure there is still an untouched zone of bone at the cavity margin to support the edge of the flap that has been reflected. This will provide a broad area of contact through which the process of healing can reattach the wound margin and develop an adequate degree of early wound strength to resist any tension during movement of the face and jaws in the period immediately after the removal of the sutures.

Mucoperiosteal flaps are relatively thin and do not possess layers which can be closed separately. Of necessity any surgically created bone cavity forms a dead space and creates a haematoma. It is important to seal this effectively from the mouth and the possible ingress of infection. Failure to achieve primary wound healing for this or other reasons leads to exposure of the underlying clot, which lyses, leaving a cavity which will be repaired slowly by 'secondary intention'.

As alveolar wounds cannot be closed in layers a valve-like closure is the best that can be achieved. Siting the incision so that there is a zone of intact bone between the cavity margin and the line of the soft tissue wound provides for such a valve-like closure. Where unavoidably the incision line crosses the cavity, eversion of the wound edge by mattress sutures creates an additional zone of tissue contact, but not as secure a closure as one supported on bone.

Provided incisions are confined to the mucoperiosteum of the alveolar process or the palate, that is the masticatory mucosa, the sutured wound is subject to little tension. The sulcus tissues in contrast are elastic and the wound edges contract away from one another, though normally not so as to create a significant tension in the sutured wound. Incisions made in the sulcus radially or at right angles to the outer aspect of the jaw are not subject to muscular pull and are readily closed with little risk of wound dehiscence during healing. On the other hand, horizontally aligned incisions in the sulcus in some parts of the mouth are subject to tension during movements of the jaws, lips and cheeks and are best avoided. If such an incision is necessary, special care is required in its closure to avoid wound breakdown.

For example, the design of flap often used when an apicectomy is performed upon an anterior tooth is a semilunar one with the convexity towards the gingival margin. The incision for such a flap should not approach closer to the gingival margin than one third of the depth of the sulcus. Such a flap suffers from all of the disadvantages mentioned above. If the incision approaches closer to the gingival margin, the remaining strip of gum may slough, because its blood supply may be inadequate, particularly after sutures have been passed through it. Furthermore, it is not always easy to predict how large the surgical cavity may be at the end of the operation, particularly if a small cyst is to be dealt with during the apicectomy, and the flap may be inadequately supported at its margin. Finally the suture line will be under tension. This can be seen as soon as the sutures are inserted because the wound edges will gape between the sutures. Some operators attempt to overcome this problem by using horizontal mattress sutures, but there is a danger with such a small wound that they will be drawn too tight and strangulate the wound margin, particularly on the gingival side. A three-sided flap which includes the gingival margin of the tooth to be operated upon and its interdental papillae is more satisfactory.

The problem of tension from muscular activity is encountered again when horizontal incisions are made either to 'deglove' the chin or to expose the anterior part of the maxilla during a Le Fort I level osteotomy. Such incisions should be made so that a generous skirt of sulcus mucosa is left on the gingival aspect. In the case of the mandible the incision should be carried out on the labial aspect of the sulcus and then obliquely downwards through the mentalis muscles to provide a sufficient thickness of tissues on the gingival side to hold sutures. A continuous horizontal mattress suture line will bring the deeper tissues together and evert the wound margin, but should not be drawn excessively tight, nor should large bites of tissue be taken at each horizontal step or the wound edge will be strangulated and slough. The epithelial edges are coadapted by oversewing with a continuous plain suture.

FLAP REFLECTION

Flaps are raised by dissecting parallel to the surface at the junction of tissue layers. Where these have similar mechanical properties, such as the junction of soft tissue layers, sharp dissection is used. Mostly dental surgeons are intent upon exposing the mandible and maxilla so that flaps are raised subperiosteally. This is done by blunt dissection with a periosteal elevator, making use of the well defined plane of mechanical discontinuity between the soft tissues and the hard bone. The attachment of the periosteum to bone varies in strength from place to place. The interdental papillae are firmly attached to the cribriform surface of the tops of the interdental septa. In the edentulous jaw this cribriform bone forms a narrow continuous strip along the crest of the ridge. Connective tissue fibres and vessels which pass from bone to periosteum resist separation by the periosteal elevator and it may be necessary to cut them with a scalpel.

The surface of the bone beyond the alveolar process can be exposed by further elevation of periosteum and overlying soft tissues, but a sufficient mesiodistal length of flap needs to be developed to permit adequate retraction and comfortable access to the bone at the operation site.

On the outer aspect of the body of the mandible several structures are encountered which require special attention. Foremost of these is the mental nerve. As the periosteum is reflected in the region of the apices of the mandibular premolar teeth, care should be taken until the foramen is found. Gentle use of the periosteal elevator will preserve the mental nerve and vessels inside their conical sleeve of periosteum.

Special care should be taken where the patient is edentulous. If the alveolar process is atrophic the mental foramen will be relatively close to the crest of the ridge. Indeed where resorption has been extreme the nerve may emerge on the crest of the residual ridge and can be seen radiating outwards beneath the mucosa.

Anterior to and below the mental foramen there are the origins of the depressor labii and depressor anguli oris muscles and the insertion of the platysma muscle. These add only a marginally stronger attachment of the soft tissues to the mandible. In contrast, the origin of the mentalis muscle below the incisors requires a substantial effort with a rougine to detach it. Indeed the periosteum is firmly attached over the whole mental eminence.

The attachment of the buccinator to the mandible is easily disrupted, but it should not be raised unless the additional access is definitely required. Once the edge of the muscle has been separated oedema of the buccal space is facilitated producing a greater degree of facial swelling postoperatively. As the body of the mandible is uncovered buccal to the second molar it should be remembered that the facial artery and vein lie immediately external to the periosteum at this point.

More posteriorly the insertion of the masseter needs to be separated to expose the outer aspect of the mandibular angle. This requires little effort until the posterior border of the ramus and the lower border of the angle are reached. However, the tough, inelastic periosteum may need to be incised by a few gentle strokes across the inner surface to permit adequate retraction of the muscle to allow work on the underlying bone.

The shape of the mandible makes surgical access to its inner aspect awkward and this difficulty is increased by strong muscle origins. The genial muscles can be detached only by cutting through their origin, close to the tubercles and of course if complete detachment is necessary, they should be reattached. The sublingual arteries enter the mandible through a single foramen just above the tubercles and if divided they must be ligated or the bleeding from them arrested with coagulation diathermy. The mylohyoid origin extends from the third molar region to the midline and is not at all easy to separate from the bone, mainly because the muscle slopes downwards and the periosteal elevator more easily perforates the thin lingual periosteum and slips over the surface of the muscle rather than lifting it from the bone. It may be detached, if this is necessary, by hooking a narrow, curved elevator beneath the posterior border and detaching it from below upwards. This should be done with care and it may damage the mylohyoid nerve producing a transient patch of cutaneous anaesthesia on the point of the chin. Naturally in the elevation of the mucoperiosteum on the lingual aspect of the 3rd molar region the lingual nerve must be safeguarded. Even the exposure of no more than the lingual aspect of the alveolar process requires care because, except in the 3rd molar region, the mucoperiosteum is thin and easily torn. Any tear in the lingual periosteum will permit blood to spread into the lax tissues of the floor of the mouth forming a bulky haematoma.

As the outer surface of the maxilla above the alveolar process is uncovered few obstacles are encountered. The buccinator attachment is barely noticed and there is only little resistance from the levator anguli oris. In contrast the depressor septi muscles form a fleshy zone over the central incisors which requires some care during flap reflection. Once the anterior bony aperture of the nose is reached the reflection of the periosteum into the nasal aspect of the maxilla impedes further mobilization of the soft tissues. Caution should be exercised high on the anterolateral aspect of the maxilla to identify and preserve the infraorbital nerve. This is done by elevating the soft tissues with a swab enclosed finger. Behind the zygomatic buttress or zygomatico-alveolar crest on the posterolateral aspect of the maxilla again the periosteum should be raised gently. It is easily stripped from the bone but care is necessary to avoid unnecessary damage to the posterior superior dental artery as it enters the bone. Exploration high up on the back of the maxilla leads to its disruption and the onset of a brisk ooze. While the haemorrhage is usually on a small scale, it can be troublesome in this corner where visibility is bound to be poor. Also a breach in the periosteum will release the buccal pad of fat, creating an even greater impediment to vision.

The mucoperiosteum of the hard palate is normally raised by incising the interdental papillae or by making an incision around the crest of the edentulous ridge. The palatal mucoperiosteum is tightly attached at the margin of such a flap so care must be taken not to use a tooth as a fulcrum for the periosteal elevator when it is raised. Initial elevation of the margin may be facilitated by using the spoon-shaped end of a curved Warwick James' elevator. The mucosa is also tightly attached to the median palatal suture and tethered to the contents of the incisive fossa. Normally a generous length of the curvature of the upper dental arch is needed to form a useful flap. However, radially placed relieving incisions can be made to limit the amount of mucosa which is raised to gain access to the surgical site. These should be short so as not to cut the greater palatine neurovascular bundle. Division of the palatine artery leads to a brisk haemorrhage which is best controlled by elevation of the posterior margin of the cut, the application of a haemostat and underrunning the vessel with a resorbable stitch which is then tied to form a ligature.

In order to raise the full width of the palate elevation is started at a premolar interdental papilla on each side and separation is carried up to and around the incisive fossa structures. The nasopalatine nerves and vessels are divided as they enter the deep surface of the flap and rarely cause trouble either with haemorrhage or postoperative loss of sensation. Posteriorly the greater palatine neurovascular bundles in the adult emerge opposite the second molars and must be preserved with care. Damage to both can result in death of the flap. Damage to one may result in cyanosis of the edge of the flap. If appropriate one-half only of the palatal mucosa may be raised by making an incision along the centre of the palate.

Access just to the centre of the palate can be made by a midline incision. The mucosa is thin, as well as tightly adherent on either side of the midline, but can be raised with care and retracted to expose the underlying bone. A V-shaped extension about the incisive fossa anteriorly increases access if this is necessary, but should not extend so far laterally as to divide the palatine vessels. Further reflection of the mucosa can be achieved by a V-shaped cut at the posterior end but the thickness of the mucosa at this site makes such an extension less helpful. In making a posterior V-shaped cut the incisions should not be carried on to the soft palate nor should they be made so as to endanger the greater palatine vessels.

INSTRUMENTATION

In general, incisions in the perioral tissues are made with a No. 15 blade. The scalpel handle is held at an acute angle with the proposed incision line but with the flat of the blade at right angles to the surface. This way much of the length of the cutting edge will be employed in making the incision and it will be deepened progressively down to the level of the tip of the blade. If the knife is held with the blade vertically in the tissues they will tend to bunch up ahead of the blade and a ragged cut will result. Where mucoperiosteum is being incised, the tissues are held steady by the underlying bone and a clean cut is easily produced. Where soft tissues unsupported by bone are being cut they must be stretched gently at right angles to the line of incision, for example on the inner aspect of the lip. Where thick tissues are to be divided, such as those over the anterior border of the coronoid process, the incision can be deepened progressively by a succession of passages of the knife. This way the direction of the cut can be controlled, divided vessels identified and picked up with artery forceps and damage to any important structures avoided. If an attempt is made to divide the full thickness in one sweep of the knife the operator will be tempted to plunge the scalpel blade in at right angles to the surface so bunching up the tissues as described above or resorting to a sawing motion, all of which will result in a ragged incision.

In order to incise the periosteum cleanly, a degree of pressure onto the bone must be maintained as the blade is advanced. After a short while this will blunt the edge of the blade. Incising over an unerupted tooth will also damage the scalpel edge and a new blade should be fitted before further incisions are made.

Loose connective tissue can be broken down by pushing the ends of the closed blades of a pair of scissors into the tissue then opening them. Performed with care this type of blunt dissection will permit vessels and nerves which are passing through such tissue to be displayed. The excessive use of blunt dissection, however, is a bad habit which will cause unnecessary tissue damage, untidy wounds and imprecise surgery.

Scissors can be used as an alternative to a scalpel to divide sheets of soft tissue, usually thin muscles and sheets of connective tissue and mostly in a direction across the fibres. They are also used to divide loose connective tissue to avoid excessive blunt dissection.

Periosteum is raised from the bone with periosteal elevators. These may have a thin rounded edge or a sharpened edge flush with one surface and the end may be curved to enable it to be applied closely to curved bone surfaces. A blade end set at an angle to the handle like a hockey stick is used in cleft palate surgery and angled Warwick James' root elevators may be used as substitutes for such periosteal elevators to raise the edges of palatal incisions.

Large bi-angled spoon excavators also form excellent miniature periosteal elevators when it is necessary to raise soft tissues from bone in a confined space such as a cyst cavity.

A periosteal elevator in which the blade ends in a sharp, straight edge is called a rugine. This chisel-like end is turned over so that the sharp edge can be applied firmly to the surface of the bone, to separate tendinous muscle insertions. The fibres of most such tendinous insertions lie almost parallel with the surface and a periosteal elevator advanced from the bone to the edge of the insertion will slip up over the surface of the tendon. The muscle insertion should be approached from the side, if possible working one corner of the rugine blade between the muscle and the bone so as to detach the tendon from this aspect. In this way even strong tendinous insertions can be raised cleanly and easily.

SUTURING

Incisions are closed and the tissues held in contact with one another to permit healing by first intention by the use of sutures. Haemostasis should be secured always before the wound is closed. While the act of suturing the wound will arrest a slight ooze from the surfaces which the stitches bring together this cannot be relied upon. If bleeding continues after the wound has been closed a haematoma will form. This may either take the form of a clot which creates a dead space in the tissues, or a suffusion of loose connective tissues with blood which later clots.

Haematomas increase the volume of the tissues, expand flaps from the underside impairing their blood supply and creating tension at the suture line. The tissues within the bite of the sutures are also excessively compressed and necrose so that the suture cuts out and the wound opens, the so-called 'burst' suture line. Secondary infection will follow. Haemostasis therefore must precede wound closure.

The cheapest sutures are undoubtedly those made from eyed needles and a suitable length of suture material cut from a reel. However, most suture materials and needles are difficult to sterilize. The needles are also difficult to clean after use and become blunt and work hardened so that they snap.

Modern sutures are prepared commercially and sterilized by gamma radiation. The needles are eyeless, with the end shaped as a tube into which the suture thread is swaged. These 'atraumatic' sutures pass through the tissues with minimal effort and damage.

Needles may be either round bodied or cutting. Cutting needles are flattened on two or more aspects behind the needle point to raise sharp edges which aid penetration of tough tissues. Round-bodied needles dilate a hole for the thread so that delicate tissues are less likely to tear and the stitches cut out. The thread also fits tightly in the hole to make a water-tight suture line in, for example, the wall of a blood vessel. Large needles may be hand held, but small needles such as are required for suturing in the mouth are held in needle holders. There should be a portion of the needle shank which has flattened surfaces which may be held by the needle holder and which prevent the gripped needle from rotating. It is a fault of some modern needles that this necessary flattening of the surface may not be present.

Needles are also either straight or have varying degrees of curvature. Suturing in a limited space is facilitated by a curved needle, so that the point can be readily seen and grasped after rotating it through the tissues. A half circle (Lane) or a ⅝ circle (Denis Browne) needle is usually chosen. These are 22 and 25 mm in length measured around the curve, and are well suited to relatively thin layers of tissue and the small 'bites' required to close them. Suture material of 2 metric (3/0) silk or polyglycollate is usually used in the mouth. Where appropriate thinner suture materials may be chosen.

The sutures may be either absorbable or non-absorbable, and monofilament or braided. The traditional absorbable suture material is catgut and despite the appearance of new synthetic materials it is still widely used. Catgut is prepared from the collagenous adventitia of lambs' intestines and is prepared either plain and simply stranded, twisted and sterilized with gamma irradiation, or treated with chromate, i.e. chromic gut, to increase its tensile strength and delay absorption. However, synthetic polymers, the polyglycollate and the polyglactin suture materials, are stronger and less irritant to the tissues. Unfortunately if uncoated these sutures may be difficult to knot securely and will spontaneously untie unless the surgeon is familiar with their behaviour and triple ties each knot. Polyglactin sutures are coated with polyglactin 370 and calcium stearate (Vicryl–Ethicon) which reduces drag.

In general, non-resorbable materials excite little tissue reaction but because they are not destroyed by the tissues are only used where they can

INTRAORAL INCISIONS AND SUTURING

be removed or buried deeply in situations where permanent support from the sutures is required and where subsequent infection of the foreign material is unlikely. They may be either monofilament or braided. Braided materials are generally more flexible and are easy to knot and so are more suitable for suturing the mucous membrane of the mouth.

Natural fibres, such as silk, with their slightly roughened surfaces hold knots better than smooth surfaced artificial fibres. However, a braided thread will act as a wick for moisture and accumulate debris and microorganisms which can irritate the wound. To prevent this, braided sutures are often coated and made water repellent with wax or silicone.

Monofilament synthetic polyesters such as polypropylene or polyamide (nylon) will not absorb and conduct liquids in this way but are more difficult to knot as they have an intrinsic springiness. Therefore only 4/0 or finer gauge monofilaments are used in the mouth.

As elsewhere in the body, catgut or other absorbable material is used for buried sutures although these are not often required during operations performed through the mouth. Absorbable sutures are also used for mucosal flap closure when operating on young children to avoid the need for suture removal, or in all age groups for suturing the inside of lips and cheek or the floor of mouth where postoperative oedema may make the sutures cut in to a degree that they are difficult to remove. Sizes 3/0 (3 metric) to 6/0 (1 metric) of catgut are chosen, dependent upon the tissues to be sewn. Size 3/0 (2 metric) braided silk or polyglycolic acid or 4/0 (1·5 metric) polyester sutures are used for mucoperiosteum.

Needle holders with narrow beaks are required to hold small, curved needles without flattening their curvature. The handles should be sufficiently long that the holding fingers do not obstruct the surgeon's view. Modern eyeless needles are difficult to hold without a ratchet type needle holder and this can be a disadvantage in awkward corners of the mouth. However, they are less highly tempered than the eyed needles and much less likely to snap if accidently bent.

The needle holder is clamped on to the needle at a position about two-thirds of the distance from its tip. If the needle is held correctly in this manner the length between the jaws of the needle holder and the point is sufficient to allow the needle to be inserted about 2–3 mm from the wound edge, and rotated through the tissues so that enough of the pointed end emerges from the wound to be gripped and drawn through. The flap is controlled with either toothed dissecting forceps or a skin hook and the edge is everted as the needle is passed. The needle point enters at right angles to the surface and it should penetrate completely through a mucoperiosteal flap to obtain the maximum grip, but emerge near the bottom of the soft tissue incision to ensure that there is no dead space left after it has been tied. Eversion of the first side of the flap enables the curved needle to travel through the tissue obliquely away from the incision to enclose a slightly larger bite on the deep aspect than at the surface.

In general the needle should be drawn out of the first side of the wound before the point is engaged in the other. Now the second side is everted with toothed forceps or a skin hook and the needle inserted from the underside of the flap. The needle is inserted into this side of the wound at the same depth that the thread emerges from the first side. Now, once the needle has penetrated into the second side the forceps or skin hook is detached from the edge of the flap and pressed against the surface of the tissues just beyond the hidden point of the needle. This action pulls the superficial tissues over the point so that the needle emerges closer to the wound edge than it would otherwise. This way again the needle embraces a greater width of tissue deeper in.

Now when the stitch is tied the wound edges are everted slightly. Eversion of the wound edges increase the area of contact and so improves the early strength of the healing wound. As the scar contracts a flat surface results. The distance of the needle punctures from the edge of the flap should be less than the depth to which the stitch penetrates into the tissues, particularly with mucoperiosteal flaps, or one edge will overlap the other as the knot is tied. Overlapping will also result if unequal depths of flap are embraced by the stitch. Excessive depth of bite in relation to width, on the other hand, results in excessive eversion and gaping of the approximated wound at the surface.

In the mouth, one side of the wound often constitutes the flap and has been freely elevated from the bone and the other side remains attached to the bone almost up to the incision. The edges of the fixed margin, however, will have been raised for a sufficient distance to permit penetration of the full thickness of the flap by the needle. Suturing from loose to fixed flap usually enables finer repositioning and reduces the chance of the suture tearing through the fixed thin tissue layers. However, comfortable suturing is important to good technique and to this end it is preferable, where appropriate, to sew from the edge further from the operator to the nearer one. A supinating action of the wrist is usually more easy to perform than the reverse.

A knot is now tied, either by hand or with instruments. If the knots are tied by hand more thread is wasted than when instrument tying is employed, particularly where the knots have to be formed towards the back of the mouth. The technique of instrument tying therefore will be described (*Fig.* 2.1). Furthermore, it is easier to see what is happening if instruments are used in the confined space of the mouth.

The needle is drawn out of the second side of the wound and the thread pulled through until a length of about 4 cm remains protruding from the entry puncture. The needle is taken from the needle holder with the index finger and thumb of the left hand. If no previous stitches have been inserted about 42 cm (17 in) of thread will hang between the needle and the wound. The excess suture is taken up into the palm of the left hand, using third and fourth fingers and the thread grasped again with finger and thumb about

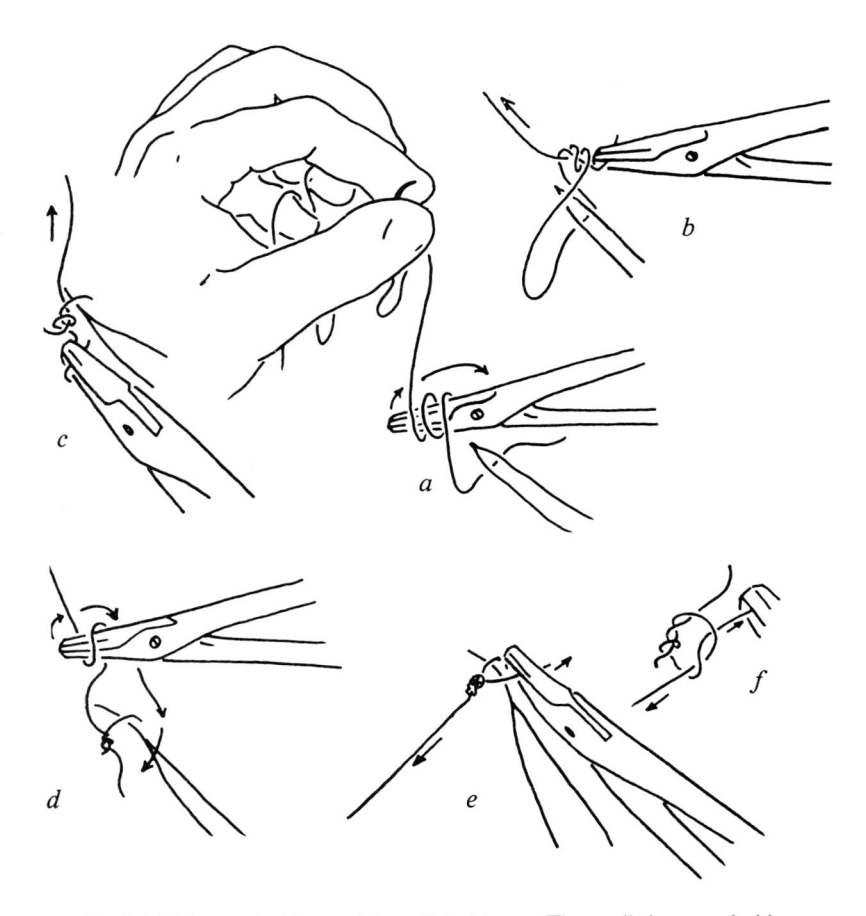

Fig. 2.1. Tying surgical knots with needle holders. *a,* The needle is grasped with forefinger and thumb of left hand and the thread drawn through to leave a short end at the other side of the wound. With a clockwise movement the needle holder picks up two clockwise turning loops of thread. *b,* The short end is grasped with the needle holders and the loops drawn off the ends of the beaks. *c,* By pulling further on the long end only the loops are tightened against the exit puncture. *d,* A single loop is twisted around the needle holder in an anti-clockwise direction. *e,* The short end is grasped again and mainly by traction on the long end of thread the second throw is tightened upon the first to complete the knot. *f,* The shape of the surgical knot.

8 cm from the wound. The beaks of the needle holder are brought across the front of the thread and rotated in a circle to pick up two loops of the thread. The short end is now gripped at its end with the needle holder and the loops slid off the beaks onto the thread by rotating the needle holders so that the beaks point towards the left and by drawing on the long end with the left hand. The short end is given a short downwards jerk which tumbles the loops into a slip knot, which is positioned just beyond the tips of the beaks and with the short length emerging from under the loops. By drawing on the long thread the knot may be made to slide down onto the tissues at the exit puncture. The short end should not be pulled as if this is done an unstable knot will result. Tension upon the long end also results in a short, short end which needs minimum trimming subsequently. The short end will emerge between the loops and the tissues and the knot will not slip while the long end only is under tension. As this first knot is tightened the left hand moves away from the operator's body and across the wound.

To form the second throw of the knot the needle holder beaks are brought across the long thread from behind and the points rotated downwards, away and to the right to pick up a single loop. The short end is again clamped but should *not* be pulled upon. The loop is drawn off the needle holder beaks and the knot tightened by traction upon the long end only with the left hand. Final tightening is accomplished by drawing the long thread towards the operator and the short end away, across the wound. A third throw will prevent any chance of a knot slipping, particularly if a synthetic suture is being used, or of the knot untying as it absorbs moisture from the saliva in the case of catgut. The loop is formed as for the first throw, but only one loop is picked up. The left hand travels away from the operator and across the wound to tighten the knot. The thread ends are held up and cut off by the assistant.

It is essential to close a wound with the correct suture tension, sufficient to keep the edges of the wound firmly together, but no more. Slight oedema of the soft tissue margins can be anticipated postoperatively and allowance must be made for this, particularly when suturing the inside of the cheek or lips or the floor of the mouth. If a suture is too tight it will cut into the tissues and produce scars at right angles to the healed incision, or stitch marks. Permanent suture scars depend more upon the tension of the sutures than upon the length of time before they are removed. To avoid irritation of the healing wound the knot should be manipulated so that it lies over the puncture point to one side of the wound. If an angled incision is used the apex between the two edges is correctly positioned first. Then the next two sutures are inserted at each mid-point between the ends of the wound and the first suture. The remaining sutures are interspaced at regular intervals.

Interrupted, simple loop sutures are used for most oral surgical procedures though where long incisions are to be closed, continuous sutures are used. Where a continuous suture has been inserted the thread is drawn out after the last penetration of the needle leaving a short loop on the other side of the wound. The mid point of this loop is grasped with the needle holder as the knot is tied, instead of the usual short end.

Mattress sutures, which may be either horizontal or vertical in design, embrace a greater volume of the tissue which increases the grip upon the wound margin and produces pouting of the wound edge. In the case of the former, the needle is introduced through one wound edge and passed out through the other in the usual manner. Then the needle is re-inserted about 3 mm further along the wound from the point of its emergence, carried back through both wound edges and tied. The vertical mattress suture is made by inserting the needle 4–5 mm from the wound margin and through the tissues in a deep bite. The needle is then re-introduced close to the wound margin and taken through more superficially in line with the previous direction of insertion, but of course in the opposite direction. The suture is then tied on the side of its original insertion. A vertical mattress will coadapt the wound margins where there is a small degree of tension and at the same time ensure eversion of the wound edges.

Absorbable sutures can be inserted to close layers below the surface, to ensure complete closure of a wound in depth, to reconstitute sheets of muscle or fascia and to eliminate potential dead spaces. The part of the suture which will persist longer than the rest and be likely to form a nidus for infection is the knot. If it lies under the outer suture line the bulk may affect the soundness of closure. For both these reasons the knot should be buried on the deep aspect of the suture line. The needle is inserted from the deep side of the layer to be sutured and reinserted from above downwards on the other side of the wound. When the knot is tied it will slip through between the approximated tissues.

The removal of sutures should be performed with care. They should be swabbed gently with chlorhexidine then each knot gripped in turn with non-toothed forceps. The external part of the suture is raised and the thread cut below the knot and flush with its point of emergence. In order to avoid a strain upon the healing wound the suture is drawn out across the wound. This draws the deep part of the suture out of the opposite puncture creating tension towards the wound rather than away from it. This prevents dehiscence of the healing wound and also draws only the previously buried part of the stitch through the wound. Never cut through a stitch in such a way that part of the contaminated external loop is drawn through the wound. Above all, avoid cutting the suture in two places so that part of the suture is left in the tissues. As the suture is divided some compression of the tissues is released and the retained segment retreats into the depths of the tissues. Even if some organisms have travelled along the suture material they do not produce a clinical infection in the ordinary way because a suture creates a wound which is drained at both ends. Leave a cut segment buried in the suture track and allow the puncture points to close so that there is no longer drainage, and a stitch abscess will result.

Sutures are normally left for 5–7 days where closure is completely without tension. Where tissues have been displaced and some degree of tension created, as in the rotation or advancement of a flap to close an oro-antral fistula, it is better to leave them for 10–14 days. Preferably sutures should be left until local tissue oedema has subsided at which time the loop will probably lie loosely over the wound and can be removed easily and without causing the patient discomfort.

CHAPTER 3

THE REMOVAL OF ROOTS

THE FRACTURED ROOT
General Considerations

A decision must be made whether to leave or remove a residual root. This requires anticipating whether the root fragment will remain asymptomatic or whether it will become infected and cause pain (non-infected roots do not cause pain), perhaps lead to an abscess and a discharging sinus, develop a cyst or interfere with a denture. Occasionally mandibular roots may even 'sink' towards the lower border creating greater problems in their removal.

If the root breaks after the tooth has become mobile the missing piece should be recovered for it is almost certain to become infected and cause pain. Conversely when the apex of a tooth with a vital pulp snaps off before the main body of the tooth has been loosened, the fragment is likely to be enclosed by the bone of the healing socket, and remain asymptomatic, and its removal can be deferred if necessary. Minute portions of root in the upper 3rd molar area are best left and put on probation, because they are often difficult to extract while the 2nd molar is still standing. Following alveolar resorption such a root lies nearer the surface and is therefore more amenable to surgical removal. Perhaps the only absolute indication for root removal is for patients for whom unpredictable local infection may become a major risk such as those who have rheumatic or congenital heart disease or who are immunosuppressed.

Forceps Removal

The narrow bladed forceps, 74N for mandibular and 76N for maxillary teeth, are invaluable for the removal of sizeable retained roots if used with care as follows:

  a. Always ensure that the blades are inserted beneath the gingiva which may have to be elevated locally first.

  b. Always obtain a grip on an identified root rather than just grip the alveolus blindly.

  c. Press the forceps well down over the root. In the mandibular molar region a small amount of alveolar bone may have to be included. This has been condemned but done with care and discretion will not damage or remove any more bone than a surgical extraction.

d. In the maxilla, apply the palatal forcep blade between the palatal and one buccal root and the outer blade buccal to the other buccal root where retained molar roots are being tackled.

e. Apply a firm continuous force with a strong grip to expand the alveolus, at the same time moving the root only through a small arc while maintaining an apically directed pressure. Rapid rocking movements although popular are likely to fracture the roots.

f. This approach is likely to remove one mandibular root or in the maxilla two roots, making the removal of the remaining one easier.

After a root has been recovered, verify that the removal is complete by fitting the tip to the previously extracted portion of the tooth. If this precaution is neglected, the surgeon may discover that he has failed to retrieve the whole of a missing root. Indeed all teeth should be inspected carefully after extraction because some have an extra root and if this is fractured and retained, its absence may be overlooked by a casual glance at the tooth.

Other Non-surgical Methods

There are a number of other manoeuvres which will enable the operator to remove a fractured root without resorting to a surgical procedure. However, too much time should not be spent in this way and if success is not soon achieved the attempt should be abandoned and a flap reflected.

In certain cases one complete root of a multirooted tooth is fractured off and retained. With care it may be possible to place a sharp pointed elevator in the empty socket and rotate it to remove first the inter-radicular septum and then the root. This is often a successful method for removing lower molar roots but is less successful in the maxilla. The distobuccal root from an upper molar may be extracted in this way provided only gentle pressure is used with an elevator inserted in the mesial socket. Unfortunately the mesial root is difficult to remove through the distal socket, as the root curvature is unfavourable for the application of an elevator from the distal aspect. Mesiobuccal roots can be elevated by introducing a Coupland chisel or straight Warwick James' elevator up the mesial periodontal membrane in order to turn the root downwards and backwards.

Elevators should not be used to remove the palatal root of an upper molar. The buccal wall of the socket does not form a satisfactory fulcrum and can be crushed by the elevating force. Furthermore there is always the danger of forcing the root into the antrum. The palatal root must be seen clearly, which usually implies the removal of both of the buccal roots and, if necessary, some surrounding bone which can be done with a bur. Then gentle dislocation with a narrow Coupland's chisel or rotation with upper root forceps should deliver the root. If an oro-antral fistula has been created this may be readily closed with sutures or by advancing a buccal flap as described in Chapter 9.

THE REMOVAL OF ROOTS

Sometimes a root apex is heard to fracture after the tooth has been loosened with forceps and it may be possible to see the apex clearly with the aid of a sucker. A probe or a thin root canal reamer or file can be introduced into the root canal and the loose apex withdrawn with its aid.

So-called apical elevators are usually too thick to use to dislodge the apical third of a tooth root from its socket, but a stout, bi-angled spoon excavator or a Cumine scaler may enter the periodontal space and topple it out. However, the movement will be a tilting one, pushing the sharp fractured edge on the other side of the root against the socket wall. This may be sufficient to prevent the operator dislodging it out of the socket. A narrow groove cut around the end of the root with a No. 1 rose-head bur may be sufficient to overcome this obstruction.

Used with discretion, these manoeuvres can neatly remove a number of small retained fragments but again it must be emphasized that unless success is achieved early, further attempts will prove frustrating and time consuming. It is then much quicker to raise a flap, cut away some buccal bone and tease out the fragment with a fine elevator. Indeed if socket surgery is performed incautiously, it can lead to roots being forced into the maxillary sinus or the inferior dental canal.

Blind elevation of a lower 3rd molar root can result in its deflection into the lingual space, through a thin or deficient lingual plate. To retrieve it, a long incision is made along the lingual gingival margin and the mucoperiosteum elevated and retracted towards the midline with a Lack's retractor. The floor of the mouth can be elevated by the fingertips of the assistant's hand placed externally just medial to the lower border of the mandible, and with good suction and light the apex should be readily seen and retrieved. Occasionally the mylohyoid muscle may have to be detached from its linear origin to reveal a more deeply displaced root.

Where immediate simple measures have failed to deliver a root, a formal surgical removal is essential. This should not be undertaken without clinical reappraisal and adequate radiographs to localize the root fragments and identify the features which might explain the problem, e.g. bulbous or hooked apices or adjacent unerupted teeth.

Accurate Localization of the Retained Root

A root may be so superficial that it becomes visible immediately the alveolar mucosa has been dried. Alternatively, an apex may be detected on probing a patent sinus, or an area of mucosal hyperplasia at an edentulous site. The brownish-yellow colour of dentine helps to distinguish the root from a sequestrum of bone. More often the position of a buried root can be determined only by a radiological examination. There is usually no problem when a standing tooth is present in the vicinity to act as a visible landmark from which to estimate its position.

Difficulty in localization arises when a root is discovered in the maxillary molar region where its situation may be either buccal or palatal and the only helpful pointer may be the root shape. In such circumstances two radiographs should be taken in planes at right angles to each other, such as intraoral periapical and occlusal films. In the edentulous jaw identifiable anatomical landmarks provide effective guides to the site of a root fragment and so avoid the need for localizing plates. The midline of both jaws is an obvious starting point. In the mandible this is marked by the median lingual foramen surrounded by its ring of dense bone. The mental foramen coincides with the mandibular premolar region while more posteriorly the external oblique ridge casts a dense image over an area corresponding to the 2nd and 3rd molars. Of importance as landmarks in the maxilla are the median suture and incisive fossa in the mid-line, the fork of the Y of Ennis (formed by the diverging limbs of the anterior wall of the antrum and the floor of the nose), and more posteriorly the superimposed V- or U-shaped opacity of the zygomatic process of the maxilla. The former corresponds to the canine-premolar region and the latter to the 1st molar position. Finally, the tuberosity identifies the 3rd molar region.

OPERATIVE TECHNIQUE FOR THE REMOVAL OF RETAINED ROOTS

The Reflection of a Flap

There should be no hesitation to reflect a flap whenever this is necessary to see the retained root clearly (*Fig.* 3.1). It is also essential to remove adequate bone to enable unimpeded elevation of the fragment along the appropriate line of withdrawal. This will avoid much frustration from repeated premature attempts to dislodge the root.

In the edentulous jaw the incision is made along the crest of the ridge or, if adjacent teeth are standing, the incision is made along their gingival margins. The flap must be ample in length and vertical depth in order to provide adequate access for surgical manipulations without damage to the soft tissues.

Where there are standing teeth the incision should be carried through the gingival crevice of the tooth on either side of the retained root and continued into the sulcus at an obtuse angle. This will produce a two-sided flap with a single relieving incision, or a three-sided flap with two relieving incisions depending upon the amount of access which is required. An entire papilla is included at each corner to facilitate closure (*Fig.* 3.1 *d*). If a flap is to be raised to remove a lower premolar root, care should be taken to identify the mental nerve at an early stage during elevation of the flap so that it can be preserved intact.

Bone Removal

What constitutes adequate bone removal can be learned only by experience but, within reason, it is better to remove rather too much bone than too little.

THE REMOVAL OF ROOTS

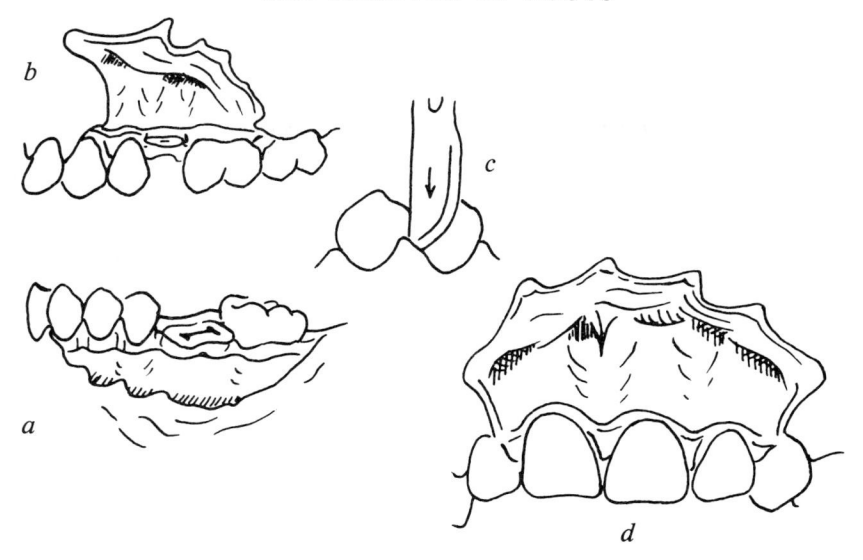

Fig. 3.1. a, An envelope flap to expose the roots of $\overline{6}$. *b,* A two-sided flap to uncover $\underline{|5}$ root. *c,* The correct way to divide an interdental papilla. *d,* A three-sided flap to uncover the upper incisor region up to the nasal floor over $\underline{|1}$.

Bone is usually cut away from the buccal aspect of a root, because this not only improves the access but brings the fragment into full view. The socket wall can be removed either with a hand chisel or gouge, a mallet and chisel, or a drill.

In general a bur in a dental drill is preferable to a chisel or gouge for the removal of bone around a buried root because if a hammer and chisel are used inexpertly the edge of the chisel may strike the root itself and fracture it at the level of the bone cut so necessitating more bone removal. Furthermore, most conscious patients undergoing surgery under local anaesthesia find the sensation produced by a mallet and chisel objectionable. If the bone surrounding the root is very hard, the mandible thin, or the root brittle then a chisel is definitely contraindicated.

When using a bur, care must be taken not to damage the adjacent teeth or to cut into the root fragment itself to a degree that weakens it and results in fracture when elevation is attempted. A No. 8 rose-head bur is excellent for the removal of the overlying buccal or labial bone. When bone has to be removed alongside the root to provide for mesiodistal movement and for the application of an elevator, a No. 4 or No. 6 rose-head should be used. Rose-head burs have two advantages over fissure burs for the removal of bone: they are more easily cooled and washed by a water or saline jet, and the site at which they are cutting is more readily seen, even where a gutter is being cut by the side of a root.

Burs are also used to separate divergent or recurved roots. A tapered fissure bur is best for this purpose. Separation of roots with a bur may take longer than splitting them apart with an osteotome, but is more certain. If the roots are shattered by the splitting blow their removal may be made more difficult. What is more, a space is created between the root ends by the bur cut permitting recurved or divergent roots to move towards one another as they are elevated. If the roots are split apart the split surfaces may still impact against one another as elevation is attempted (*Fig.* 3.2).

The least complicated but not necessarily the most successful way to remove bone from around a retained root is by means of hand gouges. A Coupland's chisel with its straight cutting edge but gouge-like blade is the most frequently used instrument of this type. The special shape of the Coupland's chisel permits bone to be removed accurately around the curved surface of a root. There are none of the problems of sterilization, lubrication and cooling associated with the use of a dental handpiece and bur when hand-held cutting instruments are used. Some patients find the pressure needed to cut the bone uncomfortable but there is none of the sharp shock and bone transmitted noise associated with the use of a mallet and chisel. Hand-held cutting tools will remove the soft, thin bone on the outer aspect of the maxillary alveolar process and on the labial surface of the lower incisor region. However, if they are to be used successfully they must be sharp. A Coupland's chisel should be sharpened after each use. In most cases the bone on the palatal side of the maxillary alveolar process and buccally in the lower molar region is too hard or too thick to be cut with sufficient efficiency with hand-held instruments. Bone on the lingual aspect of lower tooth roots is rarely removed as access is difficult. The removal of small slivers of bone one after another is the most efficient way to use a Coupland's chisel.

If the operation is performed under a general anaesthetic it may be convenient for the operator to use chisels and a mallet instead of a handpiece and bur. Two vertical cuts are made, one on either side and parallel to the side of the root. For the more mesial cut the bevel of the chisel should face distally and for the distal one, mesially. This way the remaining bone edges are not crushed. A third cut is made horizontally and joining the other two cuts at a suitable distance from the socket margin so as to expose at least a third of the length of the retained root fragment. The cuts should just penetrate the cortical bone and care should be taken not to damage the adjacent teeth, nor should the chisel strike the root as the third cut is made or it will be fractured. A gouge of suitable width can be tapped down the side of the root and between it and the outer alveolar plate, so separating the overlying bone. A gouge is also used to create a trough between bone and root on either the mesial or distal aspect. A curved Warwick James' elevator is inserted into the trough to lever the tooth from the socket. In all

THE REMOVAL OF ROOTS

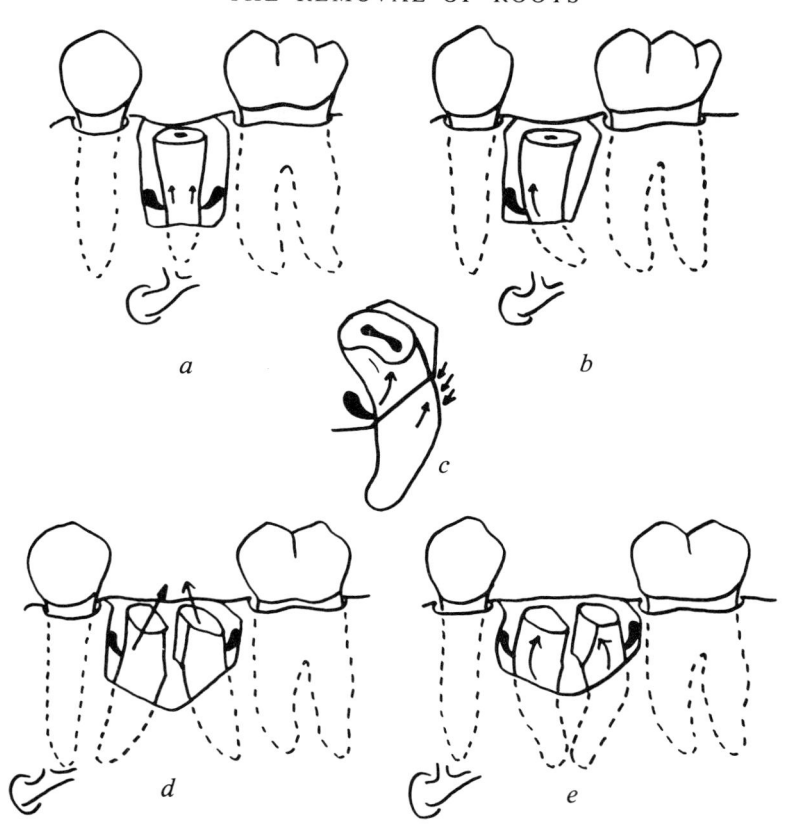

Fig. 3.2. Elevation of roots. *a,* Elevators can be applied either side of a straight root. *b,* But can be applied only to the convex surface of a curved root. *c,* Application of an elevator to the concave surface forces the convexity against the bone. *d,* Divergent roots must be separated, creating a space between them, and then elevated towards one another. *e,* A similar method is used to elevate convergent, curved roots.

cases excessive removal of buccal bone should be avoided as this will damage the foundation for a denture.

Where the retained root, such as one from a lower third molar, is situated in thick bone a gutter should be created with a rose-head bur all round the root from above. This will often permit the fragment to be dislocated with a Warwick James' elevator without the need to destroy the full thickness of the overlying buccal bone. Alveolar bone may also be conserved during the removal of small apical fragments. Instead of removing the whole length of the lateral wall of the socket to reach the root tip a window is cut in the bone overlying the apical part of the socket and access gained to the root in this way. It may be delivered laterally through the opening or it can be dislodged into the socket and retrieved from this aspect if it is a fresh socket.

If a lower premolar root tip has to be removed bone should be removed on the side away from the mental nerve.

The Application of an Elevator

The configuration of the root and direction in which it must be moved for its delivery will determine the correct site of application of the elevator. Roots may be straight or curved and the only way to establish the shape of a particular root is by radiography. The operator should always try to identify the reason why the root fractured during the original extraction. Was the impediment to success during the original extraction of the tooth relieved by the fracture leaving a readily removable root or does the obstruction still exist?

Theoretically, an elevator can be applied to any side of a straight root in order to apply the necessary dislocating force. However, if a root is curved the elevator must engage its convex aspect. If it is applied incorrectly to the concave side of the root it will not displace it from the socket but will produce a further fracture of the fragment (*Fig.* 3.2).

When dealing with multirooted teeth the roots of which all curve in the same general direction, the elevator may be applied to the convex aspect of the whole root complex. However, if the lines of withdrawal of the apices conflict, because of a divergent or recurved root pattern, then the roots must be separated before applying an elevator against the convex surface of each in turn. Occasionally the application of an extraction force to unfavourable roots in infected or resilient bone will result in successful delivery without fracture, but in the vast majority of cases, the unorthodox approach will lead to further fragmentation or to crushing of the socket wall and the formation of a dry socket. Even in the absence of a suitable preoperative radiograph, an experienced operator can often feel whether he is applying pressure to the correct aspect of the root, for on sensing the slightest resistance he will alter the position of the instrument so that the edge of the blade engages a more appropriate side of the root. Nevertheless, it is obviously more satisfactory to avoid guesswork, and obtain the relevant information about root pattern from a radiograph. The elevating force should always be modest and controlled as the application of excessive force will result in further fractures of the tooth fragment or even a fracture of the jaw. A fractured jaw is most likely to occur during the removal of deeply embedded roots in a thin mandible.

There are times when, after adequate surgical exposure of the socket, a systematic search for the root tip proves abortive. Alternative possibilities for its location should then be considered, namely dislodgement into the soft tissues, deflection into the antrum from upper posterior teeth, displacement into the inferior dental canal or lingual pouch from lower posterior teeth, loss into the mouth or on to the surgery floor, aspiration up the surgical sucker or ingestion or even inhalation. Some patients refuse to have a retained root removed. When this happens the issue should not be pressed, but an entry should be made in the case notes to this effect.

CHAPTER 4

UNERUPTED AND IMPACTED TEETH

The most common cause of failure for a tooth to erupt is a lack or loss of space in the overlying alveolar arch. A discrepancy between tooth size and jaw size is probably the result of a combination of both genetic and environmental factors. The inheritance of large teeth in small jaws appears to be aggravated by a lack of maximal jaw growth due to a softened sophisticated diet which requires minimal chewing. These factors particularly affect the 3rd molars and the canines. Sufficient space for the second premolars to erupt, especially in the mandible, can be lost because of the premature extraction of the overlying 2nd deciduous molar allowing the 1st permanent molar to drift forwards.

Maxillary central incisors may be impeded by retained pulpless deciduous incisors, or the presence of supernumeraries. Sometimes the tooth may be damaged and have a dilacerate root. Natural or traumatic displacement of the tooth germ will also lead to an impacted tooth. Less common causes include impaction against odontomes or cysts, radiotherapy, hypothyroidism and cleidocranial dysostosis.

THE IMPACTED MANDIBULAR THIRD MOLAR

Successful 3rd molar surgery is dependent upon detailed preoperative assessment and treatment planning and the skilful application of an appropriate operative technique.

The Clinical Examination

A conscious assessment of the general size and build of the patient should be made. A large patient with a massive mandible presents a different problem from a small, delicately boned person. The patient's attitude and demeanour is important and may give valuable clues as to the way he or she will respond to the stress of surgery and therefore the type of anaesthesia and/or sedation which will be required. In the context of any operative procedure, age and general fitness are important, but undoubtedly increasing age adds to the difficulty of the removal of lower 3rd molars. Compared with a teenager the young adult in the late twenties will already have bone which is significantly more difficult to cut and teeth which require more force to separate them from the bone. At a variable age between the early forties and late sixties the mandibular bone will develop a hard, brittle quality and the attachment of the teeth a rigidity which succumbs to an extraction force only after a substantial amount of investing bone has been removed. The presence of facial swelling and enlarged, tender, lymph nodes of course indicates the presence of active infection and used to preclude an operation until it had been treated. However, with antibiotic cover, postoperative morbidity in such cases is not increased.

The size of the oral cavity, the size of the tongue, the degree to which the patient can open his or her mouth, the size of the rima oris and the extensibility of the lips and cheeks all contribute to surgical access. A general inspection of the mouth reveals much about the patient's oral hygiene habits, the general state of the dentition, and the degree to which it has required previous dental care. The health of the 1st and 2nd molars may affect the decision to remove the wisdom teeth. Large crowns, inlays or amalgams in 2nd molars can be dislodged during elevation of the wisdom tooth even when care is being exercised. Teeth which are loose due to advanced periodontal disease and crowns on anterior teeth should be mentioned to the anaesthetist if a general anaesthetic is required.

Attention is then focused on each 3rd molar in turn, observing how much of the crown is visible, or palpable if it is unerupted. Partially erupted teeth should be explored with a probe to determine which is the occlusal surface (which feels rough) and which a mesial or distal surface (which will feel smooth) for at times it is not easy to differentiate horizontal, vertical and disto-angular impactions by inspection alone. If no part of the 3rd molar crown is visible, the gingival crevice distal to the 2nd molar should be explored with a periodontal probe to see if there is a pocket leading down to the crown of the 3rd molar. The depth of any visible crown below the occlusal plane and its general relation to the level of the alveolar crest is noted, as is the distance between the distal surface of the 2nd molar and the anterior border of the ascending ramus. The external and internal oblique ridges of the mandible are palpated. If the external oblique ridge is low, relatively vertical and relatively posterior to the tooth there will be thin alveolar bone buccal to the 3rd molar. If the external oblique ridge lies high and well forward relative to the tooth the thick cortex of the ridge will form the bone buccal to the 3rd molar. Similarly if the internal oblique ridge lies well back there will be thin bone both distally and lingually to the wisdom tooth and conversely an anteriorly placed internal oblique ridge carries thick bone around the 3rd molar on the lingual side.

The condition of the soft tissues over the wisdom itself is noted. Are they scarred and indented by the upper 3rd molar? Is there active pericoronitis present, or pus beneath the gum flap? Both conditions require treatment and there may be a delay before operation. A non-tender flap from beneath which a whitish, creamy material resulting from desquamated follicular epithelium can be milked is not a contraindication to surgery provided the flap is cleaned preoperatively with a sucker and povidone iodine or other suitable antiseptic introduced under it. Of importance to the future health of the gingivae around the lower 2nd molar is the relationship of the masticatory mucoperiosteum to that tooth. If there is a broad zone of gingival mucoperiosteum buccal to the 2nd molar which extends distally there are good prospects that there will be a normal gingival margin around the distal aspect after the 3rd molar wound has healed. What is more, there will be a sufficient buccal sulcus to permit ready cleansing of the gingival margin and buccal aspect of the crown of the 2nd molar. If on the other hand the gingival mucoperiosteum tapers to an end buccal to the 2nd molar then inevitably the gingival margin around the distal aspect of that tooth will be composed of mobile sulcus mucoperiosteum. Tearing of the gingival crevice will be a frequent occurrence and periodontal pocketing most likely to develop as the years go by. Furthermore there will be at most a shallow sulcus, lateral to the 2nd molar and cleansing of the buccal aspect will be difficult. In extreme cases the mucosa will ascend vertically over the buccinator muscle from the distal aspect of the 2nd molar.

The position and condition of the upper 3rd molar is checked and its occlusal relationships to the lower 3rd and 2nd molars noted. If the tooth is in a position which makes it difficult to keep clean, if it is already carious, if it does not, and will not, occlude with a tooth which is to be retained, and particularly if it is over-erupted, it should be extracted. Indeed if it bites on the gum flap of the lower 3rd molar its extraction may cut short an attack of pericoronitis permitting more latitude in the timing of lower 3rd molar surgery. Lastly, consideration should be given to its possible future use as a denture or bridge abutment.

If the lower 3rd molar on one side is considered for extraction the other side also should be examined, particularly if it is likely that the operation will be carried out under a general anaesthetic. Finally the related lymph nodes should be palpated to determine the extent of any infection.

The Radiographic Examination

Periapical radiographs are taken whenever possible because the detail which they reveal is better than with any other technique and of course most of the surgical difficulties are to be seen in a lateral view of the tooth and its related anatomy. The film should be positioned with care. In general the mesial edge of the film should not lie further forward than the mesial surface of the 1st molar for vertical, mesio-angular and disto-angular impactions. For horizontal teeth the mesial edge should not lie further forward than the middle of the first molar, but the film can be rotated so that the long lower edge slopes upwards towards the back, parallel to the mylohyoid ridge. This way a horizontal tooth will lie in the diagonal axis of the film.

An occlusal film should be taken for all difficult teeth and particularly where the tooth is completely unerupted so as to complete the two views at right angles necessary for an understanding of the problem in three dimensions. The occlusal view will provide an alternative view to the periapical film of the roots of horizontal teeth, particularly where the presence of a third root is suspected. It is essential for buccolingually placed teeth to identify which way the crown is pointing and to show the shape of the roots. It is helpful to show the thickness of the lingual alveolar plate where the 3rd molar is buccally displaced.

Rotational tomographic films have largely displaced oblique lateral jaw views because they provide a lateral rather than an oblique view and are less subject to misinterpretation. However, like the oblique lateral jaw view, rotational tomograms lack much of the valuable detail to be seen in a periapical film. They are taken particularly:

a. Where good periapical films are not possible because of difficult access for positioning the film, or where the patient will not tolerate a periapical film even with the application of a topical anaesthetic.

b. Where the tooth is so far from its normal position that it cannot be projected on to a periapical film in the mouth.

c. Where there is an associated pathological process larger than can be demonstrated on one periapical film, such as a cyst or tumour, infected bone, multiple impacted teeth or a fracture.

d. Where the jaw is thin, or weak, or where the 3rd molar is close to the lower border.

e. Where the position and relationship of the upper 3rd molar cannot be judged adequately by clinical examination.

f. To exclude latent disease elsewhere in the jaws.

Radiological Assessment

Assessment in relation to the surgical removal of lower 3rd molars means estimating how much work will need to be done at the operation and what technical difficulties will need to be overcome. When the results of the radiological assessment are added to those of the clinical assessment the operator should have a clear idea of the problems to be faced and the sequence and extent of the surgical procedures necessary to remove the tooth. All facets of the proposed operation should be mentally anticipated. The following features should be considered.

1. *The Orientation of the Tooth*

Lower 3rd molars may be mesio-angularly, vertically or disto-angularly inclined, horizontal or ectopic. Horizontal teeth may lie at various depths such as with the crown opposite the crown, or the neck, or the roots of the 2nd molar. Most are orientated in line with the dental arch with the crown forwards but some lie transverse to the arch. Whether the crown faces lingually or buccally should be determined by an occlusal radiograph. Ectopic teeth may be found in many unusual situations from the coronoid notch to the lower border of the ramus. The basic extraction movements are determined by the orientation of the tooth, but may be modified by tooth depth, root formation and bone density.

Mesio-angular teeth are first tilted distally by mesial elevation until the mesial surface of the 3rd molar is inclined upwards to clear the distal aspect of the 2nd. Buccal elevation is then applied to drive the tooth upwards, forward and lingually out of the socket.

Horizontally impacted teeth which are mesially facing are moved in a similar fashion except that the initial upwards and distal tilting movement needs to rotate the tooth through a greater angle. Where the lingual plate has been split off by the split bone technique, after mesial elevation to loosen the tooth, it is rolled out lingually by buccal application of an elevator. This technique can be applied to both mesio-angular and horizontal impactions.

Buccolingually orientated teeth are not difficult to uncover on their superior and buccal aspects. The problem often is to find a point of application for an elevator with a satisfactory fulcrum. It may be necessary to remove bone from around the tooth until a curved elevator can be introduced under the crown to raise the tooth from its socket.

Vertically orientated teeth require only slight distal tilting to release frictional contact with the 2nd molar followed by an upwards and lingual extraction movement produced by buccal elevation, provided the investing bone has been adequately removed of course to permit such movements.

Disto-angularly impacted teeth are first tilted distally by elevation applied to the mesial surface to release frictional contact with the 2nd molar as before. However, the mesial bulbosity of the 3rd molar must be displaced backwards and then upwards from under the convex distal surface of the 2nd molar in those cases where the impacted tooth lies below the general level of the occlusal plane. The second movement again results from buccal application of an elevator, but with the fulcrum of the elevator opposite the distal cusp of the 3rd molar. The crown of the 3rd molar is raised upwards and forwards so that the slope of the crown below the mesial contact point of the 3rd molar slides over the distal contact point of the 2nd molar. Further consideration will be given to the primary disimpacting and extracting tooth movements in relation to root shape and provision for a path of removal.

2. *The Depth of the Tooth*

An assessment of the depth of the tooth indicates the amount of bone which must be removed to uncover the tooth. Depth is measured first from the alveolar crest to the level of the greatest diameter of the crown, and secondly from the neck of the tooth to the greatest diameter of the root if the latter is bulbous. The level of the crest of the alveolar bone is indicated by a line which joins the surface of the retromolar fossa to the crest of the interdental septum, between the 2nd and 1st molars in a gentle, concave curve. The crest of the retromolar bone is marked in a periapical radiograph by the apex of the triangle between the bone surface and the top of the follicular space distal to the crown. Bone is usually removed to uncover the tooth completely to just below the greatest diameter of the crown and the socket widened by a guttering process down to the greatest diameter of a bulbous root.

3. *The Degree of Impaction of the Tooth*

This together with root shape indicates whether tooth division is optional as a means of facilitating the extraction of the tooth and so reducing bone removal, or whether it is obligatory.

Disto-angular and vertical teeth are usually impacted against the soft tissues and bone only. The soft tissues are simply incised to permit a favourably impacted tooth to be delivered. The major problem is usually access distolingual to impacting bone which has to be removed to free the greatest diameter of the crown.

Mesio-angular and mesially facing horizontal teeth are impacted against the 2nd molar. In general such teeth must be tilted upwards, rotating them about a point close to the apex of a single-rooted tooth or the distal apex of a two-rooted tooth until the mesial surface of the 3rd molar will clear the crown of the 2nd as it is ejected from its socket. To test whether this can be permitted by bone removal alone a line is drawn from the apex of the distal root of the 3rd molar to the tip of its mesial cusp. With this line as radius an arc of a circle is described. If this passes clear of the image of the crown of the 2nd molar elevation after simple bone removal is likely to be successful. If the arc cuts the image of the crown of the 2nd molar, tooth division will be essential if this mode of elevation is used.

With the split bone technique a varying amount of distal and lingual bone is split away. Elevation of the tooth is by application of force to the cervical enamel just under the crown of the tooth and from the buccal side. The tooth rotates about the apices and is displaced lingually and upwards. If a good occlusal radiograph can be obtained the likely success of this manoeuvre can be tested because this time the radius of the arc of movement joins the lingual edge of the distal root apex to the tip of the mesiobuccal cusp. If the mesiobuccal cusp will clear the tooth in front as the tooth rotates lingually, simple elevation will be successful; if not tooth division will be required. The types of tooth division will be considered under surgical technique.

4. *Root Shape*

This may be either favourable or unfavourable. Roots may be unfavourable in that their curvature opposes the initial distal tilting movement which most impacted teeth require. If either one or both roots curve mesially this distal tilting is prevented. Bulbous roots are obviously unfavourable and the socket must be widened down to the bulbosity to permit the root's extraction. On the other hand, the bone around large bulbous roots may be thin, particularly lingually, and easily split away. Conversely, thin spindly roots, especially those of three-rooted teeth, are often in thick bone and easily fractured. Where there are two or more roots they may either converge or diverge, locking the tooth into the bone and this again is unfavourable and often demands tooth division.

5. *Bone Removal to Form a Path of Elevation*

Bone has to be removed to provide space into which the tooth can be tilted in preparation for the application of a force dislocating it from the socket. This is usually space distal to the tooth. The tooth is mentally tilted in this fashion in relation to the radiographic image so that the amount of bone which must be removed can be judged. If the roots of the tooth curve distally the initial tilting movement is favoured, but this root curvature may now oppose an upwards movement with a lingual and forward component such as follows buccal elevation. When the upwards extracting movement still has distal component imposed upon it by the root shape, further bone removal distal to the tooth will be required or tooth division. The relationship of the mandibular canal as it curves downwards through the bone to the site of distal bone removal should be noted to avoid damage to the nerve if a substantial amount of distal bone is to be removed.

6. *Bone Removal to Permit Application of Elevators*

Usually a channel must be created down to the follicular space beneath the mesial surface of the crown, at the amelo-cemental junction. If the follicular space is narrow it must be widened to accommodate the elevator blade. The relationship of the elevator's point of access on the mesial surface of the tooth to the inferior dental canal should be considered, particularly in the case of horizontal teeth.

Another common point of application is buccally at the bifurcation of a two-rooted tooth or under the buccal bulbosity of the crown of a single-rooted one. Normally a deep pit is driven down to the point of application so as to leave a shoulder of buccal bone at a higher level which will form the fulcrum for the elevating movement.

7. *Bone Density*

This affects the ease with which bone may be removed. It may be assessed by noticing the thickness and number of the medullary trabeculae. The thickness of the mandibular cortex at the lower border will also give some indication of the density to be expected in the external oblique ridge, as will the relative radiopacity of the latter in a periapical film, given a standard exposure. Bone in negroes and patients brought up in tropical areas with high levels of fluoride in the drinking water also tends to be harder to cut.

8. *The Relationship to the Inferior Dental Canal*

This has been touched upon during the discussion of bone removal. Consideration must also be given to its relationship to the roots of the 3rd molar. If the canal is below the apex it is not at risk. If it is at the apex it may be damaged by mesially applied elevation which forces the apex down if bone removal has been inadequate. This is particularly true if the apex is bifid and grooved by the neurovascular bundle. Splitting the tooth longitudinally with an osteotome also may 'concuss' the nerve and produce a neuropraxia.

If the nerve is above the level of the apex it is usually *buccal* to the root unless the crown is lingually inclined so that the root lies buccally. A buccally placed nerve is at risk from buccal bone removal particularly during the formation of a point of application for an elevator or by a lingual extraction movement of the crown which forces the root laterally. Conversely, buccal movement of the crown may force the root against a lingually situated nerve. It is of course neurovascular bundles which either deeply groove or penetrate one or both roots which are most at risk. A marked radiolucency of the image of the canal where it crosses the root implies loss of dentine at that point. If the white lines which mark the upper and lower boundary of the canal are also missing as the canal crosses the tooth this too implies grooving and often deep grooving or perforation of the root because the greatest diameter of the canal is involved. The same may be predicted if the image of the root is narrowed where it crosses the canal.

Equally disturbing is narrowing of the image of the canal at this point. Another feature which suggests either deep grooving or perforation of the root is when the canal is looped upwards by the tooth. The implication is that the neurovascular bundle has been pulled upwards at that point as the tooth has attempted to erupt. In some instances the neurovascular bundle is embraced between the mesial root and an additional lingual root, which are fused at the apices. Because there is no reduction in thickness of the roots there will be no radiolucent mark and no radiographic evidence of the complication.

To Remove or Not to Remove

The first consideration is whether the 3rd molar has been, or is currently, involved in a disease process. Pericoronitis or food packing between the crown of the impacted tooth and the 2nd molar with the sequel of caries of either one or both of these teeth is common in young adults. In later life caries, periodontal disease or suppuration around a buried wisdom tooth are the more frequent states of affairs. Sometimes orthodontists want the 3rd molars removed if they feel that during their eruption imbrication of the anterior teeth will reappear. However, a causal relationship between incisor imbrication and 3rd molar eruption has never been firmly established. Occasionally there arises a late follicular or keratocyst. More rarely there may be an ameloblastoma present, but then the problem is not just the removal of the impacted 3rd molar but the excision of the neoplasm. The involvement of the 3rd molar by any disease is a clear indication for its surgical removal.

The more difficult decision involves the prophylactic removal of impacted mandibular 3rd molars. The reasons for removal of these teeth in late adolescence or early adult life is because the surgery involved is significantly easier at that time. In the past, in pre-antibiotic days of course, a spreading infection from a lower 3rd molar was not infrequently life threatening. This provided a strong incentive for the prophylactic removal of lower wisdom teeth. Prompt treatment with antibiotics has reduced the severity of these infections and a life threatening situation is now rare and the removal of symptomless lower 3rd molars for the younger patient is largely a matter of convenience. The surgery may be undertaken by choice at a time when there is the least disturbance to either study or career.

Pericoronitis is undoubtedly relatively common in teenagers and young adults so that the argument that the removal of partly erupted wisdom teeth will avoid this problem is valid. If the patient has reached the late twenties but has not experienced an attack, the chances that he or she will do so seem substantially reduced. Caries and periodontal pocketing, particularly affecting the 2nd molar, remain a risk, but fresh specific indications for the extraction of impacted wisdom teeth tend not to arise unless and until the other cheek teeth have been lost and the patient becomes a denture wearer. Then resorption of alveolar bone uncovers previously buried teeth and makes partly erupted ones more prominent. If they are covered by a denture, suppurative pericoronal infection or gross caries is common. The prospect that this might happen with the likelihood of tedious, lengthy surgery in an elderly patient is another reason for the prophylactic removal of these teeth. If they are still present such teeth must be removed when the other posterior teeth in that quadrant are extracted. On the other hand there is a natural reluctance for patients to agree to surgery to deal with a condition which is not troubling them. Furthermore, the dental surgeon must balance the possible advantages of prophylactic surgery against the discomforts which the patient will suffer and the possible risks of complications.

Surgical Technique—General Considerations

For general anaesthesia the patients require preoperative medical assessment as to their suitability for this type of anaesthesia and at least a haemoglobin estimation and urinalysis. Other investigations such as a chest X-ray and sickle test, etc., will also be considered. Day-stay general anaesthesia is only appropriate for straightforward surgery with minimal anticipated morbidity and good social circumstances for immediate aftercare.

It is normal to remove the teeth on one side at a time under local anaesthesia but in suitable patients, experienced operators can remove all four wisdom teeth during the same session, especially if intravenous sedation is employed. Without sedation around 45 minutes of surgery under local anaesthesia is as much as most patients find tolerable. One and a half cartridges (3 ml) of 3 per cent prilocaine with 0·03 i.u. felypressin should be used for each mandibular molar. Use of this solution permits better post-surgery clot formation and is not followed by reactionary haemorrhage as vasoconstriction wears off.

The lips, all retractors and the shanks of elevators should be lubricated with vaseline gel to prevent abrasion. Some operators have a preference for 1 per cent hydrocortisone cream. In general the operator stands on the right of the patient to remove the teeth on the right side and on the left to remove the ones on the left side. The soft tissues are stretched up over the anterior border of the ascending ramus and the incision started behind the 3rd molar and out towards the external oblique ridge. As the 3rd molar alveolar process overhangs the submandibular fossa, medial to the line of the ramus of the mandible, the incision line does not run straight backwards from the 2nd molar but is deflected laterally over the bone towards the external oblique ridge. The scalpel divides only mucosa and sub-mucosa at the commencement of the incision but cuts down onto bone distal to the position of the 3rd molar. The incision is then carried forward to the 2nd molar, over the crown of the wisdom tooth and through the gum flap. The interdental papilla distal to the 2nd molar is divided, then the incision is carried round the gingival margin of the 2nd molar up to the mesial cusp on the buccal side and down towards the sulcus through attached gingiva only. For a deeply buried tooth the papilla mesial to the second also is included in the flap.

A right-handed operator finds it more comfortable to make the incision from behind forward on the right side and from before backwards on the left. Where the 3rd molar is partly erupted the incision is made in two parts, the line of the incision being broken by the opening in the gum flap.

A periosteal elevator is inserted in the mesial relieving incision down to bone and the flap reflected distally to include the papilla between the 2nd and 3rd molars. By lifting the mucoperiosteum in a tunnel lateral to the 3rd molar the attachment of the follicle to the underside of the flap edge is displayed and cut with scalpel or scissors following which elevation of the buccal flap can be completed. The attachments of the underside of the lingual flap to the follicular or gubernacular tissues over the crown of the 3rd molar and at its distal margin are divided with a scalpel, being cautious not to pass the blade too far lingually.

Where relatively little bone needs to be removed the anterior vertical relieving incision is omitted and an envelope flap reflected (*Fig.* 4.1). Although it is not so easy to insert the periosteal elevator under the periosteum and reflect the buccal tissues, closure of the wound is easier and soft tissue healing more rapid.

A periosteal elevator is next introduced under the lingual flap, just behind the 3rd molar and the periosteum raised first in a distal direction until the firm attachment of the pterygomandibular ligament has been released. Elevation continues from this point lingually being particularly careful to

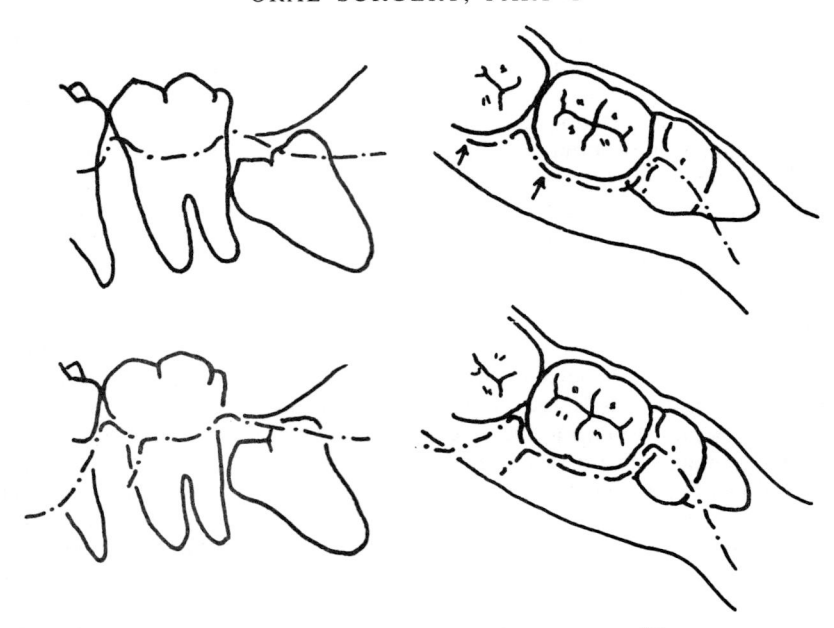

Fig. 4.1. The upper diagram shows an envelope flap incision for $\overline{8|}$. Depending upon the depth it may be finished at one or other of the two arrows anteriorly. The lower diagram shows the incisions for two-sided flaps. Either a short or a long relieving incision may be used, again depending upon the depth.

keep between the periosteum and the bone until the instrument tip drops over the internal oblique ridge. The tissues will then strip forwards to raise the whole lingual flap. This stripping movement should be performed firmly but carefully or the lingual nerve will be bruised. Retractors are placed to hold back both buccal and lingual flaps and, on the lingual side, positioned subperiostally to protect the lingual nerve.

Bone may be removed with either burs or chisels. Burs rather than chisels should be used when the patient is receiving a local anaesthetic with or without sedation or in older patients with brittle bone and at any age where the external and internal oblique ridges lie forward so that the investing bone is thick.

Bone removal is commenced with a No. 10 rose-head bur and starting at the distolingual corner, being careful of course to keep a retractor between the bur and the lingual nerve. The distal bone is removed next, being sure to cut right up to the surface of the distal root. Bone removal is continued on the buccal side, developing the cut into a semicircular trough and deepening it with a No. 6 rose-head down to the bifurcation of the roots laterally, and mesially to provide an application point for an elevator.

In general chisels may be used where the patient is young and the bone has a distinct grain, provided both internal and external oblique ridges lie well back so that the investing bone is thin.

When chisels are used the order of the procedure depends upon the amount of 3rd molar crown which is visible. If there is a substantial amount of bone covering the wisdom tooth so that the position of the distal aspect of the crown is not visible, bone is removed first on the buccal side. If the occlusal surface of the 3rd molar is clearly seen the lingual split is performed first.

The removal of buccal bone proceeds as follows (*Fig.* 4.2). Two vertical stop cuts are established, one at the mesial limit of bone removal which is made right into the follicular space, and the other at the distal limit, which is made to a similar depth, but because of its position may not end in the follicular space. The vertical extent of the anterior cut is usually 7 mm and therefore a 5 mm chisel is chosen. The bevel faces distally towards the bone which is to be removed. The 5 mm chisel is then rotated through 90° and a corner of the blade is engaged in the lower end of the anterior cut to start a third cut, joining the previous two. The bevel faces upwards and the shaft of the chisel is at 45° to the buccal side of the body of the mandible. As the chisel is tapped in it is also moved distally and the buccal bone split away from the anterior stop cut backwards. A crack will propagate backwards, ahead of the chisel edge. As soon as the split reaches the posterior stop cut the chisel is turned over, so that the bevel faces downwards and backwards. By rotating the chisel about its long axis and swinging the handle laterally the cut can be continued into the stop cut and across the back of the tooth. These cuts expose the crown of the tooth.

In preparation for the removal of the lingual plate both lingual and buccal retractors are adjusted to expose the bone distal to the 3rd molar. A chisel is placed so that its edge lies just to the lingual of the lateral ridge outlining the retromolar triangle of bone. The bevel of the chisel faces lingually and the edge lies diagonally across the jaw from the distobuccal corner of the 3rd molar to the lingual side 3–4 mm more posterior. The posterior corner of the blade should just reach the lingual surface. By increasing the angulation of the chisel the depth of the cut will be increased, and therefore the amount of lingual plate which will split away. The assistant must ensure that the lingual tissues and particularly the lingual nerve are adequately protected. The chisel is tapped into the bone across the back of the wisdom tooth cutting off the bone which forms the posterior rim to the two-sided balcony of bone which contains the tooth. When the blade is just short of the lingual side the lingual plate will often split off and move lingually. If not a twist of the chisel will complete the split. The actual edge of the chisel should not penetrate right through to the lingual side.

At this point the lingual plate will be hinging on the anterior end, where

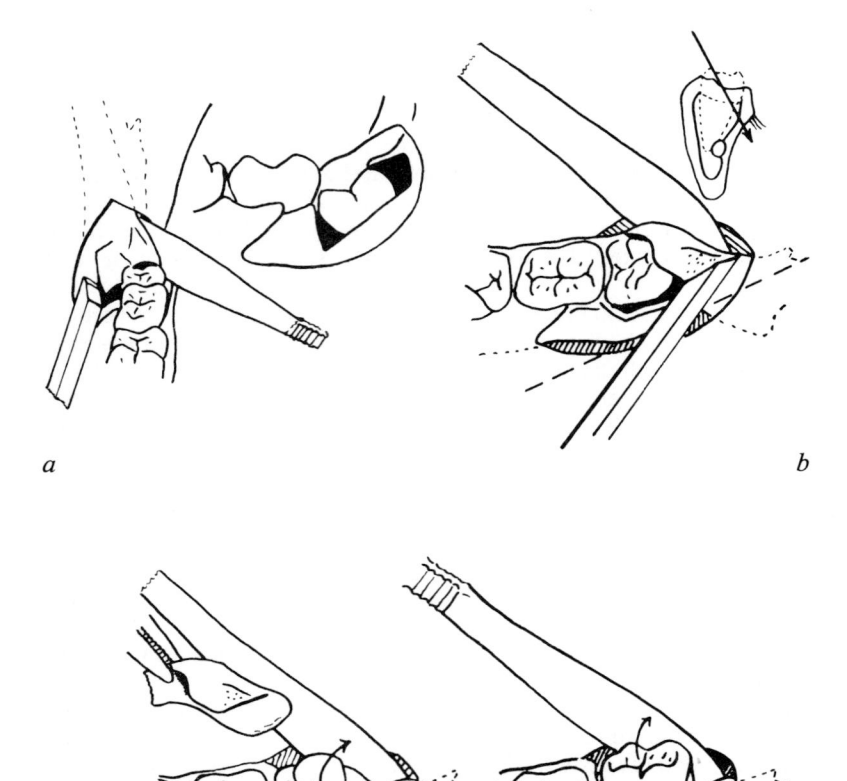

Fig. 4.2. The split lingual bone technique for removal of lower 3rd molars. *a,* After surgical exposure of the site anterior and posterior vertical stop cuts are made. These are joined by a horizontal cut which removes the buccal bone. *b,* The chisel is positioned parallel to the external oblique ridge (dashed line), just to the lingual of the buccal side of the retromolar triangle and driven through the bone to separate off the lingual plate. *c,* The lingual plate is levered up and removed. A straight elevator is tilting the tooth distally and lingually. *d,* An elevator applied buccally delivers the tooth.

the bone is thinned by the mesial root of the 3rd molar or the bulbosity of a horizontal tooth's crown. A curved Warwick James' elevator is inserted into the split and the plate levered upwards, disrupting the hinge. With great care the separated plate is withdrawn with toothed Fickling's forceps, protecting the lingual tissues as the curved, thin, knife-like posterior margin is brought out of the wound. The blade of the curved elevator is passed under the origin of the mylohyoid muscle from the lingual aspect of the piece of bone and the muscle detached, freeing the lingual plate completely. Removal of this piece of bone should expose both the distal and the lingual side of the tooth. Some vertical or disto-angular teeth are surrounded by a wide saucer of bone on the lingual edge which cannot be visualised or split off until the crown has been removed. Occasionally a large section of lingual plate and cortex may be split off running back towards the lingula. If it is possible to elevate the tooth without removal of this large piece of bone, it should be left attached to the soft tissues and allowed to heal. Failure to position the chisel at 45° across the long axis of the jaw is one cause of this occurrence.

Now it may be necessary to remove V-shaped wedges of bone mesio-buccally with a narrow 3 mm chisel to provide access for elevators. Often the use of chisels and burs can be combined to provide for the most effective removal of investing bone. One contraindication to the use of the split bone technique even in young patients is the presence of a very thick lingual plate beside a buccally inclined tooth. With adequate reflection of the soft tissues the situation will be obvious and the bone should be removed with a No. 4 or 6 rose-head bur.

The basic extraction movements depend upon the orientation of the tooth and were considered during assessment. The indications for tooth division have also been discussed. Splitting off the distal third of the crown with an osteotome will often permit a disto-angular tooth with distally curving roots to be removed without excessive bone removal (*Fig.* 4.3). Splitting off the mesial third will *not* disimpact a mesio-angular tooth as the fragments tend to impact together and the smaller fragment, being wedge-shaped, cannot be removed first (*Fig.* 4.4).

If a two-rooted tooth is eased a little in its socket it may be split longitudinally between the roots. Provided the root shape is favourable the two fragments may be elevated separately, freeing a tooth which is impacted in a mesio-angular or horizontal position. Splitting a tooth requires a sharp rather than a hard blow with a mallet and a high quality hard steel or tungsten carbide edged osteotome. For the inexperienced, division with a fissure bur avoids the risk of a fractured jaw.

If only the distal root shape is unfavourable the tooth may be delivered by inserting a tapered tungsten carbide fissure bur into the bifurcation, cutting upwards a little and then distally to separate the distal root. A tap with an osteotome across the transverse fissure of the crown will split off the distal half of the crown so that the mesial half of the tooth can be tumbled over the

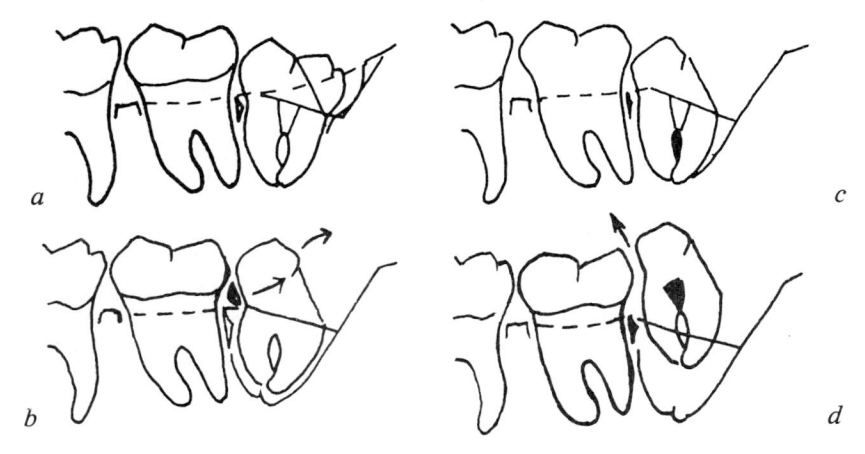

Fig. 4.3. Removal of a disto-angular 3rd molar. *a,* The crown is uncovered and the distal part split off with an osteotome. *b,* This permits access to the distal bone, previously hidden by the bulbous distal part of the crown. Sufficient distal bone is removed to permit tilting of the 3rd molar. The bone between the recurved roots is drilled away. *c,* A straight elevator is applied mesially to tilt the 3rd molar clear of the 2nd. *d,* Buccal application of an elevator drives the tooth upwards and forwards out of the socket.

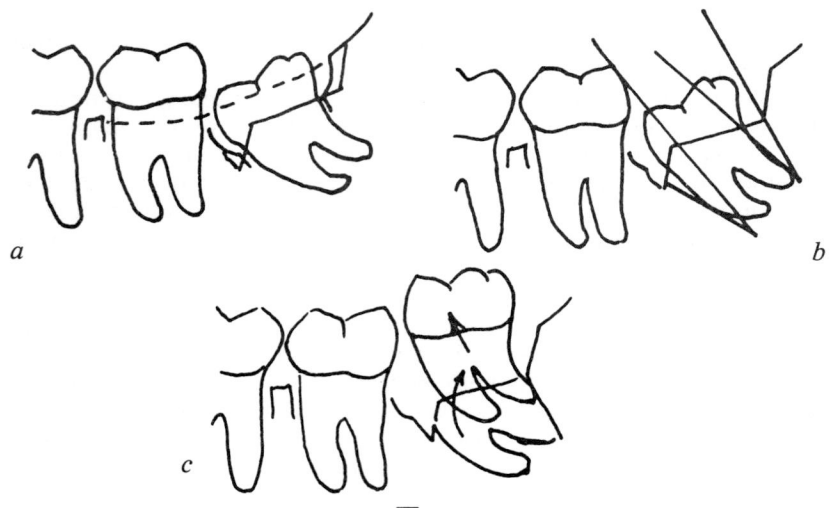

Fig. 4.4. Removal of mesio-angular ⌈8. *a,* Bone is removed below the greatest diameter of the crown and below the mesial convexity to make a point of application for a straight elevator. *b,* Bone is removed distally to permit the tooth to be tilted through a sufficient angle to clear ⌈7. *c,* It is elevated distally and then upwards first by mesial application of a straight Warwick James' elevator and then buccal application of a curved one.

UNERUPTED AND IMPACTED TEETH

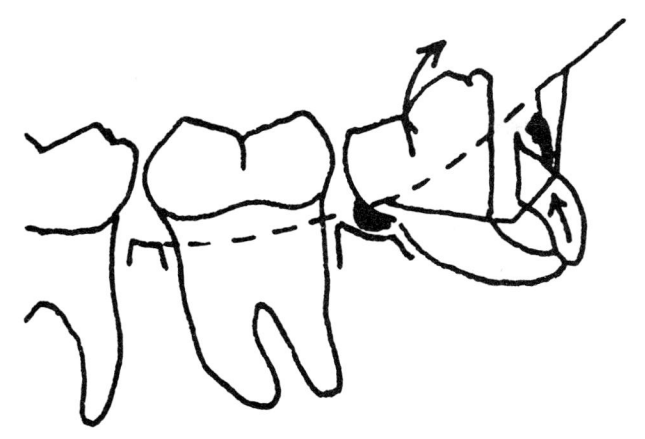

Fig. 4.5. Removal of a mesio-angular 3rd molar with recurved roots by section of the distal root.

distal root (*Fig.* 4.5). It is usually a simple matter to elevate the remaining distal root forward into the empty space created by the removal of the crown.

Dividing the tooth in its long axis between the roots will disimpact a mild mesio-angular or horizontal impacted wisdom because after the removal of the distal portion the centre of rotation of the mesial half of the crown is altered (*Fig.* 4.6). The mesial cusp now describes an arc around the mesial root apex and often will move clear of the tooth in front.

If the degree of tooth impaction is severe or if both roots are curved unfavourably the whole crown must be removed and the roots separated at the bifurcation with a bur (*Fig.* 4.7). This is particularly important if tooth fragments wedge together as soon as elevation is attempted due to the root curvature.

Tungsten carbide tapering fissure burs in an air drill are best for the separation of whole crowns. The cut should be made through the thin cervical enamel, but at a level that will leave enough of the cervix for the application of elevators. The cut should gradually approach a little closer to the occlusal surface as it travels towards the lower aspect of the impacted tooth. This will avoid the creation of a fragment which cannot be levered out of the space. The cut should provide sufficient space that the occlusal fragment can be collapsed backwards away from contact with the 2nd molar. In making this cut if the bur penetrates completely through to the lingual side of the crown it may also penetrate the lingual plate as the lower part of the cut is made, putting the lingual nerve at risk unless it is well protected by a Howarth periosteal elevator. If the bur emerges completely at the bottom end of the cut and is not controlled as the softer bone is entered

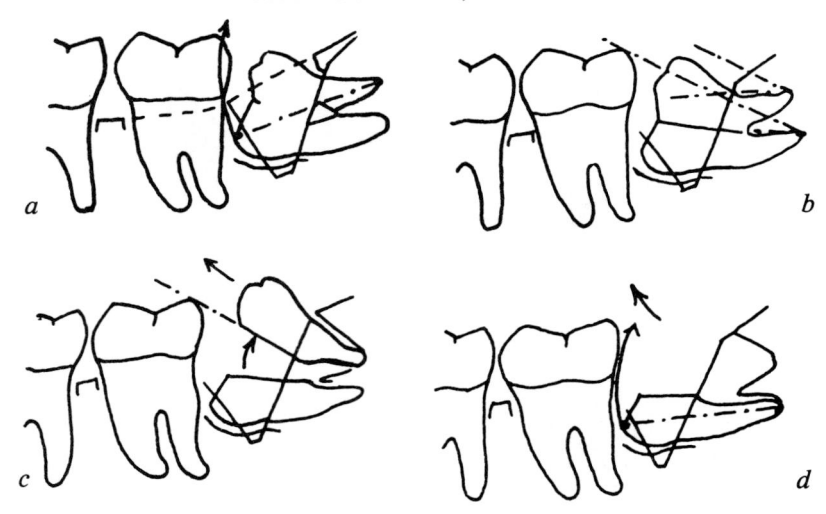

Fig. 4.6. Removal of a horizontal 3rd molar. *a,* Bone is removed to expose the crown. With later mesial elevation it would rotate about the distal apex, but the mesial cusp would not clear the distal surface of ⌈7. *b,* The tooth is divided longitudinally between the roots. The angle needed to tilt the distal half clear of the 2nd molar is determined and appropriate bone removed distally. *c,* The distal half is elevated out. *d,* The mesial half will now rotate about the mesial apex and clear the distal surface of ⌈7.

the distal root of the 2nd molar or the inferior dental nerve may be damaged.

On the other hand, if the cut does not penetrate to these surfaces and the crown is cracked off a wedge of enamel may split away from the neck of the tooth with the crown, so locking it in place. These problems can be avoided by splitting off the top half of the sectioned crown with an osteotome placed against the buccal aspect of the transverse fissure after two-thirds of the cut has been made. Then the remaining part can be cut through with better visibility.

Socket toilet should follow the completion of the extraction. The socket is irrigated with sterile normal saline, taking particular care to aspirate away all bone and tooth debris from beneath the periosteum under the buccal flap and the cut surface of the cancellous bone. If bone or tooth debris is left in the crevice between the periosteum and the buccal bone an abscess will form there three to four weeks later, perhaps with a sinus in the buccal sulcus and exuberant granulation tissue. Any sharp points or edges to the socket especially on the lingual side should be nibbled smooth with bone nibblers. If they are left they may penetrate the flap and irritate the patient's tongue until sequestrated.

UNERUPTED AND IMPACTED TEETH

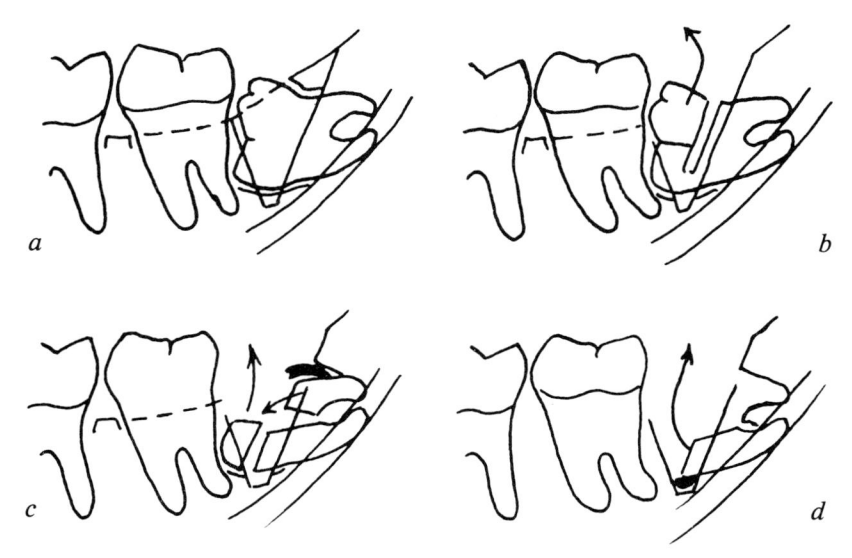

Fig. 4.7. Removal of a deep, horizontal 3rd molar. *a,* The crown is uncovered and a mesial application point for an elevator established, clear of the mandibular nerve. *b,* The crown is partly divided and the distal half split off and removed. *c,* This gives better access and visibility for the section of the mesial half of the crown. Create a wedge, narrow below, so that the fragments can be elevated out. *d,* The roots are separated and elevated out one at a time.

Suture of the flap requires some care and should be delayed until all bleeding is controlled. An envelope flap simply requires a suture between buccal and lingual flaps distal to the 2nd molar. A two-sided flap ending midway along the 2nd molar can be closed in a similar fashion, but the suture should penetrate the lingual flap close behind the 2nd molar and the buccal flap further distally. This is because the buccal flap retracts distally. Special note should be taken of the collar of gingival margin which fits against the distobuccal corner of the 2nd molar. It is easy to pick this up by mistake and suture it across the 3rd molar socket depriving the 2nd molar of the masticatory mucosa which should form the gingival margin at this point. Where the flap extends to the papilla between the 1st and 2nd molar both this and the sulcus incision will need suturing to retain the flap in place. If the wound can be closed with a single stitch any ooze will leak out from the buccal sulcus incision. Tight suturing prevents the drainage of ooze which then finds its way into the buccal space creating a haematoma. The loop of the stitch should be large enough to facilitate its removal. Sutures should be removed at around seven days postoperatively.

Complications

Some degree of pain and swelling is normal and the natural consequence of the surgery required to remove the 3rd molar. The more extensive the surgery the more the discomfort. A gentle surgical technique, gentle soft tissue retraction, care in selecting the method of bone removal, the use of sharp burs and chisels and the use of elevators with minimum force and only after proper disimpaction of the tooth or tooth fragments will minimise both swelling and postoperative discomfort. The use of substantial force to elevate a tooth crushes the bone of the fulcrum which can lead to postoperative pain and may be a factor in the production of a dry socket. While a careful surgical technique and the use of prophylactic antibiotics reduces the incidence of dry socket following the excision of impacted third molars they do not eliminate the complication, even where the extraction has not been unduly difficult. Sympathetic treatment is required.

Some operators favour the use of 10 mg of dexamethasone intravenously with the anaesthetic induction agent (or orally if using local analgesia) followed by 10 mg the following day. This will reduce the swelling and pain but not trismus without any impaired healing or other complications and may be appropriate where substantial swelling is anticipated. Doses of 10 mg of dexamethasone produce a temporary suppression of circulating cortisol which recovers within three days. However, again no complications have been noted (Al Haag et al., 1985). The same trial showed 15 minutes of ultrasound immediately and 24 hours postoperatively to be almost as effective in the reduction of postoperative morbidity.

Anaesthesia of either the lingual, mylohyoid or the inferior dental nerves is another common complication. Often the anaesthesia is due to neuropraxia and lasts only a few days to a few weeks.

There are a number of ways in which these nerves are at risk. Attention to the details of surgical technique will help to reduce the incidence of more lasting damage.

The lingual nerve is at risk:

a. From a periosteal elevator raising the lingual flap: the flap is often tough and patience combined with division of the attachment of the follicle to the underside of the flap will reduce the force used and the risk of bruising the nerve.

b. From lingual flap retractors: prolonged retraction of the lingual nerve with the other lingual tissues results in a neuropraxia even while it protects the nerve from more serious damage. Care must be taken to see that the retractor is between the nerve and the bone. It is easy to insert the retractor too far lingually and not under the periosteum.

c. From instruments used to both cut and grasp the lingual bone and from the lingual plate itself if the split bone technique is used.

d. From a suture which may under-run the nerve if a large bite of lingual flap is taken.

The inferior dental nerve is at risk:

a. During the removal of distal bone, particularly for deep disto-angular teeth.

b. During division of the crown of a horizontal tooth, particularly if it lies low in the jaw.

c. During the splitting of a tooth with an osteotome if the nerve is in contact with the root of the tooth.

d. During the mesial application of an elevator for a mesio-angular tooth where the nerve lies at the apex.

e. Where the nerve grooves or perforates the root of the tooth the risk of crushing or dividing the nerve is high. If the risk is anticipated it can be reduced by careful surgery but not eliminated.

A suppurative infection of the socket with localised osteomyelitis or fracture of the mandible, particularly where a deeply placed tooth has been tackled, are rare complications which arise from time to time.

Fracture may occur during removal of a deeply buried tooth or later when the patient starts to chew again. In the former case immobilization is recommended, if necessary with the addition of a transosseous wire. With late undisplaced fractures a soft diet, antibiotics and careful supervision may be sufficient.

It is often claimed that periodontal pocketing down the distal aspect of a 2nd molar is a late complication of 3rd molar surgery, particularly where a horizontal tooth has been removed. In this context the preoperative extent of masticatory mucosa buccal to the 2nd molar is probably more important than any damage to the cementum on the distal root of the 2nd molar or infection in the socket. Incorrect approximation of the tissues when they are sutured may result in the adhesion of sulcus tissue to the buccal gingival margin of the 2nd molar, replacing masticatory mucoperiosteum at the gingival margin and eliminating the buccal sulcus.

Persistent infection of a socket extending beyond the period normal for a dry socket suggests either the presence of a foreign body such as a fragment of enamel, or localized osteomyelitis, or, if there is redness and swelling of the overlying face, actinomycosis.

Finally patients should be warned preoperatively of the discomfort and swelling to be expected, and of any likely complications, without causing unnecessary apprehension.

THE REMOVAL OF IMPACTED MAXILLARY THIRD MOLARS

Partly erupted maxillary 3rd molars are often difficult to keep clean, particularly if they are buccally inclined when they also tend to bite into the cheek. Over-erupted unopposed upper 3rd molars tend to traumatize the lower retromolar tissues. All such non-functional teeth should be removed.

Completely unerupted upper 3rd molars can be associated with follicular or keratocyst formation but rarely cause trouble with infection and, even when partly erupted, pericoronitis is much less common than with lower 3rd molars. The risk of resorption of the 2nd molar roots is very rare in the case of lower 3rd molars but occurs from time to time with upper ones. Unerupted wisdom teeth are usually removed when the other posterior teeth are extracted and as a preparation for the provision of dentures, or if the patient is to be given a general anaesthetic for the removal of the lower 3rd molars, unless they are difficult and accidental damage to the 2nd molars or some other complication such as fracture of the tuberosity is a risk. Fully erupted teeth which are in the line of the arch may be retained even if they are functionless when the need for a distal abutment for a prosthesis is anticipated.

Unerupted upper 3rd molars are best shown by rotational tomographic films. Oblique lateral jaw films also provide a good representation of their position. While periapical films produce a more detailed image they are often unsatisfactory because of the angle of projection.

Surgical Technique

To remove an unerupted upper 3rd molar an incision is made diagonally across the tuberosity from its distopalatal aspect to the distobuccal corner of the 2nd molar and on in almost the same line up into the buccal sulcus. In most cases if a broad Coupland's chisel is introduced under the flap at the distobuccal corner of the 2nd molar it can be used to elevate, not only the mucoperiosteal flap, but also to dilate the coronal space around the crown of the unerupted tooth. If the bone is thin it can be pushed aside to form an osteomucosal flap. It is important to free the palatal cusps from the palatal tissues in the same way. A straight Warwick James' elevator is inserted into the follicular space and worked upwards mesial to the neck of the 3rd molar, following which the tooth can be elevated out. A curved Warwick James' elevator can be hooked into the same situation to disimpact a mesio-angularly impacted tooth and deflect it laterally out of the socket. The opposite forefinger is used to receive the tooth as it emerges into the buccal sulcus to prevent its loss into the pharynx.

More formal bone removal may be required to prepare the tooth for elevation. If this is so the incision for the flap is extended around the upper 2nd molar to its mesial aspect and the mesial papilla included before it is taken up into the sulcus. This provides a flap which can be retracted adequately to enable the operator to see to remove the necessary bone. Normally the answer to unexpected surgical difficulties is to improve access and vision to the maximum. However, access is rarely easy to a high impacted upper 3rd molar and inexperienced operators should avoid embarking upon tricky surgical procedures.

After the removal of the tooth the wound is irrigated in the usual way and any loose fragments of bone are removed. Unless the extended flap has been needed no suture is required.

Complications

1. Excessive bleeding which usually arises from the sulcus incision and may require prolonged compression or suture.

2. Haematoma formation may be dramatic with periorbital oedema but is of no consequence.

3. An oro-antral fistula may arise after elevation, but it invariably heals satisfactorily if the wound is sutured.

4. Displacement of the wisdom tooth into the antrum will require removal through a Caldwell–Luc antrostomy which can be carried out by extending the incision horizontally forwards in the sulcus (*see* Chapter 9).

The tooth is occasionally displaced distally into the infratemporal fossa lateral to the pterygoid plates. Here a careful experienced hand with good tissue retraction is required to remove it. Should it seem irretrievable the operator should leave the tooth until localizing radiographs and help can be obtained.

5. Fracture of the tuberosity may occur especially if the roots are hypercementosed. It is usually advisable to dissect out the fractured alveolus and tooth and close the wound primarily. Small tuberosity fragments are difficult to splint, and due to premature occlusal contact of the contained tooth cause considerable discomfort.

THE IMPACTED MAXILLARY CANINE

Upper canines more frequently fail to erupt than lower ones. In both cases malposition of the unerupted tooth is common and in some circumstances the tooth lies a substantial distance from its normal path of eruption. Failure of both upper canines to erupt properly is also a frequent occurrence.

Maxillary canines start their development at a higher level than and erupt after the adjacent teeth. With a greater distance to travel through the bone to its normal position in the arch there is an increased chance of deflection from its path. Also in a crowded arch, the additional space required for the canine may be taken up by the 1st premolar by the time that it is due to erupt. There are many other suggested causes of malposition of upper canines, most of which are not convincing or apply only in occasional circumstances. These include: disturbances of the axis of the tooth germ, scar tissue in the path of eruption, failure of the root of the deciduous predecessor to resorb, ankylosis of the deciduous predecessor and the congenital absence of the lateral incisors, the roots of which may act as a guiding influence for the canines. Rarely a maxillary canine is congenitally absent or it is transposed with the adjacent lateral incisor or premolar or it fails to erupt as part of an abnormality which results in the failure of several or many teeth to erupt.

It is wise to monitor the position and development of the maxillary canines from the age of nine onwards as part of a general assessment of the development of the adult dentition. If this is done, many future problems can be avoided. Certainly if by the age of 13 the upper canines have failed to erupt their position should be investigated. The attitude of the patient and the parents to the problem, and the patient's standard of oral hygiene should be assessed and noted. The opinion of an orthodontist is required to determine whether the tooth can be brought into a functional position. The adjacent teeth should be examined for caries and tested for vitality. The presence of a non-vital lateral incisor or heavily filled first molar might appreciably alter the treatment.

Clinical Examination

The canine may be partially erupted or there may be an obvious bulge on either the buccal aspect of the alveolar process or in the palate, which denotes its position. A palatal impaction is more common than buccal, but one can be deceived into assuming a palatal bulge is the crown of the tooth when it may well be a local bone thickening. Furthermore bilateral impactions are not necessarily symmetrical. Palpation of the maxilla through the labiobuccal sulcus may also reveal the crown of the tooth to be high in the maxilla and adjacent to the floor of the nose. Occasionally the lateral incisor may be proclined due to the presence of the canine crown lying labial to the root. Palatal inclination of the lateral can be caused by a palatally placed canine which is impacted against the apical part of its root. Rarely the root of a palatal canine may be felt on the buccal aspect as a small knob high on the side of the maxilla above the premolars. If there is no clinical evidence of an unerupted canine it may be lying within the alveolar process in the line of the arch.

Radiological Examination

Careful radiological assessment of the unerupted canine is required before deciding upon treatment because, unlike a wisdom tooth, it may be possible to uncover the tooth to permit its eruption into the arch. The position of the canine can be determined from a choice of occlusal, periapical, rotational tomographic and lateral skull radiographs. The periapical radiograph provides a detailed picture of the tooth and its surroundings and is helpful for demonstrating the degree of root formation of the canine, apical curvature, the existence of any root resorption affecting the adjacent lateral incisor and the presence of an associated cyst. The vertex occlusal projection which produces an axial view of the incisors provides buccopalatal localization of the canine and determines its relationship to the standing teeth. The same view will also reveal any rotation of the tooth about its long axis. The parallax method which uses two periapical films of the canine taken from different positions or a periapical and a standard occlusal will also establish whether the crown is lying buccally or palatally to the arch.

From the first periapical view, the relationship of the canine crown to the adjacent incisor root is noted, and compared with this relationship on a second periapical film taken when the tube has been displaced distally and re-angulated mesially to centre on the film.

If the canine appears to move away, i.e. distally, from the incisor root and in the same direction as the displacement of the tube, the canine lies palatally. Should it appear to move mesially, increasing its overlap of the incisor, the crown lies buccally to the arch and if there is no obvious change, the crown probably lies wedged in the arch between the adjacent teeth. The clinician should also assess the position of the root relative to the premolar roots in case the canine lies across the arch, with the crown on one side and the root on the other.

For surgical purposes periapical and vertex occlusal films alone will often suffice, but rotational tomographic radiographs (e.g. OPG) are advantageous for demonstrating the vertical angulation of the tooth and its height above the alveolar margin. In a lateral sinus view, or cephalometric lateral skull projection, if the image of the crown of the canine overlaps the incisors this usually indicates that the canine is labial, whereas if the tooth is behind the incisors it is either positioned in the line of the arch or is palatally situated. This view is also used for assessing the height and inclination of the buried tooth. A postero-anterior (PA) projection will provide information about the angulation of the tooth in the coronal plane, the proximity of the crown to the sagittal plane, and the relative position of the canine to the roots of the incisors, premolars, nasal floor and antrum. Periapical radiographs should be taken even when the canine is partially erupted, because marked curvature of the apex not infrequently occurs although the extraction may seem straightforward. Apical hooking should be suspected if the end of the canine root appears blunted, or indistinct as it is likely that the long axis of the curved tip is coincident with the path of the X-ray beam.

Reasons for Removing Unerupted Canines

Many completely buried canines give no trouble and often there is no reason to remove them. Indeed the surgical removal of unerupted canines, both upper and lower, carries an element of risk for the adjacent teeth and needs substantial care. They need removal:

    a. Before the fitting of full or partial dentures, but it is also prudent to remove them before the construction of a bridge in that part of the dental arch.

    b. To permit the orthodontic alignment of other anterior teeth.

    c. Where there is resorption of the root of an adjacent lateral or central incisor. If resorption is noticed in time, it may be arrested by removal of the unerupted canine. If resorption is marked, exposure of the canine and removal of the lateral should be considered.

d. Where a follicular cyst has developed.

Infection of buried canines is uncommon until the patient is edentulous and wearing dentures.

Surgical Technique

In the presence of standing adjacent teeth it is obvious that if the canine is situated buccally a buccal incision should be made and, if it is impacted in the palate a palatal approach is required (*Figs.* 4.8 and 4.9). When,

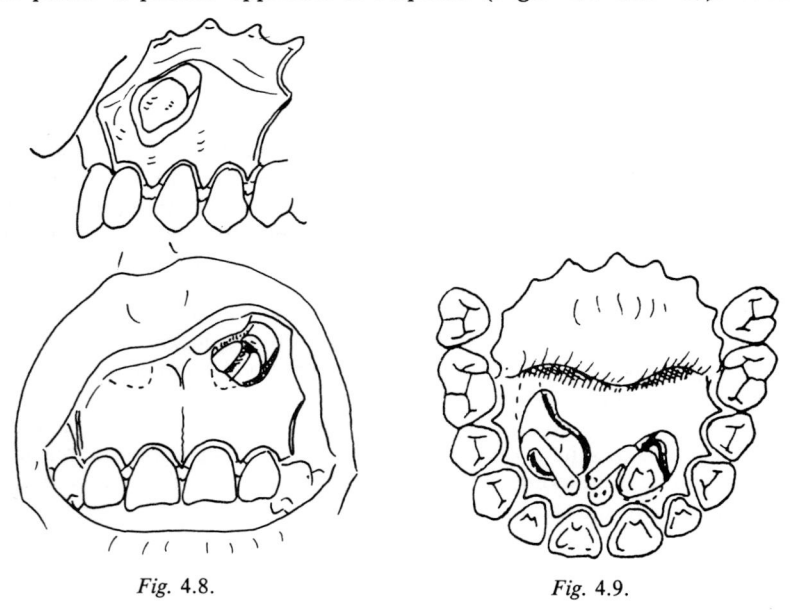

Fig. 4.8.   *Fig.* 4.9.

Fig. 4.8. Removal of labial canines. *Above.* A three-sided flap is raised and the thin bone over the crown and neck of the tooth removed. Following this the tooth is elevated out. *Below.* A three-sided flap from premolar to premolar is raised to expose bilateral high labial canines. The crown and cervical third of the root is uncovered. The neck is cut across with a thick fissure bur and the crown divided longitudinally with a thin one. It is best not to uncover the tip or to cut through to the tip. The crown is split apart and the fragments removed. Next the root is elevated out.

Fig. 4.9. Removal of palatal canines. *Right side.* A favourably placed and curved canine can be uncovered and elevated straight out. *Left side.* If the crown is tight against the incisor roots it is best separated by an oblique cut from the root. This permits it to tilt out away from the standing teeth. The root can be elevated into the crown space.

however, the unerupted canine is lying directly over the teeth in the arch, both labial and palatal flaps should be reflected from the beginning. It is also essential to expose the tooth from both palatal and buccal aspects when the long axis of the unerupted canine lies across the arch with the root on one side and the crown on the other and the root passing either above, or between, the roots of the standing adjacent teeth.

In the edentulous patient one incision made along the crest of the ridge will permit access from both aspects. Incisions in the palate should never be made directly over the buried tooth. If the sutured edges of the flap rest over a socket the suture line may break down, and in the case of a palatal socket this occasionally leads to the formation of an oroantral or oronasal fistula.

Extraction by the Buccal Approach

If the teeth are standing a horizontal incision is made around their gingival margins. It is then taken into the buccal sulcus at each end in a gentle curve for a distance of about half an inch. The flap is designed so that a complete interdental papilla is left at each corner (*Fig.* 4.8). After the flap has been raised a bony bulge may be visible or palpable indicating the site of the unerupted tooth or even a portion of its crown may be seen. Occasionally, however, there is no clinical indication of the exact position of the tooth. Sufficient overlying bone is removed therefore with either a chisel or a bur over the site of the buried canine to uncover its crown. Provided that the root formation is favourable and the canine not impacted against an adjacent standing tooth, it should be feasible to deliver it by application of a curved Warwick James' elevator. If, unfortunately, the root configuration prevents simple elevation, the root should be exposed over a good part of its length before further force is applied. If delivery of the canine still cannot be effected, the tooth must be sectioned at its neck with a bur and the two fragments teased out separately.

In a number of cases the bulge in the buccal sulcus represents the apex of the canine which may be hooked, and under these circumstances the crown will be found on the palatal aspect of the arch. If the coronal part of the tooth is then uncovered, it may be possible to apply sufficient force to the root on the buccal side to push the entire tooth through the palatal socket. If this cannot be accomplished because of a sharp apical curvature, the apex is cut off and removed buccally following which a sharp tap delivered with a straight elevator and a mallet to the flat end of the root will deliver the tooth palatally.

After the canine has been extracted, the wound is cleaned by gentle irrigation with warm, sterile, normal saline and the flap is sutured back into position. The follicular tissues need not be avulsed unless virtually detached. If left *in situ* they help to protect the roots of the adjacent teeth and never result in cyst formation. Care must be taken to ensure that bleeding has ceased before suturing, otherwise there is a risk of haematoma formation beneath the flap. Haemostasis can be achieved by firm pressure with a gauze swab.

Sutures are passed through the palatal half of the interdental papilla, between the teeth from the palatal side, through the buccal half of the papilla and back beneath the contact point and tied palatally. This avoids the unnecessary and unsightly row of knots and suture ends visible between the teeth on the buccal side. Improved flap apposition can also be achieved by using a vertical mattress suture, again commencing the suture from the palatal side. Each interdental papilla should be sutured back into place. To ensure accurate apposition a suture is placed initially through the single papilla at each end of the incision line. Then the buccal extension is closed before the remaining papillae are sutured. When inserting sutures at the buccal extremities it will be found technically easier to pass the needle through the flap first and then into the tissue on the other side of the wound which should be elevated from the bone for about 2 mm from the edge.

Attempts to suture in the converse direction may lead to a tearing out of the stitch or inversion of the wound edges. If the sutures will not pass between the teeth a bite is taken with the needle through the palatal mucoperiosteum adjacent to the interdental space and then the suture material is eased down between the teeth after which the needle is passed through the buccal half of the papilla and the suture completed.

Extraction by the Palatal Approach

The length of the palatal incision will, of course, depend upon whether one or two impacted canines are to be removed. In the edentulous case the incision as stated is made along the crest of the alveolar ridge. If two canines require extraction the incision line runs in the gingival crevice from the 1st molar region on one side to a similar position on the opposite side, but if only a single canine is to be removed the incision need extend only from the 1st molar region on the side to be operated upon to the canine region on the opposite side (*Fig.* 4.9). The mucoperiosteal flap is raised with a curved Warwick James' elevator or Howarth periosteal elevator working from each side towards the midline. When detaching mucoperiosteal flaps from around the teeth it is a mistake to prise away the flap from within the gingival sulcus because it will be damaged causing interference with gingival reattachment. Therefore, in order to lift the palatal flap as atraumatically as possible a palatal papilla is lifted from between the premolar teeth and a curved Warwick James' elevator or Ward's periosteal elevator introduced beneath its base. As the blade of the instrument, with its convexity facing the undersurface of the flap, is advanced, the mucoperiosteal tissues will peel away from the necks of the teeth. When necessary the neurovascular bundle passing through the incisive foramen should be divided with a sharp scalpel close to the bone. Clamping is unnecessary, for the small vessels do not bleed much and haemorrhage can be arrested easily by applying firm pressure with a gauze swab. The attachment of the flap to the median suture is reflected with care as the mucoperiosteum is thin in this area. The flap is retracted away from the operation site by an assistant using a Lack's retractor.

Once the palatal mucoperiosteal flap has been raised, the crown of the tooth—with or without its follicular sac—may be immediately visible. Sometimes, however, a bulge is present on the palate and there is a thin layer of bone overlying the crown. This can be shaved off quickly and cleanly by using a sharp chisel with hand pressure only. Once the neck is uncovered the general orientation of the tooth is then apparent.

The removal of bone around a canine in the edentulous individual is straightforward because of the absence of adjacent teeth. If, however, the unerupted canine is lying in close proximity to standing teeth, bone removal must be restricted to the distal and palatal aspects of the tooth. This approach will reduce the risk of damage to the roots of adjacent incisors or premolars, but some temporary loss of support of these teeth may be inevitable, after the canine has been removed, if the socket is adjacent to their roots.

When a canine is completely buried a portion of bone overlying the suspected position of the tooth is removed with a chisel or bur and the outline of the crown is uncovered. Once the lie of the tooth is ascertained, bone is taken away with either a mallet and chisel or with a No. 6 rose-head bur, ensuring that the roots of any standing teeth are left undamaged and their supporting bone is retained. Not only is it essential to expose the crown of the tooth, including the maximum convexity and the incisal tip, but often it is necessary to free the coronal part of the root of its immediate investing bone by the 'guttering' technique. If the canine has a favourable root shape and is not tooth-impacted, it should now be easy to deliver it. A sharp, hook shaped, apical curve will prevent delivery by palatal bone removal alone. Forceful elevation will then snap the apex off and attempts to retrieve it via the socket can result in its displacement into antrum or nose. Sharply angled apices like this result when the dentine papilla of the developing root impinges against the underside of the periosteum. Such an apex may raise a distinct knob on the surface of the bone high over the premolar teeth.

Alternatively, radiographs may reveal it to be in the angle between the antrum and the nasal fossa. If the apex can be uncovered through a buccal flap and amputated the remainder of the tooth can be pushed through towards the palate.

When it is judged that an adequate amount of bone has been removed from around a buried canine, very gentle leverage with a curved Warwick James' elevator should be applied to the appropriate surface (*Fig.* 4.9). Which one will depend upon whether the root is straight or curved. If there is a responsive movement from the tooth, it should be eased out of the socket, but if resistance is encountered more bone should be drilled away. During elevation it is a wise precaution to apply the fingers of the left hand to the buccal surfaces of standing incisors or premolars to support them and ensure that they do not move. Often delivery of the canine can be expedited by using two curved Warwick James' elevators simultaneously—one on each side of the tooth—with a double lifting action. Occasionally it is possible to grasp the canine with forceps and extract it with a rotary motion.

Sometimes the crown of the canine is deeply impacted against the roots of adjacent erupted teeth which may show evidence of progressive resorption. Any attempt to elevate the intact canine is likely to cause movement of, and damage to, these adjoining teeth. In such circumstances the crown should be cut off with a bur at right angles to the long axis of the tooth then it can be displaced away from the adjacent teeth and into the space created by the bur cut and lifted from the wound (*Fig.* 4.9). Once the crown is removed there is usually adequate room for the root to be brought forward and elevated. Where it is difficult to free the mesial and distal bulbosities of the crown a further vertical cut through the crown will permit the parts to collapse inwards. Once this has happened it can be removed.

When the root of the canine lies across the alveolar process between the roots of standing teeth, its apical prominence may be felt high in the buccal sulcus, and in this case both buccal and palatal flaps are raised. After exposing the apex on the buccal aspect and uncovering the crown in the palate, an attempt is made to deliver the whole tooth palatally by applying pressure to the apex. Where the root of the canine is curved the tooth may be loosened, the crown amputated and removed from the palatal aspect and the root pushed through into the coronal part of the socket.

After the impacted canine has been extracted, loose remnants of the dental follicle should be removed from the socket with a pair of toothed Ficklings forceps. The follicle should be left where it covers the root of an adjacent tooth, particularly if the latter is resorbed. After smoothing the bone edges the socket is irrigated with warm sterile normal saline to clear away any tiny fragments of bone or tooth debris.

It is important to ensure complete haemostasis before suturing the soft tissues, in order to prevent a haematoma accumulating beneath the palatal mucoperiosteal flap, as this may become infected. The flap should be correctly repositioned and moulded tightly against the palatal vault with firm pressure from the operator's fingers. Each interdental papilla is then accurately sewn back into place with the suture knots as stated on the palatal aspect. A 22 mm half-circle cutting needle is inserted squarely through the base of each papilla. If the needle is not positioned in this manner but is introduced at an angle there is a tendency for the suture to tear out.

After piercing the palatal papilla the needle is passed between the teeth so that it emerges through the corresponding buccal interdental papilla, about 3 mm from its tip. Some difficulty may be experienced in driving a needle between the teeth of young patients whose interdental crests of bone extend to the full height. However, a slim pattern modern eyeless needle will usually pass through even under these circumstances. A similar problem arises in patients who possess a gross irregularity of the anterior teeth. Where it is found impossible to slip the needle directly between the teeth in the conventional fashion, the suture is first passed through the palatal papilla and then eased down gradually between the contact points into the gingival embrasure before rotating the needle through the buccal papilla. On the rare occasions that suture material cannot be drawn past a tight contact point into the interdental space, a suitable compromise is to pass the suture through both the palatal and buccal papillae leaving the intervening portion resting above the contact point between the approximal surfaces of the two crowns.

If it has been necessary to raise a buccal flap in addition to the palatal one, suturing is performed in exactly the same manner, each corresponding palatal and buccal papilla being sewn together. A thin acrylic palatal plate, held in place by cribs on the 1st molars, will prevent the formation of a haematoma beneath the palatal mucosa.

Alternative Methods of Treatment of the Unerupted Canine
1. *Leave in Situ*
If the canine is asymptomatic and its extraction might cause loosening of, or damage to, the adjoining erupted teeth, there is a strong case for leaving it alone. But such a policy depends upon the absence of infection, abnormal and *progressive* widening of the follicular space, resorption of adjacent teeth, or irregularity of the anterior teeth which the patient wishes corrected by orthodontic treatment. The patient should be kept under annual review to verify that these complications have not arisen. If the deciduous canine remains *in situ*, its doubtful long-term retention must be stressed to the patient, although a few may remain functional throughout life. With crowding of the permanent teeth, extraction of the deciduous canine may relieve the situation, and aposition of the 1st premolar and lateral incisor can be acceptable from the aesthetic viewpoint, particularly if the lateral incisor has a large crown, and the palatal cusp of the first premolar can be ground to increase its resemblance to a canine.

2. *Surgical Exposure*
Before an attempt is made to assist the eruption of a malposed and unerupted canine into a functional position certain criteria must be fulfilled, namely:

  a. That there is adequate room in the arch to accommodate the tooth;
  b. That the potential path of eruption is unobstructed;
  c. That when eruption is completed the apex of the tooth will be near to the normal position in all planes;

d. That exposure of the crown of the tooth can be carried out as close as possible to the time at which normal eruption would occur.

The initial stage of the operation is to reflect the mucoperiosteum and trim away the bone overlying the tooth to expose the greatest coronal diameter, the incisal edge and the cingulum. Care must be taken to avoid damage to both the unerupted tooth and the adjacent standing teeth, so, preferably, bone should be removed by using a chisel with hand pressure only, but in late adolescence the use of burs may be necessary. Before replacing the palatal flap a window is excised in it corresponding to the bony cavity containing the canine crown. The flap is then sutured as usual and a pack of Whitebread's varnish on ribbon gauze or Coe-Pak should be pressed firmly into the bony defect so as to cover the exposed crown. This should be held in position with sutures and left *in situ* for 2–3 weeks to prevent granulation tissue and mucosa from overgrowing the denuded crown. After removal of the pack the progress of eruption should be observed at frequent intervals.

Following eruption of the tooth, orthodontic treatment may be required to guide it into a good position in the arch. Sometimes orthodontic traction is arranged at the time of surgery. If this policy is followed it is important that the force applied to the tooth should be a gentle one. Traction to bring the tooth downwards towards its correct position in the arch is likely to be at an angle to the long axis of a displaced and unerupted tooth. This will tend to concentrate the force at a fulcrum in the surrounding bone. If this happens localized resorption of the tooth and bone deposition may result in ankylosis which will permanently prevent eruption. The simplest technique now available is the acid etched cementation of an orthodontic bracket to the crown which may be performed at or after the operation.

In the case of the unerupted buccally placed canine the tooth may lie in the sulcus tissues. An opening created through these tissues to expose a tooth crown will soon close when the pack is removed. Furthermore if the tooth erupted into an area of non-keratinized mucosa its gingival margin attachment will be poor. Therefore a buccal flap must be raised including the attached mucoperiosteum. After carefully exposing the crown the flap margin is sutured above the crown and the bare area below covered with a pack. With care the follicle can be raised from the surface of the crown and the flap margin sutured to it.

3. *Transplantation and Surgical Repositioning*

The success rate with transplantation is highest for unerupted teeth which still have open apices because of the possibility of revascularization, and may be seven years or longer. It is essential to establish that there is sufficient space to accommodate the canine crown. This can be estimated with fine dividers using the contralateral canine as a guide. Minimal space deficiency may be overcome by grinding of the crown, but otherwise orthodontic therapy may be required to move the buccal teeth distally. Another problem encountered in late adolescence is over-eruption of the lower canine against the retained deciduous canine. This can only be treated by grinding of the incisal edge with a diamond.

The canine should be extracted carefully and transferred to the surgically prepared socket in the dental arch with the minimum of delay. It is preferable that the root surface should not be touched either with instruments or fingers as the viability of the cementum and periodontal membrane remnants will determine the success of the transplant. Should the new socket not be ready when the tooth has been delivered the latter is stored in the patient's own serum, or under the flap in order to keep the root moist. Root filling is not attempted so as to reduce handling of the tooth and apicectomy is unwise. An acrylic dummy can be prepared with the aid of an extracted tooth and after consideration of the patient's radiographs. This should be used to guide the preparation of the new socket, and to reduce the degree to which the canine itself is handled. The transplanted tooth should be splinted in its new position for a month after the operation.

In the technique of surgical repositioning, the displaced tooth is not extracted but rotated or tilted about its apex. It is usually undertaken where the tooth is fully erupted, but where the crown is out of the line of the arch. However, there must be adequate space for the canine in its correct position. Substantial skill is required to remove bone between the canine and the desired position in the alveolar process, without damage to the root of the canine. There must also be a good reason why normal orthodontic means are not used to reposition the tooth.

THE IMPACTED LOWER CANINE

Lower canines are impacted less frequently than upper ones, and they are usually buccally placed with the crown either fully or partially exposed. Some lie beneath the roots of adjacent standing teeth and with the crown positioned near the midline. A few are vertical and lingual to the incisors.

For orthodontic and aesthetic reasons it is often necessary to remove the partially or fully erupted but malposed tooth and this can be achieved by elevation with a suitable elevator or sometimes by simple extraction with specially designed forceps having one narrow blade which enables the tooth to be grasped without damaging or moving adjacent teeth. If the tooth is erupted but entirely buccal to the arch it can be grasped mesiodistally with a pair of upper premolar forceps. Should such measures fail to deliver the canine, buccal bone is removed, which will enable the extraction to be accomplished successfully.

The surgical problem is more complicated in the case of the unerupted canine deep to the apices of the standing incisors. These teeth should be localised radiographically with some care. A rotational tomographic film or a periapical film, an occlusal film taken with the central ray directed accurately along the long axis of the lower incisors and a tangential view of the chin are all essential to permit their full assessment. The deeply embedded buccal impaction can be removed after raising a buccal mucoperiosteal flap, if necessary degloving the chin, and excising the bone covering the canine until the tooth is freed sufficiently for force to be applied. Although lingual impactions can be treated in the same way via a lingual approach, access is far from easy and there is a strong case for leaving these teeth *in situ* unless associated with a pathological process. The patient should be reviewed annually. Removal is simple in later years if the individual is endentulous but unnecessary until then if no clinical disturbance is being caused.

Rarely a buried lower canine lies across the arch with the crown either buccally or lingually placed, and this may necessitate a dual buccal and lingual approach with perhaps the sectioning of the tooth and separate delivery of the fragments.

THE IMPACTED LOWER PREMOLAR

Failure of eruption of mandibular premolars is the result of lack of space, gross malposition, or retention of the deciduous predecessor. The 2nd premolar is most commonly affected due to the drifting forwards of the 1st permanent molar after early loss of the 2nd deciduous molar. Impacted lower premolars may be positioned lingually, lie in a vertical position within the arch or rarely, buccally. Occasionally they lie horizontally below the apices of the molars. The crown of the tooth may be fully exposed, partially erupted, or completely embedded.

If the tooth is unerupted, but in a superficial situation, a bulge may identify the position of the crown. Sometimes the more deeply buried premolar can be palpated lingually.

Radiographs are always necessary to determine the position of the premolar and its relationship to the roots of the standing teeth. An intraoral periapical and either a rotational tomographic or an oblique lateral jaw radiograph are the best views, together with an occlusal film to demonstrate the buccolingual position. In young patients the opinion of an orthodontist should be sought before making the irrevocable decision to extract the tooth, particularly if the 1st molar is heavily filled or grossly carious.

The reasons for the removal of partially erupted teeth are to eliminate a stagnational area or food trap and to prevent periodontal disease and caries.

If the crown of the tooth is largely erupted and presents lingually or buccally to the adjacent standing teeth, it is often possible to deliver the tooth with forceps. For instanding premolars the ideal pair of forceps is the upper roots pattern (Read's 76N). The instrument is applied from the opposite side of the mouth and rotated so that the beaks are directed downwards so as to seize the tooth mesiodistally or buccolingually. If a satisfactory purchase cannot be obtained immediately with the forceps, the judicious removal of a little investing bone may allow the tooth to be gripped firmly and delivered by rotatory or rocking movements. Slightly less accessible teeth may be delivered by expanding the bone on the lingual aspect of the root with a Coupland's chisel or by creating a narrow trough around the lingual aspect of the tooth by running a No. 4 rose-head bur backwards and forwards around the periodontal membrane. A Warwick James' straight elevator is passed through the interdental space between the adjacent teeth from the buccal aspect until its end engages on the lower part of the crown. A gentle tap or two on the end of the instrument will push the tooth out.

When the tooth is partially or completely impacted in the arch its crown will be wedged between the 1st premolar and 1st molar in the case of the malposed 2nd premolar, or between the canine and 2nd premolar in the case of the 1st premolar. Therefore, any leverage on the impacted tooth will put the adjoining teeth at risk. In such circumstances a buccal flap should be raised of adequate length to ensure good access. It should embrace at least one standing tooth on each side of the impaction together with a complete interdental papilla at each end. Adequate working space will diminish the risk of injury to the mental nerve. If, in fact, the tooth is seen to be in close relationship to the mental foramen, the patient should be warned preoperatively that temporary impairment of labial sensation may complicate the extraction. In retracting a flap in the vicinity of the nerve, undue tension should be avoided. The nerve should be identified and protected from trauma by the blunt wide end of a Howarth's periosteal elevator or a retractor while drilling or chiselling is in progress.

Buccal bone should be removed with either a chisel or a bur to uncover the cervical half of the root of the impacted premolar. The crown is then sectioned with a No. 4 fissure bur. To avoid damage to the adjacent teeth the fissure bur is sunk into the centre of the tooth at the amelocemental junction and driven through from the buccal to the lingual aspect. Having transfixed the tooth the bur is then taken mesially and distally with a sweeping stroke until the crown is just separated at its margin with the root. Once divided the crown is then displaced vertically downwards with an elevator into the space created by the No. 4 fissure bur, following which it can be delivered buccally. Next the root is elevated from its socket, the bone edges smoothed, and the flap repositioned and sutured into place.

A similar technique is employed to remove a premolar impacted lingually or buccally which resists an initial attempt to deliver it following simple removal of the lingual or buccal plate covering the crown. Sometimes the tooth is instanding and deeply embedded with the root lying buccally. In such cases the surgical approach is predominantly from the buccal but an incision along the crest of the ridge on the lingual aspect is necessary to uncover the crown and permit removal of the overlying bone. The impacted tooth should be sectioned, the crown delivered lingually and the root buccally.

However, in assessing difficult teeth serious consideration should be given to leaving them alone as tooth damage, fracture of the jaw and persistent deep infrabony pockets are possible sequelae. Impacted unerupted premolars which are present in an otherwise edentulous mandible are usually deeply placed and the jaw is often thin. If in such circumstances extraction is required, it is prudent to use a drill rather than a chisel. With a No. 8 rose-head bur, the immediate investing bone should be cut away from around the tooth to form a channel, preserving as much buccal and lingual plate as possible. Next, curved Warwick James' elevators are inserted into the gutter and applied at suitable points along the long axis of the root. With gentle rotation it should be possible to elevate the tooth up and out. Premolars with mesially or distally inclined apices may require separation of the crown from the roots before effective elevation can take place. Then the entire wound and socket should be cleared of debris and the flap replaced.

THE IMPACTED MAXILLARY PREMOLAR

An upper premolar is usually impacted with its crown palatally, but occasionally the tooth is lodged in the arch, obstructed by adjoining teeth or even by a submerged primary tooth. The crown may be wholly exposed, partially erupted or completely buried. If a sufficient amount of the coronal surface is uncovered, the tooth may yield to a simple forceps extraction or to elevation with a Coupland chisel which is forced into the socket and then levered against the root. These straightforward methods are more likely to be successful when the root is conical and the patient young. The majority of impacted premolars can be delivered only after adopting a planned surgical procedure involving the removal of palatal bone. To achieve suitable access for working on a palatal impaction an incision extending round the gingival margins from the 2nd molar to lateral incisor is necessary. The bone overlying the crown and neck of the tooth can be excised with mallet and chisel or gouge, or with burs, and further removal of the wall of the socket will expose the greater part of the root and allow an effective extruding force to be applied.

If, however, the crown is wedged between erupted standing teeth in the arch it is necessary to use a buccal exposure, to section the tooth with a bur, and dislodge the crown downwards and then outwards. Subsequent delivery of the root portion can be accomplished readily unless an apical hook is present. In the latter case drilling to a higher level alongside the root is usually necessary before the dilacerated apex can be teased out along a curved path. Naturally care should be exercised during the use of a bur for either tooth exposure or tooth division to avoid damage to neighbouring teeth. Where the impacted premolar lies across the line of the arch both buccal and palatal flaps should be used.

IMPACTED FIRST AND SECOND MOLARS

First and 2nd molars are sometimes impacted, but it is usually a comparatively simple matter to raise a buccal flap, remove bone and carry out vertical section of the tooth in order to facilitate its extraction. First molars are sometimes found vertically placed near the lower border of the mandible. In tackling these it must be remembered that the mandibular nerve is likely to cross the tooth buccal to its neck.

Exceptionally, the 1st, 2nd and 3rd molars are all impacted. It is impossible to catalogue all the possible combinations and variations of such impactions, but in practice such multi-impactions are not unduly difficult to remove. Following a careful study of the radiographs, common sense dictates which tooth should be removed first, usually the mesial of two, or the middle of three impactions. Following the removal of the first tooth, extraction of the remaining teeth is usually comparatively simple.

Where multiple molar impactions are found in young patients it is unwise to leave the teeth to correct themselves as the impacted state usually worsens. A careful estimate is made of which tooth needs to be removed to release the rest and allow eruption.

THE BURIED DECIDUOUS MOLAR

Occasionally a deciduous molar is retained in either the upper or the lower jaw, and is usually ankylosed. As the permanent teeth on each side of it erupt, they appear to stimulate periradicular alveolar bone growth, leaving the ankylosed molar completely or partially buried in the alveolar process and tightly wedged between the adjacent teeth. It is impossible to remove such teeth with forceps, even when part of the crown is visible, without fragmentation or damaging the adjacent permanent teeth. A buccal flap should be raised and the buccal aspect of the crown of the deciduous tooth uncovered. Even then it may be difficult to elevate and the crown of the tooth should be sectioned vertically through the centre, after which the anterior fragment can be elevated mesially.

SUPERNUMERARIES

Supernumeraries are principally found in the premaxillary region and are often small and peg-shaped, a type exemplified by the mesiodens which appears in the midline between, and frequently palatal to, the central incisors. Mesiodens may lie horizontally, or adopt an inverted position. Occasionally they are responsible for a dentigerous cyst. Supplemental teeth which have the size and shape of normal teeth may also develop in the upper anterior region, commonly in relationship to the lateral incisor. Supernumeraries may be single or multiple, unilateral or bilateral, and are a common cause of failure of eruption, rotation, spacing or malposition of one or more permanent maxillary incisors. The normal incisors seem to be most often displaced in a labiolingual direction. Removal of the supernumerary tooth frequently allows the abnormally placed incisor to erupt, or revert to its natural position in the arch, but orthodontic assistance may be necessary fully to correct the misalignment or malposition.

The premolar and molar areas are also sites in which supernumerary teeth may develop and in addition to the conical and supplemental varieties, other types may be present in these locations, such as teeth of conventional shape but smaller or larger in size than a normal tooth. Multicusped patterns or gross caricatures of the normal may be seen. An extra tooth in the upper 2nd or 3rd molar region is designated a paramolar if it is positioned buccally to the permanent tooth. It is often small and conical and can be fused to the adjoining molar. Fourth molars (distomolars) situated in the upper jaw may be either conical or molariform in shape. Their precise location may be either directly distal or distopalatal to the maxillary third molar. Mandibular 4th molars are usually about the same size as normal 3rd molars. A supplemental lower premolar may be difficult to distinguish from the adjacent teeth of the normal series.

Accurate localization is facilitated by taking intraoral radiographs from different angles. Periapical films will demonstrate tooth shape, the immediate surrounding, the presence of additional supernumeraries, and the vertical relationships of low supernumeraries. The principle of parallax can be applied to determine the buccopalatal relationship of the supernumerary to the adjacent teeth, but the vertex occlusal projection often provides the surgeon with more certain information in the maxilla.

For high maxillary supernumeraries additional views are helpful, namely PA jaws and lateral sinuses projections, because they demonstrate the proximity of the supernumerary to the nose. It is also useful to complete the radiographic study with a tangential view if the deciduous dentition is still *in situ,* as this view makes clear the relative positions of the erupted and unerupted teeth, particularly when the supernumerary is buccally placed.

Supernumerary teeth should be extracted only when their presence is responsible for the failure of eruption or malalignment of permanent teeth, or if they are the cause of other abnormalities. Remember that a small proportion of supernumeraries in the anterior palate are inverted, that is, the crown is directed towards the nose. Caution is necessary in recommending the surgical removal of an inverted palatally placed supernumerary which is situated close to the roots of the central incisors high in the maxilla and adjacent to the nasal floor. The roots of the supernumerary and the central incisors may be adjacent to one another and also difficult to differentiate from the surrounding bone, so that injury to the root of a permanent tooth may occur. If treatment is not indicated for a supernumerary, periodic radiological review is recommended.

The best time for the extraction of supernumeraries preventing the eruption of upper incisors is around six to seven years of age, when both central and lateral incisors are well formed, and it is unlikely that a permanent tooth will be elevated out in error. In addition, the supernumerary itself is sufficiently well developed to be easily identifiable and there is still a reasonable likelihood of the eruption of an upper central incisor.

For supernumeraries in the anterior maxillary region the surgical approach will depend upon accurate preoperative assessment, but in the majority of cases a palatal mucoperiosteal flap is reflected after making a gingival incision around the necks of the standing teeth from the 2nd premolar region on one side to the corresponding tooth on the opposite side. Usually a pyramidal labial flap need only involve the central interdental papilla for mesiodens, or from canine to canine for those in the central incisor area.

Relatively inaccessible teeth are approached from both aspects. Often bone removal can be carried out with a sharp chisel or gouge applied with hand pressure only, and limited to that immediately overlying the supernumerary. Once freed, the tooth can be turned out with a cumine scaler. During the operation unerupted permanent incisors need to be identified before uncovering the supernumerary, but, as a general rule, surgery is confined to delivery of the supernumerary, and exposure of the normal teeth if high is delayed in the hope that they will erupt naturally. If subsequently they fail to do so a pack is placed after exposure as with the unerupted canine. After adequate debridement and haemostasis the flap is returned to its original position and interrupted sutures inserted. With children plain catgut eliminates the need for removal which many fear. Primary closure is normally followed by uneventful healing and antibiotic prophylaxis is less important than in the case of lower third molar surgery.

In the case of supernumerary upper premolars and molars, periapical, rotational tomographic and occlusal films will supply all the relevant information, such as their relationship to adjoining standing teeth and their proximity to the maxillary sinus and tuberosity. Surgical access will usually be from the buccal aspect using a suitably designed flap modelled on that used for exposure of the upper 3rd molar.

DILACERATED INCISORS

Trauma to the upper deciduous incisors in childhood occasionally damages the underlying permanent incisor tooth germ, especially at the stage when only the crown is calcified, i.e. about 2–3 years. Further root development takes place at an angle to the crown producing a bent tooth which cannot erupt.

Occasionally exposure and ingenious orthodontic traction may bring such teeth into occlusion but usually they are best removed early so that the space may either be filled with the lateral incisor which ultimately can be crowned, or maintained for a partial denture or bridge.

Whenever unerupted permanent teeth have to be removed for pathological or orthodontic reasons it is absolutely essential:

a. To have the best possible radiographic assessment of the area, and

b. To identify carefully each of the unerupted developing teeth so that the wrong one is not removed.

SUGGESTED READING

Al Haag M., Coghlan K., Christmas P. et al. (1985) *Br. J. Oral Surg.* **23**, 17–23.

Andreason J. O. and Hjorting-Hansen E. (1966) Replantation of teeth I. *Acta Odontol. Scand.* **24**, 266–286.

Andreason J. O. and Hjorting-Hansen E. (1966) Replantation of teeth II. *Acta Odontol. Scand.* **24**, 289–305.

Bowdler-Henry C. (1969) Excision of the developing mandibular third molar by lateral treparation. *Br. Dent. J.* **127**, 111–118.

Brown I. D. (1981) Some further observations on submerging deciduous molars. *Br. J. Orthodont.* **8**, 99–72.

Cook R. M. (1972) The current status of autogenous transplantation as applied to the maxillary canine. *Int. Dent. J.* **22**, 286–300.

Di Biase D. D. (1969) Mid-line supernumeraries and eruption of the central incisors. *Dent. Prac.* **20**, 35–40.

Di Biase D. D. (1971) Mucous membrane and delayed eruption. *Dent. Prac.* **21**, 241–250.

Guralnick W. C. and Laskin D. M. (1980) NIH Concensus Development. Conference for removal of third molars. *J. Oral Surg.* **38**, 235–236.

Howe G. L. (1958) Tooth removal from lingual pouch. *Br. Dent. J.* **104**, 283–284.

Kural J. (1981) Infra occlusion of primary molars: An epidemiological and familial study. *Community Dent. Oral Epidemiol.* **9**, 94–102.

MacGregor A. J. (1985) *The Impacted Lower Wisdom Tooth.* Oxford, New York and Toronto: Oxford University Press.

McKay C. (1978) The unerupted maxillary canine. An assessment of the role of surgery in 2,500 treated cases. *Br. Dent. J.* **145**, 207–210.

Mortis C., Karabonta I. and Laparidis N. (1978) Extraction of impacted mandibular wisdom teeth in the presence of acute infection. *Int. J. Oral Surg.* **7**, 541–548.

Rood J. P. (1983) Degrees of injury to the inferior alveolar nerve sustained during the removal of impacted mandibular third molars by the lingual split technique. *Br. J. Oral Surg.* **21**, 103–106.

Rud J. (1970) Removal of impacted lower third molars with acute pericoronitis and necrotising gingivitis. *Br. J. Oral Surg.* **7**, 153–159.

Rud. J. (1983) Third molar surgery: relationship of root to mandibular canal and injures to the dental nerve. *Tandlaegebladet.* **87**, 619–531.

Seward G. R. (1954) Notes on dental radiography Parts II, III and IV. *Dent. Prac.* **IV**, 247–253, 312–319, 355–361.

Seward G. R. (1963a) Radiology in general dental practice VII: Radiography of lower third molars. *Br. Dent. J.* **115**, 7–9.

Seward G. R. (1963b) Radiology in general dental practice VIII: Assessment of lower third molars. *Br. Dent. J.* **115**, 45–51.

CHAPTER 5

SURGICAL PREPARATION OF THE MOUTH FOR DENTURES

Most patients tolerate the transition from a natural to an artificial dentition with reasonable ease, provided teeth are extracted and dentures constructed with skill and care. Every effort should be made at the time of extraction to conserve the remaining alveolar bone and masticatory mucosa so that, when healing is complete, the best possible foundation is created for the subsequent prosthesis. Anticipation of prosthodontic problems may allow their solution by surgical means at the time of extractions. Though more limited in extent, the surgical aspects of preparation for partial dentures are otherwise similar to those for complete dentures.

PROSTHODONTIC CONSIDERATIONS AT THE TIME OF EXTRACTION

Careful clinical examination of the teeth must precede the extractions and a record should be made of their appearance and shade, the relationship of the dental arches and the height of the lower third of the face. The size, shape and relationship of the future edentulous areas and any adverse bony or soft tissue irregularities should also be noted.

Radiographic examination of the teeth and jaws will greatly assist anticipation of surgical difficulties and complications. Rotational tomographs are particularly convenient for this purpose but more detailed intraoral radiographs should be obtained of any suspicious areas. Obviously, teeth should be extracted with minimum trauma and all debris removed from the extraction wounds.

Not all fractured roots need be removed. The disadvantage to the patient produced by destroying part of the future denture support must be weighed against the symptoms likely to arise from retention of a root fragment. As a general rule, fragments which are less than one-third of the original root length may be left *in situ* unless they were infected or have been loosened during the extraction process and would therefore become separated foreign bodies.

Rocking movements to expand the tooth sockets create a number of vertical fractures in the labiobuccal and linguopalatal plates and displace the intervening fragments outwards. These must be compressed back into place as they can result in sharp margins which will have to be removed surgically at a later date.

SURGICAL PREPARATION OF THE MOUTH FOR DENTURES

Small pieces of alveolar bone are often fractured off or extracted with the teeth and the sharp edges of any such defects can be trimmed conservatively with rongeurs. However an alveolar bone file allows just enough bone to be removed to leave a ridge which feels smooth when palpated through the overlying soft tissue. The thick gingival mucoperiosteum should be retained as far as possible, even if lacerated, since this tissue will eventually bear the load from a denture more successfully than the thin mucosa of the sulcus. Indeed it is the extent of the masticatory mucoperiosteum rather than the residual alveolar bone which defines the functional denture bearing area. Generous bone removal at this stage, although producing a smooth ridge in the short term, will probably lead to a significant reduction in bulk in the longer term. As some degree of resorption is unavoidable, extensive surgical destruction must be avoided as excessive resorption can follow surgical interference.

The gingival tissues should be replaced so as to cover any substantial areas of exposed bone after extraction, but complicated re-arrangement is usually unnecessary. Suturing the gingival margins of the sockets will hold them in place while healing takes place, helps to arrest bleeding, and also retains the shape of the compressed sockets. Sutures are best placed across the sockets midway between the interdental papillae. The interdental papillae and the crests of the interdental septa create a series of prominences along the ridges which, if recorded on the inner aspect of temporary dentures and impressed through them by mastication on the healing ridges, will become permanent. Irregularities are smoothed out whilst healing and natural resorption take place before permanent dentures are fitted. Smoothing the inside of the temporary dentures rather than the ridges helps to avoid this problem without loss of alveolar bone. Smoothing the interdental septa with a bone file and dividing the interdental papillae and interdigitating them as the sockets are sewn up, using a continuous plain or blanket suture, can also reduce the ridged effect.

IMMEDIATE DENTURES

When a complete clearance of the natural teeth is to be carried out, the provision of immediate replacement dentures should be considered to avoid both social and functional embarrassment to the patient. There are two ways of doing this, depending on the convenience to the patient and the preference of the operator.

1. Two-stage Immediate Denture Replacement

All remaining posterior teeth may be extracted and partial dentures constructed, fitted and worn until the initial healing of the ridges is complete. These dentures may be worn for some months, relined, and then used as the basis for full dentures, which are inserted following removal of the anterior teeth in a second stage. This method introduces the patient to denture wearing gradually and helps preserve the natural functional jaw relationship.

In the past, either the additional anterior artificial teeth were 'socketed', i.e. made with root-like prominences on the fitting surface, or the bulk of the upper alveolar process was reduced to provide room for a labial flange. The immediate aesthetic result of socketing the anterior teeth was very good, but unless the fitting surface was minimally contoured, permanent indentations in the ridges were created. On the other hand, alveolectomy of the upper alveolar ridge removing the outer cortical plate and much of the outer walls of the sockets promoted a destructive degree of resorption.

It is best to cover the untrimmed ridges with thin acrylic flanges and to reline these as soon as shrinkage occurs, following which the prominence of the flanges can be reduced. Where the alveolar process is bulky, the incisors may be 'socket fitted' to merely fit within the gingival margin.

In those cases in which the upper anterior teeth are proclined and the alveolar process is both prominent and unusually undercut, the less destructive technique of inter-septal alveolotomy may be employed to reshape the ridge. In this technique the interdental septa are removed with burs or straight bone shears and the labial cortical plate is fractured inwards. The bone shears are inserted across the septum into each neighbouring pair of sockets in turn and closed so as to cut through both the bony interdental septum and the soft tissue interdental papilla simultaneously. They are inserted first from the labial and then from the palatal direction and the blade points pushed as far apically as possible. In this way, a narrow wedge of bone and soft tissue is severed and removed without raising the soft tissues. A vertical cut is made with the bone shears or a narrow fissure bur through the labial plate distal to the canine socket cutting from inside the socket outwards. When these cuts have been completed, the entire labial cortical plate is fractured inwards at its base by firm finger pressure. It is best to squeeze the alveolar process between the fingers and thumbs of both hands while grasping it in a swab. In some patients it may be necessary to drive a flat chisel into the sockets, bevel facing palatally, to create a horizontal split across the buccal plate, particularly through the buttress of the anterior nasal spine. A continuous blanket suture approximates the gingival margins and maintains the new position of the labial bone. By this means, a reduction in labial bulk is obtained, but the cortical plate is preserved and resorption should not be excessive. It is often convenient to excise the upper labial frenum at the same time so that the provision of a notch for it in the denture flange is unnecessary and a point of weakness in the finished denture is eliminated.

2. *One-stage Immediate Denture Replacement*

The dentures are constructed from casts of full upper and lower impressions that have been taken carefully to ensure that the maximum denture-bearing area is included, and that muscle attachments and sulcus form are precisely recorded. The lingual sulci and tuberosity regions are often neglected. With an accurate squash bite the models are mounted on an articulator and teeth removed for denture construction. It is important that the dentures should be fully flanged to facilitate an early reline with a tissue conditioner. The flanges must not be overextended otherwise painful ulceration will occur. Similarly undercut areas should be relieved, especially the maxillary canine eminences.

The teeth are removed as described, preserving but smoothing the alveolar ridge and loosely suturing the gingiva.

The dentures are fitted immediately and checked for margin pressure points which must be trimmed.

Most patients adapt well to wearing the dentures continuously for the first two weeks, but removing them whenever possible for cleansing both the mouth and dentures.

Careful review will avoid pressure ulceration and loss of retention can be readily corrected with a soft tissue conditioner lining at about 4 weeks post-extraction and which may require repeating before a hard acrylic reline at 4–6 months.

In the first few months after the provision of full dentures, the occurrence of small pressure ulcers is not uncommon, but these can usually be induced to heal by relieving the fitting surface of the denture. Sometimes, however, small spikes or spurs may become prominent as initial remodelling of the bone occurs and these require trimming. Sequestration of small fragments may also happen and, where possible, these should be allowed to separate naturally since over-enthusiastic surgery may perpetuate the problem and lead to further loss of bone. Where there are multiple areas of discomfort, the dentures should be relined and the use of a semi-soft tissue conditioner material may be an invaluable intermediate stage. All immediate dentures have to be regarded as temporary appliances and conventional relining or replacement should be arranged after six to twelve months.

PROBLEMS PRESENTING IN ESTABLISHED DENTURE WEARERS

Surgery can only be considered when faults in denture design have been eliminated as a cause of the problem. Whilst most patients adapt well to the edentulous state and can wear properly constructed dentures without discomfort, there remains a minority who never do. This persistent denture intolerance is the basis of repeated complaints for many of which an obvious cause cannot be identified, and is usually a psychogenic oral dysaethesia (*see* p. 327). Every effort must be made to avoid unnecessary surgery even in the face of persistent patient pressure, as complaints about the results of the operation will simply be added to complaints about the dentures and will not cure the patient's unhappiness. There are, however, a number of irregularities of the denture-bearing areas which can be identified and relieved with great benefit to denture comfort.

An adequate radiographic examination is essential for accurate diagnosis in edentulous patients, as, in addition to buried teeth and roots which are relatively common, other unsuspected pathological changes may be discovered. However, great care must be taken to ensure that what is found can be related to the patient's complaints.

RETAINED ROOTS, UNERUPTED TEETH AND PATHOLOGICAL LESIONS

Retained roots are unlikely to be a source of symptoms unless they become superficially placed due to resorption of the surrounding alveolar bone. Pressure of the denture over such a root may initially cause only discomfort, but eventually ulceration occurs and infection with oral micro-organisms follows immediately. Exactly the same process may occur in relation to an unerupted tooth and, in both cases, extraction is indicated. This should be accomplished by as conservative an approach as possible, involving only the minimum removal of bone.

A sinus is often present which leads directly to the root. In some selected cases, larger roots, suitably aligned, such as those of lower canines, can be exposed, root-filled and restored so as to provide useful partial support for a denture. This approach seems to avoid the amount of ridge resorption which occurs following extraction and is said to enhance the subjective load bearing capacity of the patient.

Burrowing resorption is sometimes seen in buried teeth and radiographically resembles caries of the crown. This condition may be associated with pain and can be a rare indication for the removal of an uninfected and deeply buried tooth.

The presence of pathological lesions such as cysts or tumours in the edentulous jaws dictates the need for appropriate treatment, and although prosthetic considerations are secondary, they should not be ignored, so that the operative technique should be modified so as to retain the best possible denture foundation.

IRREGULARITIES OF DENTURE-BEARING TISSUES

Comfortable denture wearing may be impeded by a variety of bony or soft tissue anomalies.

Bony Irregularities and Prominences, Knife-edge Ridges

Irregular resorption may lead to the presence of bony prominences which tend to be covered by thin mucosa and on which the denture fitting surface bears heavily and causes discomfort. Such irregular resorption is much less common when provision of dentures is delayed for a few months after extractions or where the ridge is carefully prepared for immediate replacement.

If adjustment of the denture fitting surface does not provide relief the troublesome areas are treated by raising a soft tissue flap and reducing the prominent bone with a bone file or an acrylic bur. However, avoid removing too much bone with the latter.

The same approach may be used to eliminate inconvenient bony undercuts or to smooth knife-edge ridges.

However the subperiosteal insertion of particulate hydroxylapatite may provide a better solution to undercut and knife-edged ridges than reduction of the existing bone.

Fibrous Ridges

Flabby fibrous tissue provides a poor foundation for a stable denture and may be reduced in bulk surgically. This problem occurs most commonly in the upper anterior region when a full upper denture is opposed by natural lower anterior teeth. In such cases, consideration should be given to extraction of the lower anterior teeth as well as trimming the ridge. There is no identifiable plane of cleavage between the mucosa and the fibrous tissue so that a V-section fillet has to be removed and the wound edges sutured together.

A procedure similar to an apical repositioned flap, as used in periodontology, can provide a form of sulcus deepening and conserves the masticatory mucosa, but leaves the patient with a flattened ridge.

If a flap is raised from the sulcus sub-mucosally, but deepened onto bone when the masticatory mucosa is reached at the crest of the ridge, a pocket can be formed over the ridge. The thickened ridge mucosa can be cautiously thinned by shallow incisions in the periosteum. The edge of the labial soft tissues is raised sub-periosteally to permit the formation of a suture line with the flap margin to close the pocket. The sulcus can be resurfaced with split skin. Various calcium hydroxyapatite preparations can be used for ridge augmentation within the pocket.

Rarely, patients are seen with gross generalized fibrous enlargement of the alveolar ridges, a condition akin to hereditary fibromatosis gingivae. The surgical treatment of such cases follows the same principles, and may be done as follows.

a. Reflect a masticatory mucosa flap by dissecting parallel to the surface with a sharp blade, then excising the underlying fibrous tissue with the periosteum. The mucosal flap is then gently sutured back over the bare area.

b. Gross enlargments are pared away to produce the desired contour, with particular care to control the resulting haemorrhage. This can usually be achieved by application of a Whitehead's varnish dressing to the new surface, carried on a specially constructed plate or denture. Skin grafting is not indicated, but mucosa may be used. The mucosal epithelium is sliced off first to form thin mucosal grafts. The slivers of tissue are accumulated on a piece of tulle gras and kept moist with a sterile swab soaked in saline until the end of the operation. The plate is lined with gutta percha and an impression taken of the operation site after the fibrous ridge has been surgically reduced. The mucosal grafts supported on the tulle gras are then placed in the mould and applied to the operated area.

Frenal and Fibrous Bands

The presence of a prominent labial frenum in the upper anterior region, or less commonly in the lower anterior region, may produce problems in denture construction or may cause displacement of a denture where adequate retention is difficult to achieve. Fibrous bands running from the ridge across the buccal sulcus to the cheek regions produce similar difficulties, and, in either case, allowance for these structures prevents adequate peripheral extension of the buccal flange of the denture. The problems are worst when the frenum or band is attached at or near the crest of the ridge because the deep notch in the labial flange also weakens the denture so that a fracture may occur under masticatory stress. (For excision see following sections.)

Frenectomy

Excision of the labial frenum is a small procedure which can be done conveniently under local anaesthesia. If a second assistant is available this is beneficial as the upper lip can be held everted by a finger and thumb of both hands. Sometimes there is a brisk ooze and this also can be controlled by the assistant compressing the labial artery. The outline of the incision should be determined before the local anaesthetic is injected as this tends to balloon the tissues and distort them. A V–Y procedure is best for reducing the height of attachment of the frenum.

An incision is made on either side of the attachment of the frenum to the alveolar process and close to the frenum so that, once it is detached the bare area is as narrow as possible. The two incisions meet near the crest of the ridge and the apex of the frenum is then picked up, either by a skin hook or a stitch and is dissected off the periosteum with a scalpel.

The periosteum between the edges of the wound in the attached gingivae is incised down to bone and the mucoperiosteum lifted from the bone with a periosteal elevator for at least 0·5 cm on either side. The scalpel can be used to undermine the edges of the incisions in the sulcus in a plane over the surface of the periosteum.

A 4/0 absorbable suture is used to close the incision. The first stitch is inserted in one side of the wound towards the top of the sulcus. The edge of the mucosa is everted with a skin hook and the needle picks up the

SURGICAL PREPARATION OF THE MOUTH FOR DENTURES

periosteum under the edge. The stitch is passed from side to side through the apex of the freed frenum, through the periosteum under the other edge of the wound and then through the mucosa. As the stitch is tied the apex of the triangular shaped dissected frenum is re-located at the top of the sulcus and the wound closed at this point. Interrupted sutures approximate the mucoperiosteum over the labial aspect of the ridge as close as it will go. A single suture in either arm of the Y on the lip side of the reconstructed frenum is usually sufficient.

Excision of Fibrous Bands

A similar technique to that just described for the correction of overlarge frena has been used for the elimination of fibrous bands. However, there is usually a significant difference between the shape of the fibrous bands, found in the premolar or molar region, and the labial frena.

The 'fibrous' bands are in effect folds of sulcus mucosa which arise from a broad base on the cheek side of the sulcus. Incisions on either side of an upper labial frenum lie close together and almost parallel to one another. Incisions made on either side of a fibrous band diverge to separate a substantial triangle of mucosa. When this is advanced into the fornix of the sulcus a triangular defect is left which stretches up into a deficiency in the masticatory mucosa. Undermining the mucosa adjacent to the defect and closing it does not repair the lack of alveolar mucoperiosteum and subsequent scar contraction in the mobile mucosa raises a fresh band across the sulcus.

At first sight a Z-plasty appears to be a more rational plastic procedure with which to deal with these bands as it can be used to break webs and bands elsewhere in the body. An incision is made along the length of the band and then two others, one of which runs from the ridge end down into the sulcus and the other on the other side of the band from the cheek end, again down into the sulcus. Two triangular flaps are formed; one is used to cover the defect on the alveolar aspect, and the other that on the cheek aspect with a suture line which now lies at the bottom of the sulcus at right angles to the original band.

Unfortunately the repair on the alveolar aspect is still composed of sulcus mucosa with its mobile loose connective tissue submucosa, and the breach in the masticatory mucosa is not dealt with. Scar contraction will re-establish the fold.

If the periphery of the denture bearing area is to be improved the masticatory mucosa must be advanced down towards the sulcus at the same time as the mucosal band is re-attached. This may be done by a rotation flap of ridge mucoperiosteum which creates a new defect on the palatal aspect of the ridge surrounded by masticatory mucosa and which will heal by secondary intention with a similar mucosa, or by free palatal mucosal grafts applied to the denuded periosteum.

Excision of the Lingual Frenum

Short lingual frenum or tongue-tie is a congenital condition which occasionally causes the patient considerable inconvenience. Apart from being unable to protrude the tongue, the patient's main disability is the inability to clear away food which has become lodged in the roof of the palate or in the labiobuccal sulci. A few patients develop a lisp and occasionally if the frenum is attached to the gingival margin it may cause recession of the gingiva around the lower incisor teeth or a diastema. In the edentulous patient, a tongue-tie interferes with the stability of the lower denture by causing its displacement every time the tongue moves.

The anterior part of the tongue is tilted upwards first on one side of the frenum and then the other and a local anaesthetic solution is injected into the under surface of the tongue close to the sides of the frenum so as to avoid the ranine veins. Further solution is injected into the floor of the mouth on either side. When anaesthesia has been achieved a stitch is passed through the tip of the tongue and the frenum divided with scissors close to the under side of the tongue. As this is done the tip can be elevated and the wound stretched into a diamond shape. Sometimes there is a knob of fibrous tissue in the anterior border of the separated frenum. If this is so it is best excised. The lateral margins of the diamond are undermined with fine, blunt tipped scissors, being careful not to damage the ranine veins or the submandibular duct papillae. Two short lateral incisions may be made, one ⅓ of the way down from the top of the stretched incision on one side and the other ⅓ of the way up from the bottom on the other. This permits further elongation of the wound, and its closure as a Z-plasty by interrupted 4/0 absorbable sutures (*Fig. 5.1*). Particular care must be taken to ensure good haemostasis or a large haematoma will develop in the floor of the mouth, which if it becomes infected will lead to scarring and recreation of a tongue-tie.

Enlarged Maxillary Tuberosities

Enlargements of the tuberosity may be fibrous, bony or both, and may extend buccally, palatally, vertically, or in any combination of these planes. Lateral bulbous tuberosities with very deep undercuts will interfere with the fit of the upper denture and also lead to its displacement due to impingement of the coronoid process against the buccal flange of the denture when the mandible is opened or moved laterally. This can also cause pain in the soft tissues overlying the coronoid process. Excessive height of the tuberosity may reduce the inter-alveolar space to such an extent that there is inadequate room for the lower denture.

Bony Enlargements of the Tuberosity

Enlargements of the tuberosity, which are predominantly bony, and which do not contain an extension of the maxillary sinus, should be reduced to a satisfactory size with rongeurs, chisels, or bone burs. The tuberosity is

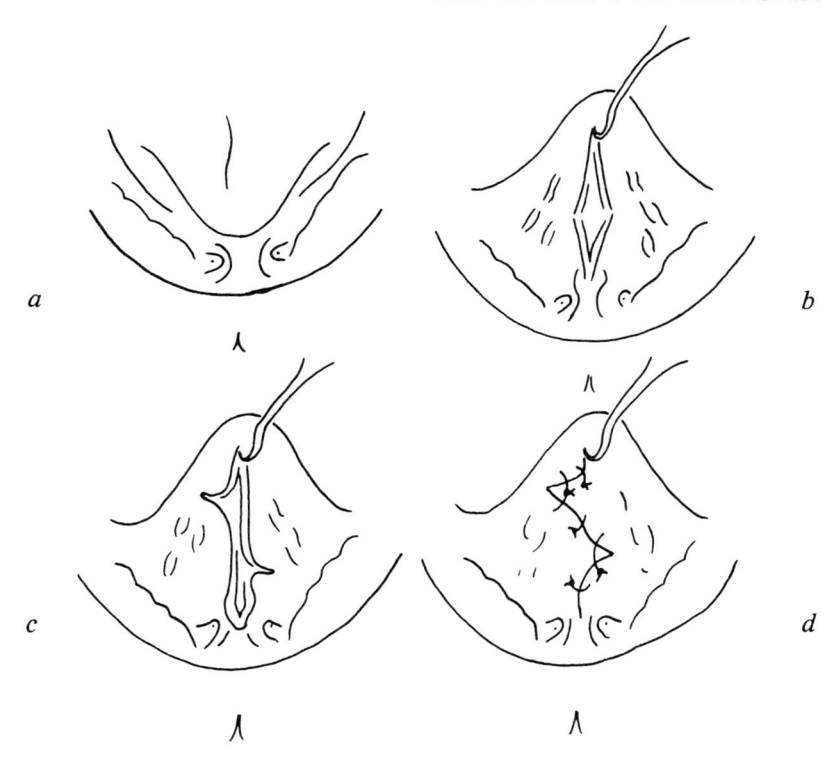

SURGICAL PREPARATION OF THE MOUTH FOR DENTURES

Fig. 5.1. Excision of short lingual frenum and tongue-tie. *a*, The preoperative state. *b*, The tip of the tongue is picked up and the frenum divided close to the under side of the tongue. The wound opens up as shown. *c*, The scarred and lumpy part of the lower end of the frenum is excised. Two short lateral incisions are made as shown, avoiding the sublingual veins. *d,* The wound is closed as a Z–plasty.

approached through an incision straight along the crest of the ridge extending from the posterior aspect of the tuberosity to the first molar region. After the bone has been reduced, the two mucoperiosteal flaps should be approximated, and any excess soft tissue trimmed off of one or both of the flaps, taking care not to reduce the extent of the masticatory mucosa on the lateral side and therefore the sulcus depth. The wound is then closed.

Preoperative radiographs are essential before reduction of enlarged tuberosities to demonstrate the proportion of bone and soft tissue and the extent of the maxillary sinus within them. Where the mucoperiosteum is of normal thickness and the enlarged tuberosity composed of thin bone over an extensive extension of the antrum reduction in size is more difficult. The mucoperiosteum is reflected to enable the operator to cut through the bone in the mid line of the ridge with a rose-head bur and then to cut out triangular sections on either side to leave interdigitating triangular segments. The antral mucosa on them should not be disturbed. They are in-fractured with greenstick fractures and the mucoperiosteum trimmed and sutured, making sure that there is a slight excess to give a tight suture line.

Fibrous Enlargements of the Tuberosity

Fibrous enlargements may be either firm or mobile and the latter type makes the construction of a satisfactory denture particularly difficult as the soft tissues can be displaced when impressions are taken.

An incision can be made along the crest of the ridge and then flaps raised with a scalpel, cutting them to the normal thickness of the ridge mucosa. The excess tissue is filleted out from under the flaps and then an ellipse removed from the edges of the flaps until they meet edge to edge and do not overlap. This technique removes both a lateral and a vertical excess (*Fig.* 5.2).

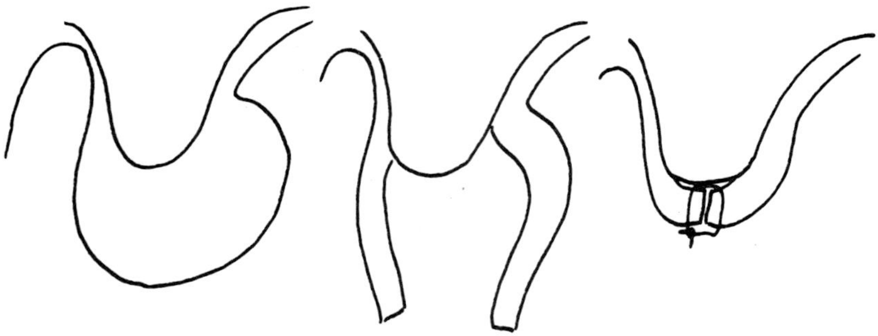

Fig. 5.2. Diagram showing reduction of fibrous enlargement of the tuberosity. The mucosa is raised by undercutting the flaps, being careful to preserve a blood supply to the flap by conserving an adequate thickness of flap, particularly palatally. The excess fibrous tissue is excised, the flaps trimmed to length and sutured.

Firm fibrous enlargements are best trimmed by paring them down with a scalpel. An acrylic base plate is prepared preoperatively. The epithelium is trimmed off first as a free mucosal graft and the pieces assembled on tulle gras, cut surface upwards. The fibrous tissue is pared to size and an impression of the new tuberosity taken in black gutta percha using the prepared base plate. The mucosal grafts on the tulle gras are placed into the impression and the baseplate reinserted in the mouth (*Fig.* 5.3). It may be retained by two bone screws driven outwards from the palatal aspect into the base of the alveolar process. Often retention is adequate without mechanical fixation. The plate is left undisturbed for 14 days.

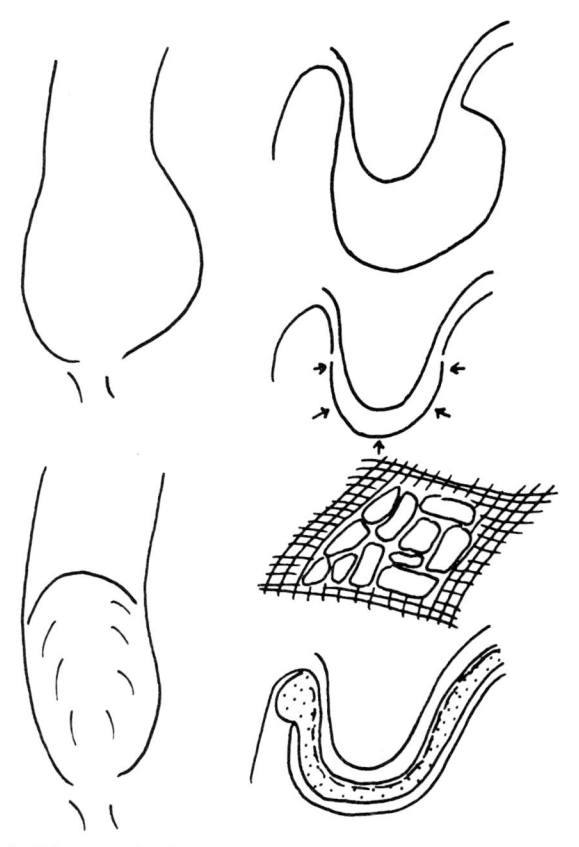

SURGICAL PREPARATION OF THE MOUTH FOR DENTURES

Fig. 5.3. Diagram showing reduction of firm fibrous enlargement of the tuberosity. The epithelium is removed as thinly as possible to form free patch grafts and the pieces assembled on petroleum jelly gauze. The excess bulk of fibrous tissue is trimmed away but *not* down to bone. The graft is supported in contact with the raw area by a GP lined acrylic baseplate.

Occasionally a relatively normal tuberosity needs to be reduced in height where there is insufficient room between the ridges in the 3rd molar region for both an upper and lower denture.

Tori

Tori are developmental exostoses, found most commonly in the midline of the hard palate but occasionally on the lingual side of the mandible in the premolar region. It may be possible to relieve an upper denture in the area overlying a small torus palatinus, but dentures tend to impinge on the larger ones and may cause ulceration. In addition, the midline relief may cause a point of weakness in the denture and lead to repeated fracture. Horseshoe shaped dentures without a palate have been used, but are rarely satisfactory. Sometimes there may be more than one bony mass in the midline, for when the torus is large it tends to become lobulated. Four lobules with a 'hot cross bun' effect is a common arrangement. Surgical exposure of this bony prominence may be made by an incision around the crest of the ridge in the edentulous patient or around the palatal aspect of the gingival margins when teeth are present. The greater palatine vessels will, of course, be contained in this large flap when it is raised.

Another surgical approach to the centre of the palate may be made through a straight incision up the midline (*Fig.* 5.4). This gives an excellent

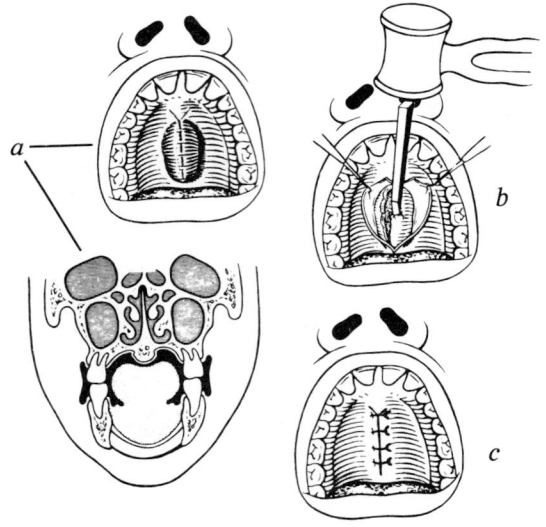

Fig. 5.4. Removal of torus palatinus. *a*, Y incision to expose torus. *b*, Removal of torus. *c*, Wound closure.

exposure of a torus palatinus, especially if the anterior end of the incision near the incisor teeth is made to diverge in the form of a Y or a T so avoiding the neurovascular bundle at the nasopalatine fossa. All incisions must, of course, be made down to bone so that the flaps raised consist of mucosa and periosteum. The mucoperiosteum overlying the torus is often thin and may easily tear during elevation of the soft tissues from the exostoses. Similarly, when excising the bony nodule, the surgeon should realize that the palatal processes of the maxillae are also thin and that any attempt to remove a torus composed of compact bone with a chisel may result in a fracture of the palate and perforation of the nasal floor. In a young patient a small torus palatinus may occasionally contain cancellous bone, and this can be chiselled off quite easily.

Usually, it is wise to remove the exostosis with a drill. A fissure bur should be employed to section the lesion so that a number of slender pillars of bone can be individually removed with a chisel. The remaining cut surface should be smoothed with a large bur. If the torus palatinus has been approached through an incision along the centre of the palate, it will be found that on replacing the soft tissue flaps over the palatal vault there is a surplus of mucoperiosteal tissue due to elimination of the bony mass. The edge of one of the flaps should be trimmed with a scalpel or scissors until there is accurate approximation, after which the wound is sutured. The sutures should be left *in situ* for seven days, but it will be found that as patients tend to use their tongues to play with sutures in the centre of the palate some may be lost earlier.

If the torus has been approached from an incision along the crest of the ridge or around the palatal gingival margins of the remaining standing teeth, a bulge in the centre of the flap approximating to the torus will be seen after the torus has been removed. This excess can be eliminated by removing an ellipse of soft tissue with a scalpel, after which the wound in the centre of the plate is sutured. The denture or a previously prepared acrylic plate may be lined in the centre with gutta percha and used to hold the flaps in close apposition to the bone surface during healing.

The mandibular torus is situated on the lingual side of the alveolar process opposite the lower canines and premolars and is usually bilateral. Occasionally it may extend posteriorly as far as the first molar region. Like the torus palatinus, the exostosis varies in size from patient to patient and may be lobulated. Lingual tori need only be excised if they cause pain or difficulty to denture wearers.

In the edentulous mandible the torus mandibularis may be approached surgically by an incision of adequate length along the crest of the ridge. If any teeth are present, the incision is made around their gingival margins.

Unlike the torus palatinus, the torus mandibularis can be removed easily with a chisel. The underlying bone is then smoothed with a bone file or large bone bur and the incision sutured. There is no necessity to tailor the flaps after the excision of the bony lump, for the bony mass is comparatively small and the surplus soft tissue is therefore minimal (*Fig.* 5.5).

Prominent Bony Attachments for Muscles

When gross resorption of the edentulous alveolar ridges occurs, the processes of the mandible to which muscles are attached, and which therefore retain a functional stimulus, do not atrophy, and tend to become relatively prominent. Dentures may impinge on these areas causing pain and ulceration, and the activity of the muscles themselves may have a displacing effect on the margin of the prosthesis. The muscles involved are

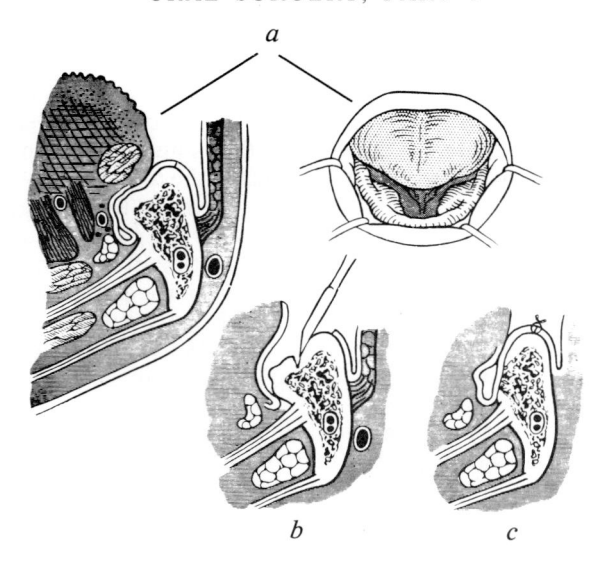

Fig. 5.5. Removal of torus mandibularis. *a*, Torus. *b*, Removal of torus. *c*, Wound closure.

the mylohyoid, which is attached to a ridge on the lingual side of the molar region, the genial muscles, attached to the genial tubercles on the lingual side in the midline, and the mentalis muscles, attached just beneath the sulcus on the labial side on either side of the midline.

Mylohyoid Ridge Resection

The surgical approach to the area is made through an incision of adequate length along the crest of the ridge and this incision usually extends from canine to the 3rd molar region where it is angled laterally onto the external oblique ridge to avoid the lingual nerve. The position of the lingual and mylohyoid nerves should be borne in mind continuously while working in the 3rd molar region.

The mucoperiosteal flap is elevated lingually with a Howarth's periosteal elevator, care being taken not to disturb the tissue on the buccal side of the incision. The mylohyoid ridge and its attached muscle are exposed and the flap held back lingually with a Lack's retractor. A chisel is positioned with its cutting edge against the base of the thin ridge where it joins the body of the mandible and a light tap with a hammer is sufficient to detach it. The separated fragment or portions of mylohyoid ridge are pulled away from the body of the mandible by contraction of the mylohyoid muscle and they are then gripped by Fickling's forceps.

At this stage it is sometimes helpful if the assistant presses upwards in the

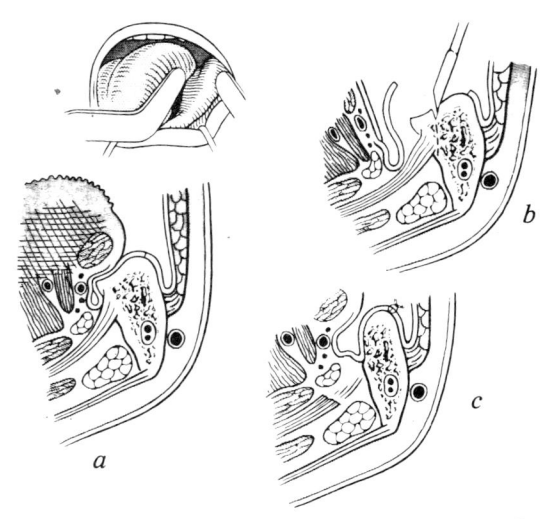

Fig. 5.6. Mylohyoid ridge resection. *a*, Prominent mylohyoid. *b*, Removal of ridge and 0·6 cm of mylohyoid muscle. *c*, Wound closure.

submandibular region to raise the detached piece of ridge so that it can be more easily grasped. Gentle traction on the Fickling's forceps is used to pull the severed ridge and attached muscle upwards out of the wound. The mylohyoid muscle, which is only about 3 mm thick, is then divided close to its ridge attachment, using long curved Mayo or McIndoe scissors.

After separation of the ridge fragment, the main mass of the mylohyoid muscle contracts back into the floor of the mouth. Any residual sharp bony edges at the site of the ridge are eliminated with a large pear-shaped bone bur. Only when the lingual aspect of the mandible feels quite smooth to the touch is the wound closed. Before suturing, the area is gently irrigated with warm saline solution to remove bone debris. Any bleeding points should be controlled by diathermy coagulation (*Fig.* 5.6).

A vacuum drain may be inserted on each side. The introducer is passed firmly against the lingual surface of the mandible anterior to the submandibular gland and out through the skin of the neck. The drain end is drawn through and the perforated part cut to a length to fit in the sublingual space. The mucosa is closed with a continuous suture to make a leak proof suture line and the neck end of the drains attached to sterile vacuum bottles. It is advisable to prescribe a course of antibiotic treatment postoperatively to prevent the development of infection.

Removal of Genial Tubercles

Where there is gross resorption, the genial tubercles form a hook-like process over which the denture rides and tilts. It has been considered unwise to divide both genial muscles and mylohyoid muscles at the same time as control of the tongue is affected. Fortunately, the intrinsic musculature prevents this even if the genial muscles are completely detached.

The surgical approach is straightforward. The incision is best placed directly over the genial tubercles, in the lingual frenum and at right angles to the line of the arch in order to avoid tension across the suture line during movement of the tongue. The incision is made down to bone, and the soft tissues and muscle attachments stripped off the bony prominence of the tubercles which can then be removed with rongeurs or a bur as is convenient. The incision is sutured and a suitably modified denture inserted.

If necessary the whole of the genial muscle mass can be displaced downwards. A 2/0 chromic catgut or polyglactin suture is passed with a fine awl from the buccal sulcus, around the mandible and through the genial muscles. The suture is removed from the awl, which is 'partially' withdrawn and then reinserted on the other side of the muscle bellies where the suture is rethreaded through the awl's eye. The end is taken back again, through the muscle and back to the labial side. This embraces the genial muscles in a mattress suture. The muscles are now detached with stout curved scissors, cutting close to the bone, and pulled down by the suture to the lower border of the residual mandible. If necessary the sutures can be removed at 14 days. Artery forceps are applied to the mattress suture below the knots in the labial sulcus and the suture ends cut off between the knots and the forceps. One artery forceps is released and the mattress suture pulled out.

Branches of the sublingual arteries enter the mandible above the genial tubercles and will be divided as the muscles are cut through. Bleeding from these and any other muscular vessels must be arrested before the muscle is pulled down and the wound closed.

Denture-induced Hyperplasia

These lesions develop following the persistent wearing of an ill-fitting denture. They are usually a consequence of gross alveolar resorption so that the denture flanges become relatively over-extended. When first seen, they are inevitably inflamed and oedematous, so, if the offending denture is radically relieved, or preferably not worn at all, there will be considerable shrinkage over a period of 10–14 days. The necessity for excision of the lesion can be better assessed following this initial phase of resolution. Lesions are most commonly found in the lower anterior region, but may occur in relation to any part of the periphery of a mobile denture. They often consist of multiple leaflets of fibrous tissue covered with relatively normal mucosa. Though they should always be examined histologically when excised, the incidence of malignant change is surprisingly small.

Each strip of hyperplastic tissue arises from the sulcus tissues by a long

SURGICAL PREPARATION OF THE MOUTH FOR DENTURES

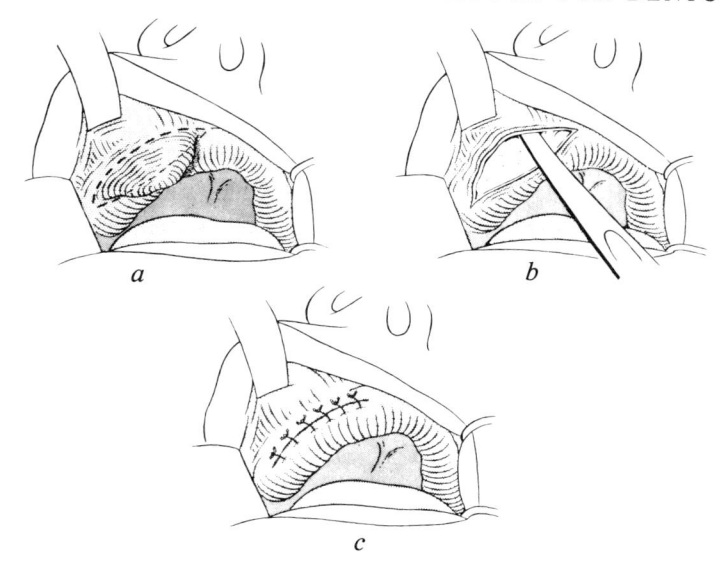

Fig. 5.7. Removal of localized mass of denture hyperplasia. *a*, Incision through mucosa only. *b*, Undermining edges of defect. *c*, Wound closure.

thin attachment. In cross section the fibrous mass is usually substantially wider than the attachment which in the other direction stretches along the length of one edge. The attachment therefore can be described as a linear pedicle. Not infrequently the mass is bifid in a longitudinal direction or there are two masses running parallel to one another and attached close together. One mass fills the space between the fitting surface of the denture and the now much reduced ridge while the other overlaps the flange of the denture.

Single or bifid granulomas can be treated by simple excision through the linear pedicle. The margins of the wound are undermined with a scalpel and any residual core of fibrous tissue from the pedicle excised down to the surface of the periosteum. Usually the wound can be closed without further loss of depth to the sulcus (*Fig.* 5.7).

Simple excision of thick fleshy lesions will leave a sizeable mucosal defect. Undermining the margins of such a deficiency and suturing it will lead to a loss of sulcus depth and increase the prosthetic difficulties.

An incision can be made on the labial or buccal aspect of the mass and the mucosa dissected off the surface as a thin layer until the ridge is reached on the other side of the mass. The fibrous core of the hyperplastic tissue is excised down to the periosteum and the flap of mucosa sutured to cover the defect. The blood supply to the mucosal flap will be too tenuous for it to survive as a flap if it has been removed in a sufficiently thin layer to permit adequate excision of the fibrous core. It should be regarded as mucosal graft which is attached along one edge. A previously fabricated acrylic plate is lined with gutta percha at the site of the excision and held in place with circumferential or per alveolar wires as appropriate. The pressure will prevent haematoma formation under the mucosa and permit it to attach as a graft.

In some patients there are multiple rows of granulomatous masses so that their individual excision is quite impractical. The entire complex will need to be excised and the resultant defect grafted with a split skin (Thiersch) graft.

Alveolar Ridge Remodelling

Following extraction of the teeth, bone is formed within the healing sockets and subsequently undergoes remodelling until there is little or no radiographic evidence of their former presence. Remodelling resorption also affects the entire alveolar process to produce, after some six to eight months, relatively stable ridges of even contour, but reduced bulk compared with the immediate postextraction alveolar processes. Further slow resorption continues thereafter which varies in rate between subjects. In some patients barely detectable changes result over many years. In others, within five or ten years all the original alveolar process has gone and in some, basal bone is also lost. Indeed the body of the mandible may be reduced to pencil thinness.

Comparatively little is known about the factors which govern the rate of this long-term remodelling and less about ways of preventing it. It is probable that masticatory forces acting on mucosal borne dentures are one cause of alveolar bone loss, hence one of the reasons for interest in overdentures. Not only do studs and copings added to the root-filled roots aid retention and the stability of the denture, but some of the masticatory force is transmitted naturally to the alveolar bone via the periodontal membranes of the supporting roots. Indeed, it may be sufficient to root-fill the roots and smooth off the cut surface, bevelling the margins. Special oral hygiene measures are necessary in all cases to ensure the health of the gingival margin and to prevent caries of the root end.

Atrophy of the alveolar bone is seen radiographically where posterior teeth in one jaw are unopposed either by natural teeth or dentures, but this is expressed as a loss of medullary bone trabeculae below and between the tooth roots. There is a thinning of the lamina dura but the crests of the interdental septa and the buccal and lingual cortical bone appears to be largely unaffected.

During the initial remodelling of the edentulous ridge sometimes a bulkiness is left at one point which will be found to surround a retained root. This has led to the suggestion that the deliberate retention of roots containing vital pulp tissue might help to preserve the size of the alveolar process and perhaps reduce long-term bone resorption. The pulps of the teeth must be healthy so tooth loss must be necessary for periodontal disease. The teeth must not exhibit excessive mobility and about half the original socket depth must remain. Single prominent teeth are not suitable as the denture is likely to rub on the resultant bulbosity. A reverse bevel incision is made to remove epithelium lining the pockets and buccal and lingual flaps reflected, those buccally to well below the level of the sulcus. Infected granulation tissue and any calculus deposits are carefully curetted away and the tooth crowns amputated with a water cooled bur. The root ends are reduced to below the level of the alveolar crests and bevelled towards the buccal and lingual aspects without damage to the socket walls. The periosteum is divided under the labial and buccal flaps well below the sulcus to permit easy advancement of the mucosa to cover the sockets and to permit tension free suture with a fine continuous monofilament suture material.

Success depends upon primary healing and failure follows exposure of the root ends and infection of their pulps. The evidence from observation of accidentally retained roots suggests that the presence of deeply buried fragments does not affect ridge remodelling and that with time a proportion of larger roots are likely to be uncovered as a result of slow bone resorption, necessitating their extraction. It seems unlikely that this technique will have more than an occasional application.

Also promising is the insertion of non-porous hydroxylapatite cones in extraction sockets. These resist resorption, but bone will be deposited on their surface so that they can be incorporated in the healed alveolar bone. Incomplete closure of the sockets does not necessarily lead to failure as they can be covered by granulation tissue at any defects in the suture line. In experimental animals bone will grow over the cones. Trials in humans are in progress in American universities and it will be interesting to see if retention of alveolar ridge bulk results in the long term.

Sulcus Deepening

As the alveolar ridges shrink over the years there is not only a loss of bone height but a reduction in area of the masticatory mucosa. The decrease in denture bearing surface increases the potential pressure to which it is subject during mastication leading to pain and probably also to a further loss of supporting bone. Although the sulcus tissues are mobile, movements of the jaws and facial muscles will still displace the periphery of an overextended denture. Also, once the ridges have lost their height, the displacing forces generated in the sulcus tissues and by mastication result in great denture instability and a succession of frictional ulcers.

Where there is bone below the sulcus which could form additional support for a denture, a sulcus deepening procedure can improve denture stability and comfort. If this additional bone is to be made available it must be covered by a mucosa which is firmly and immovably attached to the bone surface. Various attempts have been made to excise the loose submucosa from beneath the sulcus tissues and to press the mucous membrane into firm contact with the periosteum so that they become united. These techniques employ closed and open submucosal dissections utilizing compression base plates to hold the mucous membrane down onto the periosteum.

Alternatively, flaps are advanced into the sulcus leaving the exposed periosteum to granulate and heal by secondary epithelialization. Regrettably they rarely lead to a permanent gain in sulcus depth. Over the months the sulcus tissues contract back to their previous position. The most reliable technique is to line the extended sulcus depth with a split skin (Thiersch) graft taken from a non-hairy part of the arm or leg. These too contract quite markedly if they are not kept stretched for at least three months, by which time a permanent gain in sulcus depth can be assured. The best results are therefore achieved by deliberately over extending the new sulcus, but not to the extent of damaging the mental nerves, or the origins of the depressor labii inferiors or depressor anguli oris because an unnatural lack of lower lip movement will result. Nor should the new sulcus reach too far on to the point of the chin where the bulk of a denture flange becomes unsightly.

Base plates lined with black gutta percha are prepared preoperatively on models cast from overextended impressions. The dissection is carried out so that the graft–buccal mucosal junction, which scars, will sit over the denture flange assisting retention. Care must be taken not to damage the periosteum which will need to be incised around the mental nerves. If the nerves are very superficial it may be necessary to prepare to groove in the underlying bone to set them below the surface.

After the dissection the black gutta percha is heated in hot water and moulded into the depths of the new unlined sulcus. After cooling *in situ* the base plate is carefully removed, dried and sprayed with an acrylic adhesive such as nobecutaine and the split skin graft draped over the buccal periphery and undersurface. The graft is then gently inserted on this acrylic and gutta percha mould and the plates are wired in place for 10–14 days. After removal and the trimming off of the excess skin they are reinserted to keep the grafts stretched.

Dentures should be made before the operation and the flanges modified with a tissue conditioner to fit the new sulcus. They replace the temporary plates and should be worn day and night for 3 months until the skin grafts are reasonably stable. They are of course removed after each meal, cleaned and immediately reinserted. Once the grafts have matured and softened, acrylic flanges are added to replace the tissue conditioner and they are left out each night in the usual way. The technique also works well for the maxilla where the dissection is much simpler.

The best form of free graft is undoubtedly palatal mucosa which can be removed in strips, cut off as thin as possible and assembled on tulle gras. Small spaces between the pieces will epithelialize over. Such grafts are applied as described on gutta percha lined plates. This method results in fresh masticatory mucosa which is stable and does not shrink.

Unfortunately the amount of graft which can be harvested from a palate is limited so that extensive sulcus deepening procedures cannot be grafted in this way. The denuded palatal mucosa is protected with a plate and a suitable dressing until it has re-epithelialized.

Lowering of the Floor of the Mouth and Vestibuloplasty

This procedure, as described by MacIntosh and Obwegeser in 1967, in effect combines the benefits of a mylohyoid ridge resection and a lower buccal sulcus deepening procedure with a split skin graft. Ten millilitres of a 1:240000 solution of adrenaline in saline is injected into one side of the floor of the mouth so as to distend the tissues and separate the tissue planes. An additional 10 ml of sterile normal saline can be injected if required once vasoconstriction has occurred.

An incision is made at the attachment of the lingual mucosa to the inner aspect of the ridge from the 2nd molar region to the midline. A swab rolled onto a sponge holder is pressed against the underside of the tongue to open up the wound. With gentle touches of a knife the connective tissue is separated from the periosteum.

Once the lingual nerve has been identified the mucosal incision can be extended backwards and then laterally over the retromolar region. The lower end of the superior constrictor is separated from the mandible so as to free the nerve. The sponge holder is moved deeper into the wound and the attachment of the mylohyoid muscle to the mandible is separated from the bone with scalpel and scissors. Remodelling of a sharp mylohyoid ridge follows detachment of the muscle. A few of the upper fibres of the genioglossus may be divided also.

After the buccal sulcus has been infiltrated with vasoconstrictor the incison is continued on the buccal side at the junction of the attached and sulcus mucosa. The buccinator is detached in the same way as the mylohyoid, taking care to identify and preserve the mental nerve. To avoid a floppy lower lip separation of the origins of the depressor muscles should be avoided. A similar procedure is completed on the other side.

Four polyglactin sutures are initially inserted into the lingual flap and both ends are then passed under the mandible with the aid of a circumferential wire awl, entered through the submandibular skin, and brought upwards into the buccal flap. Even though resorbable sutures are used, removal is best and is facilitated with a pull-out black silk suture, knotted onto each circumferential suture in turn, above the lingual mucosa.

When the buccal sutures are tied, the two ends from adjacent sutures are knotted together so as to increase the length of buccal mucosa which takes the pull of the thread. Soft PVC tubes may also be threaded on to stop them cutting in. As the sutures are tightened the floor of the mouth and the buccal mucosa are both drawn down towards the lower border of the mandible.

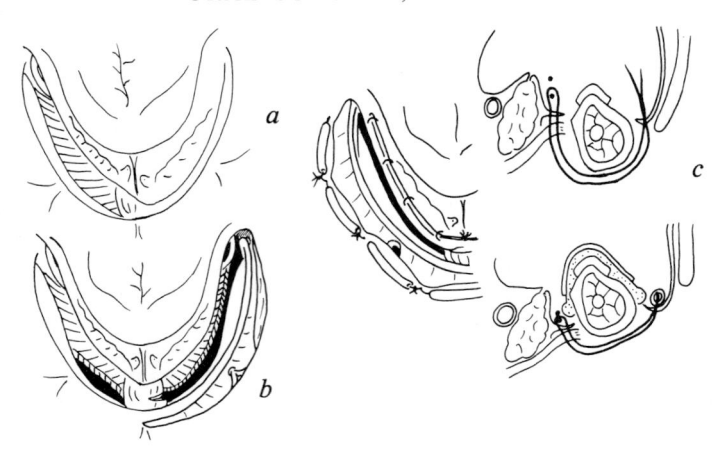

Fig. 5.8. Lowering of the floor of mouth and skin graft. *a, (Patient's left.)* The floor of mouth is incised at the lingual edge of the ridge masticatory mucosa *(patient's right)*. The soft tissues are displaced medially off the mylohyoid muscle, the lingual nerve found and preserved. *b, (Patient's right.)* The mylohyoid muscle is cut, close to the mandible. *(Patient's left.)* The entire mylohyoid is separated and the buccal mucosa incised at the lateral margin of the ridge mucopelriosteum. Mental nerve and buccinator are uncovered. *c,* The mental foramen is extended downwards to lower the nerve. Sutures are passed through lingual mucosa and muscle, around pull-out sutures. The ends are passed with circumferential awls under the mandible and through the buccal mucosa, displacing the buccinator muscle. The ends of *adjacent* sutures are threaded through soft rubber tubes and tied.

After the sutures have been tied the two pull-out threads will be tied together at the front under the tongue (*Fig.* 5.8).

The ridge remains covered with masticatory mucoperiosteum, but there is now a bare area of periosteum both buccally and lingually. The areas are covered with a skin graft applied with a black gutta percha mould on an acrylic plate, as previously described, and the plate is fastened on with circumferential wiring. The plate and the sutures are removed at 14 days. Sometimes removal of a particular suture can prove difficult, hence the use of resorbable ones. The mould should be washed and replaced until dentures, which have been previously constructed, can be modified to fit the new foundation. They should be inserted as soon as possible, preferably the same day, and worn continuously except when removed for cleaning for around 4–6 months.

Augmentation of the Bony Ridge

Where atrophy of the alveolar bone is extreme and where there is additionally loss of basal bone, sulcus extension procedures alone will not help. If the results of some of the techniques of sulcoplasty are poor those of augmentation of the bony ridges are mostly disappointing.

One of the complications of such extreme atrophy is the bilateral fracture of the edentulous, pencil thin mandible which results in a severe 'bucket handle' deformity. This can be treated successfully either by Gunnings' splints and pyriform aperture wires, or if the mandible is thick enough by miniature (Champey) bone plates applied supraperiostealy along the lower border of the mandible. The latter technique may be improved by using a submandibular approach and by inserting cancellous bone chips from the iliac crest. The use of interosseous wires at the fracture site which require severe disruption of the periosteum for their insertion, and which lack rigidity results in a delayed or mal-union.

The successful treatment of such cases with bone grafts along the mandibular lower border fixed with circumferential wires led to attempts to increase the thickness and strength of the jaw before fracture had occurred. Sulcus deepening procedures were added to this technique as a means of augmenting the foundation for a lower denture. Unfortunately the additional bone is completely resorbed within a matter of a year or so, frustrating both objectives.

Bone grafts of split and contoured rib, segments of iliac crest and medullary chips have also been used to augment and rebuild both the mandibular and maxillary alveolar ridges. Such techniques require division of the periosteum beyond the immediate base of the flaps to permit their advancement and closure of the soft tissues over the grafts. Meticulous vertical mattress suturing is required because only a one-layered closure is possible and any leak leads to infection of the grafts. Because the area of masticatory mucosa is also greatly reduced, sulcoplasties become necessary, once the grafts have become vascularized, to create the new bony denture foundation. Unfortunately, once again, much of the height gained may be lost, often within a period of two to three years. On the other hand, the width of the denture foundation is usually increased permanently. Indeed, as an alternative approach, the grafts may be added laterally to increase the width but not the height of the denture foundation.

More recently attempts have been made to increase the height of the bony ridges by sandwich grafting so that the denture bearing surface is formed by part of the original mandibular cortex, nourished during the healing process by a periosteal blood supply through attached mucosa and muscles.

A visor osteotomy has been used in which the mandible is sectioned vertically between the cortical plates. This is possible for the full depth of the mandible between the mental foramina, but further back the plane of section has to be angled medially to avoid the mandibular neurovascular bundles. The cut therefore emerges on the lingual side between the mylohyoid ridge and the lower border of the mandible. The lingual fragment was then raised up still attached to the mucosa and muscles, and the lower part at the front wired to the upper border of the outer segment. Bone chips could be packed around it to increase the bulk. Unfortunately the lingual fragment was often thin and weak, particularly posteriorly, and the result did not resist resorption.

A horizontal sandwich osteotomy with a cartilage or bone graft inserted into the resulting gap will raise the anterior alveolar crest upwards.

Hopkins (1982) refined the sandwich osteotomy by unroofing the inferior dental canal from the mental foramen backwards and freeing the mandibular neurovascular bundle as far as the ramus. This permitted a 45° oblique osteotomy to be made from one molar region to the other without fear of damage to the nerve. The upper fragment was supported on substantial blocks of bone and bone chips packed in to fill all recesses and to give contour to the reconstructed mandible (*Fig.* 5.9). He was able to report a 60 per cent residual increase in height after two years which appeared thereafter to be stable (Hopkins and Sugar, 1982). Unfortunately neural morbidity tends to be high with all these techniques. A sulcoplasty is necessary once the osteotomies have united and all grafts have been incorporated.

Problems with augmentation of the ridge with bone grafts have led to the use of non-absorbable substitutes. Calcium hydroxyapatite has proved to be an inert material which resists resorption. Two preparations have been tried: particulate hydroxyapatite and either solid or porous blocks. The particulate material is difficult to confine in a sub-periosteal pocket and problems have been experienced with ulceration and dehiscence of the soft tissues overlying blocks. Once exposed the blocks are likely to be lost. There are probably two causes for the damage to the overlying mucoperiosteum. The first is small sharp irregularities on the surface of the blocks. Second, while there is an ingrowth of tissues into the porous blocks it is rare for any circulation to be established through the block. The covering mucosa therefore remains dependent upon a blood supply from its margins.

As a result, efforts have been concentrated on stabilising the granular material. Both fibrin and collagen have been mixed with the granules to trap the particles in a paste-like matrix. When the collagen takes up moisture the initial carvable block softens and conforms to the ridge and covering soft tissues but the hydroxyapatite is held until granulations grow into the area. Vascularisation of the mass is improved but there is some loss of bulk.

Attempts to retain the granules by sutures proved ineffective but special tissue expanders create excellent closed tissue cavities into which the particulate hydroxyapatite preparations can be placed. The tissue expanders are tubular silicone bags incorporating a reservoir which has a self-sealing injection site. A space is created surgically for the tubes over the crest of the ridge and they are inflated by the injection of saline through the injection site after the expander has been inserted and the incisions sutured. Further small quantities of saline are introduced at weekly inter-

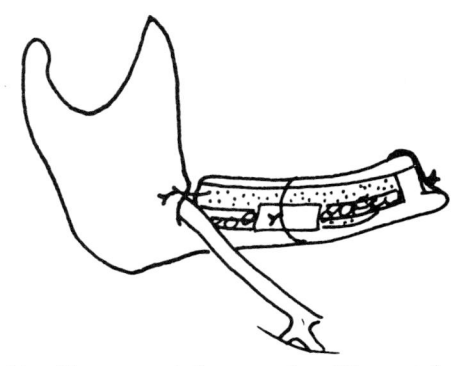

Fig. 5.9. Hopkins ridge augmentation procedure. The mental nerve and mandibular nerve are uncovered by removing a strip of bone and displaced sideways. The jaw is divided vertically from end to end of the ridge. The lingual fragment is raised and wired to the rami posteriorly. Block bone grafts support it in place and bone chips are packed into all gaps. Three circumferential wires sandwich the bone grafts in place.

vals to create a tension just short of tissue palor in the overlying tissues. These respond by stretching. After an interval of 4–6 weeks the expander is removed to reveal an encapsulated space overlying the ridge. This can be filled with particulate hydroxyapatite.

Two approaches have been made to the problem of trying to stimulate living bone around the particles so as to reduce the vulnerability of the hydroxyapatite should a soft tissue dehiscence occur at some time. Autogenous bone chips have been mixed with the granules. If this is done it must be certain that sharp fragments are not created which would damage the overlying tissues. Hydroxyapatite is inert, which is in many ways an advantage, but it does not possess osteo-inductive properties. Decalcified bone powder does have such properties due to a substance variously called osteogenin, skeletal growth factor or bone morphogenic protein. Various preparations derived from powdered decalcified bone matrix have been mixed with hydroxyapatite granules to encourage the ingrowth of bone.

PROBLEMS WITH EXTENSIVE PROCEDURES

Those patients who require the more extensive procedures tend to be elderly and may have respiratory, cardiovascular or other illness: problems which make them poor risk cases for surgery. Old people, even if fit, recover less rapidly, are more prone to complications and take longer to achieve full mobility again after an enforced period in bed.

Once patients have had all their teeth extracted they usually believe their dental problems are over. They rarely envisage trouble with dentures and certainly not difficulties that cannot be solved by prosthetic skills. The concept of a surgical solution to their problems is not accepted readily particularly if a substantial operation is proposed. The newer more conservative techniques are much more acceptable. However they require more, rather than less, surgical skill and attention to detail. There can be no guarantee that even the best of these techniques will produce a lasting improvement, and the surgeon should be wary of being over-persuasive.

IMPLANT PROCEDURES

Subperiosteal Implants

The first type of implants to have any success over a prolonged period of time were the sub-periosteal implants. Used for carefully selected patients there was the possibility that they would give service for eight to ten years. However, migration of epithelium to line the soft tissue-metal interface, periodontal abscess like infections, resorption of underlying bone and soft tissue break down with exposure of the supportive framework led to their failure.

Endosseous Implants

Many designs of endosteal implant were tried but almost universally the implant was separated from the bone by a thin layer of fibrous tissue. Retention was due to the interlocking shape of the implant and the surrounding bone. Stresses on the implants resulted in widening of the fibrous tissue layer. Once this began the increased mobility which resulted increased the rate of bone resorption until the implant was lost leaving a worse condition than before with extensive soft tissue scarring added to inadequate bony ridges.

Staple Implants

For a while the Small staple implant led the field. These implants, inserted vertically through the mandible between the mental foramina, transfixed the jaw and were attached to a plate at the lower border of the mandible. Copings and a connecting bar joined the parts protruding into the mouth. The bar at both top and bottom gave the implants a rigidity, greatly reducing destructive bone resorption.

Branemark Implants

The introduction of the Branemark system is looked upon as a watershed. Holes are drilled into the bone and successively widened. Once the correct depth and diameter has been achieved the hole in the bone is tapped. Very slow speeds for the cutters and saline irrigation to avoid thermal damage to the bone is very important. All debris is carefully flushed away. Threaded pure titanium implants are screwed into the holes with a special spanner. The implant fits flush with the top of the bone and a temporary cap screws into a threaded hole in the top. The flap for the surgery is designed so that the suture lines are remote from the implant.

The implants are left buried until healing has occurred. Healing includes growth of bone right up to the surface of the implant where the bone gains a physical attachment called osseo-integration. Several months later the tops of the implants are uncovered by removing a disc of mucosa and the caps removed. A collar is screwed into place which brings the end of the implant into the mouth. The gum heals tightly about the implant. Meticulous oral hygiene to keep the mucosa-implant interface clean is important. A variety of bridge abutments and attachments for dentures can be fixed to the collars. If the collar is tapped a clear ringing sound indicates successful osseo-integration. Even if a single fixture fails and is removed the damage is limited and localised and if remaining fixtures are insufficient a further insertion may be made following a healing period.

Obviously the depth and thickness of the bone of the jaw at any one place limits the placement of these implants; likewise the proximity of the inferior dental bundle and the maxillary sinuses. Probing the thickness of the mucosa and plotting the results on models, rotational panoramic tomograms, CT scans to give cross-sections of the jaws and hypocycloidal tomograms across mandible and maxilla with a Scanora are various ways in which the dimensions of the bone can be judged. Between the mental foramina is obviously the easiest site into which to insert implants.

Various strategies have been devised for inserting implants in difficult anatomical positions. Several new designs of implants, like the Corevent have emerged. Where there is insufficient bone it has proved possible successfully to pin bone grafts to the alveolar bone with osseo-integrated implants. The graft bone which immediately supports the implant does not seem to be resorbed in the way that occurs with other onlay grafts. New bone inducing strategies are emerging involving Gortex fabric.

Other uses for osseo-integrated implants have been developed including implants inserted through the skin to retain artificial ears, facial prostheses and obturators.

ORTHOGNATHIC SURGERY

Skilful prosthodontics can often provide useful dentures for patients with discrepancies in the relative position of the upper and lower jaw. These patients have established masticatory habits related to the malrelation of their natural teeth and can often use such dentures which reproduce this relationship within the limits of stability. However, in some instances it is impossible to make dentures which are stable enough for chewing purposes, although they may be acceptable aesthetically and for speech. Where the prosthetic problems prove insoluble it may be necessary to produce a more normal relationship of the alveolar ridges by means of orthognathic surgery.

ORAL SURGERY, PART 1
SUGGESTED READING

Block M. S. and Kent J. N. (1984) Long-term radiographic evaluation of hydroxylapatite—augmented mandibular alveolar ridges. *J. Maxillofac. Surg.* **42**, 793–796.

Block M. S. and Kent J. N. (1985) Healing of mandibular ridge augmentations using hydroxylapatite with and without autogenous bone in dogs. *J. Maxillofac. Surg.* **43**, 3–7.

Branemark P. I. (1977) Osseointegrated implants in the treatment of the edentulous jaw. *J. Maxillofac. Surg.* **42**, 793–796.

Brook, I. M. and Lamb, D. J. (1991) Management of the atrophic anterior maxilla by combined hydroxyapatite augmentation and vestibuloplasty. *Br. J. Oral Maxillofac. Surg.* **29**, 5–8.

Dugan D. J., Getz J. B. and Epker B. N. (1981) Root banking to preserve alveolar bone: a review and clinical recommendations. *J. Am. Dent. Assoc.* **103**, 737–742.

Frame, J. W. and Laird, W. R. E. (1987) Management of the mobile fibrous ridge in the atrophic maxilla using porous hydroxyapatite blocks. *Br. Dent. J.* **162**, 185–189.

Hall H. D. (1971) Vestibuloplasty, mucosal grafts (palatal and buccal). *J. Oral Surg.* **29**, 786–791.

Harle F. (1975) Visor osteotomy to increase the absolute height of the atrophied mandible: a preliminary report. *J. Maxillofac. Surg.* **3**, 257–260.

Hopkins R. (1982) A sandwich mandibular osteotomy: a preliminary report. *Br. J. Oral Surg.* **20**, 155–167.

MacIntosh R. B. and Obwegeser H. L. (1967) Preprosthetic surgery: a scheme for its effective employment. *J. Oral Surg.* **25**, 397–413.

Quale, A. A., Marouf, H. and Holland, I. (1990) Alveolar ridge augmentation using a new design of inflatable tissue expander: surgical technique and preliminary results. *Br. J. Oral Maxillofac. Surg.* **28**, 375–382.

Schettler D. and Holtermann W. (1977) Clinical and experimental results of a sandwich-technique for mandibular alveolar ridge augmentation. *J. Maxillofac. Surg.* **5**, 199–204.

Starshak T. J. and Sanders B. (1980) *Preprosthetic Oral and Maxillofacial Surgery.* St. Louis, Mosby.

Stoelinga P. J. W. Tideman H., Berger J. S. and De Kooman H. A. (1978) Interpositional bone graft augmentation of the atrophic mandible. A preliminary report. *J. Oral Surg.* **36**, 30–32.

Sugar A. and Hopkins R. (1982) A sandwich mandibular osteotomy: a progress report. *Br. J. Oral Surg.* **20**, 168–174.

CHAPTER 6

PYOGENIC INFECTIONS OF THE SOFT TISSUES

ACUTE ALVEOLAR ABSCESS

Some clinicians use the term alveolar abscess as being synonymous with a periapical abscess, while others would include periodontal or even pericoronal abscess, so using it like the lay term 'gum boil'.

Acute periapical abscess arises when organisms from an infected necrotic tooth pulp invade the periapical tissues. They usually gain access to the periradicular tissues through the apical foramina so that the infection is truly periapical, but on occasions the infection escapes through an accessory canal, an endodontic perforation, or an opening in the floor of the pulp chamber of a primary molar resulting from resorption or a fractured root. Under these circumstances the abscess develops on the lateral aspect of the root or at the root furcation. Infection from a split root characteristically presents as a mid-root sinus or a longitudinal area of resorption along the lateral border of the root.

The usual causes of infective necrosis of the pulp are a carious cavity, or contamination of a traumatic exposure of the pulp. Sometimes the initial necrosis is a sterile process, as when the apical vessels are torn by a blow on the tooth or following inadvertent chemical or thermal damage to the pulp during a coronal restoration. The necrotic pulp subsequently becomes infected via the periodontal lymphatics from the gingival crevice. Radiographic evidence suggests that the acute abscess is often an exacerbation of a pre-existing chronic periapical infection and presents initially as redness and swelling in the sulcus, usually on the outer aspect of the alveolar process. Then a fluctuant, submucosal swelling develops which bursts to produce a sinus discharging pus. The condition is painful until the pus has been released either spontaneously or surgically (*Fig.* 6.1).

Acute periodontal abscess arises in the periodontal membrane adjacent to a periodontal pocket. While in some cases, food impaction or repeated occlusal trauma appears to be the precipitating factor, often the immediate cause of the abscess is not apparent. An acute periodontal abscess produces redness and swelling of the gingival margin, interdental papilla and of the mucoperiosteum lateral to the tooth. The pain is usually continuous, dull or throbbing, variable in intensity but rarely as severe as a periapical abscess. The pus usually discharges via the gingival pocket, but may produce a sinus on either the inner or outer aspect of the alveolar process and only rarely tracks to the skin surface.

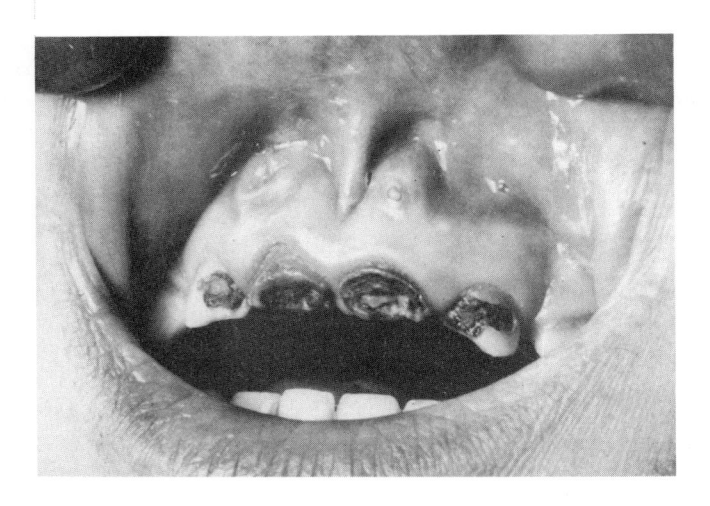

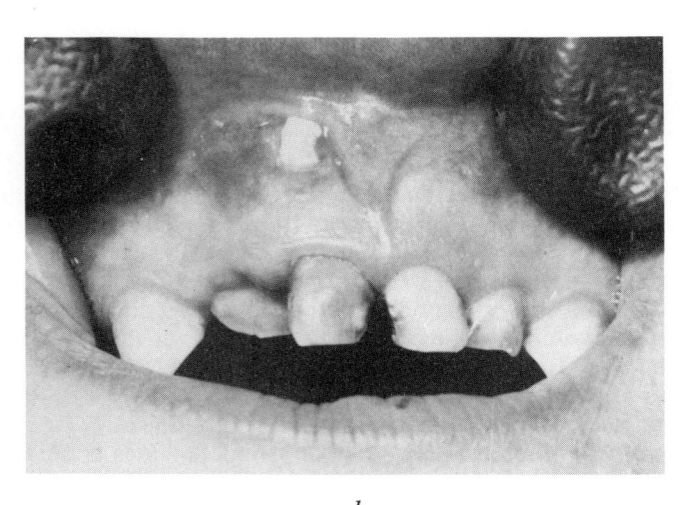

Fig. 6.1. *a*, 'Comforter' caries has destroyed the crowns of these deciduous upper central incisors. Sinuses in the sulcus over the apices due to chronic apical abscesses. *b*, A⏌ discoloured and pulpless. Mesial caries A|A. The apex of unresorbed A⏌ is being pushed out of the sinus in the sulcus by developing 1⏌ .

PYOGENIC INFECTIONS OF THE SOFT TISSUES

A pericoronal abscess arises around the crown of a partially erupted vital tooth, usually the 3rd molar, and therefore, resembles a periodontal abscess.

Abscesses may also arise in association with infected cysts, odontomes, tooth and bone fractures, subperiosteal and endosteal implants and other foreign bodies. Factors which determine whether an alveolar abscess is acute or chronic are similar to those affecting abscesses in general, namely the virulence of the organisms concerned, the general condition of the patient and the presence or absence of drainage.

Differential Diagnosis

The differential diagnosis between an acute periapical and an acute periodontal abscess is as follows. With a periapical abscess there is a tooth or root with necrotic and infected pulp, a swelling over the apex and possibly a sinus. The tooth is periostitic and later may become mobile. A periodontal abscess arises in relation to a periodontal pocket and there is a swelling or sinus in the gingival third of the alveolar process or, alternatively, a discharge from the pocket. The tooth is both tender to pressure and mobile at an early stage in the evolution of the condition but the pulp is usually vital. Periodontal abscesses are uncommon in children and an acute swelling close to the gingival margin of a primary molar is usually a periapical abscess.

Just occasionally a periodontal abscess may secondarily infect and destroy the pulp of the related tooth, or an apical abscess may discharge via the gingival crevice, but careful consideration of the clinical and radiographic evidence will usually permit a differentiation to be made.

Bacteriology

Collection of a sample of pus on a swab or in a tube will recover only aerobic or facultative anaerobic organisms, some of which are likely to be surface contaminants. This accounts for the view that streptococci of the viridans group and *Staphylococcus aureus* or *epidermidis* are the major pathogens in alveolar or tissue space abscesses of odontogenic origin. Studies in which pus has been aspirated into a syringe and cultured immediately by techniques including strict anaerobic conditions shows that while facultative anaerobes are still recovered, strictly anaerobic gram negative bacilli, including a variety of pigmented and non-pigmented bacteroides species and anaerobic gram positive cocci predominate. CO_2 dependant streptocci like *Streptococcus milleri* are also found. A mixed population of 3–4 species is usually recovered. This means that whenever specimens are taken for culture and sensitivity tests the pus should be aspirated before the abscess is incised. The sample in the syringe should be taken at once to the laboratory for culture. Where this is not possible an appropriate transport medium should be used.

Clinical Course of a Periapical Abscess

The acutely inflamed pulp produces a throbbing pain characteristically provoked by heat. Occasionally, the pain subsides with pulp necrosis especially if the infection pursues a chronic course. However, when the infection spreads into the periapical tissues from the root canal of the tooth, the periodontal membrane becomes acutely inflamed and swells, raising the tooth slightly in the socket so that it comes into premature contact with the opposing tooth when the patient bites. Thus the tooth becomes tender to bite upon, tender to percussion (periostitic), and moderately mobile as demonstrated by lateral pressure. Pus accumulates in the periapical marrow spaces where normally it is successfully walled off by a pyogenic membrane. An intense throbbing pain is experienced at this stage, but relief occurs immediately if the tooth is extracted and the pus is allowed to drain. If treatment is delayed, bone resorption permits the pus to penetrate the overlying cortex and spread out under the periosteum. The character of the pain changes from throbbing back to a dull ache and there is usually a marked diminution in its intensity.

While the pus is still confined within the bone a soft, puffy collateral oedema of the overlying tissues develops and the regional lymph nodes become enlarged and tender. With the spread of infection through the cortex, the swelling becomes more marked and the tissues immediately overlying the pus become firm and tender. Should a spreading cellulitis supervene, or a suppurative infection of a tissue space result, then an extensive firm swelling develops and the previously pinkish hue of the overlying skin deepens to a distinct red colour. It is important to distinguish between pitting collateral oedema and the firm swelling associated with a cellulitis or soft tissue abscess, for the former will resolve rapidly without additional treatment after the drainage of the intrabony pus following extraction. This is true even for children where collateral oedema can produce a sizeable swelling. A cellulitis on the other hand requires not only the extraction of the infected tooth and the drainage of any soft tissue abscess, but also prompt treatment with antibiotics.

Further Course of the Infection

Mostly, the pus burrows laterally through the adjacent cortical bone rather than disseminates through the cancellous bone which is protected by an inflammatory cell barrier. The presence of a previous bone cavity excavated by a symptomless periapical granuloma which often precedes the acute abscess and the closeness of the apices of most teeth to the labial or buccal cortex may facilitate this process. Untreated the pus will eventually discharge into the mouth or onto the face or neck. Early extraction with a course of antibiotic therapy (e.g. metronidazole, penicillin, etc.) will usually bring about resolution of the infection. Rarely, and only in circumstances to be described later, is it appropriate to leave infected teeth *in situ* until the infection 'has been brought under control'. The best method of control of any surgical infection is removal of the cause, drainage of any pus and antibiotics.

Sometimes it is possible to drain the pus through the apex of an acutely abscessed tooth by opening into the pulp canal. This is most easily accomplished in the case of single-rooted teeth such as incisors and canines and has the obvious advantage of preserving the tooth. If drainage is effected in this way antibiotics should be given to help control the infection. Any pus which has accumulated in the adjacent soft tissues should be drained. If, despite these measures, the infection persists, then the tooth must be extracted.

In the case of a periodontal abscess, it is seldom essential to remove the tooth to promote drainage unless it is either a bifurcation or trifurcation abscess. However, simple drainage must be followed by periodontal surgery to prevent recurrence.

PERICORONAL INFECTION

Pericoronitis is an inflammation of the soft tissues covering the crown of a partially erupted or unerupted tooth. The condition can only arise in association with an unerupted tooth if there is a communication between the crown of the tooth and the oral cavity. A transient inflammation of the overlying gingiva often occurs immediately preceding full eruption of the deciduous teeth. However, this rapidly subsides as the tooth erupts further.

Classic pericoronitis is likely to occur when the eruption of the tooth is impeded or unduly prolonged, usually as a result of malposition or impaction. It is because of this that pericoronal inflammation is almost invariably associated with the mandibular 3rd molar and is only seen in a small number of cases in relation to other impacted teeth such as the upper 3rd molar. Some affected lower wisdom teeth may be in a favourable position for eruption, and once the infection has been controlled, further upward movement may take place so that a normal gingival margin is attained. Fortunately, deeply buried teeth are not involved in pericoronal infection and there is rarely justification for their prophylactic removal. In fact, many patients with impacted lower 3rd molars remain symptom-free throughout their whole lifetime.

Another interesting anomaly is that bilateral concurrent pericoronitis is rare, despite the presence in many young adult mouths of two partially erupted lower 3rd molars, and when it occurs it usually implies a predisposing condition such as infectious mononucleosis or Vincent's ulcerative gingivitis

Aetiology

The aetiology of the condition is obscure. It has been postulated that food collects between the crown of the tooth and the overlying gum flap and that this constitutes a favourable site for bacterial incubation which, in turn, causes inflammation of the gum flap.

This may be true, but similar conditions prevail in other individuals with partially erupted teeth without pericoronitis supervening. Indeed it is sometimes possible by pressure on the operculum to express, from a clinically quiescent pericoronal space, a large amount of white material which is composed of desquamated epithelial cells, decomposed foodstuff, and dead and living bacteria.

Trauma to the overlying pad of gum from the cusps of an opposing tooth is an obvious aetiological agent, but in many cases it is difficult to determine whether the traumatic injury to the intervening soft tissues occurred before or after the flap became swollen by inflammatory oedema. The virulence of the bacteria within the pericoronal space must also be an influential factor and it is now recognized that these organisms are usually anaerobes such as bacteroides which have assumed a pathogenic role.

Lowering of the host resistance appears to be correlated with the development of a pericoronitis and many patients have a history of an upper respiratory tract infection such as acute coryza, pharyngitis, influenza or infectious mononucleosis. Other systemic illnesses, fatigue and emotional strain also appear to precipitate the condition.

A practical clinical classification for pericoronitis is to divide it into three categories: chronic, subacute and acute. This has the virtue of providing suitable criteria for treatment.

With chronic pericoronitis, the patient is usually asymptomatic except for the occasional mild discomfort or bad taste due to a discharge of pus from beneath the gum flap. Treatment is not sought unless the patient experiences subacute or acute exacerbations.

In subacute pericoronitis most patients experience a well localized dull pain and the gum pad is swollen, tender and red. Sometimes pus can be seen oozing from beneath the anterior margin of the gingival flap or it can be expressed by gentle pressure. There is foetor oris and indentations from the cusps of the upper 3rd molar may be observed where they impinge on the pericoronal tissues and the adjacent oedematous buccal mucosa. The patient may complain of slight discomfort on swallowing and some difficulty in opening the mouth. The submandibular lymph nodes on the affected side are enlarged and tender.

Acute pericoronitis presents with a combination of intra- and extraoral clinical features. The signs are similar to those of subacute pericoronitis except that facial swelling is common. Limitation of opening may be marked, pain is throbbing and severe and may interfere with sleep, while the majority of patients experience discomfort on swallowing. The constitutional upset may be considerable with pyrexia, severe malaise and anorexia. The regional lymph nodes are tender and enlarged. If untreated the infection is likely to spread to the adjacent tissue spaces.

Pus from pericoronitis related to a lower 3rd molar may track forwards submucosally along the inclined gutter, formed by the body of the mandible and the attachment of buccinator to the external oblique ridge. The pus will accumulate in the submucosa beneath the mucosal reflection and point opposite the 1st and 2nd molar or even the 2nd premolar. This migratory abscess may eventually discharge spontaneously via an intraoral sinus or, more rarely, track down to the middle of the lower border of the mandible just behind the depressor anguli oris muscle where, if it is not incised, it will burst through the skin. While many pericoronal infections are suppurative, some are ulcerative. Classical ulcerative pericoronitis is due to a Vincent's infection, but acute herpetic gingivostomatitis may start around a lower 3rd molar, later spreading forwards and backwards onto the fauces and soft palate.

Treatment

It is important to decide whether the related tooth is likely to achieve full eruption. Clinical examination and radiography will help to determine this. Such factors as the age of the patient and a history of previous attacks of pericoronitis will obviously have to be taken into consideration. Eruption is unlikely after 25 years of age and several previous attacks would also suggest extraction to be the best treatment.

1. If there is abscess this must be incised and drained. With antibiotic cover it may also be convenient to remove the 3rd molar at the same time. There is no evidence that this will produce osteomyelitis or disseminate the infection provided that the extraction can be accomplished without bone surgery.

2. If there is no abscess gentle irrigation of the pericoronal space with warm normal saline, using a 10 ml syringe and a needle with the point ground off, helps to dislodge food debris and other material which may have collected under the gum flap. Irrigation is continued with hot saline mouth baths over the inflamed area. The patient should be instructed to perform this ritual at two hourly intervals while at home and during work hours.

3. An antiseptic should be instilled into the pericoronal space. This can be aqueous povidine iodine or alcoholic tincture of iodine or 1 per cent gentian violet.

4. If the condition is being aggravated by an upper 3rd molar which irritates the swollen gum flap when the patient closes, then this should be relieved either by extracting the upper tooth or by grinding down the offending cusps if the tooth's retention is important as an abutment for a future bridge or prosthesis, or if it is intended to preserve the mandibular 3rd molar.

5. Antibiotic therapy such as metronidazole 400 mg, 12-hourly, phenoxymethyl penicillin 500 mg, 6-hourly, or amoxycillin 500 mg, 8-hourly, is indicated for all cases of acute pericoronitis and may be needed also for the subacute condition if the infection is unlikely to subside quickly from the use of local measures alone.

6. Ulcerative pericoronitis due to Vincent's organisms is treated by metronidazole 400 mg, 12-hourly, supplemented by gentle local measures as under (2) and (3) above, but extraction of the upper 3rd molar would be unwise until the infection is under control.

SPREADING INFECTIONS IN THE SOFT TISSUES

An infection spreading in the soft tissues from one of the foci discussed above may take the form of the following.

1. *A Cellulitis*

This is a spreading infection of the loose connective tissues. It is characteristically the result of a streptococcal infection and does not normally result in the formation of large collections of pus. Antibiotics usually arrest the spread of the infection and bring about complete resolution of the condition. However, the presence of pockets of undrained pus should always be suspected and, if present, dealt with by exploration and drainage.

2. *A Suppurative Infection*

Suppurative infections are characteristic of staphylococci, often with anaerobes such as bacteroides, and may produce large accumulations of pus which will require immediate drainage.

3. *Gangrene*

In pre-antibiotic days the pressure within tissue compartments produced by massive oedema and suppuration in response to fulminating infections could lead to necrosis of the involved muscles. In particular this was seen in the case of subtemporalis muscle infection and Ludwig's angina. Swelling of this degree is rarely seen these days, but just occasionally infection by gas-forming organisms and anaerobes occurs which results in muscle necrosis.

Soft-tissue Infections and their Spread

Infections of the soft tissues around the jaws usually originate from a periapical infection related to a tooth or root, pericoronal and periodontal infections, or a secondarily infected cyst or odontome. Occasionally the infecting organisms enter the soft tissues from a penetrating wound, especially one with a retained foreign body, following an injection with a contaminated needle or a furuncle of the overlying skin. In children a staphylococcal, facial or submandibular cellulitis may arise from tonsillar or nasal infections or during the eruption of a tooth or following loss of the deciduous predecessor. Irrespective of the original source of infection, once it has become established within the soft tissues, its further spread tends to occur in a uniform fashion.

PYOGENIC INFECTIONS OF THE SOFT TISSUES

The routes by which the infection can spread are as follows.

1. *By direct continuity* through the tissues.
2. *By the lymphatics* to the regional nodes, and eventually into the bloodstream. If infection becomes established in lymph nodes, secondary abscesses may develop. Spread into the tissues from the nodes results in secondary areas of cellulitis or a tissue space abscess.
3. *By the bloodstream.* Local thrombophlebitis may rarely propagate along the veins, entering the cranial cavity via emissary veins to produce cavernous sinus thrombophlebitis. Organisms or infected emboli may be swept away into the bloodstream leading to bacteraemia, septicaemia and pyaemia with the development of embolic abscesses.

A number of factors affect the ability of the infection to spread. These are as follows.

1. The type and virulence of the organism or organisms.
2. A failure to drain accumulations of pus. Pus contains large numbers of organisms and their toxins and drainage of an abscess usually leads within a matter of hours to a marked reduction in malaise and a fall in the patient's temperature and pulse rate. Furthermore, pus which is increasing in volume may force its way into adjacent tissue spaces rather than towards the surface.
3. The state of the patient's health generally which may be adversely affected by a virus infection, diabetes, malnutrition or alcoholism.
4. The effectiveness of the patient's immune mechanism. It takes time for the body's immune mechanisms to be mobilized to combat an organism not previously encountered. In pre-antibiotic days a failure of the white cell count to rise was of grave significance. While antibiotics now enable clinicians to attack the organisms directly new circumstances result from the use of corticosteroids and immunosuppressive drugs which impair the body's natural defences. Patients may be encountered who have a rare congenital defect such as hypogammaglobulinaemia.

The anatomical factors influencing the direction of spread within the tissues are:

1. The site of the source of the infection, i.e. upper or lower jaw, and the particular segment of the jaw involved.
2. The point at which the pus escapes from the bone and discharges into the soft tissues, e.g. labiobuccally or linguopalatally.
3. The natural barriers to the spread of pus in the tissues, such as by layers of fascia or muscle or the jaw bones themselves.

The muscles which commonly play a part in containing infections around the jaws are the myohyoid, buccinator, masseter, the medial and lateral pterygoid muscles, the temporalis and the superior constrictor of the pharynx. Even the smaller and thinner muscles of facial expression can play a significant role in determining the direction in which the infection spreads.

The fascial layers probably play a slightly less important role than the muscles in influencing the spread of infection through the soft tissues of the face and neck. One of the problems which arise when discussing the layers of fascia is that the term is used somewhat imprecisely. Last (1959) emphasized that, on the one hand, the term is used to describe tough membranes, such as the investing layer of deep cervical fascia or the prevertebral fascia, both of which are demonstrable anatomical structures and can be incised and sutured. But on the other hand, the term is also applied to thin, delicate sheets of areolar tissue, like the buccopharyngeal membrane, or such as are normally found covering the surface of many muscles. From a surgical point of view, therefore, only the investing layer of cervical fascia, the prevertebral and the pretracheal fascia, the carotid sheath and the parotid fascia need to be considered in relation to the spread of infection in the soft tissues of the submandibular region and neck.

The Investing Layer of Deep Cervical Fascia

This layer of fascia envelops the neck but splits and surrounds the sternomastoid and trapezius muscles and is attached to the skull from the external occipital protuberance in a curve along the superior nuchal line to the tip of the mastoid process. In the front of the neck it is attached to the lower border of the mandible from the chin to the angle on each side. Between the angle of the mandible and tip of the mastoid process the investing layer splits into two layers. The parotid gland lies between these two layers which become the *parotid fascia*. The superficial layer extends upwards to be attached to the zygomatic arch. In many subjects it extends forward from the parotid gland to form a thinner sheet which covers the buccal space laterally. The deep layer of the parotid fascia is attached along the base of the skull from the tip of the mastoid process as far medially as the carotid canal where it blends with the carotid sheath.

The lower border of the investing fascia is attached to the spine of the scapula posteriorly, to the clavicle and sternum, anteriorly and encloses the trapezius and sternomastoid muscles. The midline is attached to the suprasternal notch by two layers which split a short distance above it, and the space between the anterior and posterior insertions is known as 'Burn's space'. The investing layer is also attached to the hyoid bone.

The Prevertebral Fascia

This fascia lies anterior to the prevertebral muscles and extends from the base of the skull in front of the longus capitis and rectus lateralis downwards to the longus cervicis muscle at the level of the body of the 3rd thoracic vertebra. It extends laterally across the scalenus muscles in the floor of the posterior triangle of the neck.

PYOGENIC INFECTIONS OF THE SOFT TISSUES

The Pretracheal Fascia

Its superior attachment is the hyoid bone at the midline and the oblique line of the thyroid cartilage more laterally. It splits to enclose the thyroid gland and laterally it fuses with the front of the carotid sheath deep to the sternomastoid. Inferiorly it passes behind the innominate veins to blend with the adventitia of the arch of the aorta. The pretracheal fascia therefore forms a layer deep to the infrahyoid muscles.

The Carotid Sheath

The carotid sheath is not as dense a fascial sheet as the investing layer but more a multilayered wrapping of areolar tissue. It is attached to the base of the skull at the lower end of the tympanic plate and is continued downwards to the aortic arch. It will be seen that the investing layer, the pretracheal and the prevertebral layers of cervical fascia run in a vertical direction. Anterior to the prevertebral fascia there is a space which extends from the base of the skull to the diaphragm. Its upper part is the retropharyngeal space and this compartment extends inferiorly behind the oesophagus through the superior to the posterior mediastinum. An abscess in the lateral pharyngeal space therefore may extend either laterally to the carotid sheath or medially into the retropharyngeal space and thus descend into the superior and posterior mediastinum. Similarly, infection penetrating anterior to the pretracheal fascia and deep to the strap muscles can extend downwards through the superior mediastinum into the pericardial space.

It will be seen that the investing layer, the prevertebral, and the pretracheal layers of fascia potentially permit the spread of infections down the neck into the thorax. Fortunately nowadays with antibiotic therapy this is exceedingly rare.

SITES AT WHICH PUS ACCUMULATES

Pus tends to accumulate in specific regions which are referred to as tissue spaces, none of which are actually spaces until pus has been formed. Some of these potential spaces are compartments which contain structures such as the submandibular salivary gland, the buccal pad of fat or groups of lymph nodes. Normally these are surrounded by loose connective tissue which is easily stripped back by finger pressure, either at operation in the living patient, or in the cadaver to produce a cavity. Pus destroys the loose connective tissue and separates the anatomical boundaries of the compartment as it increases in volume, so creating an abscess cavity bounded by muscles, fascia and bone.

Where a muscle is attached to a bone by Sharpey's fibres, the attachment is mostly strong and tendinous, but the muscle may be in part attached mainly to the periosteum so that it and periosteum together are readily stripped from the surface of the bone. Here again a potential space exists deep to the muscle if infection gains access to this plane of cleavage. As pus forms it elevates the periosteum from the bone to form an abscess cavity until its spread is limited by the more tendinous part of the muscle.

The narrow interval between muscles also contains a layer of loose connective tissue which permits independent movement of the layers. Here again pus can accumulate to produce an anatomically defined cavity.

The important spaces and potential spaces in the vicinity of the jaws are as follows.

In Relation to the Lower Jaw
1. Submental space.
2. Submandibular space.
3. Sublingual space.
4. Buccal space.
5. Submasseteric interval.
6. Parotid compartment.
7. Pterygomandibular space.
8. Lateral pharyngeal space.
9. Peritonsillar fossa.

In Relation to the Upper Jaw
1. Within the lip.
2. Within the canine fossa.
3. Palatal subperiosteal interval.
4. Maxillary antrum.
5. Infratemporal fossa space (this is the upper extremity of the pterygomandibular space).
6. Subtemporalis muscle interval.

It is important when studying these spaces not to become over concerned with the details of their anatomical boundaries; indeed many of these compartments intercommunicate. Furthermore, none of the muscular or fascial barriers are impassable and pus will eventually penetrate them and reach the overlying skin. However, because pus normally accumulates in these well-defined areas, its surgical drainage will be facilitated by a knowledge of the relevant anatomy. In all cases it is necessary to identify and deal with the source of the infection.

POTENTIALLY INFECTED SPACES RELATED TO THE LOWER JAW
Submental Space Infections

Surgical Anatomy
The submental space lies between the mylohyoid muscle above and the investing layer of the deep fascia below and this, in turn, is covered by

PYOGENIC INFECTIONS OF THE SOFT TISSUES

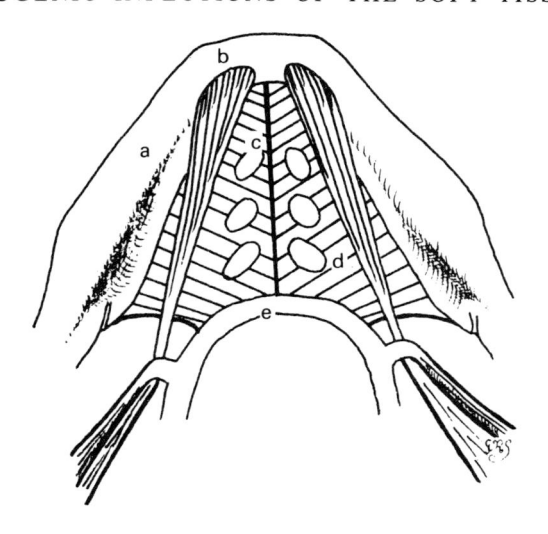

Fig. 6.2. A diagram of the submental space from below. *a,* The mandible. *b,* The anterior belly of the digastric. *c,* The submental lymph nodes in the submental space. *d,* The mylohyoid muscle. *e,* The hyoid bone.

platysma muscle, superficial fascia and skin. It is bounded laterally by the lower border of the mandible and the diverging anterior bellies of the digastric muscles over which lie the more lateral submental lymph nodes (*Fig.* 6.2). The majority of the submental lymph nodes lie within these boundaries and are embedded in adipose tissue, not loose connective tissues as is the case with the submandibular nodes. For this reason submental abscesses tend to be well circumscribed.

The submental space is usually involved secondary to infection of the submental lymph nodes following lymphatic spread from the lower incisors, the lower lip, the skin overlying the chin, or from the tip of the tongue and the anterior part of the floor of the mouth and sublingual tissues.

Signs and Symptoms
The established submental abscess forms a distinct, firm swelling beneath the chin and the patient experiences considerable discomfort on swallowing.

Treatment
Satisfactory drainage of a submental abscess can be effected by a transverse incision through the skin posterior to the crease behind the chin itself. The abscess is opened with sinus forceps and a drain inserted.

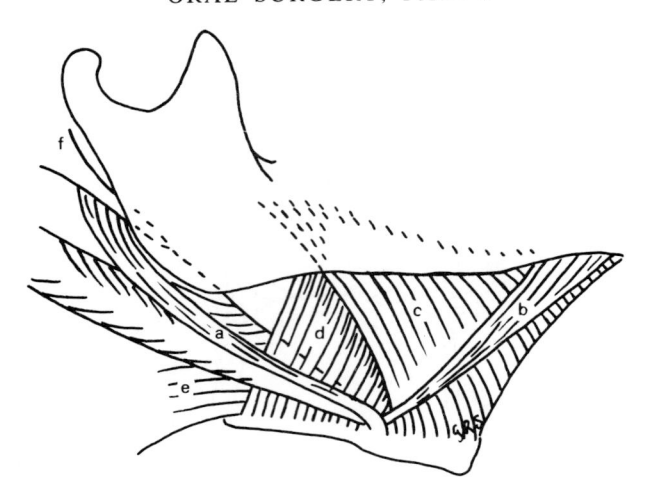

Fig. 6.3. Diagram of the submandibular space, submandibular gland and lymph nodes removed. *a,* Posterior belly of digastric and stylohyoid muscle. *b,* Anterior belly of digastric. *c,* Mylohyoid muscle. *d,* Hyoglossus muscle. *e,* Middle constrictor. *f,* Styloid process and stylohyoid ligament.

Submandibular Space Infections
Surgical Anatomy

The submandibular space is that compartment which lies between the anterior and posterior bellies of the digastric, and contains the submandibular salivary gland and the submandibular lymph nodes. The lower part lies deep to the investing layer of the deep cervical fascia and the upper part beneath the inferior border of the mandible. Anteriorly it is bounded above and medially by the mylohyoid muscle which is covered by loose alveolar tissue and fat. More posteriorly the submandibular space projects upwards under cover of the medial aspect of the mandible as high as the mylohyoid ridge. Medially the wall of the compartment is formed by the hyoglossus muscle. The C-shaped submandibular salivary salivary gland lies within the submandibular space and provides a route of communication with the sublingual space around the posterior border of the mylohyoid muscle (*Fig.* 6.3). Where the facial artery hooks around the lower border of the mandible the deep fascia is attached to the bone sufficiently above the lower border to permit the submandibular lymph nodes to overlap the mandible.

Infection from the teeth or submandibular gland may pass via the lymphatics to the submandibular lymph nodes and, as in the case of the submental space, infection of the submandibular space occurs when the lymph nodes fail to contain it. Spread of infection from the teeth by direct continuity is influenced by the origin of the mylohyoid muscle in relation to the level of the apices of the lower teeth.

The mylohyoid muscle is a thin sheet of muscle which forms the diaphragm of the floor of the mouth. It arises from the mylohyoid line on the inner aspect of the mandible as far back as the third molar tooth. The two halves of the muscle slope downwards towards each other and the posterior quarter of each is attached to the anterior surface of the body of the hyoid bone, while the anterior three quarters of each muscle meet in a midline raphe which extends from the symphysis menti down to the hyoid bone. The mylohyoid line lies near the inferior border of the mandible in the symphysial region and slopes gently upwards as it extends backward towards the region of the lower 3rd molar tooth. The apices of the roots of the lower incisors, canines and premolar teeth are, therefore, above the level of the mylohyoid diaphragm, while the apices of the roots of the molar teeth lie below the level of its attachment. Apical infection from a lower molar tooth, particularly the 2nd and 3rd, which happens to penetrate the thin lingual plate can pass directly into the submandibular space.

It is possible for infection to extend backwards from the submental space or from the submental lymph nodes via the lymphatics. Similarly infection may pass from the back of the sublingual space around the deep part of the submandibular salivary gland into the submandibular space.

It is important in assessing submandibular node enlargement due to infection to recall that the infection may originate not only from a lesion of one of the lower posterior teeth, middle third of tongue, or the posterior part of the floor of the mouth, but also from one of the upper teeth, the cheek, maxillary sinus or palate. While apical and periodontal abscesses of an upper tooth or lower posterior tooth are particularly common causes of such an infection they are not the only ones. In particular a subacute maxillary sinusitis is easily overlooked.

Signs and Symptoms

An established infection produces a firm swelling in the submandibular region. Because of the relationship of the submandibular lymph nodes and the attachment of the deep fascia to the lower border of the mandible, the swelling bulges over the lower border at the point where the facial artery crosses it (*Figs.* 6.4 and 6.5). There is invariably limitation of jaw opening and the usual systemic signs and symptoms associated with a substantial infection.

It is worth remembering that secondary deposits of a malignant neoplasm or a lymphoma in lymph nodes of the upper neck may undergo necrosis and present as a fluctuant swelling. Infiltration of the surrounding tissues by neoplasm will produce swelling and induration resembling cellulitis, except that redness of the skin, even if prevent, will not be as great as expected from an abscess. Nor will there be the degree of tenderness which would be expected. If the swelling is incised fragments of necrotic tissue will

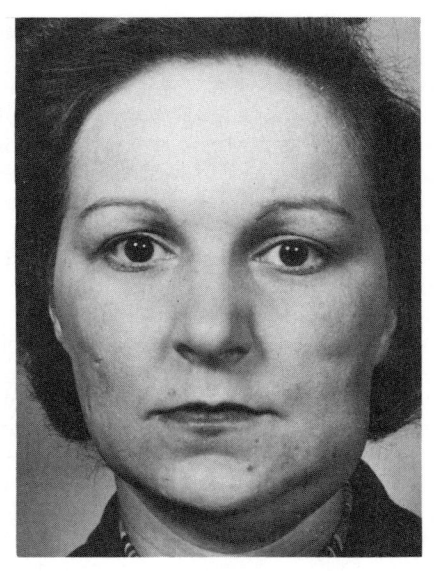

Fig. 6.4. A submandibular space infection secondary to a carious left lower molar. The way the swelling bulges over the external border of the mandible because of the position of the submandibular lymph nodes is shown.

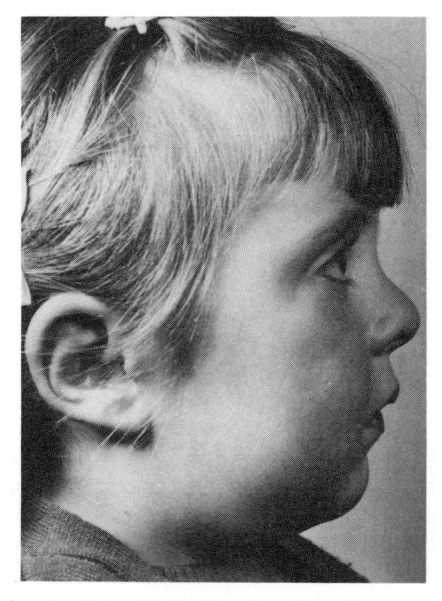

Fig. 6.5. Facial and submandibular lymph nodes enlargement and submandibular space infection secondary to an abscess $\overline{E|}$ in a child.

discharge with the liquified neoplasm. A biopsy will establish the diagnosis.

Treatment

Drainage of a submandibular abscess is effected through an incision made parallel with, but 2–3 cm below, the lower border of the mandible using, where possible, a skin crease. Skin and subcutaneous tissues are incised and then sinus forceps are pushed through the tough investing deep fascia towards the lingual side of the mandible to release the pus from the submandibular space.

Sublingual Space Infections

Infections which discharge into the soft tissues on the lingual side of the mandible at a point above the origin of the mylohyoid muscle and below the level of the mucosa of the floor of the mouth pass into the sublingual space. These infections usually arise from premolar periapical or periodontal disease or occasionally from the submandibular salivary gland. Periodontal abscesses of the lower canine or incisors may also infect the sublingual space, but periapical abscess of these teeth usually discharge labially.

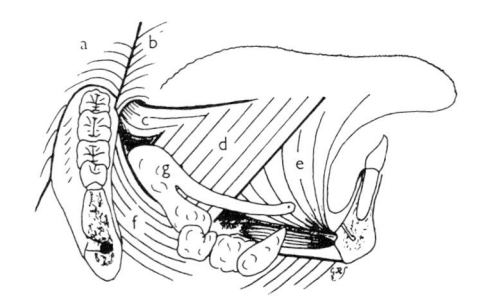

Fig. 6.6. The sublingual space has been opened up by section of the mandible and mylohyoid. *a,* Buccinator. *b,* Superior constrictor. *c,* Styloglossus. *d,* Hyoglossus. *e,* Genioglossus and, below, the geniohyoid. *f,* Mylohyoid. *g,* The deep part of the submandibular salivary gland and, more anteriorly, the sublingual salivary glands.

Surgical Anatomy

The sublingual space is a V-shaped trough lying lateral to the muscles of the tongue, including the hyoglossus, the genioglossus and the geniohyoid, and bounded laterally and inferiorly by the mylohyoid muscle and the lingual side of the mandible (*Fig.* 6.6). It is covered superiorly only by the mucous membrane of the floor of the mouth.

The infection is confined, therefore, to the connective tissue which surrounds the sublingual glands and Wharton's duct.

Clinical Features

Clinically, a firm, painful swelling is produced on the affected side in the anterior part of the floor of the mouth which raises the tongue. The oedematous tissues have a shiny, gelatinous appearance. The patient will experience pain and discomfort on swallowing, but apart from enlargement of the submental or submandibular lymph nodes there is little or no external swelling.

Infections of the sublingual space may discharge into the mouth or pass anteromedially over the hump of the genial muscles to the sublingual space on the other side. From the postero-inferior part of the space, infection can pass around the submandibular gland to enter the submandibular space (*Fig.* 6.7), or again spread posteriorly via the tunnel under the superior constrictor for the styloglossus into the parapharyngeal and pterygoid spaces. Infection may also spread via the lymphatics to the submental or submandibular lymph nodes.

The sublingual space is separated from the submental space by the mylohyoid muscle which forms a complete diaphragm within the floor of the mouth. As described earlier spread to the submental region occurs most often as a result of lymphatic spread to the submental lymph nodes. However, there are also perforating arteries which pass through the mylohyoid to form anastomoses between the sublingual arteries and the submandibular arteries which accompany the nerves to the mylohyoid. In some patients infection can spread through these apertures to the submental space.

Treatment

When the infection is only moderate in extent, antibiotic therapy combined with extraction of the responsible tooth, and the intensive use of hot saline mouthbaths, will promote satisfactory resolution of the condition. If there is gross swelling an incision to drain the floor of the mouth should be made lateral to the sublingual plica, as the only important structure at this site is the sublingual nerve which is deeply placed and unlikely to be damaged. The other important structures lie medial to the plica and include the submandibular duct, the sublingual artery and veins and the lingual nerve, and these should not be put at risk. An incision in the plica itself can result in a ranula. When both the submental and sublingual spaces contain pus they can be drained via a skin incision in the submental region, pushing closed sinus forceps through the mylohyoid muscle. Similarly when the submandibular space is involved a sublingual abscess can be reached and drained through an incision in the submandibular skin and via the submandibular space.

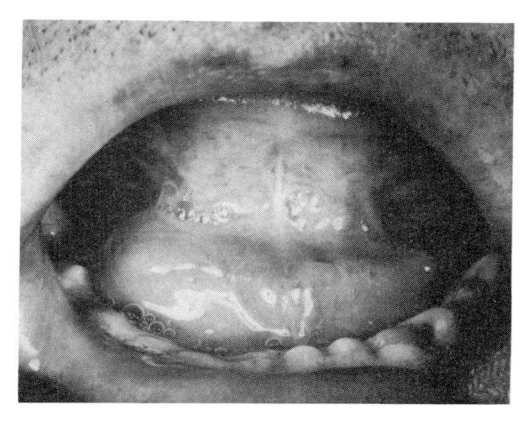

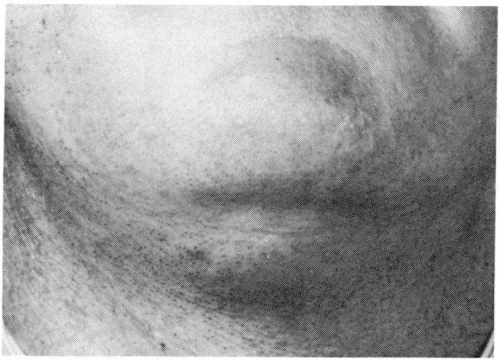

Fig. 6.7. Top. A cellulitis of the right sublingual space, spreading across the midline and originating from septic 5̅|̅ socket. *Bottom.* Enlarged submental lymph nodes secondary to the sublingual cellulitis.

Ludwig's Angina

Ludwig's angina is a clinical diagnosis and is the name given to a massive firm cellulitis affecting simultaneously the submandibular and submental regions and the sublingual spaces bilaterally (*Fig.* 6.8).

Aetiology

The complication of Ludwig's angina usually follows a submandibular space infection caused by a periapical infection or pericoronitis around the lower 3rd molar. The infection then spreads to the sublingual space on the same side, around the deep part of the submandibular gland. From there it passes to the opposite sublingual space and thence to the contralateral submandibular region. The submental space is involved by lymphatic

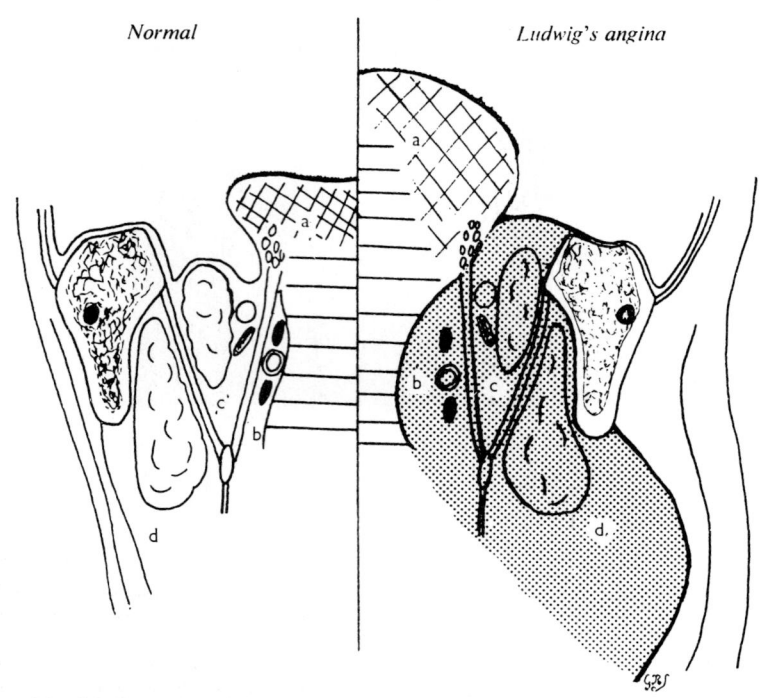

Fig. 6.8. Diagram to explain Ludwig's angina. On the left the normal side, on the right the state of affairs (bilaterally) in Ludwig's angina. The tongue, *a*, is raised by the volume of exudate in *b*, the cleft between the hyoglossus and genioglossus for the lingual and sublingual arteries and veins. *c*, The sublingual space. *d*, The submandibular space. Infection in cleft *b* has direct access to the laryngeal regions and in the sublingual space through to the pterygoid and lateral pharyngeal spaces.

spread. This serious condition can also develop in a converse manner, i.e. by spread from the sublingual spaces to the submandibular spaces.

From the sublingual spaces the infection may spread backwards in the substance of the tongue in the cleft between the hypoglossus muscle and the genioglossus and along the course of the sublingual artery. It is by this route that the infection reaches the region of the epiglottis and so produces swelling around the laryngeal inlet.

From the submandibular region the spread may rarely extend downwards beneath the investing layer of the deep cervical fascia.

Signs and Symptoms

The external clinical appearance of Ludwig's angina is of a massive firm, bilateral submandibular swelling which soon extends down the anterior part

PYOGENIC INFECTIONS OF THE SOFT TISSUES

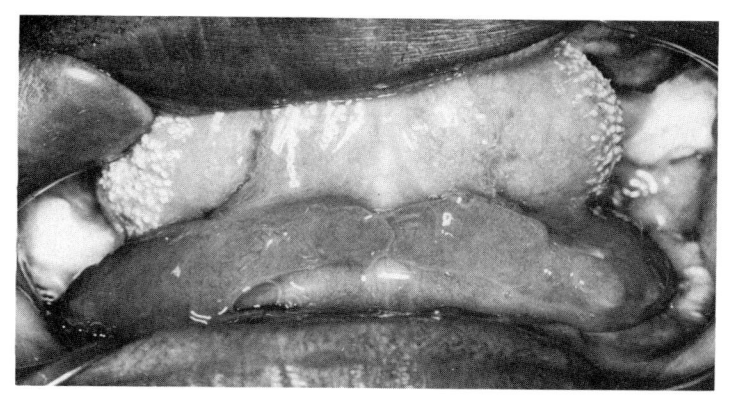

Fig. 6.9. Intraoral appearance of Ludwig's angina. The floor of the mouth is distended and the tongue forced up against the palate.

of the neck to the clavicles. Intraorally a swelling develops rapidly which involves the sublingual tissues, distends the floor of the mouth and forces the tongue up against the palate (*Fig.* 6.9). In extreme circumstances the tongue may actually protrude from the mouth.

The patient is very ill with a marked pyrexia. Deglutition and speech are difficult and progressive dyspnoea is caused by the backward spread of the infection until, in the untreated case, oedema of the glottis causes a complete respiratory obstruction. A fatal termination can occur in an untreated case of Ludwig's angina within 12–24 hours. In the past this disease carried a high mortality and even today death is a not uncommon outcome.

Treatment

Treatment is based on a combination of intensive antibiotic therapy and early intubation to control the airway, coupled with surgical drainage of the fascial spaces when pus is present. The immediate intravenous infusion of 500 mg of metronidazole and 500 mg of amoxycillin usually brings about a rapid improvement. This regime is repeated 8-hourly. (If allergic to penicillin use erythromycin lactobionate, 600 mg given slowly intravenously every 8 hours or 80 mg gentamicin intramuscularly.)

Anaesthesia

On no account should a general anaesthetic be given to such patients except by a skilled and experienced anaesthetist. Many fatalities have occurred as a result of anaesthetizing such patients, particularly when an intravenous agent has been used for induction. In such cases the patient is only maintaining the airway by the vigorous use of voluntary muscles in the region of the airway, together with assistance from the accessory muscles of respiration. If a general anaesthetic is administered this voluntary control over the airway is lost. Furthermore, as the patient becomes unconscious there is a massive increase in the oedema and the airway becomes occluded. If a laryngoscope is used at this stage the pharynx billows inwards like a bolster and it becomes quite impossible to pass an endotracheal tube. If it is imperative to give a general anaesthetic to a patient with a severe swelling of the floor of the mouth, then an endotracheal tube should be passed with the aid of a fiberoptic laryngoscope while the patient is conscious.

Established cases of Ludwig's angina can be operated upon under a combination of local analgesia and intravenous analgesia (*not* anaesthesia). It is usually possible to drain the pus after local infiltration of the skin and subcutaneous tissues overlying both submandibular regions with an analgesic solution such as 2 per cent lignocaine, with adrenaline.

A nasopharyngeal airway and a laryngotomy set should be kept ready beside the bed of any case of Ludwig's angina. The instruments for performing a tracheostomy should also be immediately available whenever an operation for drainage is performed. Immediate evaluation of the blood gases will give an additional indication of the degree of respiratory obstruction and may indicate the need for a tracheostomy even if the patient is not obviously in distress.

A tracheostomy should be performed under local anaesthesia as soon as respiratory obstruction seems likely. Even at this stage the operation will be taxing. The oedema reaches the clavicles and the tissues are brawny and inflexible. Thus the trachea is a long way from the surface of the wound and its identification is made difficult by the amount of haemorrhage from the inflamed tissues. Aspirating air with a wide bore needle and syringe from the trachea during the performance of an emergency tracheostomy ensures that the right structure is incised. A cuffed endotracheal tube may be needed instead of a tracheostomy tube because of the swelling. If the operation is delayed until venous congestion and cyanosis appears, the patient's chest will by then be heaving, so adding to the difficulty of the surgery. In an emergency a laryngotomy, opening the cricothyroid membrane, is easier to perform than a tracheostomy.

Abscess Formation in Relation to the Buccinator Muscle
Surgical Anatomy
The buccinator muscle is a wide, but fairly thin, muscle which forms a muscular sheet in the cheek. Its line of origin is horseshoe-shaped and runs along the base of the upper alveolar process from the level of the upper 1st molar distally to the tip of the pterygoid hamulus. Posteriorly it takes its

origin from the pterygomandibular raphe which unites the buccinator to the superior constrictor. At the lower end of the raphe it gains an attachment to the lateral ridge outlining the retromolar triangle. On the mandible, the attachment of the buccinator muscle follows the external oblique line to the base of the alveolar process corresponding to the lower 1st molar. The muscle fibres arising from this horseshoe-shaped line run in a generally forward direction towards the corner of the mouth where they blend with the fibres of the orbicularis oris. The fibres of the buccinator arising from the upper jaw tend to pass downwards and those from the lower jaw upwards and where these muscle bands cross over at the corner of the mouth the buccinator is thicker than it is more posteriorly. There is an important band of horizontal fibres in the inner aspect of the muscle which on contraction help to maintain the food bolus between the occlusal surfaces of the teeth. Persistent contraction of these fibres produces a linear thickening of the buccal mucosa corresponding to the line of occlusal contact.

It is important to remember that the attachment of the buccinator is above the level of the apices of the lower molars and below those of the upper molars. The buccinator muscle acts as an effective barrier to the spread of pus and this is especially true during the early stages of an abscess in the cheek. The buccopharyngeal fascia is a very delicate affair and probably plays no part in limiting the spread of infection. Pus which spreads buccally from any of the upper or lower molar teeth to perforate the outer cortex of the alveolar process can discharge into the mouth on the oral side of the origin of the buccinator muscle. Such abscesses are simple to diagnose, because the swelling is principally in the buccal sulcus beneath the mucosa and opposite the tooth of origin, while externally the facial swelling is relatively small, soft and puffy. Sometimes when the intraoral abscess is large it may reach the occlusal plane and become traumatized, but eventually it will discharge spontaneously. Evacuation of the pus is readily achieved by an incision through the overlying mucosa. Pus from periapical infection of the molar teeth which emerges from the bone above the origin of the buccinator in the upper jaw, or below its origin in the mandible, will spread to the outer side of the buccinator partition and give rise to a local buccal space abscess. Some buccal space infections originate from an infected facial lymph node.

The Buccal Space

Surgical Anatomy

This potential space is bounded anteromedially by the buccinator muscle, posteromedially by the masseter overlying the anterior border of the ramus of the mandible, and it is covered laterally by a forward extension of the deep fascia from the capsule of the parotid gland and by the platysma muscle. It is limited below by the attachment of the deep fascia to the

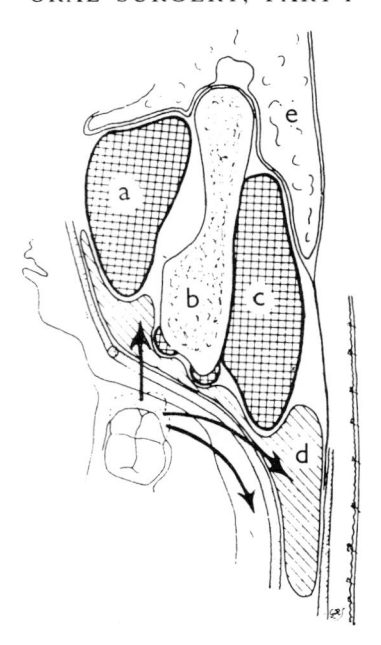

Fig. 6.10. Diagram showing the buccal space in horizontal section and the spread of infection from an impacted lower 3rd molar. *a*, Medial pterygoid muscle. *b*, Mandible. *c*, Masseter. *d*, Buccal space and the buccal pad of fat with diagonal shading. *e*, Parotid with parotid fascia extending forwards to cover the buccal space in conjunction with the platysma muscle.

mandible (*Fig.* 6.10) and by the depressor anguli oris and above by the zygomatic process of the maxilla and the zygomaticus minor and major.

The buccal space contains the buccal pad of fat and is therefore continuous posteriomedially around the fat with the pterygoid space through the interval between the buccinator and the anterior border of the coronoid process. The buccal pad of fat, of course, not only fills out the cheek but wraps around the pterygoid muscles and the temporalis tendon behind the tuberosity, as it were, to lubricate the masticatory machinery.

When a lower 3rd molar is exposed surgically blood may escape laterally due to the detachment of the pterygomandibular raphe and the adjacent bony origin of the buccinator fibres. This produces a haematoma in the buccal space. Infection from a pericoronitis of a 3rd molar can follow the same route to produce a buccal space infection (*Fig.* 6.11).

If an abscess from a mandibular tooth ultimately discharges on the skin surface the sinus track may be felt as a cord below the lower buccal sulcus. The direction of this cord will indicate the tooth of origin.

PYOGENIC INFECTIONS OF THE SOFT TISSUES

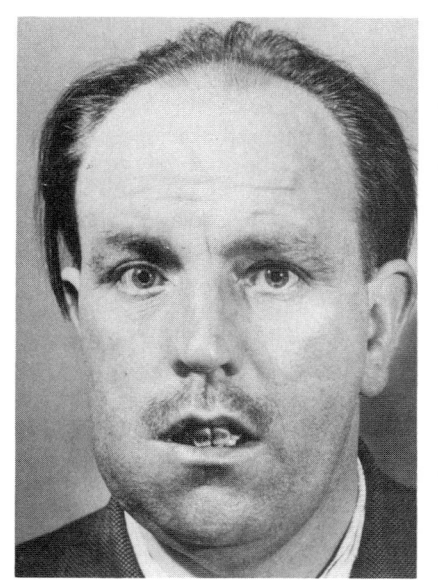

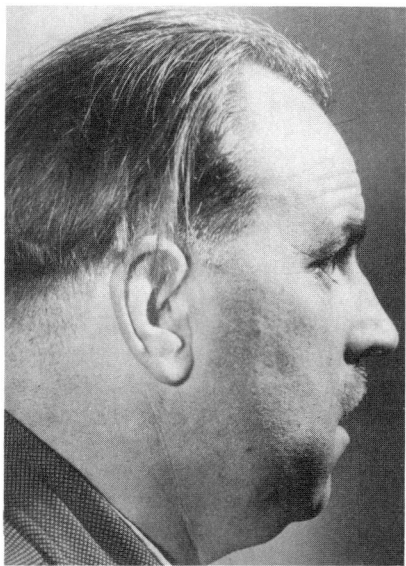

Fig. 6.11. A buccal space infection secondary to an abscess on a lower 1st molar. Observe that the swelling is just behind the angle of the mouth and reaches down to the lower border of the mandible.

Treatment

Drainage is effected by a horizontal incision low down inside the cheek through which sinus forceps are passed to penetrate the buccinator. The incision with the scalpel should not be carried through the buccinator in case the facial artery or branches of the facial nerve are divided. It should be below the parotid papilla to avoid damage to the duct. A soft corrugated rubber or polypropylene drain is essential to keep the path through the muscle open. Buccal space abscesses pointing on the face can be incised and drained through the skin, but it should be possible to drain the majority intraorally to avoid a scar.

The Submasseteric Abscess

Many anatomists have stated that the muscle consists of three heads with insertions into the ramus which are separated from each other by bare areas of bone with a space between the middle and the deep heads, termed the 'submasseteric space'. This space was thought of as providing a pathway for infection to pass upwards and backwards from the retromolar fossa region.

MacDougall (1955) examined the evidence for the submasseteric space at the bone surface and came to the conclusion that it did not exist. He based this observation on the dissection of 141 specimens of the masseter muscle together with radiological investigations following the injection of a radiopaque barium sulphate paste into cadavers, but he confirmed that the masseter muscle consists of three layers fused anteriorly but easily separated posteriorly. Although he found no submasseteric space at the bone surface, there was a potential one in the substance of the muscle between the middle and deep heads, and while the bony insertion is firm above and below, the intermediate fibres have only a loose attachment. It is possible therefore for these fibres to be separated from the bone relatively easily by the accumulation of pus at this site. As surgical exploration in cases of established submasseteric abscess has confirmed, the pus accumulates beneath the periosteum and against the bone in this area. One must assume that it tracks backwards subperiosteally to where it may erode laterally into the potential space between the muscle bellies.

Aetiology
A submasseteric abscess is by no means common and usually arises from infection in the lower 3rd molar region. Pericoronitis related to vertical and disto-angular lower 3rd molars is most likely to lead to a submasseteric abscess. The presence of the buccinator attachment probably discourages backward extension of pericoronal pus where the lower 3rd molar crown is anterior to this muscular barrier. Pus can also reach the submasseteric area if a periapical abscess from a mandibular molar spreads subperiosteally in a distal direction.

Clinical Features
In the established submasseteric abscess the external facial swelling is moderate in size and is confined to the outline of the masseter muscle (*Fig. 6.12*). The swelling does not usually extend beyond the posterior margin of the ramus or encroach on the postauricular tissues like an acute parotitis, although occasionally the postmandibular sulcus may be obscured by inflammatory oedema. Extension of the abscess inferiorly is also limited by the firm attachment of the masseter to the lower border of the ramus. Forward spread of the swelling beyond the anterior border of the ramus is restricted by the anterior tail of the tendon of temporalis which is inserted into the anterior border of the ramus. Although the swelling of a submasseteric abscess is only moderate in extent it is usually acutely tender and gives rise to an almost complete limitation of mouth opening.

The marked degree of limitation of opening is an important diagnostic feature and sometimes seems inconsistent with the amount of swelling present over the lateral aspect of the ramus. The overlying skin is only reddened in advanced cases and fluctuation cannot be elicited because the muscle lies between the pus and surface. In longstanding cases constitutional symptoms are minimal, but at the acute stage the systemic reaction includes pyrexia and malaise.

PYOGENIC INFECTIONS OF THE SOFT TISSUES

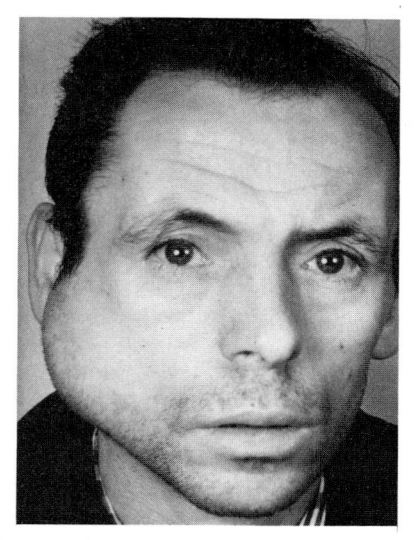

Fig. 6.12. Submasseteric abscess. Notice that the swelling does not lift the lobe of the right ear so is not due to swelling of the parotid.

Owing to the thick covering of the masseter muscle with tendinous attachments to the posterior and inferior borders of the ramus, the collection of submasseteric pus is confined against the surface of the ramus and spontaneous discharge is less likely to take place than with most other soft tissue abscesses. If the infection is particularly severe pus may discharge forwards at the anterior border of the ramus, or backwards immediately behind the angle of the mandible. But, as the point of discharge is remote from the main accumulation of pus, drainage tends to be incomplete and a residual pocket is left which gives rise to further exacerbations at a later date. A chronic submasseteric infection can persist for years punctuated by recurrent flare-ups. Each acute abscess can be drained by a skin or mucosal incision or controlled by antibiotics, but without complete resolution. Spread of the infection into the masseter muscle itself gives rise to a large multilocular abscess, the drainage of which is difficult so that treatment may become protracted.

The ramus of the mandible is more dependent upon a blood supply from the overlying muscle than the body which is to a greater extent supplied by the mandibular artery. As a result, ischaemic changes may take place in that part of the bone denuded of periosteum by a submasseteric abscess so that a low grade osteomyelitis of the lateral cortical plate occurs with sequestrum formation. The extent of bone destruction depends, of course, upon the area of bone in contact with pus together with such factors as the degree of virulence of the organism. Often submasseteric infection leads to subperiosteal new bone deposition beneath the periosteum, an important clue to the diagnosis. Such depositions are likely to be prolific in young patients in whom the osteogenic potential of the periosteum is high. Layers of new bone produce a hard swelling over the ramus, which in extreme cases may be misdiagnosed as a sarcoma. Some so-called cases of 'Garre's osteomyelitis' affecting the ramus are probably examples of this periostitis.

Radiological Examination

Unfortunately, the early, acute submasseteric abscess gives rise to no radiological abnormalities. Once it occurs, subperiosteal new bone formation is best demonstrated by a tangential postero-anterior radiograph. The new bone has an opaque linear or irregular 'fuzzy' appearance. After the infection has been cured the additional bone will gradually remodel until the ramus eventually reverts to its normal thickness. If a superficial osteomyelitis supervenes then the affected lateral cortical plate of the ramus will show evidence of bone destruction with a patchy radiolucency. If drainage is delayed, sequestrum formation may be seen. Although only the outer cortex of the ramus is affected by the osteomyelitis, when the jaw is viewed in an oblique lateral radiograph the entire thickness of the ramus appears to be involved due to superimposition.

Differential Diagnosis

Basically, swellings affecting four anatomical compartments have to be distinguished:

1. The masseteric compartment.
2. The buccal space.
3. The parotid compartment.
4. The ramus of the mandible.

1. Swellings involving the *masseteric compartment* follow the outline of the masseter muscle. Such swellings include masseteric hypertrophy which stands out on clenching the teeth and softens on relaxation. Intramuscular haemangiomas affecting the masseter can also produce an enlargement of the muscle which varies in size when the muscle is clenched and enlarges on bending the head below the waist. Sometimes in these cases phleboliths may be seen in a tangential radiograph and provide a clue to the diagnosis. Thrombophlebitis of an intramuscular haemangioma must be distinguished from a submasseteric abscess.

2. The *buccal space* is anterior to the masseter and the swelling reaches almost as far forwards as the angle of the mouth. The commonest causes of buccal space swellings are infection, haematomas and haemangiomas, and occasionally a lipoma. If thrombosis occurs in a cavernous haemangioma of the buccal space the patient can present with an acute and painful enlargement.

PYOGENIC INFECTIONS OF THE SOFT TISSUES

3. *Parotid swellings* are largely posterior to the masseter and may be due to obstruction, suppurative infections of the gland or of the related lymph nodes, mumps and cytomegalovirus infection, Sjögren's syndrome or a neoplasm. Classically the swelling extends posteriorly to raise the lobe of the ear but the anatomical extent may be less easily determined where there is considerable oedema of the overlying skin and subcutaneous tissues.

An obstruction of the parotid duct will cause intermittent enlargement of the parotid gland and the patient usually gives a history of exacerbation at mealtimes. A stone may be demonstrable by plain radiography or sialography. Acute and subacute suppurative parotitis can be more difficult to distinguish from submasseteric abscess externally, but in the case of the former, pus can be expressed from the parotid duct.

Sometimes mumps affects one salivary gland only, or one gland alone some days before the others are affected. If the parotid gland is affected again the differential diagnosis can be difficult. However, the parotid papilla will be reddened and there is usually fever and general malaise which may either precede or coincide with the glandular enlargement.

Although only one gland may be affected, frequently the other shows signs of involvement from one to five days later. The submandibular and sublingual glands are sometimes enlarged and tender. In addition the breasts, pancreas and testes may be involved. There also will be an increased serum amylase and a rise in S & V mumps antibodies.

Tumours tend to be circumscribed and non-tender and are often pleomorphic adenomas. The adenoid cystic carcinoma and malignant ones may produce a facial palsy.

4. *Ramus enlargement* is rarely difficult to diagnose as radiographs will show a developmental, cystic or neoplastic enlargement. Ramus swellings also move with the mandible as the mouth is opened.

Treatment

In the early stage of submasseteric infection it is occasionally possible to abort the condition by the removal of the causative tooth and administration of an antibiotic; benzyl penicillin or metronidazole is usually sufficient. The established submasseteric abscess must be decompressed by incision and drainage. The incision is made over the lower part of the anterior border of the ramus and deepened to bone. Forceps are then passed along the lateral surface of the ramus downwards and backwards and the loculus of pus is opened. A specimen is sent to the microbiological laboratory for examination of a stained direct film, culture and antibiotic sensitivity. The abscess is usually situated below the level of the incision and not at a point of dependent drainage, and, therefore, drainage may be inefficient. A Yeats or corrugated drain should be sewn in to keep the incision open.

The alternative approach, especially when the mouth cannot be opened, is to make a skin incision behind the angle of the mandible and to open the

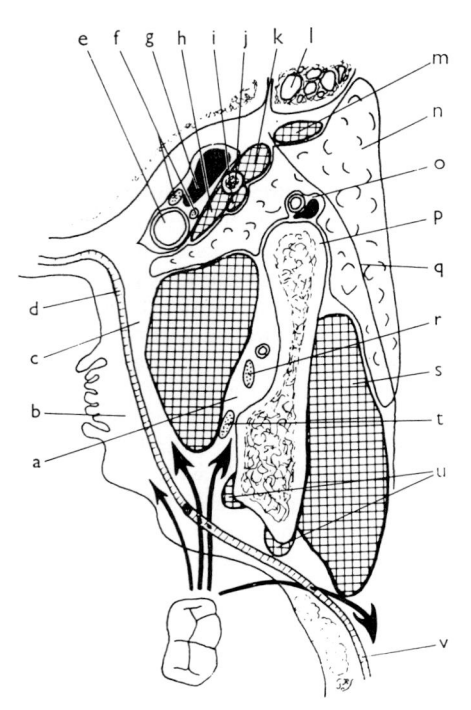

Fig. 6.13. Diagram showing the relationship of the peritonsillar, lateral pharyngeal and pterygoid spaces. *a*, Pterygoid space. *b*, Peritonsillar space. *c*, Lateral pharyngeal space. *d*, Superior constrictor. *e*, Carotid artery. *f*, Vagus nerve and sympathetic trunk. *g*, Internal jugular vein. *h*, Stylopharyngeus muscle. *i*, Styloglossus muscle. *j*, Styloid process. *k*, Stylohyoid muscle. *l*, Mastoid process. *m*, Digastric muscle. *n*, Parotid gland. *o*, External carotid and posterior facial vein. *p*, Mandible. *q*, Facial nerve. *r*, Inferior dental artery and nerve. *s*, Masseter. *t*, Lingual nerve. *u*, Tails of temporalis tendon. *v*, Buccinator muscle. (Partly after Murphy T. R. and Grundy E. M. (1969) *Dent. Prac. Dent. Rec.* **16**, 41.)

abscess by Hilton's method. A gloved finger dilates the wound further, after which a retractor can be inserted and the surface of the mandible tested with a Howarth's periosteal elevator for the presence of a sequestrum. Again a soft corrugated, polyethylene drain should be sewn into the wound. It is left in position for 24 hours at least and may need to remain 3–4 days if a recurrent abscess is to be avoided.

Infection of the Pterygomandibular Space
Surgical Anatomy

The pterygomandibular space is a compartment situated between the medial surface of the ramus of the mandible and the medial pterygoid muscle. The two heads of the latter arise principally from the medial surface of the lateral pterygoid plate and the tuberosity of the maxilla. The medial pterygoid lies at first on the medial surface of the lower part of the lower head of the lateral pterygoid muscle which it embraces with the aid of the superficial slip, and then its fibres pass downwards, laterally and backwards to be inserted by a strong tendinous lamina into the lower and posterior part of the medial surface of the ramus and angle of the mandible as high as the mandibular foramen. Between the lateral surface of the medial pterygoid and the medial surface of the ramus of the mandible run the inferior dental, mylohyoid and lingual nerves, the maxillary artery and the inferior dental artery and vein. Posteriorly the lateral pterygoid muscle forms a roof to the pterygoid space (*Fig.* 6.20) and just below the lateral pterygoid the pterygomandibular space potentially communicates with the parapharyngeal space (*Fig.* 6.13).

In practice infections do not usually spread there by this route because of the parotid gland lying tight against the back of the mandible and the medial pterygoid muscle. Infection is more likely to extend into the parapharyngeal space by passing medially around the anterior border of the medial pterygoid.

Aetiology

Infection in the pterygomandibular space may be introduced by a contaminated needle used for an inferior dental nerve block injection. It can also spread to this area from the lower 3rd molar region, especially when pericoronitis develops around the crown of a lingually inclined disto-angular tooth. In other instances the infection originates from the upper 3rd molar or follows a posterior superior dental injection.

Abscess in the Pterygomandibular Space

Even well established infections of the pterygomandibular space do not cause much swelling of the face and such swelling as is visible involves the submandibular region and buccal space. However, there is a severe degree of limitation of opening and dysphagia and on palpation tenderness can be elicited in the swollen soft tissues medial to the anterior border of the ramus of the mandible.

Usually the abscess tends to point at the anterior border of the ramus and drainage can be effected easily by an incision down the anterior border, after which a pair of sinus forceps can be directed into the plane between the ramus and the medial pterygoid to enter the space.

Occasionally an infection in this area may spread upwards along the medial surface of the ramus to produce an abscess in the infratemporal fossa and beneath the temporalis fascia. It can also pass anteriorly between the front of the ramus of the mandible and the buccinator into the buccal space, and antero-inferiorly below the lower border of the superior constrictor along the styloglossus into the submandibular space. Indeed, if there is difficulty in reaching the pus via an incision down the front of the coronoid process within the mouth, sinus forceps can be passed upwards and backwards deep to the mandible through an incision in a skin crease in the submandibular region.

Lateral Pharyngeal (Parapharyngeal) Space Infection

Surgical Anatomy

The lateral or parapharyngeal space, which is also known as the 'pharyngomaxillary' space, is a potential cone-shaped space or cleft with its base uppermost at the base of the skull and its apex at the greater horn of the hyoid bone. Its medial wall is the superior constrictor muscle with its covering sheet of buccopharyngeal fascia, together with the styloglossus, stylopharyngeus and middle constrictor and the lateral wall from above downwards consists of fascia covering the medial pterygoid, the angle of the mandible and the submandibular salivary gland. More posteriorly it is closed laterally by the parotid gland and the posterior belly of the digastric muscle. The posterior border of the space is the prevertebral fascia and the upper part of the carotid sheath lies within it.

The boundary walls of the lateral pharyngeal space do not permit easy communication with the adjacent spaces. Infection passes most easily between the lateral pharyngeal space and the submandibular space by tracking along the styloglossus muscle. There is also a weak zone in the posterior part of the fascia around the submandibular salivary gland, medial to the stylomandibular ligament, and rupture of a submandibular abscess through into the parapharyngeal space at this point results in the rapid onset of respiratory embarrassment.

Some surgeons include a downward continuation of this compartment around the carotid sheath as far as the thoracic inlet. Thus they would include the inferior constrictor and oesophagus in the medial wall, the lateral lobe of the thyroid as an anterior relation, and the sternomastoid and superior belly of the omohyoid in the lateral wall.

Aetiology

The lateral pharyngeal space may become infected from an abscess extending backwards from the lower 3rd molar area or more commonly one passing laterally from a tonsillar abscess. Infection can also spread backwards into it from a sublingual or submandibular space infection as described above.

A rare cause of parapharyngeal infection is the surgical displacement of a lower 3rd molar distally under the lingual flap and backwards into the lateral pharyngeal space. Similarly a 3rd molar root may be dislodged into it through a hole in the lingual plate. Displaced teeth or root fragments should be removed as soon as possible after the accident in order to avoid possible abscess formation. Following retrieval of the dislodged object, a prophylactic antibiotic should be administered until the risk of infection has passed.

PYOGENIC INFECTIONS OF THE SOFT TISSUES

A five-day course of phenoxymethyl penicillin 500 mg, 6-hourly, or metronidazole 400 mg 12-hourly, would be appropriate.

Signs and Symptoms

The pyrexia and malaise can be considerable in the case of lateral pharyngeal abscess, more so than with many other infections around the jaws. Pain on swallowing is extreme and there is some limitation of opening, but the latter is not severe unless the pterygomandibular space is involved as well. The tonsil and the lateral pharyngeal wall are pushed towards the midline, but the soft palate is not greatly disturbed. Usually there is little swelling of the side of the face, but there may be some at the lower border of the parotid gland and this is probably due to enlargement of the nodes in this region.

Infection of the lateral pharyngeal space is extremely serious owing to the intimate relationship of the carotid sheath. Thrombophlebitis of the internal jugular vein may occur as a complication and if pus in the lateral pharyngeal space is left undrained for any length of time the common carotid artery may become eroded with fatal consequence. Inequality of the pupils due to involvement of the cervical sympathetic can be a warning of such a disastrous sequel.

Treatment

Early intensive therapy is given with intravenous metronidazole and benzyl penicillin (or erythromycin, gentamicin or cefuroxime) followed by drainage. For drainage of such an abscess, an inhalation anaesthetic is given cautiously by an experienced anaesthetist. The head-down position must be used, because the abscess may burst as the tube is passed. A sucker is essential and the ability to pass a nasotracheal tube blind can be a great asset since visibility with a laryngoscope can be limited by difficulty in opening the jaws to their maximum. If the patient's mouth can be opened wide an intraoral incision medial to the anterior border of the ramus is the most direct drainage route. If this is not possible a skin incision is made 1 cm below and behind the angle of the mandible and then sinus forceps followed by a finger are inserted into the space between the submandibular and parotid glands and passed medial to the mandible and upwards along the inner aspect of the medial pterygoid muscle into the lateral pharyngeal space. A drain is inserted in either case.

Peritonsillar Abscess or Quinsy

Surgical Anatomy

A peritonsillar abscess is a localized infection in the connective tissue bed of the faucial tonsil between it and the superior constrictor muscle. Acute infection penetrates from the depth of a tonsil crypt or the supratonsillar fossa, but may occasionally be a complication of acute pericoronitis associated with a lower 3rd molar. In the latter case the abscess points near the lower pole of the tonsil.

Signs and Symptoms

There is acute pain on one side of the throat radiating to the ear. Dysphagia is experienced and, although the patient finds it difficult to open the mouth, the actual limitation of opening may not be pronounced. Speech becomes awkward, especially in bilateral cases, and the peculiar muffled 'hot potato in the mouth' voice is characteristic. Owing to the extreme pain experienced on attempting to swallow, saliva may run out of the mouth. The patient looks and feels ill, is anorexic and becomes rapidly dehydrated unless remedial measures are taken.

The fully developed abscess causes a tense swelling of the anterior pillar of the fauces, and a bulge of the soft palate on the affected side which in extreme cases reaches the midline and pushes the uvula downwards and forwards until it impinges against the opposite tonsil. The inflamed tonsil may protrude from behind the anterior pillar, but sometimes it is masked by oedematous tissue which covers it anteriorly. The tongue is coated and there is marked foetor oris. Oedema may eventually affect the base of the tongue, epiglottis and aryepiglottic fold. In 3–5 days the mass often becomes fluctuant and, if allowed to pursue its natural course, finally ruptures by pointing, usually through the anterior tonsillar pillar. Foul pus discharges for several days and the symptoms and signs gradually abate.

Treatment

This involves antibiotics and incision. The abscess is incised using a guarded knife and sinus forceps which are inserted into the most prominent part of the soft palate where fluctuation is maximal. A mouth prop should be used to prevent unexpected closure while the knife is in the mouth. The opening can be carried out under local analgesia, initially using a lignocaine spray but reinforced by 2 per cent lignocaine and adrenaline infiltrated into the mucosa at the site of the incision. If general anaesthesia is used the anaesthetist must be experienced in this type of case and good suction must be available to prevent aspiration of the pus. Induction and the passage of the tube should be with the patient in the head down position, because the abscess may be ruptured as the anaesthetist attempts to pass the tube.

Differential Diagnosis

Some confusion could possibly arise in the differentiation of pterygo-mandibular and lateral pharyngeal space infections from a peritonsillar abscess, especially when either of the former is pointing along the anterior border of the medial surface of the ramus. *Table* 6.1 therefore summarizes the differences between the physical signs produced by these conditions.

PYOGENIC INFECTIONS OF THE SOFT TISSUES

Table 6.1 Differential diagnosis

Space	Pterygo-mandibular	Lateral pharyngeal	Peritonsillar
Anatomy	Between mandible and medial pterygoid	Between medial pterygoid and superior constrictor	Between superior constrictor and mucous membrane
Limitation of opening:	Extreme	Moderate	Some
External swelling	Little	None	None
Swelling in mouth and throat	Some over medial aspect of anterior border of ramus	A good deal of pillars of fauces but little of soft palate	Pillars of fauces and most of soft palate

POTENTIALLY INFECTED SPACES RELATED TO THE UPPER JAW

The Upper Lip

Infections at the base of the upper lip usually occur as a result of an abscess of the upper incisors or canines. The pus forms on the oral side of the orbicularis oris muscle and tends to point in the vestibule (*Fig.* 6.14).

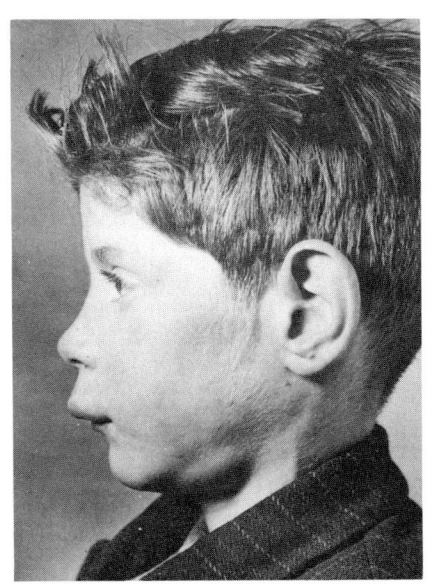

Fig. 6.14. Child with acute alveolar abscess on |1 with oedema of the upper lip. There is a markedly enlarged submandibular lymph node on the same side lying lateral to the lower border of the mandible.

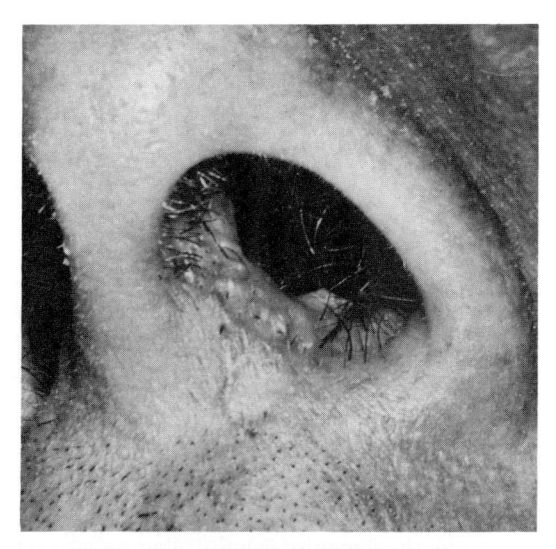

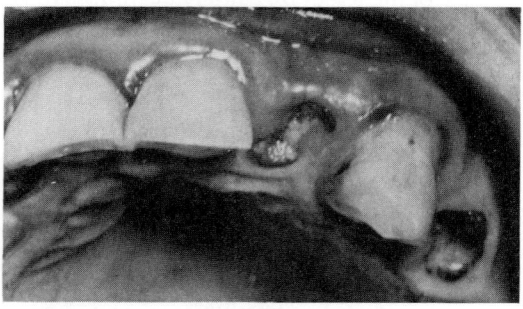

Fig. 6.15. An abscess from |2 root pointing in the nostril where it could be mistaken for a nasal furuncle. Pressure on the end of |2 root caused pus to ooze out of both the root canal and the sinus in the nose. This clinical picture occurs rather more often with the upper central incisors.

Because of the bulk of the muscles taking origin beneath the anterior nasal spine, abscesses from the central incisors point towards the apex of the lateral incisor. Rarely they will point in the floor of the nose and be mistaken for a boil of the nose (*Fig.* 6.15). Infections of the lip on the outer surface of the orbicularis oris muscle usually occur as a result of a skin infection such as a furuncle.

Infections in the area of the upper lip including the incisors and canines may rarely give rise to an orbital cellulitis or a cavernous sinus thrombophlebitis by passing from the superior labial venus plexus to the anterior facial vein and then in a retrograde direction via the ophthalmic veins to the cavernous sinus. This pathway is facilitated by the fact that these veins have no valves. Cavernous sinus thrombophlebitis used to be a fatal condition before antibiotic therapy (*see later*).

Treatment

All abscesses in the region of the upper lip should be treated by a combination of antibiotic therapy and drainage. Incision of the abscess can usually be made in the vestibule and the offending tooth is either opened and drained or extracted.

Differential Diagnosis of Swellings of the Upper Lips

1. *Trauma:* Any blow on the upper lip can produce a swelling of the tissues which may be of considerable size. If the upper incisors have been damaged and the patient is seen a day or two after the injury, it may be difficult to decide whether infection has supervened. Surgery such as an apicectomy in the upper incisor region may be followed by substantial local swelling again raising doubts about the occurrence of postoperative infection. Either postoperative or post-traumatic oedema will start to subside after 48 hours whereas the physical signs will worsen if infection is present.

2a. *Hypersensitivity reaction:* Allergic swelling of the upper lip may result from contact with a substance such as a lipstick or toothpaste which excites an allergic response or arise as a feature of angioedema (*Fig.* 6.16). Some part of the swelling following endodontic therapy would appear to be a hypersensitivity response to opening through the apex of the infected tooth. The enlarged lip is soft and non-tender and will reduce in size with antihistamines.

b. *Other oedematous swellings:* There are a number of uncommon causes of oedematous swelling of the upper lip including the Merkerson–Rosenthal syndrome. This syndrome is considered to include a swollen lip, fissured tongue and facial palsy. Biopsy of the lip will reveal non-caseating Langhan's giant cell granulomas which if associated with neuropathy are likely to be sarcoid, but if associated with granulomatous bowel disease is then Crohn's disease.

3. *Cysts and neoplasms:* Cysts of the jaws can produce a swelling in the vestibule which extends towards the upper lip and may cause enlargement of the lip especially if infected. Any odontogenic cyst in the upper incisor region or a nasopalatine cyst is capable of involving the labial tissue. The nasolabial cyst which lies against the bone between the ala of the nose and the upper lip will produce a prominent swelling in the region of the nasolabial fold. Occasionally a pleomorphic adenoma or muco-epidermoid carcinoma may arise in the labial tissues. These are usually firm in consistency, but sometimes a cystic variety is encountered. If a malignant salivary gland neoplasm involves the overlying skin, it may produce a red

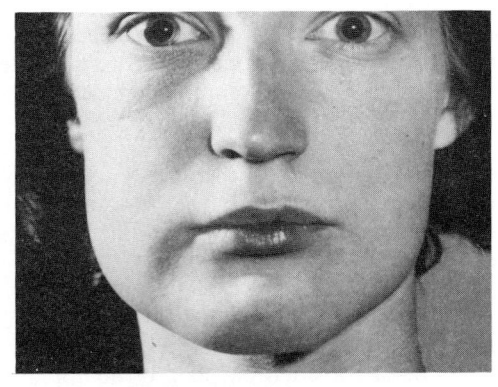

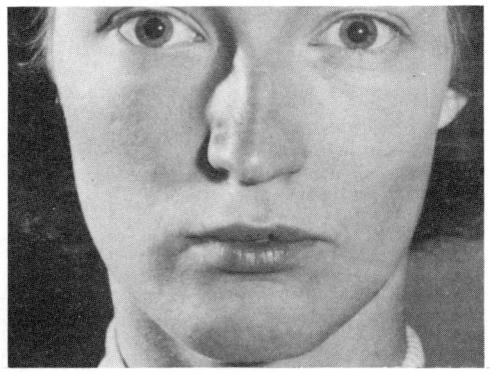

Fig. 6.16. Angio-oedema. The patient is subject to transient swellings in various parts of the face similar to the one shown above top. The picture below was taken 24 hours later.

coloured swelling with prominent dilated small vessels, and should there be an accumulation of mucus, or necrosis of the centre of the lesion it may closely resemble a pointing abscess. In all these cases the length of time the patient has had a swollen lip should correct the erroneous first impression.

The Canine Fossa

A periapical abscess which discharges buccally from an upper canine or first premolar may lead to an accumulation of pus in the canine fossa, deep to the muscles of facial expression moving the upper lip (*Fig.* 6.17).

Surgical Anatomy

If the canine root is relatively short, pus from a periapical abscess will emerge from the bone below the origin of the levator anguli oris and will

PYOGENIC INFECTIONS OF THE SOFT TISSUES

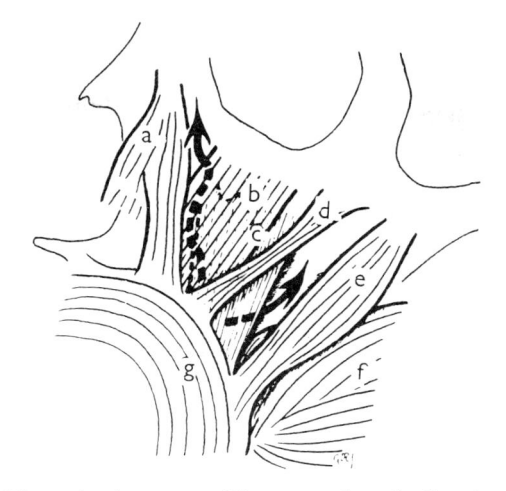

Fig. 6.17. The canine fossa space. The arrows show the direction the pus will take from the apex of the canine and from the apices of the premolars. *a*, Levator labii superioris alaeque nasi. *b*, Levator labii superioris arising above the infraorbital foramen. *c*, Levator anguli oris (dotted outline) arising below the foramen. *d*, Zygomaticus minor. *e*, Zygomaticus major. *f*, Buccinator. *g*, Orbicularis oris.

tend to point in the upper buccal sulcus, because the buccinator muscle has no attachment to the bone anterior to the 1st molar.

The levator anguli oris takes origin below the infraorbital foramen and the levator labii superioris above the foramen and overlaps the anguli oris. If the pus does not point in the buccal sulcus it tends to travel up the medial border of the levator anguli oris, deep to the levator labii which it cannot penetrate. It then emerges between the levator labii superioris and the levator labii superioris alaeque nasi to point below the medial corner of the eye.

If the root of the canine is long or the origin of levator anguli relatively low, pus from a periapical abscess may emerge above the origin of the levator anguli oris. In these circumstances it can only escape to the surface between the levator labii superioris and the levator labii superioris alaeque nasi.

Clinical Appearances

There is considerable oedema of the cheek and upper lip even if the abscess points in the buccal sulcus. If pus accumulates in the canine fossa then the nasolabial fold is often obliterated and the swelling of the upper lip produces a drooping of the angle of the mouth. Oedema of the lower eyelid heralds pointing of the abscess below the medial corner (*Fig.* 6.18).

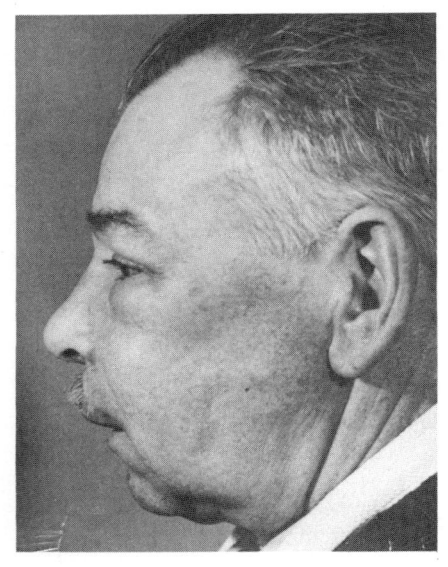

Fig. 6.18. Swelling of the left cheek and medial corner of the lower eyelid resulting from an abscess on the upper left canine.

Treatment
There is again an obvious risk of cavernous sinus thrombosis as a complication of these infections and early effective drainage is important, but should be carried out without unnecessary trauma. Antibiotics should always be prescribed.

Differential Diagnosis
Facial swelling due to an abscess from an upper tooth has to be distinguished from a carbuncle and from acute maxillary sinusitis which occasionally may cause infra orbital oedema with swelling of the lower eyelid. Swelling of both lower and upper eyelids may accompany acute ethmoidal sinusitis which may extend and become an orbital cellulitis. Acute frontal sinusitis produces oedema of the forehead and involves only the upper eyelids. Acute nasolacrimal dacryocystitis following stenosis of the duct can produce an inflammatory swelling below the medial canthus of the eye, not unlike that produced by a pointing canine abscess, but there will be redness of the lower conjunctival fornix and probably a purulent exudate there.

Abscess Involving the Upper Molar Teeth
Abscesses involving the upper molar teeth usually point in the buccal sulcus, but occasionally pus from a palatal root or a periodontal pocket in

PYOGENIC INFECTIONS OF THE SOFT TISSUES

the trifurcation may point on the palatal side. More rarely pus may discharge into the maxillary antrum giving rise to an enigmatic acute or subacute sinusitis. Buccal abscesses from upper molar teeth produce very little swelling of the face if they discharge below the attachment of the buccinator. If the pus discharges into the soft tissues above the attachment of the buccinator to reach the buccal space, a moderate swelling of the affected side of the cheek occurs. Although this type of abscess can point on the face below the zygomatic bone, it usually accumulates eventually in the buccal sulcus, and therefore drainage is carried out through an intraoral incision.

Subperiosteal Abscess in the Palate

The mucoperiosteum which covers the palate is made up of mucosal and periosteal layers which are bound together so strongly that they cannot be separated. It is attached to the periodontal membranes of the surrounding teeth and to the median suture line. The periosteum is attached to the underlying bone by Sharpey's fibres and small blood vessels and their attachment produces a roughness of the bone surface best seen on a dried skull. No actual space exists between the mucoperiosteum and the underlying bone, but the periosteum between the gingival margin and the midline can be stripped up comparatively easily during surgery and also by pus when it accumulates between the bone and the periosteum.

Although the attachment to the necks of the teeth is relatively strong, in the case of long standing infection the pus may eventually lyse the connective tissue and seep through the gingival crevice alongside a tooth. Pus rarely tracks across the centre of the palate and usually remains confined to the side of the focus of infection because of the attachment to the median suture. As the apex of the lateral incisor is often closer to the palatal bony surface, this tooth is the most common source of a palatal abscess followed by a periodontal abscess from a palatal pocket or an apical abscess from the palatal root of a multirooted tooth.

The many reasons for necrosis of the lateral incisor pulp include: caries, unlined cavities, blows and fractures, and infection through a developmental cingulum invagination. Abscesses originating from this tooth may migrate and point as far posteriorly as the soft palate, so that whenever the source of a palatal abscess is in doubt the lateral incisor must be the prime suspect and it should be tested for vitality.

Signs and Symptoms

Pus beneath the palatal mucosa produces a circumscribed fluctuant swelling which is usually confined to one side of the palate. The swelling may sometimes show little obvious distension of the tissues, but nevertheless, extends for a considerable distance beneath the thick mucoperiosteum. There may be little tendency for the abscess to discharge

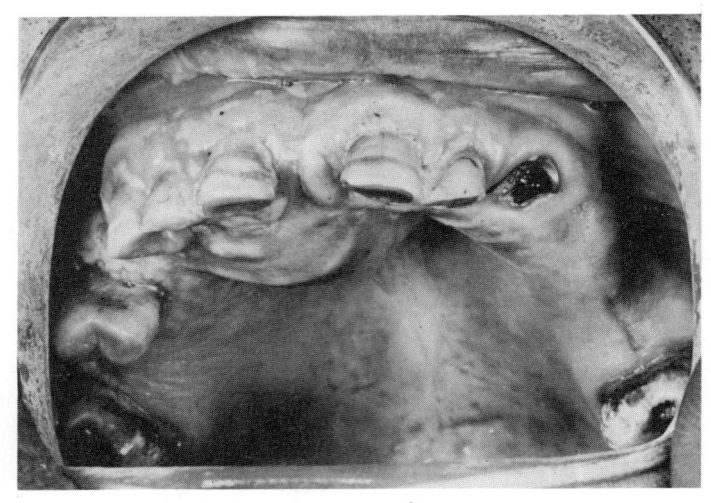

Fig. 6.19. A palatal abscess arising from $\underline{2|}$ which is carious distopalatally.

spontaneously, although pus may well up at the sides of adjacent teeth if it has been neglected for a period of time (*Fig.* 6.19).

Differential Diagnosis
Some painful, tender, fluctuant, palatal swellings are due to infected dental cysts and this diagnosis should be suspected if the swelling transgresses the midline. Otherwise the diagnosis of palatal abscess should present no difficulty, but occasionally a large, fluctuant mucous extravasation cyst or cystic pleomorphic adenoma or muco-epidermoid carcinoma may cause confusion, especially if it is in close relation to an obviously infected tooth or root. Some carcinomas from the maxillary sinus or malignant lymphomas also present as fluctuant palatal swellings. A gumma of the palate now rarely seen could also cause confusion in diagnosis.

Treatment
Incision of a palatal abscess should be carried out in an anteroposterior direction to avoid dividing the greater palatine vessels. The responsible tooth must be treated at the same time. To prevent the accumulation of a haematoma in the abscess cavity, which may progress to a further abscess, the lateral edge of the incision should be gripped with the tips of mosquito artery forceps. A knife blade is run round the tip, removing a small piece from the mucosa, and a short length of ribbon gauze drain is tucked loosely into the cavity and sutured to one edge of the wound for 24 hours. When the drain is removed there will be a cavity between the mucoperiosteum and the bone but the tongue will soon press the mucosa back into place.

PYOGENIC INFECTIONS OF THE SOFT TISSUES

Periapical Abscesses in Relation to the Maxillary Sinus

The apices of the roots of many of the upper teeth are in a close relationship to the floor of the maxillary sinus. The particular ones which are related vary from patient to patient depending upon the size of the maxillary sinus and upon the length of the roots. Ones most frequently related are the apices of the 2nd and 1st molars followed by the 3rd molar, 2nd and 1st premolars and canine. Despite this, pus from an abscess of one of these teeth usually discharges onto the alveolar surface, although radiographs often show mucosal thickening in the overlying antrum. If pus does enter the antrum the features of an acute sinusitis will follow with facial pain especially on bending, engorgement of the nasal mucosa with obstruction and a nasal discharge.

Beware of diagnosing an acute pulpitis in a tooth made periostitic due to an overlying acute sinusitis. An infected pulpless tooth or a minute oroantral fistula following an extraction may give rise to a chronic sinusitis with recurrent subacute episodes which may defy diagnosis. Advanced periodontal disease may also result in chronic maxillary sinusitis, with mucosal thickening and sclerosis of the bony floor.

Radiology

The earliest change is thickening of overlying antral mucosa or polyps seen on a periapical, rotational tomographic or lateral occlusal film. An empyema produces an opaque sinus with a fluid level best seen in an occipitomental radiograph, but the opacity may be seen also in a standard occlusal radiograph.

It is worth noting that a rotational tomographic film will only give a vertical 'cut' of the antrum and is therefore unreliable in providing information about the state of those parts which lie laterally to the cut.

Treatment

Some discharge of pus will have taken place via the nose and in most cases extraction of the infected tooth will lead to drainage of the remainder which has accumulated below the level of the osteum. Provided that the defect in the antral floor is small and the infection controlled with antibiotics, the socket should heal normally and seal the fistulous orifice. Even a larger fistula will often close spontaneously with antibiotics, frequent irrigation with warm saline and a protective acrylic plate which prevents food debris entering the sinus. If this is not successful a formal antrostomy through a Caldwell–Luc approach with removal of polyps, and intranasal antrostomy and closure of the fistula with a flap will be required.

The Infratemporal Fossa

Surgical Anatomy

The infratemporal fossa space forms the upper extremity of the pterygo-

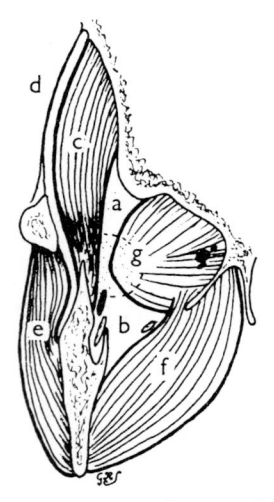

Fig. 6.20. Diagram of the pterygomandibular and infratemporal spaces in coronal section. *a,* Intratemporal space. *b,* Pterygomandibular space. *c,* Temporalis muscle. *d,* Temporal fascia. *e,* Masseter muscle. *f,* Medial pterygoid muscle. *g,* Lateral pterygoid muscle (dotted outline); position of the lateral pterygoid tendon.

mandibular space. It is bounded laterally by the ramus of the mandible, the temporalis muscle and its tendon, medially by the lateral pterygoid plate and superiorly by the infratemporal surface of the greater wing of sphenoid. It contains the origins of the medial and lateral pterygoid muscles and the lower head of the lateral pterygoid can be said to mark the border between the pterygomandibular and infratemporal spaces. It is traversed by the maxillary artery and contains the pterygoid plexus of veins. Pus can extend upwards under the origin of the temporalis muscle from the lower part of the infratemporal fossa, and also around to the lateral side of the muscle, under the temporal fascia.

It will be seen that this space is actually continuous in its anterior part with the upper part of the pterygomandibular space but is separated from it by the lateral pterygoid muscle posteriorly. Infection usually reaches the infratemporal space from the upper molars while the pterygomandibular space is more often affected by infection from the lower jaw (*Fig.* 6.20).

Clinical Features
Subacute infections due to contaminated needles may follow injections in the tuberosity area and produce relatively slight physical signs apart from trismus which must be distinguished from limitation of opening due to a temporomandibular joint disturbance.

PYOGENIC INFECTIONS OF THE SOFT TISSUES

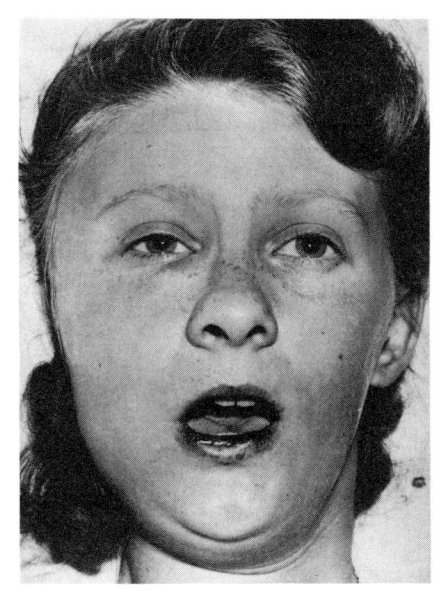

Fig. 6.21. Patient with a severe infratemporal, pterygoid and buccal space infection which followed an injection in the upper right molar region. There was anaesthesia of the tongue on the right, but no swelling of the tongue and inability either to open or close the mouth. The right temporal muscle is bulged to an extent that the position of the zygomatic bone is marked by a depression. Temperature was 104 °F with drying and cracking of the lips.

Acute infratemporal fossa infections tend to follow infections of upper 3rd molars, particularly those which are partially erupted, and occasionally from local anaesthetic injections with contaminated needles. The infection spreads upwards deep to and lateral to the temporalis muscle. Limitation of opening is marked, as with a pterygomandibular space infection, but there will be bulging of the temporalis muscle. This may not be obvious as the muscle and overlying fascia contain it, but the swelling may be detected as a filling out of the hollow behind the zygomatic process of the frontal bone (*Fig.* 6.21).

Pus may also spread upwards beneath the origin of the temporalis muscle itself almost to the lower temporal line to form a subtemporalis abscess. The situation is similar to that found with a submasseteric abscess, and in preantibiotic times, if drainage was delayed the temporalis muscle and surface of the skull would be found to be necrotic. In acute infections the patient is very ill and has a high temperature.

Infections of the infratemporal fossa are always serious owing to the presence of the pterygoid plexus of veins. Emissary veins connect these with the cavernous sinus through the sphenoidal emissary foramen (of Vesalius), the foramen lacerum, foramen spinosum and the foramen ovale. Infection from the pterygoid plexus can therefore spread to the cavernous sinus. It can also spread directly through the other foramina in the infratemporal fossa into the middle cranial fossa. Thus on rare occasions headache, irritability, photophobia, vomiting and drowsiness will indicate intracranial infection.

Treatment
Antibiotics must be given promptly. Benzylpencillin 600 mg, 8-hourly, together with metronidazole 500 mg, 8-hourly, is a suitable intravenous regime which can be followed by phenoxymethyl penicillin 500 mg, 6-hourly, and metronidazole 400 mg, 12-hourly, by mouth. Drainage of the infratemporal fossa can be effected through an incision buccal to the upper 3rd molar following the medial surface of the coronoid and temporalis upwards and backwards with closed sinus forceps. A soft drain must be sutured in. In severe cases drainage through an incision at the upper and posterior edge of the temporalis within the hairline may be necessary also. The sinus forceps are passed downwards, forwards and medially to the pus. Again a soft drain is inserted.

Course
Prolonged limitation of opening may follow these infections. In most cases the range of movement increases in time with the aid of active exercise. If jaw exercises and manipulation do not seem to increase the opening, temporalis myotomy or excision of the coronoid process may improve matters.

Cavernous Sinus Thrombophlebitis
This serious condition becomes recognizable by the appearance of marked oedema and congestion of the eyelids, and injection and oedema of the conjunctiva due to impaired venous return. This may develop into a pulsating exophthalmos where the carotid pulse is transmitted through the retrobulbar oedema. At this stage ophthalmoplegia is detectable and if the retina can be visualized, papilloedema with multiple retinal haemorrhages will be seen. Untreated the thrombophlebitis will spread to the opposite side giving rise to bilateral signs.

Cavernous sinus thrombophlebitis will require energetic antibiotic therapy and heparinization to prevent extension of the thrombosis; however, a neurosurgical consultation is essential as a matter of great urgency.

PYOGENIC INFECTIONS OF THE SOFT TISSUES

THE USE OF HEAT IN THE TREATMENT OF SOFT-TISSUE ABSCESSES

Poultices were applied to extensive infections of the soft tissues in pre-antibiotic days in order to induce local vasodilatation by means of their heat and the rubifacient substances which they contained. It was hoped that the increased blood supply would help the tissues overcome the infection. In the case of suppurative infections they appeared to hasten suppuration and encourage the pus to point under the poultice where it could be readily drained.

Poultices probably increase the spread of a cellulitis. Furthermore, if poultices are applied after pus has formed beneath the deep fascia, the increased oedema and exudate which they induce could worsen the patient's condition. Incisions for drainage are often delayed by this practice. Consequently the application of heat externally to infections of the floor of the mouth and neck has come to be regarded as a bad measure, and with the establishment of effective antibiotic treatment and early and efficient drainage has virtually disappeared. Hot salt water mouth baths still provide comfort and to a degree improve oral hygiene but, like poultices, probably have only a small therapeutic effect. If a cellulitis does not resolve rapidly with antibiotic treatment, but the disappearance of constitutional signs and symptoms suggests that the causative organisms are sensitive, then ensure that there is no undrained pus somewhere which has been overlooked.

THE SURGICAL DRAINAGE OF ABSCESSES

Successful surgical drainage of an abscess depends upon a knowledge of the applied anatomy of the part and therefore an understanding of the probable location of the accumulation of pus in the tissues, together with good surgical judgement concerning the proper time to instigate drainage. It is most important to recognize when pus has formed and to drain it at once. If the incision is carried out too early little or no pus is found, but this is no longer considered harmful to the patient. On the other hand, if incision is delayed until an abscess from a deep space presents as a fluctuant swelling then the pus may invade hitherto uninfected tissue spaces, or discharge spontaneously and produce a disfiguring external scar. Unfortunately the value of antibiotics may encourage surgeons to delay unnecessarily incision and drainage.

Immediate incision and drainage are required:

1. Where there are signs of pus beneath the deep fascia:
    a. A localized dusky redness appearing in the general redness of the firm swelling;
    b. A localized area of tenderness over the centre of the swelling;
    c. Pitting oedema in the middle of a previously firm swelling;

d. A sharp rise in the temperature, particularly if the patient is having antibiotics.

2. Where the involved compartment is inaccessible, such as the pterygomandibular and lateral pharyngeal spaces, and in the case of submasseteric and infratemporal fossa infections where it may be impossible to elicit the classic signs of suppuration. If pus is left in these situations tissue necrosis may supervene. Therefore a lack of local improvement with adequate doses of antibiotics, a recurrence of pyrexia or a sudden increase in temperature and severe limitation of opening are some of the indications for drainage of these sites.

3. With Ludwig's angina and other serious and rapidly evolving infections of the floor of the mouth and upper neck, early incision and drainage of the relevant tissue compartments is essential. However, early extraction of causative teeth and the use of metronidazole to eliminate anaerobes including bacteroides has greatly reduced the incidence of these cases.

Patients under treatment for acute inflammatory soft-tissue swellings should be seen daily. In a proportion of cases the infection will be halted and the swelling will subside as a result of the administration of antibiotics and the extraction of the causative tooth. In others the signs of suppuration or the need for incision as discussed above will become apparent. Patients with infections causing substantial swelling of the floor of the mouth or side of the pharynx need admission to hospital so that early incision and drainage can be instituted and more frequent observation of their progress made possible. Patients with dangerous or rapidly progressive infections should be under constance surveillance, preferably in an intensive care unit, for the onset of respiratory difficulty and impeding obstruction can take place with surprising rapidity.

With prolonged antibiotic treatment some modest-sized abscesses may be virtually sterilized, but this does not lead to a satisfactory outcome. At best the pus is walled off to produce a pultaceous mass, but an accumulation which can still be drained. Later invading macrophages and granulation tissue will convert the whole into a tumour-like mass called an 'antibioticoma'. Aspiration of pus with a wide bore needle and syringe is one way to obtain a specimen from which obligate anaerobic organisms may be cultured. Small superficial abscesses may be drained in this way and of course this is easy to carry out with an abscess in the buccal sulcus. However, without free continuous drainage, as achieved by incision, the abscess may refill within 24–48 hours. This is certain to happen if the tooth causing the infection has not been effectively dealt with. Where an abscess points beneath the skin as a red shiny swelling in a conspicuous position aspiration may be tried as a means of avoiding the scar of an incision, but such an abscess often heals with puckering and subcutaneous scarring so that the aesthetic benefit is marginal. Treatment of any scar should be delayed for at least 6 months because a slow improvement will occur.

PYOGENIC INFECTIONS OF THE SOFT TISSUES

Prompt drainage when pus forms avoids the temptation to prolong antibiotic treatment perhaps with exotic and potentially toxic drugs and reduces the opportunities for the emergence of resistant strains.

Success in the treatment of a cellulitis becomes apparent with a fall in the patient's temperature, a reduction in malaise and toxaemia, the relief of pain and a decrease in the swelling. The first sign of such a decrease is often the appearance of fine wrinkles in the overlying skin where previously it was tense, red and shiny.

Technique of Incision and Drainage

Incisions for the drainage of pus vary according to the location and may be made in either the skin of the neck or face or in the mucosa of the mouth. Abscesses in the sulcus are just under the surface with no structures of importance in between and the incision is made with a scalpel straight through into the abscess cavity.

In general incisions are placed over the point of maximum fluctuation, or over the most direct route to the pus, so that dependent drainage is achieved. However, this is not always essential as the tissues will contract around an abscess and push the pus out even if the opening is at the top. Indeed, it is common experience that pus will even well up the root canals of the lower incisors when they are opened to drain a periapical abscess. Since there are no structures of consequence in the subcutaneous tissues the incision may be made bodly through the skin and into the subcutaneous tissues.

The siting of the incision is guided by the direction of Langer's lines and the skin creases. Once this incision has been made the scalpel is discarded because if pus has not been found at this depth further deepening of the wound is achieved with sinus or artery forceps to avoid damage to important underlying structures. Closed forceps are pushed through the deep facia and advanced to the pus. In a man the investing layer of cervical fascia can be quite tough and a controlled effort may be required to penetrate it.

Pus will discharge up the sides of the forceps as soon as the abscess cavity is entered, whereupon the forceps are opened in a direction parallel to adjacent important structures. The hinges of the sinus forceps must be external to the wound or the path through the tissues will not be stretched and enlarged by the movement of the forceps blades. Where the patient is very thin, it must be remembered that the subcutaneous tissue will contain little fat, and even with oedema, therefore, the distance to the platysma will be small. In such subjects particular care must be taken to incise no deeper than the subcutaneous fat to avoid inadvertent damage to the mandibular branch of the facial nerve.

Some pus should be aspirated into a syringe through a wide bore needle for culture and sensitivity tests before the incision is made. Pus on a swab may be used to make a smear on a microscope slide but is of limited use otherwise because the predominant organisms are likely to be anaerobic. The specimen is taken promptly to the laboratory. Where specimens have to be sent a distance to the laboratory or cannot be cultured immediately then the microbiologist will provide bottles of transport medium. All postal regulations must be observed.

After a large abscess cavity has been adequately opened, the surgeon should insert a gloved finger into the space and explore its extent. This confirms that the whole abscess cavity has been drained and that no additional loculi of pus remain. Gentle probing with the finger will break down the walls of any loculi and allow the pus enclosed within them to be evacuated.

A soft 'Yeats' or corrugated drain is then inserted using the sinus forceps to carry the end into the depths of the cavity and the part external to the wound is sutured to one edge of the incision. A sterile safety pin has been traditionally used to prevent the drain being lost in the wound but this is unlikely in the facial region. The drain is left until little pus accumulates in a dressing left for 24 hours. Long drains should be shortened for a further 24 hours before final removal. Adhesive wound closure strips may be used to approximate the skin edges at this stage to improve the appearance of the final scar.

With intraoral abscesses, the operation may be performed in miniature and mosquito artery forceps used instead of sinus forceps. In some situations in the mouth medicated ribbon gauze soaked in Whitehead's varnish may be adequate as a drain and more comfortable than a soft plastic one. All intraoral drains must be anchored with a stitch to prevent them being swallowed or aspirated.

Occasionally where a large cavity exists it may be better to suture a soft plastic tube or quill into the dead space and irrigate it 4-hourly with saline solution until the effluent becomes clear. Drainage may continue in between irrigations into a small collecting bag sealed to the skin surrounding the incision wound. Usually within 3–4 days it is possible to remove the tube and replace it with half inch ribbon gauze again soaked with saline solution, but changed four times daily until the wound closes. This classic technique is particularly important when resistant microbes have been reported and should be used in conjunction with a simple antibiotic regime such as metronidazole.

SINUS FORMATION

The majority of abscesses will burst spontaneously if they are neglected for a sufficient period of time. However, this is an undesirable occurrence especially when the abscess discharges through the skin, for not only may the sinus appear in a location unfavourable for drainage, but the resulting scar is always puckered, thickened, and depressed and more obvious than in

PYOGENIC INFECTIONS OF THE SOFT TISSUES

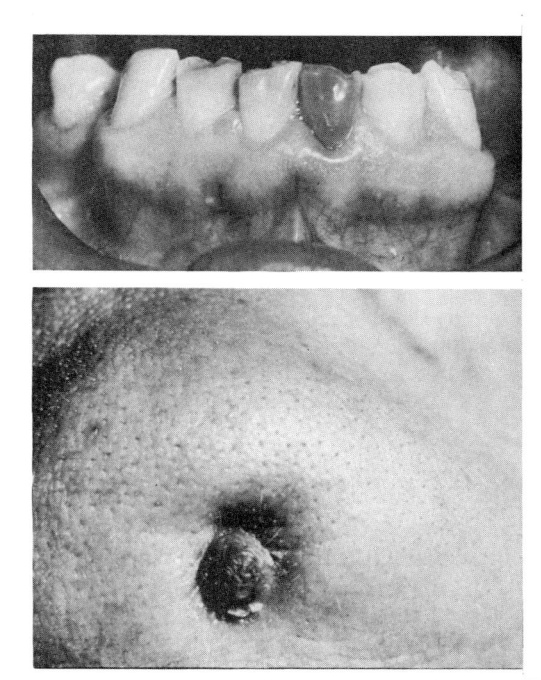

Fig. 6.22. A submental sinus resulting from a chronic abscess on 1̅|. The anterior teeth have been fractured as a result of a fall and 1| is dark brown in colour and pulpless.

cases where elective surgical incison and drainage has been carried out. Furthermore, the sinus will become chronic unless the original source of infection is removed and it will be subject to exacerbations and remissions with attempts at healing during the quiescent phase. When these sinuses are sited on the face or neck their appearance is quite characteristic and a focus of infection such as a buried tooth or root must be sought and eliminated. (*Fig.* 6.22.) Not infrequently a lack of understanding of dental pathology may lead to repeated excision of facial sinuses because of persistent infection.

The clinical appearance of sinuses on the face varies according to the phase of the infection. During an active phase they are open and discharging small quantities of pus, but during a quiescent phase they heal over. Occasionally, it is possible to insert a silver probe along the tract as far as the bone. In an active phase the tissue immediately surrounding the sinus exhibits signs of inflammation and may be tender, but after pus has been drained the sinus tends to heal over until another exacerbation of infection causes it to burst open again. If the buccal sulcus between the sinus and the jaw is palpated a firm, fibrous cord representing the sinus track may be felt. The position of its attachment to the jaw may indicate the site from which the pus is draining.

It is essential to consider chronic actinomycosis where a sinus persists in the absence of intra-alveolar disease. Usually but not invariably actinomyces may be cultured from the pus which should also be examined by a direct Gram-stained smear. In such cases long-term penicillin or tetracycline therapy is required given continuously, for example, for 4–6 weeks.

Very occasionally if the abscess drains into the mouth as well as on to the skin surface a fistula will form from the mouth to the outside of the face through which saliva escapes. However, persistent inflammation with salivary fistula should suggest the possibility of an unrecognized malignant neoplasm.

Sinus Excision

An elliptical incision is made round the external orifice so that on closure the scar lies in Langer's lines without puckered ends. Using McIndoe's scissors the tract is followed to its source, usually on the bony surface of the mandible. Some deep soluble catgut or polyglycolate sutures are inserted to eliminate the dead space and the skin wound is closed with careful eversion of the edges using interrupted 4/0 proline or other monofilament sutures. If there is a through and through wound into the buccal sulcus, the oral defect is closed with black silk sutures at the conclusion of the operation.

SUMMARY OF THE MANAGEMENT OF PATIENTS WITH SPREADING INFECTIONS

1. *An acute abscess with collateral oedema:*
    a. Extraction of the tooth alone is normally adequate treatment.
    b. If root-canal therapy is to be undertaken, open the pulp chamber to drain the abscess through the root canal and administer antibiotics.
    c. Establish local antibiotic or antiseptic treatment in the root canal as soon as possible and then seal the opening into the pulp chamber.
2. *Cellulitis or tissue space abscess:* Administer antibiotics to help eliminate local infection and prevent its spread elsewhere. Extract the tooth of origin or establish effective root-canal treatment but only if this is reasonable. Incise and drain where there is:
    a. Fluctuation as in the case of a local abscess;
    b. When there is localized pitting oedema with tenderness;
    c. When localized dusky redness and a sharp rise in temperature suggests a tissue space is involved.

PYOGENIC INFECTIONS OF THE SOFT TISSUES

SUGGESTED READING

Birn H. (1972) Spread of dental infections. *Dent. Pract.* **22**, 347–356.

Bosley A. R. J., Murphy J. F. and Dodge J. A. (1981) Septicemic Haemophilus Influenzae and facial cellulitis in infants. *Br. Med. J.* **282**, 22.

Frankl Z. (1949) The sub-mandibular space and parapharyngeal spaces: their topography and importance in oral surgery. *Oral Surg.* **2**, 1131–1139; 1270–1285.

Last R. J. (1984) *Anatomy: Regional and Applied,* 7th ed. London: Churchill.

Lewis, M. A. D., McFarlane, T. W., and McGowan, D. A. (1990) A microbiological and clinical review of the acute dento-alveolar abscess. *Br. J. Oral Maxillofac. Surg.* **28**, 359–366.

McDougall J. D. B. (1955) The attachments of the masseter muscle. *Br. Dent. J.* **98**, 193–199.

Von Ludwig W. (1837) Über eine hene Art von Halsentzundung. *Württemb. KorrespBl.* 6, Nr. 4, Schmidts. Jahr 15, 925.

CHAPTER 7

INFLAMMATORY DISEASES OF BONE

The bone of the jaw is remarkably resistant to infection. This is illustrated by the common acute alveolar abscess, where infected exudate induces resorption of the overlying cortex and penetrates the periosteum to discharge into the mouth or facial tissues without spreading laterally through the bone itself. Persistent or spreading infective inflammation of bone appears to require an element of ischaemia or infarction in addition to bacterial infection.

Pathological resorption is mediated by inflammatory agents such as the prostaglandins PGE2 and PGI2, the lymphokine osteoclast activating factor (OAF) and possibly monocyte cell factors (MCF), all of which activate directly or indirectly the osteoclast. One of the well recognized features of bone destruction is the associated local bone regeneration which is thought to be stimulated by a protein breakdown product of bone matrix called human skeletal growth factor (HSFG). This coupled effect of bone formation in association with bone destruction is an essential feature of most bone pathology and can be seen for instance in the sclerotic areas around the apices of chronically inflamed, pulpless teeth or the involucrum of osteomyelitis.

LOCALIZED OSTEITIS

Osteitis is a term used to describe a localized small scale infection of bone. The distinction between an osteitis and a localized, low-grade osteomyelitis is arbitrary. Periapical and periodontal abscesses are considered under soft tissue infections (Chapter 6).

ACUTE ALVEOLAR OSTEITIS

Acute alveolar osteitis, 'dry socket', alveolitis sicca dolorosa, or fibrinolytic alveolitis is a well recognized painful complication of dental extractions in which the blood clot disintegrates exposing an infected necrotic socket wall. This is characteristically associated with a fetid odour. The average incidence appears to be 3 per cent of all extractions and may be as high as 22 per cent of 3rd molar extractions under local analgesia, but these figures will vary with the skill of the surgeon and the prophylactic measures used. There might be a slightly greater incidence in females than males and the peak age range is 20–40 years. Few cases are seen in children and the elderly. Mandibular teeth appear to be three times more prone than maxillary teeth.

The aetiological factors responsible for acute alveolar osteitis may be divided into vascular and infective.

Several possible reasons for the loss of the clot from the socket are advanced. A popular concept is that the clot is washed out of the socket by the patient. This idea is not tenable since within a short time of the extraction the clot adheres quite firmly to the socket wall. Patients are usually advised not to rinse out the mouth during the first 24 hours after the extraction, not because of the risk of dislodging the entire clot from the socket. but because they might start the socket bleeding again. If the clot were to be forcibly removed from the socket at this time, the result would be further haemorrhage, not an empty socket.

Infection and fibrinolysis of the clot is another common suggestion. A variety of organisms can be cultured from dry sockets including fusiform bacilli, spirochaetes, diplococci and streptococci. Support for the infective cause of clot destruction comes from the degree to which antibiotic prophylaxis and careful preoperative toilet of the tooth and oral cavity can reduce its incidence. For instance 200 mg metronidazole, 8-hourly, for 3 days can produce a significant protection against dry socket, suggesting that anaerobes may play an important role.

However, infection may not be the only cause of clot lysis because alveolar osteitis may occur irrespective of the care and skill of the operator or of the trouble taken to prevent infection of the extraction wound. It has been suggested that extraction trauma as well as subsequent infection of the socket activates plasminogen to plasmin which causes lysis of the fibrin clot. Investigations have demonstrated the presence of both tissue activators and plasmin in the alveolar bone adjacent to affected sockets, and stable tissue activators are present in the connective tissue type of marrow characteristic of the jaws in the age group 20–40. However, an inhibitor of fibrinolysis, tranexamic acid, failed to prevent the occurrence of alveolar osteitis. This was considered to be due to inadequate local concentration of the drug in the alveolar bone.

Predisposing Factors

A number of conditions may predispose to acute alveolar osteitis. The incidence of alveolar osteitis after extractions for which a local anaesthetic with a vasoconstrictor has been used appears to be greater than after a general anaesthetic, although not all investigators have found this to be so, particularly in relation to the removal of 3rd molars. In theory, vasoconstrictors may temporarily inhibit the vascular component of the inflammatory reaction and tend to favour the establishment of a local infection. Similarly, when excessive vasoconstriction is used the socket may be open to contamination by saliva for some time before bleeding occurs.

Excess trauma during a forceps extraction is associated with an increased tendency to dry socket. This may result from the crushing and devitalization of the socket wall and thrombosis of the underlying vascular plexus. Such trauma would also increase the release locally of plasminogen activators. Similarly conditions with sclerotic and relatively avascular bone are also prone to socket infection. In some otherwise normal jaws a socket may be related to a localized mass of sclerosed bone. Sclerotic masses may involve much of the alveolar process in long established Paget's disease and the entire jaw may exhibit increased density in osteopetrosis and some other rare skeletal diseases. In Paget's disease hypercementosis of the teeth further increases the difficulty of extractions and the resultant crushing of the adjacent bone. Incidently, it is only the sclerotic masses in Paget's disease which are less vascular than normal. The rest of the abnormal bone is markedly more vascular. In jaws which have received a therapeutic dose of irradiation the blood supply is reduced due to obliterative endarteritis. Furthermore, where there are additional local or systemic factors the possibility of extension to an osteomyelitis is a possible complication. Pre-existing infection in the form of acute or chronic periapical and periodontal disease seems to be of little importance, but the extraction of teeth during an acute ulcerative gingivitis is an invitation to trouble.

Other factors which might predispose to a dry socket are those which influence vascular function, such as the oral contraceptive pill and smoking. A significant higher incidence of dry socket occurs in smokers, especially those who smoke after the extraction.

Clinical Features

The patient usually presents within 2–4 days of the extraction complaining of a boring, persistent, dull pain which is well localized to the socket, but may radiate to the ear or other parts of the face. In some cases the pain is exceptionally severe. This is attributed to the release of kinins as a result of the action of plasmin activators on kininogen present in the alveolar process.

The gingival margin of the socket is usually swollen and dusky red. The socket itself is either devoid of clot, or contains a brown, friable, sometimes foamy clot which is easily washed out. Food debris may have accumulated in the socket which, with the disintegrating clot, produces a foul taste and smell. If this material is washed away the bone of the socket wall is seen to be bare and it may be extremely sensitive if touched. If the gingival margin about the socket has already contracted it can be difficult to examine the socket and appreciate that it does not contain a normal clot. The regional lymph nodes may be tender and can be enlarged. There is rarely a pyrexia.

The critical time for development of a 'dry socket' is during the first four days after an extraction because at about the third day granulation tissue starts to invade the clot. From this time therefore loss of the clot will no longer expose bare bone. Often there is no frank sequestration of bone, but from time to time exuberant granulations form and small pieces of the socket wall or parts of the inter-radicular septum separate and are discharged with small amounts of pus. Occasionally a complete ring, or even a 'thimble' of socket wall is sequestrated. After a period of some 7–14 days granulation tissue lines the socket and gradually fills it up.

Radiographs will show the outline of the socket and should be taken to confirm the absence of a retained root, foreign body or a loose, fractured fragment of septal or alveolar bone.

Preventive Measures

1. Preoperatively, scale and clean the teeth and improve oral hygiene as far as is practical including the use of chlorhexidine gluconate mouthwash, if possible, starting several days before the extractions.

2. Execute the extraction carefully with minimal manipulation of the tooth.

3. Where a dry socket may be anticipated, such as following the extraction of a lower 3rd molar, give a 5 day course of metronidazole 400 mg b.d. postoperatively. Tetracycline 250 mg taken 6-hourly for a similar period is also effective.

Various cones containing sulphonamides, antifibrinolytic agents such as tranexamic acid (AMCA) or the propyl ester of parahydroxybenzoic acid (PEPH) have been tried prophylactically but there is no evidence that they are better than general measures which leave the socket undisturbed to heal spontaneously.

Treatment

Because the patient may be suffering severe pain sympathetic and prompt treatment is required. All disintegrating clot and food debris should be irrigated away with warm saline and a suitable dressing should be inserted in the socket. Such a dressing may contain a topical local anaesthetic to relieve pain and a non-irritant antiseptic to inhibit the growth of bacteria and fungi. It should also protect the bone from the irritation of food debris accumulating in the socket. Finally, it should dissolve slowly or extrude as healing progresses, so that it is neither incorporated in the granulation tissue nor prevents it filling the socket.

A suitable paste is composed of the water-soluble waxes; polyethylene glycol, 4000–5·10 g, polyethylene glycol, 1500–5·10 g, incorporating lignocaine hydrochloride, 2·0 g, domiphen bromide (Bradosol), 0·5 g, distilled water, 20 ml. The material is warmed slightly to soften it so as to permit it to be inserted painlessly. Ribbon gauze moistened with Whitehead's varnish is a useful alternative.

Packs containing eugenol or other essential oils, zinc oxide and cotton wool relieve pain but the eugenol devitalizes more bone and healing is delayed. Dry sockets which have persisted for weeks, lined with yellow-brown bone and which show no signs of healing have usually been dressed liberally with eugenol containing dressing.

The use of inert hydrophilic dextron polymer beads, Dextranomer (Pharmacia (GB) Ltd), appears both to relieve pain and encourage rapid healing but the socket has to be dressed daily with the fine beads alone or in glycerine and then sealed with Orobase gel. The preparation probably absorbs exudate and toxins, relieving pain and inflammation and does not interfere with healing.

Irrigation and dressing of the socket should be repeated as often as is necessary to control pain. In severe cases this may mean daily for several days. In addition for severe cases an analgesic sufficient to control pain and night sedation are essential and metronidazole 400 mg b.d. should be prescribed for 5 days.

OSTEOMYELITIS

This condition is now rare in Western European countries indicating not only the value of antibiotics and early treatment but the importance of predisposing factors such as poor nutrition, chronic debilitating illnesses and gross untreated dental disease. Most cases seen are in alcoholics with malnutrition, drug addicts, diabetics and patients with impaired immunity due to the need to take steroids or cytotoxic drugs. Special problems such as follow the use of therapeutic irradiation and in Paget's disease will be discussed separately.

For a true osteomyelitis to occur the infected exudate must spread throughout the cancellous spaces of the bone producing thrombosis of the nutrient vessels with ischaemia, infarction and sequestrum formation.

Until old age the main blood supply to the mandible is the central inferior dental artery with its centrifugal distribution anastomosing with the peripheral periosteal vessels which enter through Volkmann's canals. Parts of the ramus and coronoid process are supplied by additional small nutrient arteries but are dependent to a substantial extent upon small vessels entering the cortex from muscle attachments. In elderly subjects the mandibular arteries may be occluded. When the central vessel is divided, or thrombosed through the spread of bacteria and their toxins, ischaemia then infarction will take place. This is a rare problem in the maxilla which has predominantly cancellous alveolar bone with a thin cortex and a rich plexiform blood supply.

Experimentally, sequestrum formation in rabbits' tibias by *Staphylococcus aureus* has been prevented by treatment with the non-steroidal anti-inflammatory analgesic indomethacin which inhibits prostanoid (prostaglandin-like substances) formation. This was probably due to the inhibition of thomboxanes normally synthesized and released by the infection, and which are potent platelet aggregation factors and therefore could be responsible for the thrombosis and infarction.

INFLAMMATORY DISEASES OF BONE

Osteomyelitis of Infancy

This condition which occurs sporadically affects infants only a few weeks old and the maxilla almost exclusively, hence the alternative term, maxillitis of infancy. The causal organism is the *S. aureus* which is thought to be introduced from an infected nipple or incipient breast abscess or contaminated feeding bottles. Access may be through a break in the mucosa, perhaps over the eminence caused by the maxillary first deciduous molar tooth germ. However, the conjunctiva and lacrimal sac or the nose may be alternative primary infective sites.

Clinical Features

The condition shows considerable variation in severity. There is fever, anorexia and a swelling or redness below the inner cathus of the eye in the lacrimal region which leads to marked oedema of the eyelids on the affected side. Later a frank orbital cellulitis may supervene. A sinus may also open below the inner canthus of the eye. The alveolar process and palate in the first deciduous molar region often become swollen and pus discharges intraorally through one or more sinuses. Eventually, if untreated, sequestra including tooth buds may be discharged after two or three months.

The oral manifestations help to distinguish the early condition from dacryocystitis neonatorum, orbital cellulitis, and ophthalmia neonatorum. Acute cellulitis of the face without bone involvement produces a grossly swollen dusky red cheek usually in older infants of between 6 months and 1 year of age. A similar presentation is also possible with infantile cortical hyperostosis, but again in older infants.

Treatment is by energetic antibiotic therapy with flucloxacillin and amoxycillin and surgical drainage. Removal of sequestra should only be undertaken when they have completely separated, since overenthusiastic intervention will result in unnecessary loss of teeth and considerable deformity in later life. Hypoplasia of the deciduous teeth which are not sequestrated is usual and at least some degree of underdevelopment of the affected side of the maxilla must be expected. Varying degrees of disturbance to the adult dentition will occur.

Flucloxacillin 125 mg and amoxycillin 125 mg may be given by nasogastric tube 6-hourly. Erythromycin stearate or lactobionate may be given as an alternative. A swab should be taken to confirm the bacteriological diagnosis. Adequate fluid intake is important and the child should be barrier nursed to prevent to spread of the staphylococcal infection to other patients.

Other Childhood Bone Infection

Infection of the middle ear will penetrate its thin bony floor and enter the temporomandibular joint space where it is usually confined. Destruction of the meniscus and fibrocartilage surface of the condyle takes place leading to an irregular proliferative osteitis of the condylar head and ankylosis. The antibiotic therapy is as already described.

Osteomyelitis of both mandible and maxilla in children can arise following cancrum oris. This necrotizing infection of the facial tissues appears to be confined to tropical countries where the predisposing factors are malnutrition or a virus infection such as measles and malaria.

The principal infective agents are bacteroides especially melaninogenicus associated with *Borrelia vincentii* and anaerobic Gram-negative fusiform bacilli, and the treatment therefore is metronidazole. The additional use of penicillin or erythromycin for the aerobic organisms will be determined by culture where possible.

ACUTE PYOGENIC OSTEOMYELITIS OF THE MANDIBLE

Aetiology

The most common cause of pyogenic osteomyelitis of the mandible is odontogenic infection and the organism is primarily *S. aureus*. Once sinuses are formed a mixed infection is usually found. Osteomyelitis can also occur by direct extension from a source of infection other than the teeth, such as middle ear disease or a boil on the chin. More rarely the jaw infection is due to haematogenous spread from a distant focus and this tends to occur in children.

As stated previously, delay in surgical and antibiotic treatment for a preexisting infection together with some underlying predisposing factor are important in the aetiology.

Clinical Features

Following a periapical abscess with or without surgical intervention the patient experiences a severe, deep seated pain over the affected part, where an indurated swelling of moderate size develops. If, as is often the case, the premolar and molar region is involved, loss of sensation occurs in the lower lip in the area supplied by the mental branch of the inferior dental nerve. This is pathognomonic of thrombosis of the inferior dental vasa nervorum and a rise in pressure from oedema in the inferior dental canal and must be distinguished from a simple alveolar abscess discharging through the mental foramen.

A number of teeth may become tender to percussion and loose in the affected segment of the jaw and eventually pus discharges through sinuses in the alveolar process, up the periodontal membranes of adjacent teeth, and also externally onto the face. The lymph nodes draining the area are enlarged and tender. There is a pyrexia but the adult patient may not feel particularly ill, which is in marked contrast to the effect of osteomyelitis of the long bones. Following drainage of pus as a result of sinus formation the temperature tends to fall and the pain eases. If the condition is not treated a protracted chronic state ensues characterized by acute exacerbations at irregular intervals.

Radiology

Radiographs of the affected area appear virtually normal until osteomyelitis has been present for about 1–3 weeks. Then the bone takes on a mottled appearance due to widening of the medullary spaces and enlargement of Volkmann's canals. Gradually resorption around the periphery of the infarcted area of bone separates it off as a sequestrum. The granulation tissue between the living and dead bone produces irregular lines and zones of radiolucency. This results in the characteristic moth-eaten radiographic appearance of established osteomyelitis. Subperiosteal new bone, the involucrum, can be seen as a fine linear opacity or as a series of laminated opacities like an onion skin, parallel to the surface of the cortex. This is seen at the lower border or may be best outlined on the buccal cortex by an occlusal film. Where the new bone is superimposed upon that of the jaw a delicate fingerprint or orange peel appearance adds to the loss of radiographic definition of the original underlying bone structure. The deposition of subperiosteal new bone is particularly marked in children and adolescents. Later, substantial fragments of dead bone, especially thick cortical bone, may be separated from the adjacent bone by well demarcated radiolucent zones and may even become displaced from their original position. Sequestra are often prevented from spontaneous discharge through sinuses in the overlying soft tissues by the enveloping involucrum and come to lie in granulation tissue and pus filled cavities between the involucrum and the surviving mandibular bone. At this stage there is a risk of pathological fracture (*Fig.* 7.1).

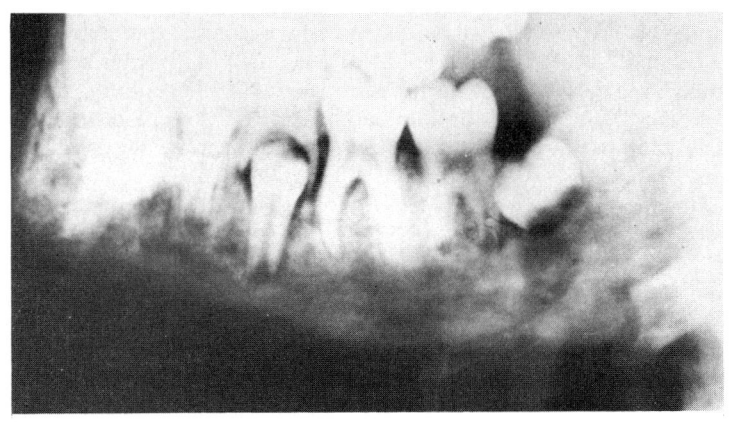

Fig. 7.1. Oblique-lateral radiograph showing extensive osteomyelitis in the mandible of a child of 10 years.

In pre-antibiotic days several clinical types of acute osteomyelitis were seen, the extent of the lesion probably related to vascular factors. Massive, diffuse infections frequently involved the whole of one side of the mandible, the whole of one side together with the mental region as far as the opposite mental foramen, and in extreme cases involvement of the whole of the jaw (*Fig.* 7.2). Localized osteomyelitis tended to follow two patterns, vertical

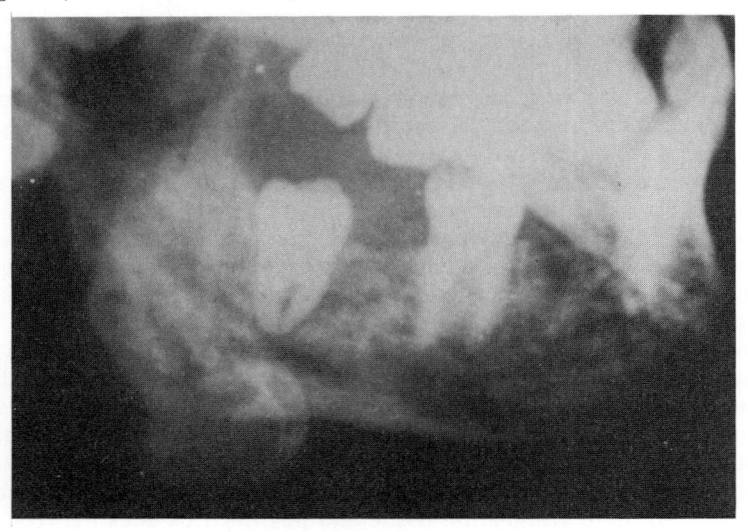

Fig. 7.2. Osteomyelitis affecting the whole of one side of the mandible in an adult.

and alveolar. In vertical osteomyelitis a short segment of the body of the mandible was involved in full depth from alveolar crest to the lower border (*Figs.* 7.3 and 7.4). In the alveolar form a segment of alveolar bone and the subapical bone down to the inferior dental canal would separate, containing the sockets of perhaps three or four teeth (*Fig.* 7.5). As with other infections the early administration of antibiotics modifies the natural evolution of the disease.

Treatment

In the early stages, the clinical and radiological course of an alveolar abscess and an incipient odontogenic osteomyelitis are the same. The treatment appropriate to an alveolar abscess is therefore employed. In many cases this will be sufficient to arrest what, with hindsight, was an early case of osteomyelitis. This should be extraction of the infected tooth with incision and drainage. It is rarely necessary to drill holes in the mandible as with long bones to establish release of the pus as the socket provides a supplementary exit.

INFLAMMATORY DISEASES OF BONE

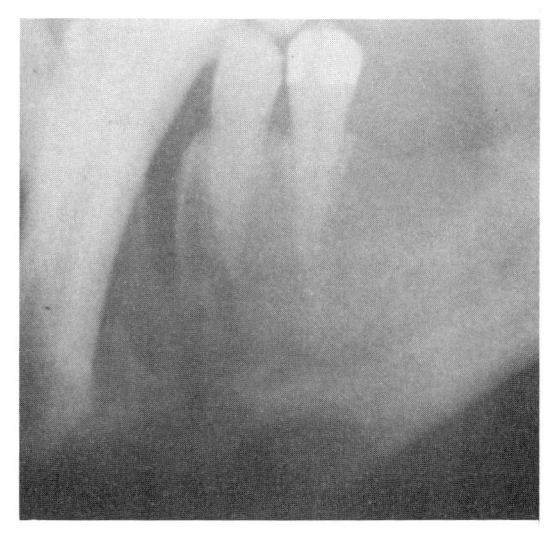

Fig. 7.3. Osteomyelitis spreading vertically downwards from a lower canine socket. Subperiosteal new bone (involucrum) encloses a granulation filled cavity at the lower border containing a sequestrum of cortex.

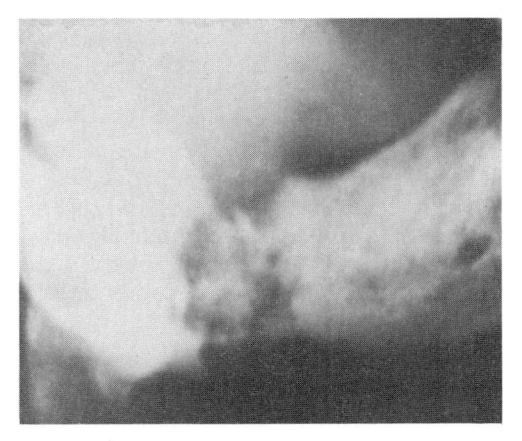

Fig. 7.4. Vertical osteomyelitis spreading through the mandible from a 3rd molar socket. Only involucrum (seen in an occlusal film) maintains continuity of the jaw. There is a sequestrum almost separated.

As it is not practical to wait for the identification of the responsible organism and the determination of its antibiotic sensitivities, a swab should be taken when draining the pus but before commencing the antibiotic therapy.

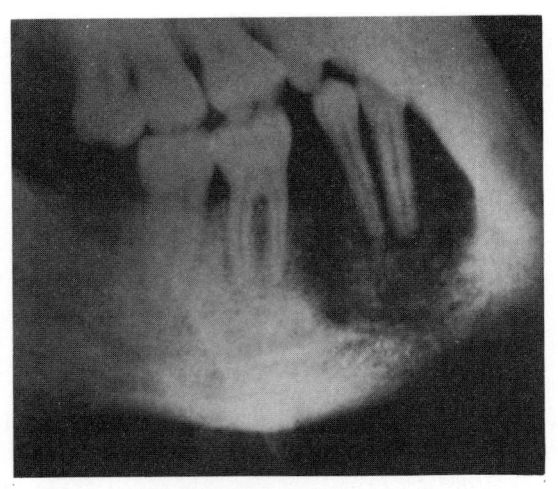

Fig. 7.5. Localized osteomyelitis with a sequestrum of alveolar bone containing a mandibular canine and premolar.

A broad-spectrum bacteriocidal antibiotic is best combined with one resistant to staphylococcal penicillinase until the organism and its sensitivities are known. Amoxycillin (500 mg, 8-hourly) and flucloxacillin (250 mg, 6-hourly) may be preferred. For patients who are allergic to penicillin, erythromycin or a cephalosporin alone, or in combination with sodium fusidate 500 mg, 8-hourly, may be used. Some clinicians advocate the use of clindamycin 300 mg, 6-hourly, because of its ability to diffuse widely in bone. It has the advantage of being effective, not only against staphylococci and streptococci, but also against the anaerobic bacteroides which can be the cause of a persistent, low grade chronic continuation of the disease. This drug should be stopped promptly if diarrhoea occurs because of the risk of pseudomembranous colitis developing (*see also* Chapter 8).

There is no simple indication for the best duration of antibiotic administration, but in early acute cases treatment should be maintained for a minimum of 2 weeks and may be continued for up to 8 weeks depending upon the severity of the infection and its response to treatment. With this type of conservative management even cases which have progressed to the stage where early radiographic changes are seen will resolve with drainage as the only treatment.

Once extensive osteomyelitis is apparent radiographically sequestrectomy will be required and should be undertaken through an intraoral or submandibular incision depending on the site of the sequestrum.

The bony cavity is saucerized with an acrylic bur so that when the wound is closed the soft tissues eliminate any dead space. Generous irrigation of the bone with sterile saline is important. Primary closure of the soft tissue wound is carried out with a Yeates drain or suction drainage and antibiotics are administered for a minimum of two weeks postoperatively or until all evidence of infection has subsided. Provided that all infected and necrotic bone is removed healing is uneventful.

Before sequestrectomy consideration should be given to the need to splint and immobilize the mandible to support it so as to avoid a surgical fracture, or to avoid displacement of the fragments if a pathological fracture already exists. Any form of fixation appropriate to the dentition and site of fracture may be used. General supportive treatment is important. Fluid and food intake must be maintained. Feeding may be carried out by fine bore nasogastric tube if the mouth and teeth are tender and jaw movement restricted and painful. Anaemia, diabetes and malnutrition will need specific attention.

'Chronic following on acute cases' usually have a sequestrum *in situ*. As a result, pus is discharged through sinuses which pass through cloacae in the involucrum onto the surface of the oral mucosa and facial skin. While a free flow of pus occurs, patients are relatively symptom-free and have little pain, but at irregular intervals they suffer acute exacerbations of the infection. Bouts of pain and swelling occur which last for three or four days and then subside when the abscess discharges, following which the condition becomes quiescent again. In the absence of surgical intervention to remove the dead bone, this chronic phase can be lost indefinitely.

CHRONIC OSTEOMYELITIS

Presents with minimal pain and discharge, although the mandible is invariably enlarged by the deposition of subperiosteal new bone at the site of inflammation. One characteristic feature is the preservation of mental and labial sensation.

The patient is usually over forty and may give a history of difficult extraction perhaps with retained infected roots. Often the patient is edentulous and the involved segment of mandible is composed of sclerosed bone. Sometimes there is evidence that this predated the initiating extraction and the onset of chronic osteomyelitis. Other times the sclerotic bone forms and spreads with the infection.

There is a combination of resorption and bone deposition both subperiosteally, thickening the cortex, and in the medulla producing zones of sclerosis, as a result of a low grade infection centered in a multitude of small abscess cavities.

Radiology

Radiographs show irregular radiolucencies superimposed on areas of sclerosis and abnormally thick trabeculation. There is more of an overall moth-eaten appearance than in acute osteomyelitis which differs by virtue of its sequestrum formation.

Treatment

Prior to definitive treatment it may be desirable to explore a readily acessible cavity and enucleate the granulation tissue in it under local anaesthetic to establish the bacteriology and its sensitivity and also to provide a biopsy for histopathological examination. This may not only help by supplementing the bacteriological investigation by revealing, for example, tuberculosis, but will exclude an infected neoplasm which may resemble a chronic osteomyelitis.

Surgery is required to remove roots and sequestra and decorticate the infected medullary area because zones of sclerosed infected medullary bone rarely become demarcated and sequestrate naturally. Bone removal should be done generously with a saline cooled acrylic bur until an area of healthy bleeding bone is established. An intraoral approach is usually the most appropriate but the wound must be drained to prevent haematoma formation. Copious irrigation is necessary before closure. If the soft tissues cannot be closed without leaving a dead space or because of rigid fibrosis, the wound is packed with 2-inch ribbon gauze moistened with Whitehead's varnish.

Completely separated sequestra lie in granulation tissue and are easily recognized at surgery once any overlying subperiosteal new bone has been breached. Necrotic but unsequestrated cortex has a dirty white colour compared with the yellowish hue of living cortical bone. As the removal of dead cortex approaches normal bone the cutting should cease from time to time. If the cortex is viable tiny red bleeding spots will appear on the cut surface after a minute or two. The dense sclerosed medulla is removed until the inside of the opposite cortex is reached and normal cancellous bone found at either end. Granulation tissue from cavities in the bone should be conserved for diagnostic purposes. Some is fixed and sent for histological section. Other samples are placed unfixed in small sterile containers and sent to the microbiologist. A chronic non-suppurative osteomyelitis from which a positive culture is not obtained in this way is probably due to obligate anaerobes.

Occasionally a chronic intramedullary abscess is encountered. The medullary bone has an open cancellous structure as there is no living tissue to deposit new bone. It is grey in colour, does not bleed when cut, contains a pasty whitish material and is friable. All necrotic tissue must be removed until fresh bleeding bone is encountered and specimens sent for diagnosis as above.

On rare occasions when it is apparent that the full thickness of the segment of jaw is involved and a conservative approach has failed to bring about a cure, consideration should be given to resection of the involved part. When the healed wound is infection-free secondary bone grafting can be undertaken. During the resection only the soft tissue related to the dead bone should be elevated, lest adjacent living cortex is devitalized. Antibiotic therapy will be determined by the culture results but as anaerobes and in particular bacteroides are important pathogens, metronidazole 400 mg, 12-hourly, should be included in the regime.

Chronic external sinuses may also require gentle irrigation. This can be done daily with Eusol (calcium hypochlorite 1·25 per cent and boric acid 1·25 per cent) or Milton's solution (stabilized 1 per cent sodium hypochlorite solution—Richardson Merrell). Furthermore, where the bacteriology shows a predominance of exotic antibiotic-resistant micro-organisms it is advisable to stop all antibiotics except metronidazole and irrigate and pack daily as described above.

Specific infective forms of chronic osteomyelitis include, tuberculosis, syphilis, yaws and actinomycosis. These should receive the same surgical treatment but with the appropriate medication. As would be expected, tuberculosis may require therapy for up to a year, and actinomycosis for 2–3 months.

POST-IRRADIATION MORBIDITY AND OSTEORADIONECROSIS

All the tissues of the face and mouth are affected by irradiation, i.e. bone, teeth, muscles, salivary glands, skin and its appendages. Actual necrosis of tissues as a result of therapeutic irradiation is a rare event with modern methods of treatment. True osteoradionecrosis therefore is uncommon. Bone may be damaged by therapeutic radiation from both external and implanted sources, such as caesium needles used in the tongue, or more rarely from absorbed radioactive substances which become trapped within the mineral component of the bone.

Substantial damage was common with older forms of radiotherapy with an appreciable incidence of radionecrosis. With high energy sources giving greater penetration of bone and a more uniform dose between bone and soft tissues and with the use of multiple portals of therapy, the risk has been reduced. However, in some centres the increased tolerance has encouraged the use of higher tumour dosage leaving the bone equally at risk.

The pathological changes appear to be identical irrespective of the nature of the source of irradiation, resulting in endarteritis obliterans, ischaemia and a reduction in the viable osteocyte population. The resultant picture is that of hypovascularity of all elements of the bone, including the marrow and periosteum as well as the investing soft tissues. In addition there appears to be a failure of osteoclast activity; whether this is related to the impaired blood supply or lack of osteoblast stimulation is unknown.

Ionizing radiations destroy malignant neoplasms by damaging the chromosomes so that cell division is imperfect or impaired. As the malignant cells are dividing more often than host tissue cells a greater proportion succumb and the tumour regresses. Normally, resting osteocytes are stimulated to activity by bone damage and start to divide rapidly in order to repair an injury such as a tooth socket. If in the past some of these osteocytes have suffered radiation injury, cell division may be imperfect and the osteocytes will die.

These changes make the bone vulnerable to trauma and infection producing initially a localized osteitis which fails to heal and then tends to spread as a chronic ischaemic necrosis through bone which is incapable of endosteal or periosteal repair and prey to infection. Thirty or more percent of cases appear to arise spontaneously suggesting that repair and replacement of the damaged bone failed without any traumatic or infective stimulus. In such cases a zone of radiolucency appears with no clinical signs of infection or communication with the mouth. If soft tissue dehiscence and infection is avoided a return to normal appearances may occur, but the time scale is years rather than months.

The irradiation also induces an inflammatory response in the soft tissues with erythema, desquamation and then pigmentation of the overlying skin such as is seen with sunburn but with a longer time scale. Similarly there is an erythema of the oral mucosa with desquamation within the zone of maximum dose. Here the denuded surface is covered by a yellow fibrinoid exudate which in a well planned treatment is sharply defined at the margins and closely related to the tumour. If the salivary glands are within the fields of irradiation, salivation is suppressed and a scanty, sticky secretion covers the teeth and gums. The patient adopts a soft, semi-liquid diet rich in carbohydrate exposing the teeth to a high caries risk. The acute mucosal and skin changes resolve within a few weeks but salivary flow may be suppressed for 12–18 months or even permanently.

Following therapeutic irradiation pre-existing periodontal disease is exacerbated, but there is also a degree of atrophy of the periodontal membrane even where the gums are healthy and gingival recession occurs without pocketing which exposes the necks of the teeth. A combination of xerostomia, a soft, cariogenic diet and a degree of neglect of oral hygiene measures leads to widespread caries affecting the smooth surfaces of the crowns of the teeth and the exposed necks as well as fissures and contact areas. Furthermore, in the absence of saliva recalcification of early (white spot) enamel lesions cannot occur. This is the so called radiation caries.

Following treatment the healed oral mucosa tends to be atrophic and delicate, easily damaged by friction and slow to heal if it is ulcerated. Dentures must be constructed with great care and should be left out whenever reasonable. Cotton wool rolls used to control saliva during dental treatment should be slightly moistened so that they do not adhere to the mucosa.

The overlying skin shows similar changes: atrophy, loss of sweat glands and hair follicles and telangiectasia. Where the masticatory muscles have been heavily irradiated fibrosis may render them inextendable. When the temporalis, medial pterygoid and masseter are involved marked extra articular ankylosis is the result. As this is not due to muscle spasm the term trismus is not appropriate. Oral hygiene and dental treatment are rendered additionally more difficult as a result. Where the temporalis is maximally affected an intraoral coronoidectomy with stretching under a general anaesthetic can be considered.

A common cause of osteoradionecrosis is the extraction of teeth from the irradiated area and, as prevention is easier than cure, this should be anticipated. Once postirradiation caries has become established its control by restorative measures is usually very difficult.

Prophylaxis

Any teeth in the area due to receive the full therapeutic dose should be extracted before treatment is started together with any teeth for which the prognosis is poor. Unless the dentition is generally healthy and well cared for and the patient likely to be motivated and able to maintain a high standard of oral hygiene a clearance is, in the long term, the best policy. Certainly this should be the case where the teeth are neglected. Tact and understanding is necessary in explaining the need for these measures to a patient who is likely already to be under severe mental stress.

The extractions should be carried out as soon as possible after histological confirmation of the diagnosis and a decision on treatment policy, including the need for irradiation, has been agreed. If a general anaesthetic is to be given for an examination to enable the full extent of the neoplasm to be determined, the extractions can be carried out at the same time, but local anaesthesia, with sedation if appropriate, is quite satisfactory. Every effort must be made to ensure rapid and trouble-free healing. There may be a delay in the start of treatment of around 10 days because of the extractions but this is fully justified and often will occur anyway while a mask is made and external beam irradiation planned or while radioactive isotopes for implantation are ordered.

Prominent interdental septa and sharp or splintered socket margins should be trimmed as remodelling resorption of the alveolar process will not occur after irradiation. Fractured inter-radicular septa should be removed and the soft tissues carefully sutured. Unerupted and deeply buried teeth are probably best left *in situ*. Difficult, caries-free but partially erupted lower 3rd molars may create a dilemma if it is thought that their removal will result in troublesome wounds, protracted healing and, as a result, delay the start of treatment. There is a further difficulty if the surgery is likely to disrupt the neoplasm, opening up tissue planes to contamination which may have to be taken into account with the tumour therapy. Their retention, if the patient survives for any length of time, is of course also likely to lead to problems.

As far as possible the mouth should be cleaned up before the extractions, sloughing malignant ulcers are freely irrigated, and infected and necrotic tissue sucked away. Penicillin or metronidazole should be given immediately before the extractions and afterwards for 5–7 days. During radiotherapy an 0·2 per cent aqueous chlorhexidine mouthwash will help to keep down secondary infection of any ulcerated mucosa and will reduce plaque accumulation and caries. Supervised tooth cleaning with the aid of a mirror and the regular services of an oral hygienist will do much to prevent the deterioration in cleanliness of the remaining teeth which otherwise occurs.

Meticulous oral hygiene using a fluoride toothpaste is essential, and the use of a daily fluoride mouthwash also adds protection. Dietary advice can both reduce the intake of food and drink with a high dextrose content and improve nutrition.

Another means of protection is the cementing of vacuum moulded acrylic or cellulose butyrate acetate splints onto the teeth with a fluoride containing cement and which remain in place until an adequate salivary flow is restored which may take up to two years. Unfortunately, cervical caries may develop unnoticed with this regime.

Sometimes in the months immediately after radiotherapy there will be a limited break down of the ridge mucosa to expose a patch of bone a few millimetres across. This should be left to sequestrate and only lifted off when quite loose, although this may take many months. If a sharp spike is exposed in this way the point can be nibbled away with bone nibblers.

Should a tooth need extraction from a previously irradiated part of the jaws this must be done as follows:

1. The mouth should be carefully cleaned and the patient given a preoperative dose of metronidazole 400 mg.

2. A local anaesthetic not requiring a vasoconstrictor, or one with felypressin as vasoconstrictor, should be chosen so that there will be free bleeding from the socket.

3. The gingiva are painted with povidone-iodine.

4. A simple extraction is done with great care, being particular not to remove the clot from the socket by the use of suction. The extraction of multirooted teeth may be made easier by dividing them with a tapered fissure bur, being certain that all debris is removed before the actual extraction. Resistant teeth can be weakened by cutting into the periodontal membrane with a No. 2 rose-head bur under a water spray.

5. Mucosal flaps should not be raised as this may kill the underlying cortex but long prominences and sharp points at the margin of the socket are removed and the mucoperiosteum sutured.

6. Mucosal flaps should be avoided, while in general limited envelope mucosal flaps may be raised carefully from the alveolar margin only but the alveolar bone should be trimmed generously before they are closed over it.

7. Metronidazole is continued for 10 days or until the wound has healed.

INFLAMMATORY DISEASES OF BONE

N.B. The problem of postextraction osteoradionecrosis can be avoided by root filling non-vital teeth, even if the crowns are not to be restored.

The Recognition and Treatment of Osteoradionecrosis

Osteoradionecrosis may start as a dry socket, or an area of painful exposed bone in the base of denture ulceration, or spontaneously. It is seen not uncommonly in the lingual cortex of the mandible adjacent to the site of a neoplasm of the lateral border of the tongue or floor of the mouth which has been treated with a radioactive implantation technique. Radium needles in particular resulted in this state of affairs because of their proximity and continuous radiation. The exposed yellow necrotic bone fails to separate, and either spontaneously or as a result of injudicious surgical interference further mucosal breakdown exposes more dead bone and small quantities of pus are discharged. Radiographs reveal the characteristic moth-eaten appearance of devitalized bone which slowly extends through the mandible. Only small fragments separate after a period of very many months and never involve all the dead and infected bone. True sequestration of the non-vital from vital tissue does not take place. Attempts at local excision simply extend the area of dead bone. As the osteogenic periosteum is destroyed by the radiotherapy no involucrum of subperiosteal new bone is formed (*Fig.* 7.6), and if pathological fractures occur substantial displacement of the bone ends follows with little chance of union occuring. Protruding bone ends may be trimmed and the site packed with ribbon gauze soaked in

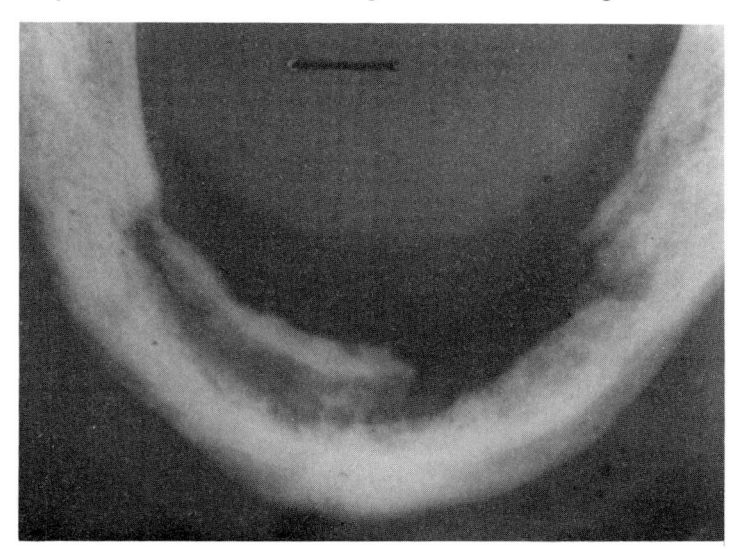

Fig. 7.6. Radionecrosis of the anterior part of the mandible. Slow sequestration of the lingual plate. Notice that there is no subperiosteal new bone forming an involucrum.

Whitehead's varnish to give some stability. If there are teeth present in both jaws intermaxillary fixation will reduce the degree of further displacement of the fragments.

Histological examination of the bone shows widespread ischaemic necrosis with no microbial or inflammatory infiltration in the deeper parts. Active infection is not always present but acute or subacute episodes should be controlled with antibiotics after culture and sensitivity tests. Co-trimoxazole (trimethoprim 80 mg and sulphmethoxazole 400 mg) twice a day is a useful regime, but courses of antibiotics should not be prolonged as this leads to overgrowth of resistant microbes and without any clinical benefit. Local irrigation of suppurating cavities and the maintenance of local hygiene with hot saline or perborate mouthwashes will make the condition more tolerable for both patient and relatives.

Exposing the patient to a pure oxygen environment at 2·4 atmospheres pressure for 2 hours a day for 4–8 weeks will increase the concentration of oxygen in the plasma and tissue fluids (hyperbaric oxygen). This encourages granulation tissue and leucocytes to migrate into the zone of necrosis, facilitating the separation of sequestra and enhancing bone healing. During treatment cyanosis is abolished in tissues which are normally marginally oxygenated and creates an adverse environment for anaerobic organisms. Some patients suffer severe pain with osteoradionecrosis and this is relieved.

This treatment is not without risk, particularly if the proportion of time during which the patient is exposed to hyperbaric oxygen is increased or if higher pressures are employed. Pulmonary congestion can occur and oxygen toxicity is manifest by convulsions which usually are preceded by twitching of the lips. There can also be problems in keeping pressure in the middle ear within acceptable limits. Furthermore, not all patients will tolerate being enclosed in the treatment tank and emphysematous pulmonary disease is a contraindication to its use. Enthusiasm for some other uses of hyperbaric oxygen has waned and in practice there can be difficulty in finding a unit willing to offer facilities for this treatment.

While patience and a conservative management is appropriate for small areas of osteoradionecrosis there are several good reasons why this approach is not suitable for extensive lesions. The patient may be committed indefinitely to a burden of sepsis, and pain which is in some cases severe, an objectionable taste and smell, and orocutaneous fistula and pathological fracture. Therefore there are several alternative surgical treatments for osteoradionecrosis. These are as follows.

a. Excision of the affected segment of the mandible and accepting the deformity which results. This may be reasonable where the posterior part on one side is involved and where the bone of the chin at least as far back as the canine region can be left. The bone is approached by the most direct route and sectioned well beyond the infected and necrotic segment. The cut in the bone must be made as close as possible to a point where the soft tissues are still attached. The sharp edges at the bone end are rounded off and the soft tissues sutured over the bone end. Muscle is best for this purpose, and a temporalis flap if available will provide vascularity and help fill the dead space. The rest of the wound is closed carefully in layers with drainage. The soft tissues may be oedematous and friable and tight suturing is to be avoided.

b. Trimming away exposed and necrotic bone until the line of attached soft tissues is reached and bringing in a simple vascular flap to cover and revascularize the area. Again a temporalis muscle flap is ideal and only part of the muscle may be necessary to fill the defect.

c. Excision of the affected segment and subsequent free bone grafting of the defect. Considerable care is necessary to provide adequate soft tissue cover. Again, bringing in a well vascularized muscle flap such as temporalis or pectoralis major to wrap around the graft and over the bone ends will improve the chances of success.

d. Excision of the necrotic bone and scarred and poorly vascularized soft tissue and effecting a repair with a composite flap. This may be a pedicle flap, for example, a pectoralis major myocutaneous flap incorporating rib or sternum as the osseous component, or a free flap attached by microvascular anastomosis, such as the forearm–radius flap. Surgical healing will also be enhanced by further hyperbaric oxygen therapy if available.

Sometimes the initial exposure of the irradiated bone results from ulceration of a recurrent neoplasm. The proliferating and necrosing malignant tissue may not be recognized immediately amid the granulation tissue and suppuration surrounding the dead bone. In other cases after a substantial interval what may be a fresh squamous cell carcinoma arises in the mucosal margin adjacent to the necrotic and infected bone. Clinicians should be on the lookout for a combination of osteoradionecrosis and an active malignancy as this clearly demands urgent surgical treatment.

ASEPTIC NECROSIS OF BONE

It is possible surgically to deprive substantial pieces of bone of their blood supply so that they are, in effect, attached bone grafts. If the masseter is stripped from the mandible during an Obwegeser–Dalpont sagittal split osteotomy much of the buccal cortex after the split is in this condition. Parts of the facial skeleton must also have at most a tenuous blood supply after the extensive degloving required for craniofacial surgery. In general this does not affect the outcome provided that immobilization and soft tissue coverage is achieved with early reattachment of the soft tissues by avoiding haematomas. Infection in such cases can be disastrous. Cancellous bone is less likely to suffer in this way and any ischaemic cancellous bone will be revascularized.

Bone necrosis can occur in sickle-cell disease. This is a haemoglobinopathy principally of negroes where the abnormal haemoglobin HbS when hypoxic produces elongated erythrocytes which aggregate and obstruct capillaries and arteries. This may occur spontaneously in the homozygote sickle disease and rarely in the heterozygote.

Episodes of pain and swelling will suggest local bone infarction and should be prophylactically treated with antibiotics and analgesics in the first instance. In sickle-cell disease the continued haemolysis tends to 'overwhelm' the reticuloendothelial system and the patient may also be more susceptible to infections. Surgery is only required if infection supervenes converting an aseptic necrosis into osteomyelitis. Pus is drained and sequestra removed in the usual way and if done under a general anaesthetic an adequate haemoglobin level and full, assured oxygenation are required.

Herpes zoster may rarely, when it involves the inferior dental nerve, give rise to infarction of the dental pulps and/or the body of the mandible with subsequent infection and osteomyelitis. This appears to be usually a complication of the elderly, of cytotoxic chemotherapy and neoplasia. Treatment is symptomatic.

CHEMICAL NECROSIS

Bone necrosis due to exposure to phosphorus, mercury or bismuth either from industrial processes or drug therapy is fortunately rare and largely of historical interest.

Arsenic trioxide is still occasionally used by dental practitioners to devitalize inflamed painful pulps. If it accidently extrudes into the periodontal space it leads to necrosis of the adjacent alveolar process and sequestration. Similarly, inadvertent injections of phenol, hydrogen peroxide and the like have been the cause of chemical necrosis of bone and treatment includes adequate irrigation and debridement of the area and prophylactic antibiotics. Some root-filling pastes if they are extruded beyond the apex have a similar effect.

Intraoral haemangiomas involving the buccal and palatal mucosa must never be treated with sclerosants such as sodium tetradecyl sulphate. Successful sclerosis of the vascular abnormality will also devitalize the adjacent alveolar bone and teeth, which will gradually become sequestrated.

OSTEOMYELITIS DUE TO NON-PYOGENIC ORGANISMS

Syphilitic Osteomyelitis

Infection by the *Treponema pallidum* may affect the bones in syphilis in both the secondary and tertiary stages, and also in cases of congenital syphilis, but nowadays, in countries where treatment for syphilis is freely available, skeletal disease of syphilitic origin is seldom seen.

Pathology

The reactions of bone to the presence of the *Treponema pallidum* are essentially similar to those of other tissues, though modified by its special anatomical and physiological characteristics. At the site of the lesion there is a chronic, inflammatory granulomatous and necrotizing periarterial infiltrate accompanied by partial destruction of bone. As the disease progresses the vascularity of the area becomes diminished and the bone tends to become sclerosed. Osteosclerosis with new bone formation is more common than osteoporosis and rarefaction.

Neonatal Syphilis

In neonatal syphilis the involvement of the skeleton takes place approximately at the end of the fifth month of intrauterine life and the characteristic bone changes are present at birth. Gummatous destruction of the nasal septum and hard palate are common and the characteristic saddle-shaped nose is due to subsidence of the bridge of the nose, a condition which is often associated with perforations of the palate. However, not all perforated palates are the result of congenital disease; palatal perforations also occur in the late stages of acquired syphilis. In the cranium there may be a diffuse osteitis or multiple periosteal nodes, usually grouped around the anterior fontanelle. Radiologically, the cranium has a worm-eaten appearance due to subperiosteal gummas and in the absence of treatment as the patient becomes older, separation of circular sequestra from the base of ulcerating gummatous lesions may lead to complete perforation of the bone.

Acquired Syphilis

In acquired syphilis bony changes are seldom seen before the tertiary stage and the palate, nose, skull and tibia are the bones most commonly affected. The changes take the form of periosteal and central gummata (*Fig. 7.7*). Bone is resorbed at the site of the gumma producing a radiolucency with a poorly defined margin. The central necrotic mass is rubbery in consistency, and later becomes cheesy. The overlying tissues may break down to form an abscess or an ulcer with a characteristic 'punched out' margin and yellowish, sloughing base. At this stage secondary infection with pyogenic organisms may be responsible for a more extensive bone necrosis and sequestrum formation.

Syphilitic osteomyelitis of the jaws is not easily distinguished from pyogenic osteomyelitis on clinical and radiological examination. Unless a gumma is seen or evidence of tertiary syphilis found elsewhere in the body and particularly signs of involvement of other bones by syphilis, the diagnosis may be missed unless serological tests are carried out.

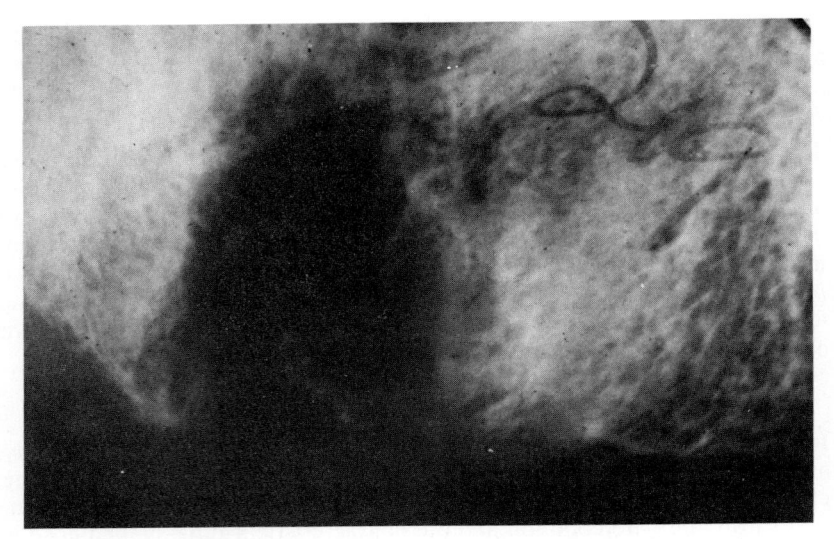

Fig. 7.7. A gumma of the maxilla involving the alveolar process in the premolar region. Tiny sequestra in the slough.

Pathological fracture often develops but rapid improvement usually occurs with penicillin or erythromycin therapy.

Yaws

A sclerosing osteomyelitis and periostitis may be seen in patients from the Caribbean area who give a history of yaws in childhood. This condition occasionally affects the jaws where, like syphilis, the diagnosis should be suspected if osteomyelitis is accompanied by much sclerosis and pursues an unusual course. Unfortunately, the serological tests for syphilis are also positive in yaws. Treatment is penicillin.

Tuberculosis

Tuberculous osteomyelitis of the jaws is rare.

Pathogenesis

Infection of bone by the *Mycobacterium tuberculosis* is usually brought about by metastatic haematogenous spread and is almost always secondary to a primary focus in the respiratory or alimentary tract. In England prior to World War II 7% of milk supplies for human consumption contained tubercle bacilli and much bone tuberculosis at that time was bovine in origin. However, in countries such as the United Kingdom where tuberculosis in cattle is now largely eradicated the human bacillus is responsible for such bone infections as are seen.

INFLAMMATORY DISEASES OF BONE

Tuberculous osteitis occurs when blood-borne bacilli lodge in cancellous bone, especially in the epiphysis of long bones, the phalanges, and the dorsal and lumbar vertebrae. It usually starts in the metaphysis of a bone and causes widespread destruction. Large subperiosteal cold abscesses form and may burrow long distances towards the surface along muscle planes. It destroys the epiphysial cartilage and so infects the neighbouring joint, but the temporomandibular joint is virtually never involved.

There are recorded cases in which it has been suggested that the localization of a tuberculous embolus in bone may be determined by trauma, but this is very difficult to prove.

Localized osteomyelitis may follow tooth extraction performed on tuberculous patient. Active tuberculous infection of tooth sockets is seen, both in patients with pulmonary tuberculosis with a positive sputum and in patients who have an active infection in cervical lymph nodes. The infected socket, unlike the normal dry socket, is relatively painless. The attention of the clinician is drawn to the situation because the socket fails to heal and continues to discharge small amounts of watery pus. Over a period of weeks a substantial amount of bone destruction occurs to produce a granulation tissue filled bone cavity submucosally at the site of the socket. There is no sequestrum formation and no florid exuberant granulations such as might accompany a pyogenic infection of the tooth socket. The diagnosis is usually confirmed by biopsy of the soft tissue forming the socket wall. If the infection in the mandible is left untreated it may spread into the soft tissues and form an indolent, chronic, facial sinus.

A superimposed pyogenic infection may cause difficulty in establishing the correct diagnosis. The onset is insidious and pain is not a prominent feature in the early stages. There may be limitation of opening and if an extensive area of the mandible is involved a pathological fracture can occur. Tubercle bacilli may be seen in biopsies or smears from exudate from the sinuses, but culture is a lengthy process as a means of diagnosis.

Treatment consists of local surgery and antituberculous drug therapy.

Salmonella

Bone infection as a late complication of typhoid or paratyphoid fever and other forms of salmonella infection is rare. Classically, typhoid osteomyelitis affects the vertebrae giving rise to 'typhoid spine' but long bones may also be affected. Occasionally typhoid or paratyphoid bacilli are involved in infection of the bones of the jaws, and this is more common in cases of sickle cell disease.

Actinomycosis

Cervicofacial actinomycosis of the soft tissues is not uncommon and the organism responsible for the condition in human beings is the *Actinomyces israeli*, while a similar disease, lumpy jaw in cattle, is attributed to another organism, *A. bovis*.

'Actinomyces' is the generic term given to a group of organisms which represent the higher bacteria, a number of which are pathogenic for man. These organisms are Gram-positive filaments which tend to branch and mat together in an amorphous matrix designated the 'mycelium'. A mycelium of this type is found in the pus of actinomycotic lesions, in the form of a granule, described as the 'sulphur granule', and represents a single colony of the actinomyces organism. The mycelium in the tissues tends to be surrounded by peripheral Gram-negative clubs, which radiate outward in the shape of a ring. This appearance explains the expression 'ray fungus' which is applied to *A. israeli* or *bovis*.

A. israeli is a normal inhabitant of the mouth and can be isolated from crypts of tonsils, carious teeth, salivary calculi, and the gingival crevice and it is probable that most cases of actinomycosis are endogenous. Colonies are reported from time to time in histological preparations of cysts and in the root canals of teeth without evidence that this was part of a clinical infection.

Other commensal actinomyces such as *A. viscosis* may also become pathogenic. It is also important to establish there is not superimposed infection by *Staph. aureus,* or *Actinobacillus actinomycetemcomitans.*

Actinomycotic osteomyelitis of the jaws is rare but may present as:

1. A periostitis as a result of the involvement of adjacent soft tissue.

2. An actinomycotic osteomyelitis in which the mandible is thickened and honeycombed by narrow tracts in which the fungus is embedded in granulation tissue (*Fig.* 7.8). Eventually sequestration of the bone occurs. The disease may resemble pyogenic osteomyelitis both clinically and radiographically or such a proliferative mass of indurated soft tissue and

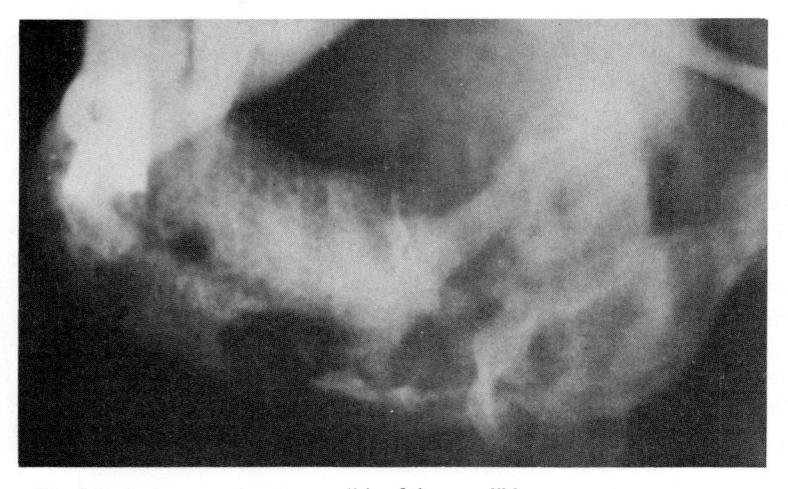

Fig. 7.8. Actinomycotic osteomyelitis of the mandible.

subperiosteal new bone forms around the jaw that the whole may be mistaken for an osteogenic sarcoma or lymphoma.

3. A chronic infection of a fracture and produce a chronic facial sinus.

Radiology

There are no specific diagnostic features of actinomycosis of the jaws and the lesion usually appears as irregular areas of bone destruction, as is seen in suppurative osteomyelitis, or as a massive periostitis. Cases have been reported which produced a single bone cavity resembling an odontogenic cyst radiographically.

Diagnosis

The diagnosis of actinomycosis often results from the microscopic examination of a specimen of pus, but if the condition is suspected the bacteriologist may culture the organism with the appropriate media. Sulphur granules are rarely present when the patient has already received antibiotic therapy.

Treatment

Treatment entails prolonged antibiotic therapy with penicillin, e.g. 500 mg of phenoxymethyl penicillin, 6-hourly, or 500 mg amoxycillin, 8-hourly, by mouth for some 6–8 weeks or for several months as necessary. Tetracycline 250 mg, 6-hourly, is a suitable alternative preparation and is active against the actinobacillus. Surgical intervention will be required to remove any sequestra which have formed.

CHRONIC HYPERTROPHIC OSTEOMYELITIS

This is a descriptive term from pre-antibiotic days, but a few similar cases can still be seen. After many years of chronic osteomyelitis the radiographic appearance comes close to resembling that seen in Paget's disease of the mandible. The original cortex is lost, there is much subperiosteal new bone and even hypercementosis of the involved teeth. With recurrent flares of infection the case comes to resemble osteomyelitis secondary to Paget's disease and only serial radiographs showing the evolution of the disease permit a differentiation.

Similarly during the healing phase of extensive osteomyelitis in the child the woven bone of the involucrum, together with new bone deposited to replace the destroyed part of the jaw, can produce a radiographic appearance closely resembling fibrous dysplasia, and only the history, together with the slow return to normal architecture, enables a distinction to be drawn between the two conditions.

ORAL SURGERY, PART 1

GARRE'S OSTEOMYELITIS AND NON-SUPPURATING SCLEROSING OSTEOMYELITIS

Garre (1893) described gross subperiosteal thickening of long bones resulting from mild irritation or infection. It is difficult to be more precise about Garre's osteomyelitis because his description (1893) predates the clinical use of X-rays in 1896 so there is no descriptive radiology of his patients. However, the name has been applied by a number of modern writers to cases of osteomyelitis of the mandible in which there is a marked periosteal reaction (*see also* Periostitis below). Since in most of these cases the patient is a child or adolescent a vigorous deposition of subperiosteal new bone is to be expected as a response to infection or trauma, or indeed to any inflammatory condition and so has no special significance.

The mass can mimic a tumour in radiographs and in infective cases may even have a subperiosteal sun-ray trabeculation rather than the expected concentric laminated appearance.

With the decline in acute and chronic, and chronic following acute suppurative osteomyelitis, chronic non-suppurative osteomyelitis has emerged as a more distinct and troublesome entity. Acute episodes in which there is swelling of the face and an easily palpable, tender, periosteal reaction over the affected part of the jaw are accompanied by substantial pain and a mild degree of malaise. Administration of systemic antibiotics leads to subsidance of symptoms, but after a variable period of time they recur. By trial and error antibiotics are found to which the infection responds because, in the absence of suppuration no organisms are cultured. Tetracycline, clindamycin metronidazole and ampicillin tend to be antibiotics to which the infection responds suggesting that anaerobes are involved. Prolonged courses of antibiotics, decortication, and decortication with implantation of gentamicin impregnated polymethylmethacrylate beads along with systemic gentamicin are regimes which have had both successes and failures. Initially the radiographic changes are minimal. Even the obvious, palpable periosteal reaction is difficult to demonstrate radiographically. With time a dense sclerosis develops with small patches of radiolucency. At operation the affected bone is delineated by ragged, thin layers of periosteal new bone which flake away from the surface. Success in controlling the condition depends upon its early recognition and prompt decortication. Gentamicin beads are inserted and intravenous gentamycin must be given. In some cases in which early aggressive treatment has not been used relapses of a tolerable severity may occur at quite long intervals over many years.

Antibiotics and intermittent decortication control these but the chance of eradicating the infection has been lost. After many years the attacks may die out. In some patients severe, demoralising recurrences are frequent despite decortication and prolonged courses of antibiotics. Resection, followed by secondary bone grafting is then the only chance of cure.

INFLAMMATORY DISEASES OF BONE

OSTEOMYELITIS IN PAGET'S DISEASE

Almost always osteomyelitis in Paget's disease affecting the jaws follows periapical infection, tooth extraction or other forms of surgery of the alveolar process such as an alveolectomy. The risk is present once sizeable 'cotton wool' masses of sclerotic bone appear in relation to the apices of teeth. Infection of such a mass as a complication of a periapical abscess or 'dry socket' is seen from time to time even if antibiotics are used as part of the treatment of these conditions. Surgical trimming of the bulky, enlarged alveolar processes may be undertaken for aesthetic reasons and to make possible the fitting of reasonable sized full upper and lower dentures. Great care must be exercised, if this is done, not to leave dense bony nodules at the cut surface or to permit haematomas to collect beneath the flaps and become infected.

If osteomyelitis becomes established the safest course is to wait until the infected bone has completely separated, so that is may be enucleated from a bed of granulation tissue. There is a risk with premature attempts at sequestrectomy of infecting adjacent sclerotic masses, starting a fresh cycle of localized osteomyelitis.

OSTEOMYELITIS IN OSTEOPETROSIS (ALBERS–SCHÖNBERG'S DISEASE)

Several entities are now known to produce the characteristic dense bones of this condition. There is either an absence of osteoclasts or a failure for these cells to be produced in a timely fashion to effect remodelling resorption. There is blurring of the corticomedullary bone border, reduction or obliteration or marrow spaces and poor remodelling of the external contour of the bone. Phagocytosis and repair of dead bone are grossly impaired. Because of the reduction in bone marrow secondary anaemia and extramedullary haemopoiesis is often found with enlargement of liver and spleen.

An intractable osteomyelitis is highly likely to complicate a periapical abscess and tooth extraction. Once established nothing short of total resection of the involved bone may control the infection, with all the consequences which ensue from such a decision. Management of these patients is similar to that of heavily irradiated patients except that the control of caries presents fewer problems.

CORTICAL OR SUBPERIOSTEAL OSTEOMYELITIS

Cortical osteomyelitis is the consequence of a sizeable accumulation of pus being confined beneath the periosteum. It is usually a complication where the pus accumulates beneath a muscle attachment such as with a submasseteric or subtemporalis muscle abscess (*see* pp. 145, Chapter 6). It may also occur when infection from a boil on the chin involves the outer cortical plate of the mental region of the mandible.

Blood vessels entering the cortex from the periosteum are thrombosed and destroyed and infection penetrates the cortex via Volkmann's canals. The full thickness of the cortex and the immediately subjacent medullary bone are involved. It is important to distinguish this entity from intramedullary osteomyelitis for which it may be mistaken if only rotational tomographic or oblique lateral radiographs are studied. A PA jaws view for ramus infections and tangential and occlusal films of the chin will demonstrate that only one cortex is involved.

PERIOSTITIS

Periostitis refers to a reactive response of the periosteum which is characterized by the deposition of subperiosteal new bone. Mostly the term is used for such a response where it forms part of a reaction to infection in the underlying or overlying tissues. This is often infection within the bone which may induce osteoblastic activity by the adjacent periosteum by some unknown stimulus, or by exudate directly spreading to involve the periosteum and raising it from the cortical surface. Infection in the parosteal soft tissues will also invoke a similar response, as in the earlier stages of submasseteric abscess or where lymph nodes adjacent to the bone are infected or where the mucoperiosteum is chronically inflamed.

Inflammation of the periosteum as part of the response to trauma to a bone or to the parosteal tissues will result in a similar reaction, particularly where the periosteum is raised from the bone by a haematoma. A similar response seen where the bone has been weakened internally by the presence of a cyst or neoplasm or raised from the surface of the cortex by neoplastic tissue is referred to simply as a periosteal reaction and this term may be used in relation to a traumatic cause also.

Initially a thin shell of new bone is deposited by the periosteum over the surface of the subperiosteal accumulation of pus or blood. If the cause is a haematoma or if the pus is drained and replaced by blood a reactive mass of bone is deposited as the haematoma is organized. The cycle may be repeated in the case of a chronic infection with subacute episodes, resulting in a multilayered onion skin lamination, best seen in an occlusal radiograph. This is in contrast to the radial 'sun-ray spicule' appearance produced characteristically where malignant bone neoplasms raise the periosteum and where the tumour bone is deposited in relation to blood vessels which pass from the marrow spaces via Volkmann's canals.

The proliferative reaction is particularly well seen in children where the most common cause is periapical infection. Where the infection is of long standing the swelling may become large enough to be misdiagnosed as an osseous or fibro-osseous tumour (*see* Garre's non-suppurative osteomyelitis above). If due to a periapical infection of the lower 1st molar in children the enlargement is usually mid-body in location whereas haematogenous metastatic infections tend to involve the angle of the mandible or incisor region.

Radiology

Only if there is a substantial thickness of new bone will there be a change in radiopacity in an oblique lateral projection or rotational tomogram and an appreciable difference in the textured quality of the image. The initial deposits of subperiosteal new bone will be overpenetrated and not seen but later the normal bone contours are rounded out and thickened. Subperiosteal new bone is best seen where the rays pass tangential to the surface of the bone as in occlusal and PA jaws views, and in taking the film exposure should be reduced. Initially there is a linear opacity parallel to the cortex and later a fuzzy mass, usually with a smooth lateral contour or the onion skin lamination referred to above.

Investigations

Specimens will be required for microbiology and for histopathology as there is always a possibility of a granulomatous infection, lymphoma or neoplasm.

Treatment

Treatment is essentially of the underlying condition. Removal of the sources of the infection, such as a diseased tooth or root, the drainage of pus and treatment with antibiotics will bring about resolution of the condition and resorptive remodelling of the mass.

Denture Periostitis and Pulse Granuloma

This is a chronic periostitis occuring in edentulous mandibles of denture wearers. It may start as an area of inflamed mucosal thickening often under the buccal flange of the denture where it rests in a groove between the residual alveolar bone and the external oblique ridge. A supraperiosteal or subperiosteal abscess may develop and later a sinus either in the sulcus or on the face. Sometimes a root fragment is present and its removal with drainage of the abscess brings about resolution. In many cases there is no such cause.

    A considerable smooth rounded elevation of the periosteal tissues occurs increasing the irritation from the flange of the denture and a vicious circle is set up. In time a mass of subperiosteal new bone will be demonstrable by occlusal radiography.

    The condition usually occurs in fit middle-aged patients who have worn comfortable dentures for many years. The cause is considered to be food particles implanted into the submucosal tissues, thereby provoking a foreign body reaction. Leguminous pulse seeds, i.e. fragments of beans, peas, lentils or peanuts, have been demonstrated in the submucosa producing a granulomatous reaction. The seeds are recognized as 100μ cellulose bodies containing clusters of starch granules which may be stained with iodine and PAS.

Treatment

Initially the dentures, which have probably been worn day and night, are left out completely for at least two weeks. Often this brings about resolution. Any pus is drained and antibiotics given. If the condition fails to resolve within reasonable time it should be explored and the granulation tissue curretted and excised so as to remove the foreign material. A biopsy will be obtained which may confirm the diagnosis.

Occasionally a similar clinical presentation results where there is a malignant neoplasm present, characteristically a lymphoma which has passed through the cortical bone from the medulla but without causing sufficient bone resorption for its presence to be suspected.

The excess new bone usually remodels, but can be trimmed surgically if it fails to do so. New dentures are made and the patient instructed to wash them and the mouth thoroughly after each meal and not to wear them at night.

INFANTILE CORTICAL HYPEROSTOSIS—CAFFEY'S DISEASE OF BONE

This rare condition affects infants of less then six months of age, often at around three months. The child becomes irritable and ceases to take an interest in food. There is a low fever of about $38°C$ ($100\cdot4°F$) and a marked anaemia occurs. Swelling develops around the eyes and often bilaterally over the mandible. Other swellings may affect a limb over the long bones, the clavicle or even the scapula. The nasal bones and bones of the skull are occasionally involved. The child's general illness, temperature and the bony swellings suggest acute osteomyelitis. There is a markedly raised white cell count with a predominance of polymorphonuclear leucocytes and a raised ESR. If the rami of the mandible are involved parotitis may be suspected.

The swellings have a deep, woody, hard and tender component which is fixed to the underlying bone and produced by the periosteal reaction. The overlying soft tissues are oedematous but freely mobile and lack the induration and dusky redness associated with acute osteomyelitis. Nor are they bruised in appearance as would follow trauma. The regional lymph nodes are not enlarged as would be expected if the condition was infective in origin.

Histologically there is acute inflammation with deposition of subperiosteal new bone. The bony trabeculae and fibrous tissue extend out beyond the periosteum into the surrounding soft tissue and muscle. There may be a thrombocytosis with a danger of hypercoagulability or a thrombocytopenia.

INFLAMMATORY DISEASES OF BONE

Radiology

Some two to three weeks after the swellings have become evident suitable radiographs will demonstrate the subperiosteal new bone and this is frequently deposited in layers. There may be a substantial degree of destruction of the original bone.

Treatment

The general condition of the infant slowly improves though there may be relapses and new bones involved. During some three to six months the affected bones are remodelled except where the epiphyses are involved. Mostly spontaneous cure has occurred within nine months of the onset but occasionally it may take two years.

Several writers have drawn attention to a familial incidence suggesting inheritance by an autosomal dominant gene. Although bacteria or a virus have been suggested no organism has been isolated.

In the absence of a known cause rational treatment is difficult. Massive doses of prednisolone for a desperately ill child have been used and also penicillin. Analgesics and general supportive treatment including treatment of the anaemia are important.

NON-ACCIDENTAL INJURY IN INFANTS

There can be a resemblance between the presentation of these infants and those with Caffey's disease. The battered baby may present with widespread traumatic periostitis often associated with avulsed or loosened teeth. The infant may also sustain intracapsular condylar fractures with pain and disturbed occlusion. The long bones suffer fractures, dislocations and epiphyseal cartilage damage.

Treatment

Admission to hospital for careful assessment is of primary importance. The lesions usually require minimal active treatment. However, although usually presented as an accident it is important to realize this problem is the result of psychopathological parental trauma and the case should be reported immediately to the general practitioner and through him to a responsible social worker. Without intervention the child may be killed.

NEOPLASTIC DISEASE

It is often forgotten that metastatic carcinoma, especially from prostate, neuroblastoma, lymphomas or local primary neoplasms such as Ewing's sarcoma may produce swelling of a bone with pain and pyrexia, bone destruction and periosteal reaction and may simulate an osteomyelitis. In any patient where the progress of the disease is in any way atypical, or the response to antibiotics poor, a biopsy should be done with tissue sent for both histological and microbiological investigation.

SUGGESTED READING

Alling C. C. (1959) Post-extraction osteomyelitic syndrome. *Dent. Clin. North Am.* 621–636.
Barba W. P. and Freriks D. J. (1953) Familial occurrence of cortical hyperostosis in utero. *J. Pediatr.* **42**, 141–146.
Birn H. (1973) Etiology and pathogenesis of fibrinolytic alveolitis ('dry socket'). *Int. J. Oral Surg.* **2**, 211–267.
Boerema I. (1964) Hyperbaric oxygen. *Proc. R. Soc. Med.* **57**, 817–818.
Bradley J. C. (1972) Age changes in the vascular supply of the mandible. *Br. Dent. J.* **132**, 142–144.
Brull M. J. and Feingold M. (1974) Autosomal dominant inheritance of Caffe's disease. *Birth Defects* **10**, 139–146.
Caffe J. (1957) Infantile cortical hyperstosis: a review of the clinical and radiographic features. *Proc. R. Soc. Med.* **50**, 347–354.
Caffe J. and Silverman W. A. (1945) Infantile cortical hyperostosis. Preliminary report of a new syndrome. *Am. J. Roent.* **54**, 1–6.
Chapotel A. B. (1930) Tuberculose mandibulaire. *Rev. Odont.* **51**, 444–448.
Coffin F. (1973) The control of radiation caries. *Br. J. Radiol.* **46**, 365–368.
Cohen M. M. (1949) Osteomyelitis of the maxilla in the newborn. *Oral Surg.* **2**, 50–52.
Dearden W. F. (1901) The causation of phosphorus necrosis. *Br. Med. J.* **2**, 408–411.
Garre C. (1893) Uber besondere Farmen und Folgezunstande der akuten Infektionen Ostoemyelitis. *Beitr. Klin. Chir.* **10**, 241–245.
Grime, P. D., Bowerman, J. E. and Weller, P. J. (1990) Gentamicin impregnated polymethylmethacrylate (PMMA) beads in the treatment of primary chronic osteomyelitis of the mandible. *Br. J. Oral Maxillofac. Surg.* **28**, 367–374.
Heslop I. H. (1968) Syphilitic osteomyelitic of the mandible. *Br. J. Oral Surg.* **6**, 59–63.
Heslop I. H. and Rowe N. L. (1956) Metastatic osteomyelitis involving the maxilla and mandible. *Dent. Pract. Dent. Rec.* **6**, 202–206.
Holman G. H. (1962) Infantile cortical hyperostosis: a review. *Q. Rev. Pediatr.* **17**, 24–31.
Jarrett A. S. (1946) The risks of high pressure oxygen therapy. *Proc. R. Soc. Med.* **57**, 820–823.
Juniper R. P. (1982) Caffe's disease. *Br. J. Oral Surg.* **20**, 281–287.
Kennon R. and Hallum J. W. (1944) Modern phosphorous caries and necrosis. *Br. Dent. J.* **76**, 321–330.
Lewars P. H. D. (1971) Chronic periostitis in the mandible underneath artificial dentures. *Br. J. Oral Surg.* **8**, 264–269.
MacGregor A. J. (1968) Aetiology of dry socket: A clinical investigation. *Br. J. Oral Surg.* **6**, 49–58.
Mainous E. G., Boyne P. J. and Hart G. B. (1973) Elimination of sequestra and

healing of osteoradionecrosis of the mandible after hyperbaric oxygen therapy. *J. Oral Surg.* **31**, 336–339.
Major G. S. and Bononi S. (1939) Osteomyelitis of the jaws following acute mercury poisoning. *Am. J. Orthod.* **25**, 82–84.
Marx R. E. (1983) Osteoradionecrosis. A new concept of its pathophysiology. *J. Maxillofac. Surg.* **41**, 283–288.
Marx R. E. (1983) A new concept in the treatment of osteonecrosis. *J. Maxillofac. Surg.* **41**, 351–357.
Marx E. (1922) Eye symptoms due to osteomyelitis of the superior maxilla in infants. *Br. J. Ophthalmol.* **6**, 25–26.
McCash C. R. and Rowe N. L. (1953) Acute osteomyelitis of the maxilla in infancy. *J. Bone Jt Surg.* **35B**, 22–26.
Meng C. M. (1940) Tuberculosis of the mandible. *J. Bone Jt Surg.* **22**, 17–19.
Ritzau M. (1973) The prophylactic use of tranexamic acid (cyclokapron) in alveolitis sicca dolorosa. *Int. J. Oral Surg.* **2**, 196–198.
Rood J. P. and Murgatroyd D. (1980) Metronidazole in the prevention of dry sockets. *Br. J. Oral Surg.* **17**, 62–70.
Rowe N. L. and Heslop I. M. (1957) Periostitis and osteomyelitis of the mandible in childhood. *Br. Dent. J.* **103**, 67–68.
Rud J. (1970) Removal of impacted lower third molars with acute pericoronitis and necrotising gingivitis. *Br. J. Oral Surg.* **7**, 153–159.
Smith G. (1964) The present position of hyperbaric oxygen therapy. *Proc. R. Soc. Med.* **57**, 818–820.
Weiss R. W. and Lewis T. M. (1969) Infantile cortical hyperostosis: a study to determine if residual deformities exist in mandibles. *J. Dent. Child.* **36**, 441–445.
Winiker-Bland E. and Biederman F. (1969) *Rontgendiagnostik in der Kiefer-Gesichts-Chirurgie.* Ch. 9, p. 22. Berlin: Volk und Gesundheit.

CHAPTER 8

THE CONTROL OF INFECTIONS

Chemotherapeutic agents were originally antimicrobial drugs which were manufactured entirely by chemical synthesis. Antibiotics were substances which had been synthesized by living organisms. Once the chemical structure of these antibiotics was known, and the way in which they interfered with microbial reproduction or metabolism was understood, the way was open for the modification of the original molecule either to enhance its effectiveness or to increase the range of susceptible organisms. In some cases chemical synthesis has replaced biological methods of production. The sulphonamides are still referred to as chemotherapeutic agents but all the others are now generally classed as antibiotics irrespective of their current method of preparation.

The term chemotherapy is also now used for the drug treatment of malignant neoplasms. Paradoxically some of the drugs come from biological sources. In this chapter synthetic anti-infective agents, with the exception of the sulphonamides, will be grouped with those from a biological source as antibiotics.

The following groups of anti-infective agents will be discussed:

1. Antibiotics
2. Sulphonamides
3. Antifungal agents
4. Antiviral agents
5. Vaccines and antisera
6. Disinfectants (antiseptics).

THE PRINCIPLES OF ANTIBIOTIC THERAPY

1. Antibiotic therapy is no substitute for surgery. Pus must be drained, infected teeth extracted or their pulpal dead space eliminated by root-canal therapy. Similarly foreign bodies and infected non-vital tissues such as sloughs or sequestra must be removed. Attempts to treat such conditions by antibiotic therapy will lead to prolonged or recurrent infective states with a gradual replacement of common sensitive organisms by uncommon insensitive ones.

2. The antibiotic used should be appropriate to the anticipated organisms, e.g. whereas most oral organisms are susceptible to benzyl-

penicillin, osteomyelitis caused by penicillin resistant *Staphylococcus aureus* will require flucloxacillin, sometimes combined with sodium fusidate. Narrow-spectrum antibiotic therapy avoids superinfection with resistant organisms which follows the indiscriminate use of a broad-spectrum drug.

3. Where possible samples of pus, saliva, blood, urine, etc., should be examined for the infective organisms which are tested against a range of antibiotics for maximum sensitivity. Where this is impossible it may be necessary to guess the appropriate drug from previous clinical experience. Similarly such a blind choice may be employed after taking the specimen but prior to obtaining the result from the microbiology laboratory.

4. As host defence mechanisms assist the antibiotic in eliminating microbial pathogens, bactericidal drugs are not always essential, except in the management of infective endocarditis or with immunosuppressed patients.

5. Antibiotics should not be used as diagnostic agents in the management of clinical problems, such as enigmatic pain where there is a temptation to assume the cause to be an undiagnosed site of infection. This is then treated with serial courses of antibiotics, each one producing short periods of placebo relief but ultimately a complex confusing picture. Similarly they should not be used blindly as antipyretics.

6. Bacterial resistance may result from inadequate antibiotic therapy, i.e. too small a dose for too short a time, or superinfection with other organisms, particularly where inadequate surgery has been carried out—for instance, a failure to remove dead tissue or eliminate a pus-containing dead space.

7. Apart from the right choice of drug, the appropriate dosage, mode and frequency of administration are important. With severe infection a loading dose, i.e. a larger initial dose is useful. Many antibiotics are well absorbed from the gut even in very ill patients. However, initial administration intramuscularly or intravenously ensures an adequate blood level. It is unfair to prescribe frequent intramuscular administration particularly when the intravenous route can be used with a patient receiving intravenous fluid. The drug should not be changed until adequate time for evidence of effectiveness or ineffectiveness has been allowed, i.e. 48–72 hours. Similarly after successful resolution of the infection, treatment should be continued for a further 48–72 hours.

8. Two or more antibiotics should not be used simultaneously unless antagonism has been excluded.

9. Where a patient is hypersensitive to a drug, i.e. develops a rash to penicillin, an alternative drug must be used. However, it is important to establish that a description of 'allergy' is a true one. Often a patient acquires the label of being allergic after attributing manifestation of the illness to the drug. A failure to confirm true allergy may exclude the patient from valuable therapy.

ANTIBIOTIC PREPARATIONS
Penicillin

The penicillins are still the least toxic and clinically the most useful group of antibiotics. Many can be given by mouth as well as intramuscularly or intravenously and are bactericidal in action. They are principally active against Gram-positive and Gram-negative cocci, most Gram-positive bacilli, *Actinomyces israeli* and *Borrelia vincenti*. Resistant microbes include most strains of *Staphylococcus aureus*, some strains of *Neisseria gonorrhoea*, *Streptococcus faecalis* and occasional strains of '*Strep. viridans*'.

Benzylpenicillin (penicillin G, crystalline penicillin)

An aqueous solution may be administered intramuscularly or intravenously for most orofacial infections. The maximum concentration in the serum is reached within 15 to 30 minutes of injection using an intramuscular dose of 300–600 mg (500 000–1 000 000 units). This may be given 12-hourly. The frequency of injection can be reduced by using long acting depot preparations containing procaine penicillin such as Triplopen (Glaxo)—penicillin G 475 mg. Although benethamine penicillin's action is considered to last over a period of 72 hours the blood level is low and therefore this preparation is best given intramuscularly daily. It is useful as a single preparation is best given intramuscularly daily. It is useful as a single injection prophylaxis against endocarditis. Unfortunately, the procaine component may induce an allergic reaction which would be indistinguishable from that to the penicillin itself.

Phenoxymethylpenicillin (penicillin V) is acid resistant and therefore can be taken by mouth. A satisfactory blood level may be achieved by 500 mg, 6-hourly, taken half an hour before meals.

Amoxycillin

Amoxycillin is a broad-spectrum antibiotic which has superseded ampicillin. It is acid resistant and therefore can be given by mouth. Its range of activity includes not only Gram-positive organisms but Gram-negative bacilli and anaerobes other than bacteroides fragilis. The dose can be 500 mg, 8-hourly, orally or intramuscularly. It can also be given intravenously. It is used principally for lower respiratory tract and urinary infections, but it has also become invaluable as a high dose (3 g) oral endocarditis prophylaxis when given 60 minutes prior to surgery because of its excellent absorption and minimal side effects (*see* p. 222).

Flucloxacillin

Flucloxacillin is acid stable and can be given orally, intramuscularly or intravenously. The usual dose is 250 mg, 6-hourly. It is not destroyed by penicillinase (beta-lactamase) producing *Staph. aureus* for which it should be exclusively employed. In severe staphylococcal endocarditis, pneumonia or osteomyelitis it is given in high dosage, sometimes with fusidic acid or gentamycin.

Carbenicillin

Carbenicillin is used for serious Gram-negative infections and is active against *Proteus vulgaris* and some *Pseudomonas aeruginosa,* dose 2 g i.m. or i.v., 4–6-hourly. For severe septicaemia 30 g may be infused intravenously over 24 hours with 1 g probenecid orally 8-hourly in order to reduce renal excretion and so maintain blood levels. Newer similar penicillins such as ticarcillin and piperacillin are now available and may be given with an aminoglycoside such as gentamicin or tobramycin. However, when resistant strains of *P. aeruginosa* or Klebsiella appear in the orofacial region it is often due to a lack of adequate surgery and the indiscriminate use of broad-spectrum antibiotics, as for instance with infected bone grafts with discharging sinuses. Here no antibiotics, or simply metronidazole with the use of frequent hypochlorite packs, is preferable to 'heavy weight' antibiotics.

Adverse Reactions

Penicillins are remarkably free from toxic effects and despite their widespread use, fewer than 5 per cent of patients suffer hypersensitivity reactions. Such reactions occur most commonly in atopic individuals, i.e. those who give a history of eczema, asthma, urticaria and other food or drug allergies. The allergen is the penicillin nucleus and is therefore common to all members of the group.

Sensitivity usually manifests itself as an erythematous maculopapular rash or irritant urticaria. Angioedema and anaphylaxis characterized by bronchospasm, laryngospasm and hypotension are exceedingly uncommon.

Where the use of the drug is highly desirable and a history of allergy uncertain, a trial dose using an oral preparation may be acceptable.

Occasionally patients with infectious mononucleosis suffer an erythematous rash when administered ampicillin or amoxycillin. This is a specific drug reaction and does not imply hypersensitivity under other circumstances.

Clavulanic acid

Available as 125 mg potassium clavulanate in combination with 250 mg amoxycillin it protects the beta-lactam antibiotic from destruction by some beta-lactamase producing bacteria such as *E. coli,* Klebsiella and other Gram-negative bacilli.

Cephalosporins

This large family of antibiotics with low toxicity and wide range of activity are in some respects related to penicillin and have a beta-lactam nucleus. They exert a bactericidal effect by interfering with cell wall synthesis and are usually active against all common Gram-positive cocci including penicillinase-producing strains of staphylococci. Action against Gram-negative bacilli is variable and if these organisms are important, sensitivity testing is required. Cefuroxime is active against both *Staph. aureus* and *Haemophilus influenzae*.

Some cross sensitivity (up to 10 per cent) may occur in patients allergic to penicillin, although this is only a contraindication to use when a clear history of penicillin allergy is obtained. Adverse effects include urticarial rashes and nephrotoxicity.

There is some controversy as to the clinical value of this large family of drugs. It may be argued that narrow-spectrum specific antibiotics are often effective in most situations.

Dosage is Cerufoxime 750 mg i.m. or i.v., 8-hourly; orally cephalexin 250–500, 6-hourly, given half an hour before food.
half an hour before food.

Erythromycin

This important macrolide antibiotic has an antibacterial spectrum similar to penicillin. Its activity may also include *Staph. aureus*. There is no apparent cross hypersensitivity in individuals who are allergic to penicillin and it is therefore a useful alternative drug. Its action is bacteriostatic but at higher blood levels bactericidal activity is produced. Toxic effects are low although gastrointestinal irritation consisting of nausea, abdominal pain with occasional vomiting and diarrhoea may also occur.

Erythromycin estolate causes jaundice.

Erythromycin stearate 500 mg (Erythrocin 500; Abbott) may be given 12-hourly. Erythromycin succinate suspension is useful in children or adults with intermaxillary fixation 250–500 mg, 6-hourly. Erythromycin stearate is a useful oral loading dose for the prophylaxis of endocarditis in adults who are allergic to penicillin.

Erythromycin lactobionate may be administered intravenously 300 mg, 4–8-hourly.

Metronidazole

This is a narrow-spectrum antibiotic active specifically against anaerobes. With improved culture techniques there has been an increased awareness of the pathogenic role of anaerobes such as bacteroides either alone or in conjunction with other organisms in the production of soft tissue infections. It is active against bacteroides, *Clostridium difficile* and some protozoa such as trichomonas and *Giardia lamblia*. It has proved highly effective in

THE CONTROL OF INFECTIONS

the management of most oral surgical infections in addition to acute ulcerative gingivitis.

Metronidazole is well absorbed when taken by mouth and can be given either 400 mg, 12-hourly, or 200 mg, 8-hourly. An alternative regime, particularly when the oral preparation is impossible postoperatively, especially with intermaxillary fixation, are suppositories 0·5–1·0 g t.d.s. Metronidazole intravenous infusion 500 mg, 12-hourly, is also very useful. The drug penetrates abscesses well and crosses the blood–brain barrier.

The side-effects include an unpleasant metallic taste, nausea and gastrointestinal upsets but very rarely rashes. Prolonged use, i.e. more than 30 g, may produce a reversible neuropathy. Some patients experience an 'antabuse' effect with alcohol.

Aminoglycosides

These antibiotics are bactericidal and are most effective against Gram-negative bacilli, but as they are poorly absorbed from the gut are best administered by injection. Unfortunately, the principal toxic effect is to the eighth nerve, producing vestibular damage or deafness which may be preceded by headache, nausea, vomiting, nystagmus and ataxia. Therefore, blood levels should be monitored, especially if renal excretion is impaired.

Streptomycin Sulphate

Streptomycin sulphate is given intramuscularly and can be painful. Dosage is 1 g a day as a single dose or 0·5 g twice a day. Gentamicin: serum peak concentrations should be maintained at not greater than 5 mg/l, but trough levels should preferably not fall below 1·5 mg/l.

This antibiotic is active against *Pseudomonas aeruginosa, E. coli,* proteus and resistant staphylococci but is probably best reserved for Gram-negative septicaemia in combination with penicillin or with metronidazole. It is not active against anaerobes. Its principal use is as an adjunctive prophylactic antibiotic in the prevention of high-risk endocarditis. The dose is 3 mg/kg body weight a day given intramuscularly in 3 equally divided doses if renal function is normal, or 80–120 mg as a stat dose.

Neomycin

Neomycin is used topically or to decontaminate the gut. It is of value as a cream for cutaneous *Staph. aureus* infections but resistant strains are possible with widespread continued use.

Tetracyclines

Tetracyclines have the broadest antimicrobial spectrum. They interfere with bacterial protein synthesis but unfortunately are bacteriostatic and resistance to them frequently develops. They are active against many

Gram-positive and Gram-negative pathogenic bacteria strains except for those of *Pseudomonas aeruginosa*.

The tetracyclines are probably best used for minor infective conditions in penicillin allergic oral and antral cases. Being only partially absorbed from the gut, sufficient concentrations remain in the intestine to alter the flora which may give rise to local complications such as discomfort, diarrhoea and suppression of vitamin K synthesis. Additional problems include heartburn, nausea and vomiting due to gastric mucosal irritation, skin rashes and photosensitization.

Absorption is reduced by chelation to calcium in dairy products, and even more so with antacids and iron preparations. The plasma half-life varies considerably with the tetracycline and is increased in renal failure except for doxycycline which is not eliminated by the kidney and therefore may be used with impaired renal function.

Superinfection may occur with *Candida albicans* producing a sore mouth or thrush in addition to a black hairy tongue, diarrhoea and pruritus ani. Further superinfection with staphylococci, proteus or pseudomonas causing a fulminating fatal enteritis is also possible if used in heavy prolonged dosage. Oral, anal and vaginal superinfection may be avoided by concurrent nystatin or amphotericin tablets and vaginal suppositories. There is no firm evidence that vitamin B preparations may prevent or arrest alimentary tract symptoms. Tetracyclines are selectively chelated by the calcium of growing bones and teeth both in the foetus and children causing yellow or brownish discoloration of the enamel and in some cases enamel hypoplasia. Therefore tetracycline therapy should be avoided in children until twelve years of age.

Dosage is tetracycline capsules or tablets 250 mg, 6-hourly. Demeclocycline is more readily absorbed from the gut and excreted more slowly and therefore 300 mg may be given 12-hourly. Similarly doxycycline 100 mg daily may be used.

Parenteral administration is best by intermittent intravenous infusion of 1 g of tetracycline or oxytetracycline in 0·9 per cent sodium chloride each 24 hours, divided into 2 or 4 doses each infused over 5–10 minutes. Intramuscular injections are painful.

Chloramphenicol

Chloramphenicol is a broad-spectrum antibiotic with good tissue and CSF penetration. It is chiefly active against *Haemophilus influenzae,* pertussis, salmonellae and other coliforms. Its use is limited by a tendency to cause an idiosyncratic fatal aplastic anaemia which occurs in about 1 in 50 000 treatments. Bone marrow depression which is dose related is also possible. In neonates circulatory collapse, the so-called Gray's syndrome, can occur due to failure of the liver to conjugate the drug and of the kidney to excrete it producing toxic high plasma levels. However, it is still useful for certain conditions such as head injuries particularly where skull fractures involve the petrous temporal bone and external auditory meatus where it may be given with metronidazole.

It is well absorbed from the gut and concentrations in the CSF in the absence of inflammation are 50 per cent of the plasma levels. However, where there is meningeal inflammation the concentration approximately equals those of the plasma. Administration by intravenous infusion is possible, but absorption is poor by the intramuscular route.

Dosage is chloramphenicol capsules 500 mg orally, 6-hourly. Medication should not extend beyond 14 days. Intramuscular or intravenously 1 g may be given every 6–8 hours.

Chloramphenicol eye ointment introduced into the conjunctival sac is valuable in preventing infection where there has been local trauma or surgery and should be applied 6-hourly.

Clindamycin and Lincomycin

Clindamycin is a chlorinated derivative of lincomycin. They both have similarities in antibacterial spectrum of action to benzylpenicillin but are also effective against staphylococci and bacteroides.

The drug is well absorbed and widely distributed throughout the body except the CSF. Unfortunately, it may not only produce diarrhoea but also a devastating pseudomembranous enterocolitis due to superinfection with *Clostridium difficile.* Under these circumstances the drug must be stopped immediately and the patient treated with oral vancomycin or metronidazole. The fluid and electrolyte balance must be carefully maintained. Occasionally a colostomy is necessary in the management of this condition, therefore the drug should not be employed without careful consideration.

It may be useful in staphylococcal bone and joint disease where the infecting strain of *Staph. aureus* is resistant to other antibiotics and the patient is allergic to flucloxacillin.

Dosage is 150–300 mg, 6-hourly, orally; 0·6–2·7 g daily in 2–4 divided doses i.m.; or 15–40 mg/kg daily in 3–4 divided doses by slow i.v. infusion.

Fucidin

Fucidic acid is a steroid antibiotic used mainly against penicillinase-producing staphylococci. It is valuable for overwhelming staphylococcal infections and is best used in combination with erythromycin, flucloxacillin or rifampicin.

The drug penetrates bone and abscesses well and so has an obvious application in osteomyelitis. Another use is as a gel or ointment for staphylococcal infections of the skin, but this should be avoided in hospital in-patients to present the risk of generating and spreading resistant strains of *Staph. aureus.* It is administered by mouth 500 mg, 8-hourly, and is well absorbed, but can cause gastrointestinal disturbances.

Vancomycin

Vancomycin is a bactericidal drug active against Gram-positive cocci. It is not absorbed by the gut and has to be administered intravenously, but because of nephrotoxicity and eighth nerve damage it has limited use. This should be preceded by an antihistamine such as chlorpheniramine maleate 10 mg intravenously to prevent troublesome histamine release.

The main indications include the prophylaxis or treatment of *Strep. viridans* endocarditis where previous antibiotic therapy or allergy contraindicates other drugs (*see* p. 223). It may be given by mouth 0·5 g to 1 g, 6-hourly, in the management of pseudomembranous colitis due to *Clostridium difficile* which can arise following antibiotic therapy with such drugs as clindamycin.

SULPHONAMIDES

Sulphonamides inhibit the bacterial synthesis of folic acid from para-amino benzoic acid, a compound for which they act as a competitive inhibitor. By combining the sulphonamide, sulphamethoxazole, with trimethoprim, an agent which inhibits the conversion of folic to folinic acid which is important for the bacterial synthesis of DNA and RNA, a bactericidal combination co-trimoxazole is produced from two bacteriostatic agents. Co-trimoxazole (Bactrim or Septrin) is active against *Strep. pyogenes* and most staphylococci and haemophili. It is also useful in managing intermittent acute episodes in post-irradiation osteomyelitis in osteoradionecrosis, or *Actinobacillus actinomycetemcomitans* in mixed actinomycotic infections with penicillin.

Prolonged therapy may lead to macrocytic anaemia due to the inhibition of conversion of folic to folinic acid and rarely the sulphonamide may produce marrow depression or selective blood dyscrasia. Allergic reactions are uncommon but include rashes, exfoliative dermatitis, Stevens–Johnson syndrome, fever, hepatitis, serum sickness-like syndrome, polyarteritis nodosa and peripheral neuritis.

Tablets consist of trimethoprim 80 mg and sulphamethoxazole 400 mg (paediatric tablets contain 20 mg and 100 mg respectively). The dose is 2 tablets 12-hourly, these may be dissolved in water and are therefore useful with patients in intermaxillary fixation. Intravenous and intramuscular formulations are also available.

Sulphadiazine, because of its ability to penetrate the blood–brain barrier and achieve high CSF levels, is commonly used in the prophylaxis of post-traumatic meningeal infection which is discussed on p. 224. A loading dose of 3 g is followed by 1 g, 6-hourly, for 7–10 days, depending on the control of the CSF leakage. The drug may be given intravenously 1 g, 6-hourly, but in order to prevent crystalluria and renal damage a fluid intake of at least 2 litres a day must be maintained.

THE CONTROL OF INFECTIONS
ANTIFUNGAL DRUGS

Nystatin is used topically for oral candida infections and can be given as an oral pastille or suspension 6-hourly, but has probably been superseded by amphotericin B. This is usually given as lozenges 10 mg or a suspension 6-hourly. These drugs are poorly absorbed from the gut and therefore require to be given intravenously for systemic mycotic infections. However, this should be undertaken by a specialist in the management of such conditions.

Alternative antifungal agents which may be applied topically include miconazole and clotrimazole. These are both imidazoles which inhibit the synthesis of ergosteral which is a component of fungal plasma membrane but which is not required by mammalian cells. They prevent candidal yeasts developing hyphae and enhance their phagocytosis. However, it is worth noting that the most common oral fungal infection by *Candida albicans* is invariably secondary to some underlying factor such as iron deficiency, diabetes, dehydration, steroid treatment, cytotoxic drug therapy or radiotherapy, or an immune deficiency. Where possible these conditions will also require attention.

ANTIVIRAL DRUGS

Idoxuridine is a competitive inhibitor of thymidine which is necessary for the synthesis of DNA. It is therefore useful in the control of DNA viruses such as herpes simplex, herpes zoster and vaccinia.

Idoxuridine 5 per cent dissolved in dimethyl sulphoxide penetrates the skin but must be applied frequently, i.e. 1–2 hourly. Idoxuridine 0·1 per cent in purified water is used for oral mucosal and eye lesions.

Topical application is contraindicated in pregnancy in case the absorbed drug has a teratogenic effect on the foetus.

A valuable antiviral drug which again is effective against herpes simplex viruses I and II and varicella zoster virus is acyclovir. Acyclovir is phosphated to the monophosphate by viral coded thymidine kinase and then converted to the active triphosphate by cellular enzymes. Thus the active form is only found in infected cells. Acyclovir triphosphate acts as an inhibitor and substrate for herpes-specified DNA polymerase, so preventing further viral DNA synthesis. A few herpes viruses do not convert acyclovir to the monophosphate and are resistant to the drug.

Zovirax cream contains 5 per cent acyclovir in a white aqueous cream base and is applied to herpes labialis lesions 5 times a day for 5 days. Preferably it should be applied as soon as prodromal itching and burning appears and before vesicles form. The earlier in the evolution of the lesion it is applied the greater the benefit in shortening the episode. The interval between and frequency of new lesions is also reduced.

ORAL SURGERY, PART 1

THE CLINICAL MANAGEMENT OF INFECTION

Soft-tissue infection, alveolar abscess, sialoadenitis, pericoronitis and postoperative infections—many of these infections not only contain the commonly recognized streptococci and lactobacilli, but also anaerobes such as bacteroides, fusobacteria and veillonella. The role of these anaerobres in oral infections has been well observed in acute ulcerative gingivitis and in cancrum oris where *Bacteroides melaninogenicus* may be an important pathogen. Hence with appropriate surgical management a choice may be made between the narrow-spectrum anti-anaerobe metronidazole and penicillin given by mouth or parenterally if oral administration is not reliable or possible. The acute phase of severe infections can be treated with intermittent intravenous antibiotics, given as a bolus 6-hourly for the first 48–72 hours.

Erythromycin, a cephalosporin or tetracycline may be satisfactory alternatives. Where possible culture and sensitivity should always be carried out to confirm the appropriate antibiotic therapy, but, an immediate Gram-stained direct smear can be of considerable value before culture and sensitivity results are available.

Osteomyelitis

Acute osteomyelitis is now an uncommon condition in most European countries and is usually caused by β-lactamase secreting staphylococci which require the use of flucloxacillin, or erythromycin with or without fusidic acid or clindamycin. With adequate surgery antibiotic therapy should not be necessary for more than 2 weeks after drainage or removal of any sequestrum.

Chronic osteomyelitis requires thorough debridement of necrotic bone enabling central areas of dead space to be drained. This process of decortication should be supplemented by metronidazole and any appropriate antibiotic suggested by the microbiology.

Inadequately treated osteomyelitis, especially if the patient is receiving long-term broad-spectrum antibiotics, will give rise to colonization with exotic resistant organisms requiring even more exotic antibiotics. It may be wise to discontinue all antibiotic treatment except for the use of metronidazole and employ traditional surgical techniques such as antiseptic packs intraorally, e.g. Whitehead's varnish (iodoform ether varnish BPC) or bismuth iodoform and paraffin paste on ribbon gauze. When packs are used they should be changed as frequently as possible. Extraorally, sinuses should be irrigated and packed with hypochlorite solution (Eusol or Milton solution) on ribbon gauze. The external packs should be changed 2–4 times daily. Surprisingly good results may be achieved with this simple technique, particularly where sophisticated laboratory facilities are not available. The same regime applies to infected bone grafts which may be saved by such methods.

Osteoradionecrosis is a chronic ischaemic necrosis without the benefit of viable bone forming or bone removing vascular granulation tissue. Hence the separation of the dead from living bone is exceedingly slow and in many cases does not take place. The patient may be untroubled by the presence of a sequestrum protruding through the mucosa which can be trimmed and left as a protection for the underlying vital bone. Sinuses can be packed, whilst providing antibiotic therapy such as metronidazole, penicillin or co-trimoxazole for acute infective exacerbations. If infection is eliminated healing may be enhanced with hyperbaric oxygen, although this requires at least two hours at 2 atmospheres of oxygen 5 times a week for 4 weeks and is often difficult to arrange.

More radical therapy involves the excision of the necrotic bone leaving a defect and deformity. However, revascularization of the area using a temporalis muscle flap appears to be of significant value. This technique may also enable bone defects to be grafted with cancellous bone which will require to be secured in place using either lower border wires and prolonged (8 weeks) intermaxillary fixation or a bone plate and 4 weeks intermaxillary fixation. However, it is important to achieve good soft tissue coverage with a perfect intraoral seal using either two layer closure or vertical mattress sutures. Where soft tissue coverage is not available locally a vascular anastomosed 'free' composite flap such as the forearm radius flap, or an iliac crest flap based in the internal circumflex iliac artery, can be invaluable for reconstruction.

Actinomycosis

Cervicofacial infections by *Actinomyces israeli* are uncommon but should be suspected when a circumscribed area of cutaneous inflammation persists. Cases appear to follow surgery or the inappropriate treatment of a surgical condition such as an infected tooth with short courses of antibiotics. This chronic condition may occasionally also harbour in addition *Actinobacillus actinomycetemcomitans* or be a combination of *Actinomyces viscosis* and *Staph. aureus*.

Any underlying surgical problem must be dealt with, and the patient treated with continuous phenoxymethyl penicillin 500mg, 6-hourly, amoxycillin 500mg, 8-hourly, or tetracycline 250mg, 6-hourly, for at least 30 days. Co-trimoxazole may be required in addition for the actinobacillus or fusidic acid or flucloxacillin for the *Staph. aureus*. The poor penetration of the sulphur granules which may be identified by Gram staining and the slow rate of division of the organism determine the length of treatment. Anaerobic culture for 10 days may be required for identification.

Actinomycotic periostitis or osteomyelitis may require considerably longer therapy lasting for 3–6 months which can only be gauged by the clinical response.

Sinusitis

The establishment of drainage is essential and may be facilitated where the problem is merely due to congested mucous membrane by inhalations of Friars Balsam, Tinct. Benz. Co. or Karvol capsules. *Strep. pneumoniae, Haemophilus influenzae, Staph. aureus,* anaerobes and viruses may be the causative organisms and initially amoxycillin or erythromycin should be tried. However, the antibiotic therapy of persistent infections should be reassessed with culture and sensitivity testing and any surgery for correcting drainage should be carried out.

PROPHYLACTIC ANTIBIOTIC THERAPY

The concern as to whether prophylactic antibiotics should be used for clean minor oral surgery procedures is based on the fear that resistant strains of organisms may arise in such patients and by cross infection spread to other patients and persist in hospital units. In general this problem only arises when broad-spectrum drugs are used for long periods of time on in-patients. It is particularly likely to arise when other important considerations such as early wound drainage and debridement, careful appropriate surgery and aseptic technique both within the theatre and ward have been ignored. In any surgical situation the possibility of the spread of difficult resistant strains of bacteria from patient to patient must be considered against the possibility of avoidable morbidity.

Guidelines

One important rule is the use where possible of narrow-spectrum antibiotics for the shortest period of time. Metronidazole has been shown to be highly effective in preventing dry socket, and reduces wound breakdown and postoperative morbidity in 3rd molar extractions when given for 3–5 days postoperatively. Similarly the same narrow-spectrum antibiotic has reduced wound breakdown and fistula formation following major resections.

The loss of a bone graft is a surgical disaster, therefore a combination of metronidazole and flucloxacillin or a cephalosporin such as cefuroxime against cutaneous staphylococci and Gram-negative bacilli, immediately preoperative and postoperatively for at least 72 hours, has been of great value. Another regime would be metronidazole and erythromycin.

However, such a regime is no alternative to general surgical cleanliness. Hands should be washed before patients are examined and particularly when moving from patient to patient in a ward. The patient should have a Savlon bath and hair wash early in the morning of the operation day. Teeth should be scaled and polished about a week before the operation and tooth brushing supervised in the ward to see that it is effective. Chlorhexidine mouth washes and Hibitane pastilles to suck before the premedication will reduce the bacterial count in the mouth which can be swabbed out with

THE CONTROL OF INFECTIONS

Physomed when the patient is on the theatre table. Here also the skin is washed again with Savlon solution, dried and meticulously prepared with povidone-iodine solution. Efficient towelling and theatre technique with careful wound closure and suction drainage to prevent haematoma formation are all important. The application of antibiotic powder to bone grafts merely kills off the osteoblasts and reduces the graft viability as does its preservation for more than 1 hour in normal saline (*see* Bone grafting below). A 1 g suppository preoperatively or an infusion of 0·5 g metronidazole i.v. prior to taking the graft should give the bone adequate protection against anaerobic contamination when being manipulated into the mouth wound. Similar precautions apply to skin grafts.

Feeding by fine bore or 12 FG nasogastric tube for 5–7 days postoperatively appears to make an important contribution to intraoral wound healing in major oral surgery. Careful aseptic management of wound dressings and tracheostomy patients on the ward is crucial. Where a tracheostomy stoma is slow to close and continues to discharge, twice daily cleansing with 0·1 per cent aqueous hibitane or hypochlorite solution with a hypochlorite soaked gauze pack is preferable to systemic antibiotics which will rapidly encourage superinfection. Surface infection of moist unhealed wounds, especially those which are granulating and not yet fully covered by epithelium, is inevitable but can be controlled by simple local measures. The infection subsides as the wound heals. Patients with intractable infections with resistant organisms or immunosuppressed patients must be isolated and barrier nursed.

Bacterial endocarditis prophylaxis in patients with defective heart valve disease is an area where empirical attitudes create conflicting recommendations. It is well recognized that many vulnerable patients with defective valves do not suffer endocarditis either following dental extractions or from the evident bacteraemia during mastication, which occurs in the presence of periodontal disease. It is equally baffling when an endocarditis due to oral *Streptococcus viridans* arises in edentulous patients. Despite these enigmas which indicate a currently unrecognized aetiological factor or factors, every care should be taken to identify and protect such patients from a condition which, once established, is difficult to treat successfully. The maintenance of good oral hygiene and the application of 0·5 per cent chlorhexidine or povidone-iodine solution to the gingival margins before dental treatment will reduce the severity of any bacteraemia.

Bactericidal antibiotics should be given in adequate dosage immediately prior to surgery, and continued for the period during which the bacteraemia is anticipated, plus sufficient additional time to destroy those organisms which have been arrested at vulnerable sites.

The patients at risk are those with:

1. Congenital heart disease, apart from uncomplicated atrial septal defects.

2. Rheumatic valvular disease, including that associated with Sydenham's chorea.
3. Prosthetic heart valves and those who have had other forms of cardiac surgery, including those who have pacemaker electrode wires *in situ*.
4. Previous episodes of infective endocarditis.
5. Mitral valve prolapse.

Frequently unrecognized risks are bicuspid aortic valves in the young and degenerative aortic valvular disease in the old. Functional systolic murmurs which are common in children and adolescents do not usually signify heart disease. However, in the absence of a specialist cardiologist's opinion, prophylaxis must be considered to be both useful and harmless.

The main causative group of organisms from oral sources is viridans streptococci. Surgical procedures which create the risk include extractions, scaling, gingivectomy and root-canal therapy. Where a non-vital tooth is considered to be essential for preservation in a low risk patient, root-canal therapy and orthograde root fillings possibly combined with minimal apicectomy and if necessary a retrograde root filling can be carried out. Theoretically the risk to the patient is reduced if this is done in one session, but with high dose amoxycillin cover this is not essential (*see below*).

PROPHYLACTIC REGIMES

Prophylactic regimes as recommended by a Working Party of the British Society for Antimicrobial Chemotherapy (1990) are as follows.

1. Oral Regimes

   a. Amoxycillin 3g 1 hour preoperatively, preferably under supervision. For children under 10, half the adult dose, and one quarter of the adult dose for children under 5.

   b. Where the patient is allergic to penicillin or has received penicillin therapy within the previous month, erythromycin stearate 1·5g 1 hour before the procedure and then 500mg six hours later. As before half doses for children under 10 and quarter-doses for those under 5. If preferred Clindamycin may be used in a 600 mg oral dose one hour before procedure. For children under 10 the dose is 6 mg/kg body weight orally at the same time interval.

2. Parenteral Regimes

Alternative prophylactic parenteral regimes which may be more useful in hospital practice prior to a general anaesthetic are as follows:

   a. Amoxycillin 1g in 2·5ml of 1 per cent lingnocaine hydrochloride (instead of sterile water) given intramuscularly before induction of the anaesthetic followed by 500mg orally six hours later to maintain an adequate blood level. Children under 10 should have half the adult dose.

b. All high-risk adult patients, i.e. those with a previous history of bacterial endocarditis or prosthetic heart valve replacement and who are to be given a general anaesthetic, should be given intramuscular amoxycillin prior to surgery as recommended above together with gentamicin 120 mg given by i.m. or i.v. injection followed by 500 mg amoxycillin by mouth six hours later. In children under 10 who are considered to be high-risk patients, half the adult dose of amoxycillin and 2 mg/kg body weight of the gentamicin.

c. All adults who are allergic to penicillin or who have had penicillin in the previous month and require a general anaesthetic should have vancomycin 1 g by slow intravenous infusion over 20–30 minutes followed by gentamicin 120 mg intravenously before the induction of the anaesthetic. This should be preceded by chlorpheniramine maleate 10 mg intravenously as vancomycin may cause an unpleasant histamine release producing a pruritic rash. Children under 10 should be given vancomycin 20 mg/kg and gentamicin 2 mg/kg, also intravenously.

It is important never to give prolonged antibiotic therapy prior to surgery otherwise opportunist resistant organisms will colonize the mouth. However, repeated short courses of say amoxycillin separated by a month do not appear to cause this problem and should be used for a series of endodontic or periodontal treatments.

In all cases it is important that povidone-iodine be interfaced into the gingival crevice of the teeth under treatment as this reduces the size of the bacteraemia resulting from trauma to the gingival margin.

Prosthetic Heart Valve Patients

Although prosthetic heart valve patients may not be exposed to a higher risk of endocarditis than those with congenital defects or rheumatic heart disease, they do have a greater mortality from this disease and of course may also be on anticoagulant drugs. Particular care should be taken with regard to their dental assessment. With a poor dentition where extractions are anticipated for periodontal disease a dental clearance with the provision of dentures preoperatively is probably the wisest policy.

Coronary Artery or Vein By-pass Patients

Patients who have had coronary artery or vein by-pass operations and those with implanted pacemakers do not appear to represent a special risk for endocarditis.

Arterial Graft Patients

Arterial grafts, particularly those involving the aorta, do not appear to pose a great risk of infection from dental sources. However, an appropriate preoperative dental assessment is wise and within six months of the procedure prophylactic antibiotic cover should be prescribed.

Cardiac Transplant Patients

Cardiac transplants, although rare procedures, involve the suppression of immunity and the long-term administration of drugs which predispose to infection such as corticosteroids and azathioprine. Thus dental disease should be carefully eliminated prior to such surgery and extractions should be carried out taking into consideration the anti-rejection regime together with the use of anticoagulants.

Joint Replacement Patients

The risk of infection of a prosthetic joint must be low because there is no clear evidence to support a connection with dental treatment. The possibility has even been raised that penile prostheses are at risk. Where there is pressure from the patient or surgeon Cephradine 1 g orally or Clindamycin 600 mg orally may be given one hour before treatment of an infected site. Staphylococci, possibly beta-lactam antibiotic resistant, are the main targets of prophylaxis.

Post-traumatic Meningitis

The risk of meningitis following fractures involving the base of skull is difficult to evaluate and much controversy exists in this area as to whether prophylaxis is necessary. It would seem logical to assume that prophylaxis is desirable especially where a cerebrospinal fluid leak has been established. Although it has been traditional to use sulphadiazine because of its ready penetration of the blood–brain barrier this drug is bacteriostatic and it is likely that some of the organisms against which the patient needs protection are resistant to this drug, especially those from the external ear. Furthermore, following trauma and hence inflammation of meninges, amoxycillin or erythromycin probably penetrate into the CSF adequately and provide appropriate bactericidal action.

A more appropriate regime for severe skull fractures, and in particular those compounded into the external ear which may be colonized by staphylococci and Gram-negative bacilli, is a combination of chloramphenicol 0·5 g, 6-hourly, and metronidazole 400 mg, 12-hourly, which should be used especially during the surgical procedure. However, the risks associated with the use of chloramphenicol must be weighed against the danger that the patient faces from the injury and from meningitis, and is small with short-term usage.

Intermaxillary Fixation

Intermaxillary fixation presents problems of drug administration which can be overcome easily as follows:

1. Although most antibiotics may be given intramuscularly it is kinder to the patient to administer them as an intravenous bolus at the required time intervals. This is facilitated both during and immediately after operative procedures when the patient is receiving intravenous fluids. Of course care should be taken to check that the addition of the particular drug to the

infusion solution is appropriate. Drugs such as metronidazole may be given as a 20-minute piggyback infusion.

2. Most antibiotics are available in a syrup form and can be delivered through a nasogastric tube or orally. Metronidazole can also be administered as a rectal suppository 1 g, 8–12-hourly, or children 0·5 g, 8–12-hourly.

Viral Hepatitis

The two most common causes of viral hepatitis are the hepatitis A (HAV) and hepatitis B (HBV) viruses. Although they cause similar illnesses their epidemiology differs. The less common hepatitis C resembles hepatitis B.

HAV contains RNA and is shed in the faeces in large quantities and infection follows ingestion of contaminated food. It has an incubation period of 30–35 days. In the week prior to icterus, the virus is probably also shed in the urine and saliva. Subclinical infections are rare, the mortality rate is low and specific antibodies (anti-HAV) confer life-long immunity.

HBV is a hepa-DNA (DNA containing) virus usually contracted by parenteral inoculation, although infection via mucous membranes such as the conjunctiva may occur. The incubation period is about three months and arthralgia and urticaria may precede the jaundice. The acute illness may be short, perhaps two or three days, and 'flu' like but accompanied by anorexia. This is followed by a prolonged period during which there is a variable degree of malaise with episodes of toxaemia. Frank skin jaundice does not always occur, with the only indication of its presence being dark, frothy urine and a yellow tinge to the sclera. The liver is enlarged and tender and there is a gastrointestinal disturbance. The nature of the infection may be overlooked in some cases and of course subclinical cases occur.

The most important route of transmission is contamination of cuts or scratches on the surgeon's hands by infected blood. However, infection can also be carried in other body fluids, including saliva where the virus may be present in minute quantities, especially if the saliva is mixed with blood.

Sources of Infections

1. *Patients with acute hepatitis type B.* These patients may be infectious for a few weeks before hepatitis is clinically detected. The infection will usually be eliminated soon after the end of the illness, probably within 2–3 months. Dental treatment may be deferred until the patient is shown to be free of infection by testing for the disappearance of HBsAg and the appearance of anti-HBs antibody. HBsAg is a fragment of the viral coat which was formerly called 'Australia antigen'.

2. *Carriers.* A small number of patients become carriers of hepatitis B virus after acute infection. Carriers often do not give a history of hepatitis with or without jaundice and are apparently healthy, although some may have abnormal liver function as shown by biochemical tests. A past history of jaundice (which possibly was obstructive) is not by itself an indication for

HBsAg testing. The presence of the 'e' antigen, HBeAg, a fragment of the viral core, indicates high infectivity.

Incidence of Carriers

In the British population, the carrier rate is approximately 1 : 1000, but there are recognizable groups who have considerably higher carrier rates, and in some countries outside Europe and North America the general carrier rate is very much higher than in Europe and may be as high as 10 per cent.

Special categories in which the carrier rate may be especially high are:

1. Patients from countries other than Western Europe, North America and Australasia, especially from the Far East.
2. Drug addicts.
3. Mentally handicapped children living in institutions.
4. Promiscuous male homosexuals.
5. Patients who have had multiple blood transfusions (particularly if these have been given abroad), or who have received multiple injections of pooled blood products (e.g. haemophiliacs).
6. Patients who are heavily tattooed, particularly in circumstances in which the equipment may have been inadequately sterilized between clients.
7. Patients with chronic liver disease.

Recognition of HBsAg Positive Patients

The presence of HBsAg in the blood is always associated with a risk of transmission of hepatitis B infection. The test for this antigen is easily available. Approximately a quarter of HBsAg positive patients are also positive for HBeAg.

The patients with only surface antigen (HBsAg) are much less likely to transmit their infection than those with both HBsAg and HBeAg. However, while it is recognized that presence of HBeAg indicates high infectivity, it is not thought that this should alter the treatment offered to carriers in general. While patients in the special categories should always be treated with care to prevent cross-infection, the only way to determine the presence of infection is to test for HBsAg. This test can easily be obtained for patients who might be carriers, but it will not be required if the history is of a HAV infection.

Operative Procedures

1. *Precautions to control cross-infection and infection of staff with hepatitis virus, applicable to all patients.* Infection carried by infected instruments and materials should be controlled by routine autoclaving of all instruments between each patient. Note that chlorhexidine and many other commonly used disinfectants are not effective against viruses.

THE CONTROL OF INFECTIONS

For protection the operator must avoid the contamination of his skin with blood. Blood should be regarded as a dangerous material. It is preferable now that gloves should be worn as a routine even when examining mouths. They must be worn regularly during exodontia and for the surgical treatment of patients and are essential on all occasions when handling patients from high-risk groups—*see* (2) below.

2. *Precautions applicable to detected carriers of hepatitis B antigen (HBsAg).* Detected carriers are probably less dangerous than the much larger number of undetected carriers. There is no justification for refusing treatment of HBsAg or HBeAg positive patients, but special care can and must be taken to avoid infection of staff and other patients.

The following suggestions are made:

    a. Infected patients should be treated in a single chair surgery.

    b. Turbine handpieces should not be used for surgical operations as infected aerosols may be formed. Conventional handpieces should be run more slowly, and 'splashy' procedures avoided.

    c. The operators should wear gowns, gloves, surgical masks and spectacles as eye protection.

    d. After the operation, all used instruments should be put in a marked sterilization box for separate cleaning and then autoclaving. Small aliquots of any consumable materials should be dispensed beforehand and the surplus discarded. Blood contaminated swabs should be disposed of in specially coloured bags and doubly bagged. All linen should be bagged for sterilization and laundering.

    e. Where disinfectants are used to clean surfaces and floors, a 10 per cent dilution of household bleach (e.g. Domestos) is recommended (*see* Sterilization and disinfection *below*).

3. *The protection of patients at special risk.* It is important that patients on immunosuppresive drugs, particularly patients having renal dialysis and who are not carriers, should not be infected during any surgical procedures, and treatment of these patients may be best supervised by the dialysis treatment centre staff who are known to be free of infection themselves.

Some renal dialysis patients may have become carriers in which case they should be treated as detected carriers.

Accidents

Any accident involving the penetration of the skin and contamination of the wound with blood from any patient known to be infected with HB virus should be reported at once to a microbiology laboratory. The suspected patient must have a blood examination to determine the possible presence of HBsAg.

In cases of accidental infection of staff from patients shown to be HBsAg positive, hepatitis B immune globulin must be administered as soon as possible, certainly within 2–3 days.

Immunity of Staff

It is known that about 10 per cent of dental surgeons have developed immunity to hepatitis B through previous contact with the virus. Several satisfactory hepatitis B vaccines are available, some produced by genetic engineering technology. They require a series of three intramuscular doses. Dental students, hygienists and dental surgery assistant students should seek active immunisation at the commencement of their training. Any practitioners who are not immune from a previous infection should be actively immunised.

Sterilization or Disposal of Instruments etc.

1. All non-disposable instruments should be cleansed of all traces of saliva, blood or serum and rinsed and sterilized in an autoclave, e.g. at 134°C for 3 minutes, or by hot air, e.g. at 160°C for 1 hour.

2. After use, all used disposable instruments should be placed in an impervious container (for sharp instruments this should be of metal or thick cardboard) and incinerated or, if appropriate, autoclaved.

Disinfection

1. All instruments that cannot be sterilized by heat should be disinfected by immersion in a suitable disinfectant solution (*see below*) for at least 1 hour. This is less satisfactory than sterilization by heat.

2. All working surfaces should be disinfected after use by wiping with disinfectants containing 1 per cent of available chlorine, or, if made of metal, with aldehyde disinfectants.

3. Bulky equipment cannot be sterilized by heat and hypochlorite solutions will corrode metal equipment, so the latter must be disinfected with an aldehyde disinfectant.

Disinfectant Solutions

1. Hypochlorite solution containing 1 per cent of available chlorine. The solutions available through retail outlets contain 10 per cent of available chlorine (e.g. Chloros, Domestos) and are diluted one part of solution in nine parts of water for use.

2. Aldehyde solutions:

   a. Glutaraldehyde 2 per cent. Cidex is a 2 per cent solution to which an activating powder is added before use to make a buffered alkaline solution which is stable for 14 days.

   b. Formaldehyde 4 per cent. A 10 per cent dilution of formaldehyde solution BP (Formalin) should be diluted appropriately.

AIDS

AIDS, the acquired immune deficiency syndrome, was first recognized as a new, serious medical problem in the USA at the end of 1980 and cases have been reported in the UK and other countries from 1981 onwards. It is possible that the disease originates in central Africa where it affects heterosexual individuals of both sexes, spreading to the USA, perhaps via Haiti. A substantial percentage of the early UK patients had travelled in the USA and Caribbean. Some patients acquired the infection from blood products prepared in the USA and others direct from sub-Saharal Africa. The number of reported cases is increasing rapidly.

In 1983 a lymphadenopathy associated virus (LAV) was isolated at the Pasteur Institute, and in 1984 the human T-cell lymphotrophic virus III (HTLV-III) was isolated at the National Cancer Institute in the USA. In the same year an AIDS-associated virus ARV was identified at the San Francisco School of Medicine. These have proved to be variants of a single heterogenous RNA virus which shows differences in the outer envelope and is now designated the human immunodeficiency virus (HIV).

Homosexual and bisexual men form the largest group of patients, with intravenous drug addicts next in frequency. Recipients of multiple blood transfusions or infusions of blood products comprise a small, but significant group at risk, together with the female partners of bisexual men and babies born to women with AIDS.

In most cases the initial infection is symptomless, but a glandular fever-like illness may occur. It is just possible that some acquire immunity and recover completely. The majority become asymptomatic carriers. At this stage they are said to be infected with the HIV and, after an initial interval, will test positive with appropriate laboratory tests. The degree of risk for these that they will eventually develop clinical AIDS is still uncertain but substantial. A varying period of between 5 and 8 years elapses after infection before the appearance of the clinical conditions which categorise them as suffering from AIDS. Some develop the persistent generalised lymphadenopathy (PGL) syndrome, suffering a minor degree of malaise and weight loss and have symmetrically enlarged groups of lymph nodes together with a hepato-sphenomegaly. PGL patients later progress to AIDS.

The onset of clinical AIDS is a serious matter. The patients become lethargic, lose weight and have night sweats. They often present with opportunistic infections or with Kaposi sarcoma. Some develop lymphomas. These infections occur because the numbers of T-lymphocytes are reduced and in particular the OKT4 helper T-cells are depleted.

Of the opportunist infections *Pneumocystis carinii* pneumonia (PCP) is the most important. Patients with PCP develop a non-productive cough, shortness of breath and fever, then become markedly hypoxic and die unless treatment is given. Confirmation of the diagnosis is not simple, but requires bronchial lavage and transbronchial biopsy. The multiflagellate protozoa is seen in stained specimens. Treatment is by high dose i.v. co-trimoxazole for 3 weeks or pentamidine intramuscularly. The protozoa may persist in the lungs after clinical recovery with relapse in the ensuing months. Cytomegalovirus, mycobacterial and cryptococcal infections also occur, either as chest or CNS infections.

AIDS patients may present to the dentist with oral Kaposi sarcoma, widespread oral and pharyngeal candidiasis or severe ulcerating herpes simplex infections. Kaposi sarcoma can be seen unrelated to AIDS in middle-aged and elderly Eastern Europeans and Africans. Kaposi sarcoma occurring in young men almost always means AIDS. The tumours are a reddish or purplish colour and either raised or flat. They are often multiple, affecting the skin, gastrointestinal tract and oral mucosa. 'Epulides' or 'fibro-epithelial polyps' of unusual appearance should be treated with respect. Leucoplakia of the oral mucosa affecting young individuals is also suspicious, particularly hairy leucoplakia affecting the side of the tongue.

If the diagnosis of AIDS is suspected the patient should be referred urgently to a consultant physician, but it is wise if the patient is not told of the suspected diagnosis until it is proved.

Affected individuals develop antibodies to the virus, though the virus may be recoverable from blood or secretions for months before the antibodies appear. Various tests for antibodies, notably an enzyme-linked immunosorbent assay (ELISA) are available.

The HIV uniquely prevents a successful deployment of the body's defences by its effect upon the patient's immune system. The variable composition of the outer envelope suggests that development of a useful vaccine will be difficult. Despite treatment of opportunist infections and tumours the prognosis for the patient with developed AIDS is poor with few surviving more than two or three years. Drugs are now appearing which seem to improve the condition of those with AIDS and if given to those with an HIV infection, delay the onset of AIDS. These drugs have substantial side effects.

The virus can be recovered from the blood, plasma, saliva and seminal fluid of affected individuals and the mode of infection is probably similar to that of hepatitis B, but with a lower risk of infectivity. The most common modes of transmission are via semen and mucosal abrasions during homosexual activities or via the shared hypodermic syringes and needles of drug addicts. Blade razors and toothbrushes which might be contaminated with blood also constitute a risk to other users.

Normal social contact, airborne droplets, domestically clean cutlery and crockery and toilet facilities do not seem to carry a risk of transmission. There does not appear to be much risk of transmission by saliva and a lower risk than hepatitis B following accidental needle punctures.

Prevention

Known or suspected cases should be treated with all the precautions used in the treatment of hepatitis B carriers (*see above*). The present prevalence of the disease in the population is low but the number of cases is increasing.

THE CONTROL OF INFECTIONS

Unsuspected cases present a potential hazard to dentists so that well-fitting rubber gloves should be worn as a routine particularly during any procedure which may shed blood, as a protection against a variety of infections not solely hepatitis B and AIDS. Such gloves need not be sterile, but should be washed in the same way as the uncovered hands would be for the intended procedure. Glasses will protect the conjunctive from splashes and masks are used for aerosols. Care should be exercised as a habit to avoid accidental puncture of the skin with sharp teeth, needles, ends of wire, etc. As a profession we have become too unconcerned about touching undiagnosed oral lesions with ungloved hands since the virtual disappearance of ulcers in the mouth due to syphilis.

Dental surgeons often have practical hobbies which result in minor cuts, scratches and abrasions of the hands. Again, practitioners should be more careful, so reducing the incidence of damage to the hands, wherever possible. If the hands are scratched or cut, waterproof dressings should be applied before the gloves are put on for dentistry until they are healed.

While the development of an effective treatment or a vaccine must present great difficulties, some measures can help to reduce the spread of this disease. Extra precautions to prevent transmission via transfused blood and blood products are already being taken. A change of attitudes and a reduction in promiscuous sexual activity and in particular, homosexual sexual activity is an obvious preventive measure. So also would be a substantial reduction in intravenous drug abuse.

Tetanus

This is an uncommon infection in Britain and occurs when a deep or heavily soiled wound is infected by the anaerobe *Clostridium tetani*. The organism and its spores are ubiquitous in soil and the faeces of horses and cows, etc. Its insidious onset, ususally 3–21 days after wound infection, produces widespread muscle spasms including trismus, dysphagia and opisthotonos and is difficult to diagnose and treat. Death from exhaustion and respiratory failure may occur in the region of 60 per cent of cases outside specialist centres, hence prevention is of the utmost importance.

Preventive measures in appropriate trauma patients are as follows.

1. Careful toilet and debridement of all wounds especially deep or penetrating ones, removing dead tissue and foreign bodies.

2. Patients who (*a*) have not previously had tetanus toxoid immunization and who therefore are not immune, or (*b*) those for whom the last dose was given more than 10 years previously, or (*c*) those who are unaware if they have been, should be given immediate passive immunization with human hyperimmune tetanus immunoglobulin.

3. Active immunity should be ensured by giving tetanus toxoid. Therefore (*a*) the immune patient will be given a booster dose of 0·5 ml tetanus toxoid unless he or she was immunized during the previous year.

(b) Non-immune patients should be given 0·5 ml absorbed tetanus toxoid deep subciutaneously into one arm at the same time as 250 units of human tetanus immunoglobulin (HTIG) is administered intramuscularly into the other arm. The tetanus vaccine dose should be repeated after 6–12 weeks then after a further 4–12 months.

4. Antibiotics should be considered an ancillary measure but are also required. Amoxycillin 500 mg and flucloxacillin 250 mg will control the *Clostridium tetani* and any associated penicillinase-producing organisms. Erythromycin or clindamycin may be necessary in allergic cases.

DISINFECTANTS

This group of antimicrobial agents is usually used for the decontamination of inanimate objects, such as working surfaces or instruments. Less irritant preparations, the so called antiseptics, are available for the skin. Unfortunately in most cases increased efficiency is related to increased toxicity. If they are to be of value, certain important limitations must be recognized:

a. The object to be disinfected must be thoroughly cleaned of debris, blood or pus, etc., which will inactivate many agents.

b. Many antiseptics only retain their efficacy when stored in concentrated form and in some cases at particular temperatures, and dilute solutions for use must be freshly prepared. Dilute solutions not only lose their antimicrobial potency but become contaminated and actually grow bacteria and yeasts. Absorbent stoppers for bottles such as corks must not be used as these will become colonized by organisms which are resistant to the particular agent and a source of contamination for dilute solutions. Sealed sachets help to overcome this problem.

c. The appropriate concentration and period of exposure to the agent is required for adequate disinfection.

Alcohols

Isopropyl and 70 per cent ethyl alcohol are effective against most Gram-negative bacteria on clean surfaces in 30 seconds. They are not active against spores and fungi but are useful for skin preparation prior to venepuncture and for working surfaces.

Aldehydes

Glutaraldehyde and formaldehyde are active against most Gram-negative bacteria, spores, viruses (including hepatitis B) and fungi, but require up to three hours exposure. Both are irritant and toxic, glutaraldehyde less so but needs to be alkaline; 2 per cent glutaraldehyde solution is useful for fibreoptic and other non-autoclavable instruments but must be rinsed off completely with sterile water before they are used.

THE CONTROL OF INFECTIONS

Diguanides

Chlorhexidine is active against *Staph. aureus* and some Gram-negative bacteria but not spores, fungi or viruses. It can be made up in alcohol or with cetrimide. As it is readily inactivated by soap, pus, plastics, etc., its value for disinfecting equipment is limited.

Its principle use is for cleaning skin and mucous membranes, e.g. 0·5 per cent chlorhexidine in 70 per cent alcohol or chlorhexidine with cetrimide (Savlon or Savlodil, ICI) or a 4 per cent solution with detergent (Hibiscrub) as a preoperative scrub. Alternatively chlorhexidine–alcohol–glycerine solution (Hibisol) can be used for rapid hand antisepsis.

As a 0·2 per cent aqueous gluconate solution or 1 per cent gel it can be used for the suppression of oral plaque and postoperative infection.

Halogens

1. Hypochlorites are active against bacteria, spores, fungi and viruses, including hepatitis B virus. Unfortunately they are readily inactivated by blood, pus and dilution. Eusol, calcium hypochlorite and boric acid or sodium hypochlorite with sodium chloride (Milton) diluted prior to use are valuable as a cleansing agent for wounds and sinuses. Hypochlorite packs must be changed frequently, 2–4 times a day. Strong solutions are used for cleaning blood contaminated surfaces.

2. Iodophors and iodine are active against bacteria and spores and some viruses and fungi, but can be inactivated by blood and pus. Iodine may cause a skin reaction. Both are useful as a 1 per cent alcohol solution for skin disinfection. The aqueous detergent iodophor solution (povidone-iodine) is used as a surgical scrub.

Phenolics

Hexachloraphane is the most useful of this group, especially as a skin cleansing agents against *Staph. Aureas,* but has limited activity against Gram-negative bacilli. Used as a 3 per cent solution or a surgical scrub (Phisomed).

Quaternary Ammonium Compounds

Compounds such as cetrimide are anionic detergents active against staphylococci. They are easily inactivated, especially by water and soap, etc., and can become contaminated by pseudomonas. Probably best used as a mixture with chlorhexidine (Savlon).

SUGGESTED READING

Cawson R. A. (1983) Antibiotic prophylaxis of infective endocarditis. *Br. Dent. J.* **154,** 183–184.

DHSS (1986) *Acquired Immune Deficiency Syndrome AIDS, Booklet 3. Guidance for Surgeons, Anaesthetists, Dentists and their Teams in Dealing with Patients Infected with HTLVIII.* DHSS, CMO(86)7 April, 1986.

Dinsdale R. C. W. (1985) *Viral Hepatitis, AIDS and Dental Treatment.* London, British Dental Journal.

Field, E. A., and Martin, M. V., (1991) Prophylactic antibiotics for patients with artificial joints undergoing oral and dental surgery; necessary or not? *Brit. J. Oral Man-Frc. Surg.* **29,** 341–346.

Innes A. J., Windle-Taylor P. C. and Harrison D. F. N. (1980) The role of metronidazole in the prevention of fistulae following total laryngectomy. *Clin. Oncol.* **6,** 71–77.

Kaziro G. (1984) Metronidazole (Flagyl) and *Arnica Montana* in the prevention of post surgical complications, a comparative placebo controlled clinical oral trial. *Br. J. Oral Surg.* **22,** 42–49.

Lindemann R. A., Henson J. L. (1982) The dental management of patients with vascular grafts placed in the treatment of arterial occlusive disease. *J. Am. Dent. Assoc.* **104,** 625–628.

Little J. W. (1980) Dental management of patients with surgically corrected cardiac and vascular disease. *Oral Surg. Oral Med. Oral Path.* **50,** 314–320.

MacFarlane T. W. and Follett E. A. C. (1983) hepatitis B vaccine. *Br. Dent. J.* **154,** 39–41.

MacFarlane T. W., Ferguson M. M. and Mulgrew C. J. (1984) Post-extraction bacteraemia. Role of antiseptics and antibiotics *Br. Dent. J.* **156,** 179–181.

McGowan D. A. (1982) Endodontics and infective endocarditis in hospital dentistry. *Int. Endodont. J.* **15,** 127–131.

Millard H. D. and Tupper C. J. (1960) Sub-acute bacterial endocarditis: a clinical study. *J. Oral Surg.* **18,** 224–229.

Okell C. C. and Elliott S. D. (1935) Bacteraemia and oral sepsis: with special reference to the aetiology of sub-acute endocarditis. *Lancet.* **2,** 862–872.

Rood J. P. and Murgatroid J. (1980) Metronidazole in the prevention of dry sockets. *Br. J. Oral Surg.* **17,** 62–70.

Samaranayake, L. P., Scheutz, F., and Cottone, A. (1991) *Infection Control for the Dental Team.* Copenhagen, Manksgaard.

Shanson D. C. (1982) *Microbiology in Clinical Practice.* Bristol, Wright.

Thornton J. B. and Alves J. C. M. (1981) Bacterial endocarditis. *Oral Surg.* **52,** 379–383.

Watkinson, A. C. (1982) Primary herpes simplex in a dentist. *Br. Dent. J.* **153,** 190–191.

Working Party of the British Society for Antimicrobial Chemotherapy (1990) The antibiotic prophylaxis of infective endocarditis. *Br. Dent. J.* **169,** 69–71.

CHAPTER 9

SINUSITIS, OROANTRAL FISTULA AND REMOVAL OF A TOOTH OR ROOT FROM THE MAXILLARY SINUS

SINUSITIS

Sinusitis may be primarily an allergic condition or due to an infection. Upper respiratory tract allergy can occur seasonally as hay fever or non-seasonally as allergic rhinitis. In the latter case the allergies tend to be house dust mite, or animals. The mucous membranes of the upper respiratory passages are swollen and pale and an excess of clear mucus is produced. If drainage of secretions from the maxillary sinus is obstructed discomfort will be experienced and the swollen mucosa with or without a fluid level will be seen in an occipitomental radiograph. Stagnant secretions are likely to become infected and bacterial sinusitis will supervene which, depending upon the circumstances, will be either acute or chronic.

With an acute upper respiratory tract virus infection a similar sequence is seen. During the acute infection the nasal mucosa will be found to be swollen and red. With the onset of secondary infection purulent secretions will be seen, particularly by posterior rhinoscopy. Acute bacterial maxillary sinusitis occurring under these circumstances is usually bilateral, but may persist on one side if drainage from that side is impeded due to a deviated nasal septum.

A unilateral maxillary sinusitis with an obviously odorous pus is suggestive of an odontogenic infection and this has been discussed elsewhere. Another and more sinister cause of a unilateral chronic suppurative sinusitis is a maxillary carcinoma. If the neoplasm fungates into the nose it may obstruct the orifices of all the sinuses on the side to produce the radiographic appearance of a unilateral pan sinusitis.

Radiographic Features

Because the radiopacities of oedematous mucosa, mucus and pus are similar no distinction can be made on the density of the radiographic image. Swollen mucosa can be visualized in an occipitomental radiograph while outlined by an air filled cavity. A thin or thick mucosa thickening may be distinguished, or if the layer is no longer uniform, but heaped up, a polypoid thickening. A single rounded mucosal image which can be seen in tilted views to 'flop' from side to side is a mucosal cyst. These need to be distinguished from odontogenic cysts which have an unvarying shape and a denser margin as they are covered by a thin layer of periosteal bone on the antral aspect.

Mucus or pus which is still draining via the ostium will show a fluid level provided the occipitomental radiograph is taken with the head vertically. The appearance is sufficiently characteristic that rarely is it appropriate to take a second radiograph with a lateral tilt to confirm the presence of fluid. Once the sinus is filled with swollen mucosa and either mucus or pus a completely opaque image will be seen. It must be remembered, however, that oedema of the overlying cheek will also produce a unilateral difference in opacity which must not be mistaken for opacity due to replacement of the air in the antrum by soft tissue and fluid.

Also a carcinoma will initially produce a detectable thickening of the mucosa. Then, as the tumour enlarges, complete opacity will be produced, either because the neoplasm fills the antrum, or because it occludes the ostium impeding the drainage of secretions. In time of course a carcinoma will destroy part of the bony wall making the diagnosis all too obvious.

The detailed diagnosis and management of these conditions is usually the province of the general medical practitioner or ENT surgeon, but their diagnosis and differential diagnosis is of concern to dentists should their patients be afflicted.

OROANTRAL FISTULA

The accidental production of an oroantral communication is probably a relatively common occurrence during the extraction of maxillary posterior teeth. Extractions of 1st and 2nd molars are most likely to be complicated by the production of a breach of the floor of the sinus. Such incidences also occur during the removal of 3rd molars, 2nd premolars, occasionally 1st premolars and even canines, depending upon the size of the maxillary sinus and the length of its floor within the alveolar process. The close relationship between the sockets of these teeth and the antrum is more frequent when the teeth are impacted or unerupted. There is a male predominance of 2 : 1 with a peak age distribution in the third and fourth decades perhaps because the sinuses tend to be larger and the alveolus denser in men. These figures are, of course, related to the frequency and the age at which tooth extraction is required as well as to variations in anatomy.

With increased size, the maxillary sinuses extend downwards into the alveolar process between the palatal and buccal roots of the teeth and into the interdental bone. When the bony floor of the sinus is viewed from above the roots of the teeth raise oval swellings on the buccal and palatal aspect respectively, the apices of the roots and supporting periodontal membranes being separated from the sinus by a thin layer of bone. Anteroposterior extension of the sinus carries the cavity into the tuberosity and palatally to the canine and even the upper incisors. It is likely that minor cracks and defects in the floor of the maxillary sinus are created during the rocking movement of tooth extraction fairly frequently, but that spontaneous healing occurs and neither patient nor operator is aware of the fact. Indeed in some cases it may be that the bone is naturally deficient at some point. In other instances the roots may be hypercementosed and bulbous or the two buccal roots of a molar may come together at the apices embracing the inter-radicular bone so that segments of socket wall are torn off during the extraction. A rough extraction technique will increase the size of such fragments and the chance that the maxillary sinus will be opened.

The bone between the tooth and the antrum may be destroyed by disease. A periapical granuloma or cyst is frequently the cause of such bone destruction but advanced local periodontal disease can destroy the whole of the socket bone. When the tooth is extracted the granulation tissue tends to adhere to the tooth roots. If it also adheres to the sinus mucosa a hole may be torn in the lining creating an opening right into the antral cavity.

Sometimes when a tooth is extracted an opening is produced into an unsuspected dental cyst, creating a diagnostic dilemma. The reason for the fistula may be apparent if there is an obvious discharge of cyst fluid rather than air or mucopus such as might escape if an opening is made into an inflamed sinus. Neoplastic destruction of alveolar bone can have a similar result and may present following spontaneous tooth loss. Where there has been a reason to take preoperative radiographs some of these problems will be anticipated. If a difficult extraction is anticipated a mucoperiosteal flap should be raised and an attempt made to minimize damage to the antral floor either by surgical bone removal or separation of the roots of the tooth. A two-sided flap can be used making a single relieving incision which starts at the mesial papilla of the tooth to be extracted, so that the flap can be converted if necessary by a second distal relieving incision into one suitable for advancement to cover a fistula. Such an approach is also appropriate if a fistula has healed spontaneously but a root remains to be removed from the socket.

The first clue to the occurrence of a fistula is likely to be the recognition of the antral floor being attached to the roots of the extracted tooth. The appearance of the thin, smooth, curved plate of bone is quite characteristic. Preservation of the integrity of the delicate lining mucosa, if it has not been breached already, is important as it prevents contamination of the sinus cavity and reduces the chance of subsequent sinusitis.

Where it is believed that complete perforation already exists it is reasonable to instruct the patient to occlude the nostrils and blow gently so as to produce an air stream passing from sinus to mouth, perhaps with bubbling of blood in the socket. Blood trickling from the nostril on that side also confirms the presence of a complete opening and an antrum filled with blood. The temptation to explore the socket with suckers and probes to establish the size of the opening should be resisted as this merely disturbs the newly established clot, risks breaching a possibly intact lining and may carry infection into the wound.

If a fistula is created during the surgical removal of a root a characteristic hollow sound will be produced by the sucker due to an echo from the sinus. If the defect is large it is possible to observe whether the lining is inflamed, swollen and polyphoid or thin, delicate and normal in appearance. Any mucus or pus should be aspirated but irrigation is probably harmful if drainage is impaired.

The safest surgical action at this stage where the floor of the antrum has been breached is to place a horizontal mattress suture across the mouth of the socket and to tie it firmly. Normally contraction of the gum margin greatly reduces the size of the socket opening during the first 24 hours. With a mattress suture present the mouth of the socket will virtually close in this time, supporting the clot within. Where there is a large defect, and the buccal mucosa is untorn and where the operator is reasonably experienced, a buccal advancement repair can be undertaken as a primary procedure.

Radiographic Features

Periapical, oblique occlusal or rotational tomographic radiographs will demonstrate the defect in the bony floor of the antrum, but are not essential unless a fractured root fragment is still present. An occipitomental radiograph will record the state of the sinus at this stage but the floor of the antrum cannot be visualized. Immediately following the creation of the opening little will be seen except some local swelling of the lining unless there has been a haemorrhage into the antrum or the sinus has been irrigated when there will be either opacity or a fluid level. Generalized mucosal thickening or opacity, particularly if bilateral, signifies pre-existing sinusitis. The rarer possibility of a pre-existing cyst or malignant neoplasm must always be borne in mind as a cause predisposing to the creation of a fistula.

Persistence of Fistulae

Now a further set of factors needs to be considered which prevents the successful healing of the socket and results in the production of a persistent fistula. Healing of the fistula depends upon the establishment of a clot within the defect and the maintenance of its integrity and freedom from infection until it has been invaded and replaced by granulation tissue.

If the defect is small and at the bottom of a deep socket it is likely that the blood clot will be well supported and that the part immediately over the defect will be successfully and completely invaded by granulation tissue. This is best seen in 3rd molar fistulae which invariably close spontaneously.

If there has been a substantial loss of height of the socket as a result of advanced periodontal disease, and particularly in the case of a 1st molar socket, then the bony defect is likely to be wide in proportion to the shallow depth of the socket. A thin layer of clot will be supported only at the periphery and lysis of the centre is likely long before the granulation tissue has penetrated that far. Without a scaffold of fibrin the granulations are unlikely to reach across and occlude the opening. Also if there is a preexisting infection in the antrum, mucopus will drain through the opening from the start and impede the formation of an occluding clot.

Even if a clot is formed, if infection is present above or develops in an antral haematoma, the vital clot in the opening will be destroyed. Similarly if the clot in the socket is destroyed by the formation of a dry socket the odds are against the granulation tissue sealing the opening. The insertion of foreign materials such as packs, pastes, haemostatic sponges or antibiotic cones all destroy the integrity of the clot and jeopardize spontaneous closure. The granulation tissue needs also to be attached to all aspects of the bony wall of the socket. If it is unable to attach to one aspect because of a retained root of a multirooted tooth or the exposed surface of the root of an adjacent tooth, there is likely to be a continuing communication between mouth and antrum.

Some operators like to construct a simple plate to cover the defect and to protect and support the clot and developing granulation tissue. Such plates are obviously useful in preventing food debris entering the antrum through a large unhealed fistula where they will constitute a source of infection, but it is doubtful if they are useful when used to cover a fresh socket. As already advocated, with the help of a mattress suture the gingival margin soon contracts, greatly reducing the exposed surface of the supported clot.

In the larger defect, where this is unlikely to happen, given reasonable surgical skill on the part of the operator it is better to cover the defect by advancement of a buccal mucosal flap. From time to time it is advocated that small sheets of inert and self-adhesive material should be used to protect the organizing blood clot, but the value of these is also doubted.

The Chronic Fistula

If the creation of an oroantral communication is unrecognized, untreated or spontaneous closure does not occur, then a chronic fistula becomes established. Contamination of the antrum with infected oral fluids and food debris leads inevitably to chronic sinusitis. When the residual defect is very small—and some are only pin-hole in size—the consequences may be slight and symptoms only arise following an acute upper respiratory tract infection. The mucopurulent phase is more marked on the side with the fistula, a purulent maxillary sinusitis develops and persists when all other signs of the illness have subsided.

Conversely with very large defects, though reflux of food, drink and saliva is an obvious nuisance to the patient, it may allow such free drainage of secretions from the sinus that any infection is readily drained and symptoms are slight. Occlusion of the opening during the day time with a dental plate reduces contamination of the sinus and prevents the embarrassment of soup and drinks escaping from the ostium and down the nose. However, in the case of a full denture, retention may be adversely affected by the opening.

Fistulae of intermediate size tend to be both a nuisance and a source of recurrent symptoms. The patient suffers intermittent episodes of pain and local tenderness along with a chronic, foul-tasting discharge. Drainage may be obstructed by an oedematous lining or by polyps which can prolapse through the fistula into the mouth. Prolapsed polyps can be quite large, become fibrosed and even covered by stratified squamous epithelium on their surface. At this stage they can be mistaken for an epulis until, as the lump is excised, the opening into the antrum becomes apparent. If the correct diagnosis is suspected the pedicle of the tumour can be explored with a blunt periodontal probe. It will slip up between the pedicle and the ridge mucosa into the antrum, and can be passed right round the pedicle, indicating that the mass has come down through the opening.

Where a fistulous opening is partially blocked by swollen mucosa, a polyp or purulent granulation tissue, excision of this tissue promotes drainage of the antrum and makes it possible regularly to irrigate the sinus cavity with warm water or saline. This, along with a single course of penicillin, if there is a lot of pus, aids resolution of the sinusitis, prior to surgical closure. To avoid food entering the now widely open fistula, which would be counter-productive, an acrylic plate or simple vacuumed plate can be made to cover it. Care is required whenever impressions are taken with an oroantral fistula to prevent the impression material entering the sinus. If the material sets hard it may lock the impression in place and if it is readily torn, a fragment may be left in the antrum. A sizeable patch of tullegras placed over the fistula will prevent alginate impression material entering the opening while providing an impression sufficiently accurate for the purpose.

It should be remembered that a carcinoma of the antrum can present through a tooth socket and may even have been the cause of pain or tooth mobility which led to the extraction. As always, any excised soft tissue should be examined histologically. Good periapical, occlusal and occipitomental radiographs should reveal irregular bone destruction and opacity due to a soft tissue mass if a malignant neoplasm presents in this way.

Irrigation of the maxillary sinus is best carried out with a 20 ml syringe and a soft plastic catheter, which should pass readily through the opening without occluding it, in case the swollen mucosa prevents the escape of the irrigation solution through the ostium. The patient should hang the head forward so that the solution can run out of the nose and out of the mouth and not back into the pharynx.

Once the infection is controlled, a few fistulae may close spontaneously, particularly in the 3rd molar region. In general, however, the object of the treatment is to bring the patient to operation with the maxillary sinus in as healthy a condition as can be achieved. Where progress cannot be observed directly as through a large fistula, serial occipitomental radiographs will monitor an improvement.

SINUSITIS, OAF AND ROOT IN ANTRUM

Surgical Closure of an Oroantral Fistula

The patient should be warned that even the most promising of operations may fail and a fistula be re-established. Re-operation after past failures at the hands of other operators should be approached with due humility! As far as possible a flap should be raised which will cover not only the fistula but a ledge of bone which will support the suture line. The flap should have a good blood supply and should be handled gently and not grasped and crushed with dissecting forceps. It should lie in its new position without tension. There should be good haemostasis because a haematoma creates tension, delays healing and provides a nidus for infection. Failures occur where these precepts are neglected, but also because for anatomical reasons it is not always possible to carry out a fault-free operation.

Three types of repair are used as described below.

The Buccal Advancement Flap

The most useful is by a buccal advancement flap. This is a Y–V advancement in that a Y shaped wound is created which is sewn up as a V after advancement of the tissues between the arms of the Y. Advancement is possible after careful division of the inelastic periosteum on the deep surface of the flap, but depends upon the elasticity of the mucosa and submucosa so that the repair is not entirely tension free, which is one reason why it may break down.

Other problems are where teeth are still present on either side of the fistula and there is not room to create a ledge of surrounding bone. If the roots of the teeth are exposed in the fistula, the flap will not attach to the root surface and will fail. Teeth not supported by alveolar bone must therefore be extracted before closure is attempted. Sometimes there is recurrent bleeding from the incision in the periosteum which leads to a haematoma in the sulcus. Also the distal end of the flap is often quite narrow and its blood supply is easily impaired by the retaining sutures.

This flap may be used to close an established fistula, a newly created opening at the time of the extraction or to close a fistula in combination with exploration of the maxillary sinus to remove a displaced root. The procedure for closing an established fistula will be described first (*Fig. 9.1*), then the modifications appropriate in the other circumstances. In the majority of cases the procedure is not stressful and may be performed under local anaesthesia, but access may be improved if an endotracheal general anaesthetic can be used. The injection of a vasoconstrictor facilitates the surgery even if a general anaesthetic is used.

There is less chance of a reactionary haemorrhage if felypressin is the vasoconstrictor rather than adrenaline, and although the reduction in ooze is not so great it is adequate for the procedure. Between 2 and 3 ml of local anaesthetic solution containing felypressin is given buccally so as to anaesthetize the tissues for at least two teeth anterior to the fistula and two posterior. Between 0·5 and 1 ml of solution is injected palatally. The patient

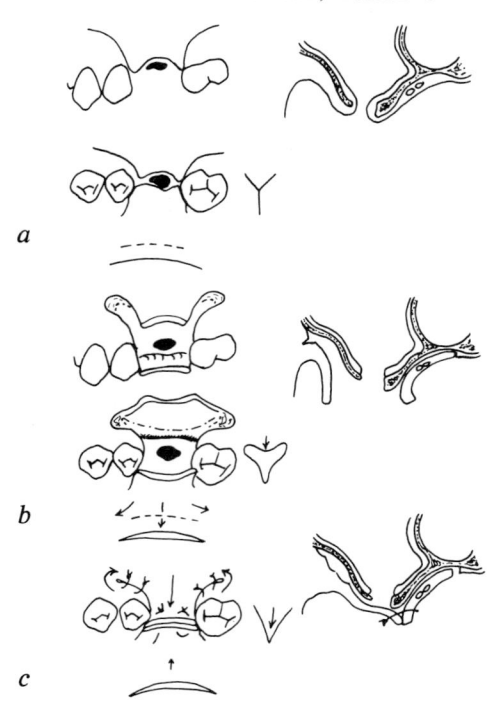

Fig. 9.1. Closure of oroantral fistula by buccal advancement (Y–V) flap. Diagrams of a fistula: lateral view of the alveolar process, below a plan view, right the fistula in section. *a,* The margins of the fistula are excised and the buccal flap outlined. An incision is made close to the mid line of the palate, and short relieving incisions at either end of the operative area on the palatal side. *b,* The palatal mucosa is undermined beneath the periosteum. The buccal flap is raised, held taut and the periosteum incised above the level of the sulcus. The palatal mucosa is raised at the edge of the defect. *c,* Plan view only. The buccal flap is advanced and sewn in eversion against the palatal mucosal edge.

is positioned so that the operator has a clear view of the operative field without stooping. Effective suction and a good assistant are essential.

In the case of a chronic fistula a rim of mucosa should be excised from the edge of the opening with a No. 11 scalpel blade exposing a rim of bone to act as a supporting shelf for the flap. At this stage, the palatal margin of the opening should be undermined for 2–3 mm to ease later suturing. Two short relieving incisions opposite the buccal ones will permit eversion of the palatal wound margin.

Two divergent buccal incisions are then made up towards the buccal sulcus. The ends of the incisions are turned in a curve outwards parallel with the top of the sulcus. Where the gap between adjacent teeth is narrow the gingival papillae at each end are included in the flap. Where there is at least the width of a molar socket the mesial and distal interdental tissues are left undisturbed. The size and shape of the flap is designed with coverage of the fistula after advancement in mind.

The buccal flap is reflected, subperiosteally, undermining the tissues well up above the sulcus. The end of this flap is grasped, either gently with toothed dissecting forceps or better still with skin hooks and everted and pulled so as to tense the inelastic fibrous periosteum which lines its undersurface. This tense lining layer is then *lightly* incised from distal to mesial, curving the cut upwards, well above the level of the sulcus at the centre of the flap.

Following this, the flap, which now consists at its base of extensible mucosa and submucosa only, can be easily advanced over the defect. Any difficulty in extending the flap fully is usually due to tethering at one or other edge of the periosteal layer and can be cured by completing the cut. Care should be taken to examine the periosteal surface of the flap before the incision so that the cut is placed to avoid any obvious vessels. Furthermore the periosteal incision should only *just* divide that layer. Any small bleeding point should be grasped precisely with mosquito artery forceps and crushed. The corners of the distal end of the flap are now trimmed a little with a sharp blade to fit the defect.

The flap is then sutured into position. Two plain sutures are placed bisecting the mesial and distal angles of the flap and holding these two points in position against the palatal gingiva. Next a horizontal mattress suture is inserted between them to evert the wound margin and ensure a broad area of apposition of the tissues. It must be tied without undue tension or the ischaemic margin will necrose and fail to heal. Further sutures can be placed to close the buccal limbs of the incision.

Sutures must be placed carefully and should embrace only sufficient tissue to hold the flap securely in place, so minimizing damage to the delicate flap; 4/0 (1·5 metric) synthetic absorbable sutures should be used. If non-absorbable sutures such as silk or proline are used they should not be removed in less than two weeks as it takes this time for a firm, strong attachment to develop.

Where the gingival papillae are included in the flap it should be wide enough to evert a little against the abutting teeth. In cases without neighbouring teeth, the procedure is similar except where the margin of the fistula is excised, mucosa can be removed mesially and distally to create a distinct shelf of bone on which the flap can rest. A broad end to the flap can be created of thick masticatory mucosa and all wound margins raised enough to facilitate suturing. Bone buccal to the fistula may be trimmed if the neighbouring ridge areas have resorbed so as to improve the lie of the flap.

During the initial healing period, the patients must be advised to avoid movements which stretch the cheek or activities such as nose-blowing or forceful mouth-rinsing which produce a pressure difference between the two sides of the wound.

Inhalations in steam and a suitable antibiotic are prescribed. The use of a steam inhalation such as menthol and benzoin 6-hourly directly moistens the airway and stimulates serous gland activity preventing crusting of blood and mucus, and patients also find its use comforting. Amoxycillin 500 mg 8-hourly, is a suitable antibiotic with doxycycline 200 mg first day and 100 mg daily as an alternative.

Some operators extend the anterior limb of the incision and explore the sinus itself through a Caldwell–Luc opening in the canine fossa, removing polypoid lining and establishing an intranasal antrostomy through which a drain such as a Yeats tubing or a Jacques catheter is inserted to prevent the accumulation of an antral haematoma which prejudices the success of the fistula closure procedure.

A simple method for establishing an intranasal antrostomy is to pass heavy curved artery forceps into the nose along the floor and laterally into the antrum. A length of ½inch ribbon gauze can then be inserted (from within the antrum) between the open tips of the forceps, grasped and then partially pulled back out through the nose. A slicing action grasping both ends of the gauze will create a smooth margined defect in the medial antral wall. A tubular drain is then drawn in a similar manner from antrum out of nose and sutured to the alar margin with one retaining stitch. The drain is removed in twenty-four hours.

Where this procedure is to be used to close a fistula at the time of its creation some variation is appropriate. The operator must not forget to explain the proposed procedure to the patient and the reason for doing it. Additional local anaesthetic injections will be necessary to increase the anaesthetized area and to ensure adequate painless operating time. Where a flap has been reflected to retrieve a root a two-sided flap has been advocated. This is more easily retracted without trauma to the tissues than a three-sided flap. A narrower flap is needed to repair the fistula than would be proper if only the root were to be removed which makes retraction even more difficult.

Where the operation needs to be combined with an antrostomy through the canine fossa to remove a root from the antrum, the part of the mesial buccal incision which curves forwards up into the sulcus is extended to the lateral incisor region.

The Palatal Transposition Flap

A finger-like strip of palate containing the greater palatine vessels is raised and the end rotated laterally and transposed over or under the intervening mucosa onto the ridge and the fistula. Because the flap has an axial artery its blood supply is ensured irrespective of its length. Success or failure hinges upon correctly estimating the length of flap required and not making it too short. Also the palatal tissues are thick and stiff and resist being twisted to

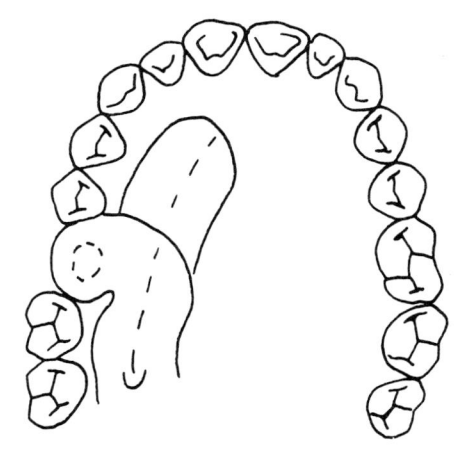

Fig. 9.2. Closure of an oroantral fistula with an arterialized palatal flap. The diagram illustrates the importance of an adequate length of flap.

lie in the new position. On the other hand they are tough and hold sutures well (*Fig.* 9.2).

Such a flap is used where there have been previous unsuccessful attempts to close the fistula using a buccal flap and the buccal mucosa in scarred and unsuitable for further surgery. Sometimes too the opening of the fistula may be towards the palatal aspect of the ridge. In these circumstances a palatal flap is more convenient.

The fistulous tract is excised as before and a shelf of bone established around it if possible. Any granulations or polyps at the mouth of the fistula are removed. A flap is outlined on the palate following the course of the palatine artery and shaped to include the vascular bundle on the deep surface. The flap curves towards the incisive papilla and so has a convex buccal margin and a concave palatal one. It must be turned laterally to cover the fistula and the length of the shorter palatal edge governs its ability to do this. Failure to recognize this will mean that the flap will be too short. It may be possible to incise around the margin of the fistula and then raise the soft tissue edge of the tract in continuity with the antral mucosa. If this is so it can be inverted into the antrum with a purse-string-like suture, but if the tissue is scarred this manoeuvre may not be easy. A single stitch is passed through the buccal side of the wound, then through the tip of the palatal flap, under the divided vascular bundle back through the tip and again through the buccal mucosa. This forms a mattress suture which also occludes the cut artery.

The flap is drawn into position but the suture is not yet tied. As the flap rotates buccally it will override a triangle of palatal mucosa which must be excised. When this has been done the mattress suture is tied and others placed to hold the flap in position. Coe Pack dressing or ribbon gauze and Whitehead's varnish is placed over the bare bone of the donor area and retained firmly with tie over sutures. It is difficult to use an acrylic plate for this purpose because of the way the palatal flap folds at the hinge as it is rotated into place. The rotation of this thick peninsula flap may be difficult for posteriorly placed fistulae and so its conversion into an island flap is worth considering.

After the flap has been raised, the greater palatine vessels on the undersurface of the base are identified and gently dissected free from the overlying musoca with McIndoe scissors. The scissors are then passed between vessels and submucosa and kept there for protection whilst the mucosa is transected with a sharp No. 15 blade. The flap is now pedicled on the blood vessels which can be carefully dissected back to the foramen allowing easy rotation of the flap to be sutured into place. A pattern made from the suture wrapping foil can be very useful in outlining the exact shape and size of the flap to be raised (Henderson, 1974).

Rotation Flaps

A palatal rotation flap is only possible in the edentulous subject. A substantial part of the palatal and ridge mucosa anterior to the fistula and up to the midline of the palate is raised and rotated backwards to cover the opening. The fistula is excised to create a triangular defect with a ledge of

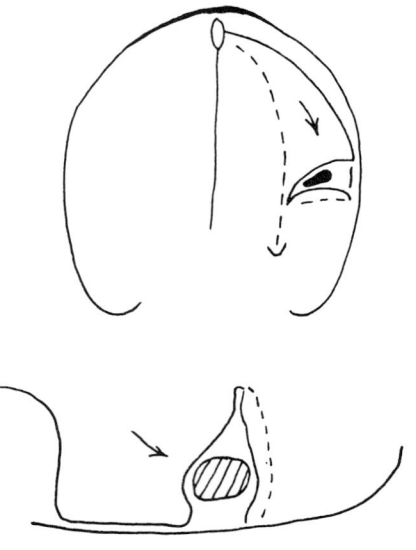

Fig. 9.3. Diagrams illustrating a palatal rotation flap and a buccal rotation flap. In each case the fistula is excised, the defect triangulated and a large flap of tissue with adequate blood supply is moved sideways to cover the opening.

bone distally. An incision is carried forwards from the base of the triangle on the crest of ridge. At first the incision swings a little buccally, then follows the crest of the ridge to the lateral incisor region, radially across the palate to the midline and then back down the midline of the palate to beyond the fistula. The whole of the outlined palatal mucosa is raised and undermined posteriorly until the flap can be displaced backwards to cover the opening. It is sutured into place around the margins.

For a large buccal opening where there is no tissue for an advancement flap a buccal rotation flap is used. The fistula margin is excised and the surrounding mucosa raised from the bone. Sometimes it is possible to turn in flaps from the margin to form an inner layer. A vertical buccal incision is made well forwards of the fistula and curved forwards at the top of the sulcus in the usual way. A large rectangular flap must be outlined which is considerably wider than the fistula. By undermining well up onto the maxilla and dividing the periosteum it will be possible to rotate the flap backwards to cover the opening (*Fig.* 9.3).

DISPLACEMENT OF A TOOTH OR ROOT INTO THE MAXILLARY SINUS

While creation of an oroantral fistula is often inevitable, the displacement of a tooth or root into the sinus occurs only as a result of the operator's actions and is usually avoidable. In the much rarer case of a whole tooth being displaced, unerupted 3rd molars, 2nd premolars or canines are most at risk. When general anaesthetics for tooth extraction were less sophisticated than today, cases were occasionally recorded of erupted teeth being forced into the sinus by excessive pressure from a gag used to open the unconscious patient's mouth. Otherwise, displacement of whole erupted teeth is unlikely except in severe maxillofacial injury.

Displacement into the antrum of unerupted teeth occurs during their elective removal when force is substituted for skill and where patience has been lost. The prudent surgeon is always aware of the possibility of this problem arising and will plan his operation accordingly. Good quality radiographs should show the position of the tooth relative to the antrum. Generous reflection of soft tissues and removal of overlying bone ensure good access, and force should be applied only in directions calculated to dislodge the tooth towards the mouth, and of course away from the sinus.

When displacement has occurred, the position of the tooth should be demonstrated by radiography in more than one plane, for example, using a rotational tomogram, or a lateral sinus view together with a postero-anterior jaw or occipitomental view and an occlusal view. It is usually necessary to open the sinus anteriorly by the classical Caldwell–Luc approach through the canine fossa which overlies the biscupid apices in order to recover a sizeable object such as a whole tooth. This provides much better vision and access than an approach via the defect through which it originally entered.

The canine fossa is reached through a horizontal incision through mucosa and periosteum in the upper buccal sulcus commencing at the zygomatic buttress opposite the 1st molar and running forwards to the central incisor. The tissues are reflected off the surface of the bone until the infraorbital foramen and infraorbital nerve are identified. A window of about 1·5 cm diameter is made with a chisel, gouge or bur in the anterolateral surface of the maxilla and care must be taken not to approach too close to the apices of the bicuspid teeth or the infraorbital nerve. The aim is to avoid premature penetration of the antral lining which lies beneath the thin bone (*Fig.* 9.4).

Once the lining is exposed, it is opened with pointed scissors or scalpel, and the cavity entered. Good lighting is essential and, if available, a fibreoptic probe is most useful. When the tooth is found, it may be lifted out with the sucker or grasped with a toothed Fickling's forceps or other suitable forceps and withdrawn. Irrigation with saline, inspection of the recesses of the sinus with a tiny laryngeal mirror, or insertion of a gloved finger may help to locate a tooth lodged in an awkward position. Grossly polypoid antral lining should be excised, but stripping of the entire lining should not be attempted. Once haemorrhage has ceased and after a final irrigation, the incision is closed with black silk sutures. A five-day course of inhalations and an antibiotic should be given as previously described on p. 244.

Displacement of a fragment of root is much more common and more difficult to avoid, but, again, poor surgical technique is often a contributory factor. It is the palatal roots of upper 1st and 2nd molars which are dislodged most frequently into the maxillary sinus, followed by the buccal roots of the same teeth, the roots of the 2nd premolar, the 3rd molar, the 1st premolar and occasionally the canine. When the root of an upper molar is retained following an extraction, examination of the socket may reveal the creation of a fistula in which case any unwise manoeuvre will soon displace the complete root into the sinus. Even in the absence of such a discovery, a close relationship of the roots of upper 2nd premolar and the 1st and 2nd molars to the sinus floor should be assumed.

If a root fragment is to be removed, the application of force with forceps or an elevator in an apical direction must be avoided. In general a mucoperiosteal flap should be raised and sufficient bone removed to give good access to the root and to allow its elevation in an outwards and downwards direction.

Fig. 9.4. Removal of a tooth or root from the maxillary sinus. *a*, Incision in the buccal sinus. *b*, Chiselling through the outer bony wall of the maxillary sinus. *c*, Lifting off the outer plate of bone. *d*, Incision through the lining of the maxillary sinus. *e*, Separating the edges of the incision to expose the sinus. *f*, Tooth removed from the sinus with forceps. *g*, Closure of the wound.

SINUSITIS, OAF AND ROOT IN ANTRUM

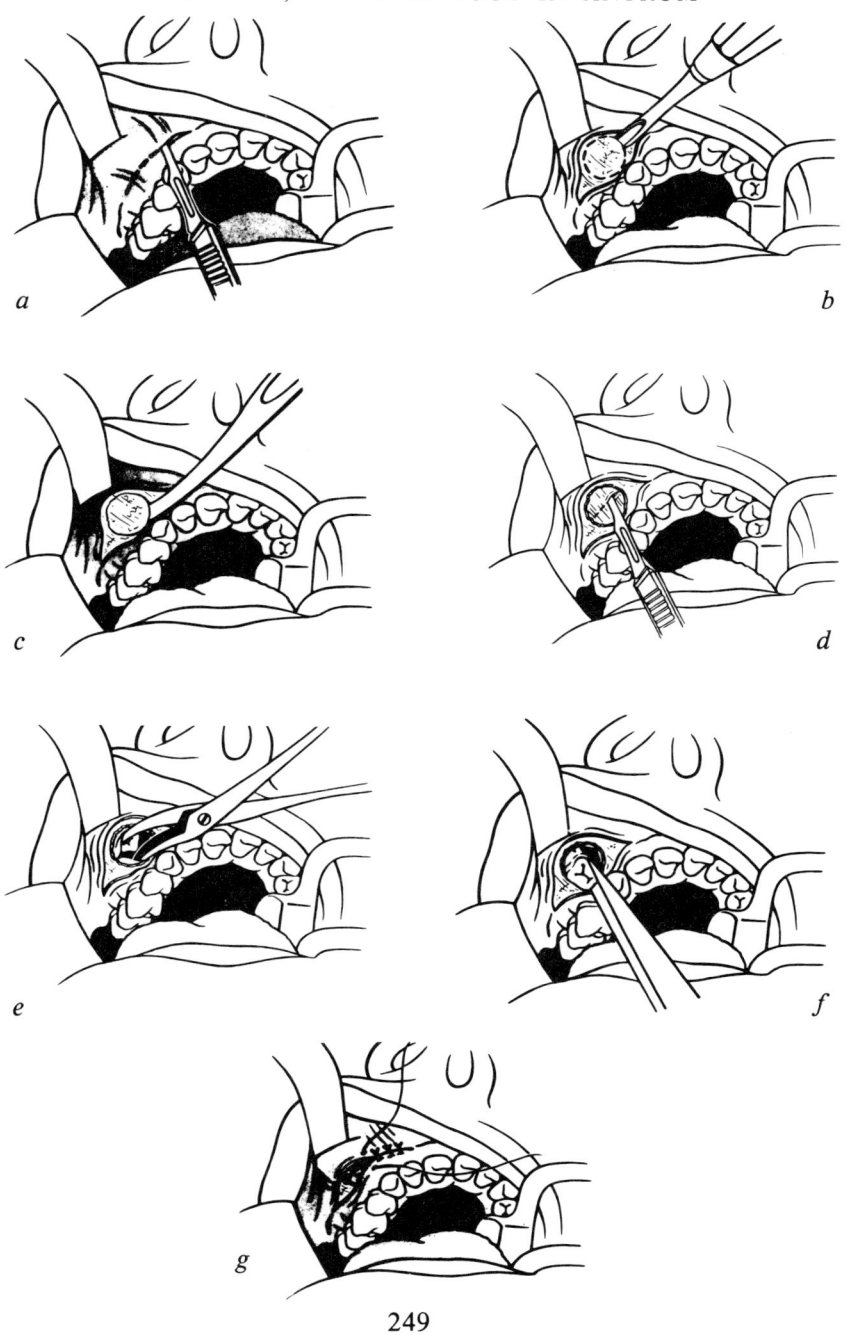

If, despite these precautions, a root is displaced into the sinus then every sensible effort should be made to remove it without delay. If the root has just 'popped' through into the antrum in response to a small force it is reasonable to assume it is close to the socket and to explore the adjacent part of the sinus on that assumption. It is probably wise to take a radiograph at this stage. A periapical radiograph of the socket and an oblique occlusal view are the most useful in these circumstances. While the films are being developed the problem and the proposed course of action are explained to the patient and additional local anaesthetic solution is injected to take account of the wider operative field, to allow for a more prolonged procedure, and to enhance vasoconstriction.

If a flap has already been raised the original incision may need to be extended forwards in the sulcus and backwards at the gingival margin so as to permit reflection of the soft tissues well above the level of the apical part of the socket. The bone over the apical half of the socket and of the antral wall just above it is removed freely using a large rose-head bur with light pressure. The defect is then explored with the sucker tip, gently elevating the antral lining from the floor of the sinus, immediately over the socket. The root may be picked up at this stage by the sucker, or at least located, especially if the antral lining is still intact. If it is not found and there is an obvious tear in the lining this is widened and the sucker tip advanced into the sinus cavity. During both manoeuvres the sucker should be directed mostly towards the location of the root as seen in the radiograph. In the absence of success, the patient should be instructed to pinch the nostrils and to blow, thus creating an airstream from the sinus into the mouth, which may carry the root with it. If this also fails the antrum is irrigated with normal saline while continuing to move the sucker tip around the cavity.

Mostly one or other of these measures will retrieve the missing root, but if they are unsuccessful attempts to locate it should not be unduly prolonged so as to exceed the patient's tolerance. It is wiser to suture back the flap, to take a further periapical and oblique occlusal film as a record of the current position of the root, and to arrange for a further exploration through a Caldwell–Luc approach under a general anaesthetic. Sometimes the problem is that the maxillary sinus is chronically infected and the root is trapped in folds between polyps. Once a root has been pushed in and the sinus has been opened, swelling of the mucosa can occur quite rapidly.

Immediately before the further exploration another set of periapical and oblique occlusal films should be taken, together with lateral sinuses, occipitomental and postero-anterior jaw views which will all help to locate the root tip. Rotational tomographic films will not demonstrate the root if, as may be the case, it lies outside the trough of sharpness. While the removal of the root at this stage hardly counts as a surgical emergency, nevertheless the attempts should not be unduly delayed. Problems with infection tend to arise if several days pass before the root is removed.

SINUSITIS, OAF AND ROOT IN ANTRUM

Spontaneous expulsion of a root from the maxillary sinus is described from time to time; presumably it is carried out of the ostium by the cilia on a stream of mucus. Usually the root is sneezed out of the nose or coughed out of the pharynx but there would appear to be a chance of inhalation, though the risk must be small.

From time to time roots are discovered in the antrum without a history of their displacement. Investigation of recurrent sinus infections may lead to such a discovery. Sometimes there is a complete absence of symptoms, perhaps because the root is between the lining and the bony wall. If the sinus appears healthy radiographically the question is bound to be raised whether it needs to be removed. On balance it is probably wise to do so in a fit patient because of the risk of future infection or spontaneous expulsion.

In longstanding cases every effort should be made to reduce any active infection before the operation. As before the root should be localized radiographically just before the patient is premedicated. The choice of approach and design of the flap will depend upon whether the root is still close to the original socket or remote from it and probably within the antral cavity, and whether there is a patent oroantral fistula which also needs repair. If the root is close to the original socket or to a fistula it is probably best to approach it directly by the local removal of bone. If it is away from the original socket a Caldwell–Luc approach is used.

In such cases it is of course necessary to be reasonably certain that the object seen in the radiograph is a root and that it is in the antrum. Apart from the general shape the detection of a root canal or a root filling is the clearest indication of the nature of the image. Small bony excrescences and ridges arising from the sinus floor or wall can closely mimic a root, but will not have a root canal. Taking a further radiograph from a slightly different position may alter the appearance of the image enough to make it clear that is is not a root.

Antroliths which are formed from calcified inspissated mucus may be mistaken for roots. As they tend to increase in size by accretion of fresh material on their surface and also give rise to infections, to mistake one for a root and to remove it will benefit the patient rather than otherwise. A root which remains in its socket will have a lamina dura and periodontal membrane space image about it in radiographs and will be correctly orientated in relation to the alveolar process. One which is displaced into the antrum is likely to lie at an unusual angle and will not be surrounded by a lamina dura. Where there is doubt exploration should be avoided rather than that the operator should chase a possibly non-existent fragment.

In the past, much was made of the distinction between a root lodged between the sinus lining and the bony wall and one free in the cavity with advice that the patient should shake the head between radiographs and any change in position noted. As a root inside the cavity may be trapped in folds in the swollen lining or simply stuck to the wall by mucus, a failure of the root to move in this way does not mean that it is not in the cavity. Roots high in the antrum are usually lifted up by swollen mucosa and are in the cavity, as are ones which are a distance from the socket of origin. Those still close to the socket may be under the lining but equally can lie just inside.

FRACTURED TUBEROSITY

A fracture of the maxillary tuberosity usually occurs during a forceps extraction of a resistant upper 2nd or 3rd molar, but may also happen during distal elevation of an impacted 3rd molar. Almost always there are marked alveolar and tuberosity extensions of the maxillary sinus so that the supporting bone is quite thin.

The cause of the difficulty with the extraction may be no more than bulbous roots or recurved roots which embrace the inter-radicular bone. An unerupted 3rd molar which is tightly impacted against the 2nd may be sufficient to require the operator to exert more than average force during the attempted extraction of the latter. In extreme cases there is false germination between the 2nd and 3rd molars, the latter being disto-angularly inclined, so that the roots of the two teeth are united by cementum. Resorption of the distal aspect of the 2nd molar in response to the presence of a high mesio-angularly impacted 3rd molar can also result in the two teeth becoming interlocked. Hypercementosed molar roots in a thickened Paget's alveolar process also predisposes to a large tuberosity fragment being separated.

extraction of the molar is not easy, unusual fragility of the bone is probably the major predisposing factor, especially when there is no obvious abnormality of the tooth being extracted. In many ordinary patients quite substantial force has to be applied to dislodge an upper molar tooth, but without a fracture occurring. Indeed, in the majority of cases in which there is a mechanical problem, either the crown fractures from the roots, or the surgeon fails to move the tooth with the use of forceps and elevators. Where the bone is eggshell thin the canals for the posterior superior dental vessels and nerves constitute a line of weakness through which the buccal part of the fracture can take place.

The exodontist is immediately aware that the tooth and tuberosity bone are moving together between the supporting finger and thumb. Furthermore, although the tooth moves freely in a buccopalatal direction it is not delivered from the socket by buccal movement. It is important that no attempt should be made to twist or manipulate free the tooth and the fractured fragment as this will tear the mucous membrane. Severe tears can lead to sloughing of the tissues and a large oroantral communication. The greater palatine vessels may even be torn with substantial blood loss.

The simplest course of action is to dissect out the entire tuberosity. An incision is made backwards from the distal surface of the last molar, over the tuberosity. The molar is grasped with extraction forceps and the fragment steadied while the buccal mucoperiosteum is elevated off the bone. The tooth is tilted a little buccally and the palatal mucosa also is raised from the fractured fragment. If a retractor is placed under the buccal flap and the tuberosity tilted palatally it is usually possible to separate the antral lining, so freeing the entire fragment. If the antrum has been opened it should be sucked out and emptied of blood, and a damp swab packed into the wound for 5 minutes to effect haemostasis.

It is usually a simple matter to suture the buccal and palatal flaps together to achieve a sound closure of the wound. While the soft tissues tend to shrink, subperiosteal new bone is deposited which will provide a satisfactory, if smaller, tuberosity from the point of view of the prosthetist.

Consideration can be given to the alternative policy of splinting the fractured fragment until it has united and then removing the tooth or teeth in it surgically at a later date. If the reason for extracting the tooth is an acute abscess this is unlikely to be wise, but if there is no acute infection and the patient has not been in pain this approach may be worth considering. It is particularly applicable if the piece of bone which has fractured off is large so that its loss will affect denture construction.

However, in making the decision to splint the fragment thought must be given to the surgical problem which will be posed by the eventual removal of the tooth or teeth. Sufficient bone will have to be removed at the time of the extraction, not only to overcome the mechanical difficulty which contributed to the fracture, but enough to make the extraction so easy that the bone is not once more fractured. If this means the cutting away of a great deal of the alveolar process the benefit to be expected from splinting the fragment may not be achieved.

SUGGESTED READING

Henderson D. (1974) The palatal island flap in the closure of oral-antral fistulae. *Br. J. Oral Surg.* **12,** 141–146.

CHAPTER 10

SURGICAL ENDODONTICS

INFLAMMATION AND NECROSIS

Inflammation and septic necrosis of the dental pulp arises most commonly as a result of a carious lesion penetrating the dentine as far as the pulp chamber. Organisms may also reach the pulp through the deficient enamel and dentine in the depths of a cingulum invagination or dens en dente, a fracture of the crown which exposes the pulp, or an inadvertent traumatic exposure during cavity preparation. Just occasionally a deep, infected periodontal pocket will cause thrombosis of the apical vessels and infection of the pulp.

Inflammation of the pulp and sterile necrosis may follow thermal irritation from inadequately cooled rotary cutting instruments, chemical irritation from certain restorative materials, or a blow to the tooth which tears the periapical vessels or fractures the root. A pulpitis may follow chronic trauma resulting from mastication on an inadequately contoured filling. If necrosis follows chronic inflammation of the pulp there may be few symptoms and little to suggest the onset of periapical inflammation. A necrotic pulp which initially was sterile may become infected as a result of organisms reaching it. In the absence of an open communication with the mouth the most likely route is from the gingival crevice and via the veins and lymphatics in the periodontal membrane.

Radiographic Considerations

Initially radiographic changes are minimal. An acute pulpal infection spreading to involve the periapical tissues will cause oedema of the periodontal membrane, elevating the tooth in the socket and widening of the periodontal membrane space in the radiograph. The difference is subtle and hardly adequate evidence on its own for a firm diagnosis.

The first indication of bone destruction is loss of the periapical lamina dura. For this to be appreciated a sharp image of the apex and periapical bone must be achieved. If the apex is pointed, and therefore the apical end of the socket is a segment of a sphere of small radius, insufficient lamina dura will be tangential to the X-ray beam to produce a linear image and the lamina dura will not be seen in the radiograph even though the tooth is normal. Conversely, if the root is broad and flattened it is possible for part of the lamina dura at the apex to be destroyed and a linear image still to appear in a radiograph. Thus early radiographic changes must be interpreted only in conjunction with other evidence as to the nature of the disease.

The tracery of cancellous bone trabeculae seen in clinical radiographs represent those which lie tangential to the X-ray beam. Destruction of cancellous bone results in the disappearance of some of these thin linear images but no detectable change in the overall radiopacity of the part. The loss of the trabeculae immediately outside the lamina dura can only be detected as a local change in trabecular density if a previous film is available for direct comparison. Also, experiment suggests that loss of the apical lamina dura is more readily appreciated when these adjacent bony trabeculae have been destroyed. A complete absence of trabecular markings will only occur when all the trabeculae have been destroyed, up to and including those which are attached to the insides of the adjacent cortices.

As the two cortical plates are responsible for most of the radiopacity of the alveolar process, a detectable loss of radiopacity signifies that one or both cortical plates is resorbed. This may be a saucer-shaped depression on the inside of the cortex which will produce an ill defined circular image with a gradually increasing radiolucency towards the centre or a dark, sharply defined image when the cortex is perforated.

If longitudinal sections are prepared through the teeth and alveolar process radially to the dental arch, it will be seen that the lamina dura is fused with the buccal and lingual cortical plates for a substantial distance below the alveolar crest. With the exception of the lower molars up to two-thirds or three-quarters of the labial aspect of the socket is fused with the cortex. This brings the majority of the apices close to the labial or buccal cortex with the result that cortical bone destruction and a periapical radiolucency occurs relatively early in the evolution of an inflammatory periapical lesion.

When a tooth is radiographed during the early days in the development of an acute periapical abscess and is found to have a substantial degree of periapical bone destruction this suggests that the acute episode has followed a previous symptomless chronic one. Paradoxically, chronic low-grade infection will cause increased bone formation on the surfaces of the adjacent cancellous trabeculae at the expense of the marrow spaces to produce a surrounding zone of bone sclerosis. Therefore the degree of periapical radiolucency depends upon the thickness of cortical bone which has been destroyed and whether this radiolucency has a well defined or ill-defined margin depends, not upon the activity or chronicity of the inflammatory process, but whether the cortical plate has been perforated or merely thinned out over the granuloma. Nor is there any reliable radiographic criteria, other than size, to differentiate between a periapical cyst and a granuloma. Beyond an arbitrary diameter of, say, 1 cm it is likely that the lesion is a cyst rather than a granuloma and the larger the lesion, the more likely.

Treatment

The lack of vitality of a tooth should always be confirmed by electrical and thermal pulp tests before root-canal therapy is commenced because of the following.

1. It is not always easy to interpret the widening of the apical periodontal membrane space or loss of the periapical lamina dura. A number of anatomical arrangements will produce radiographic burn-out of the edge of the apex and apparent widening of the periodontal membrane. A natural foramen superimposed over the apex of a tooth may also simulate periapical radiolucency.

2. A number of other pathological processes other than infection may destroy periapical bone.

The first choice of treatment for a non-vital tooth is orthograde endodontic therapy to (*a*) remove necrotic pulp remnants, (*b*) drain any exudate and eliminate active infection, (*c*) ream out the inside of the canal to an adequate size for instrumentation, to achieve a circular cross-section and to produce a suitable taper towards the apex, and then (*d*) obliterate the dead space within the tooth with a suitable root filling.

Successful root treatment and root filling is followed by a resolution of the inflammatory reaction in the periapical granuloma and its replacement by bone or a fibrous scar. In the majority of cases the normal bony anatomy of the apical part of the socket is restored. In some cases a uniform space in the bone remains over the apex filled with mature fibrous tissue with little or no inflammatory cell infiltration. This type of healing is more likely to be seen where there has been some form of periapical surgery. It is normally considered that once a periapical cyst has formed treatment by endodontics alone will not be sufficient and that additional surgical treatment of the cyst will be required. However, there is considerable radiographic evidence that even quite large cysts have healed following no more than efficient orthograde endodontic treatment.

The commonest cause of failure of endodontic treatment is a root filling which does not seal the apical third of the root canal. Such a case presents as a persistent discharging sinus in the sulcus, or a recurrent subacute abscess with pain and swelling. The proper treatment for such a tooth is removal of the faulty root filling and further orthograde endodontic treatment. There are fewer chances of technical error with orthograde treatment especially due to accessory canals than with the placement of a retrograde root filling. The patient is also saved the additional stress and discomfort associated with a minor surgical procedure.

However, there are circumstances where an orthograde root filling is not possible and the management will have to be surgical. These are as follows:

a. Where it is not possible to prepare mechanically and fill the apical third of a root canal because it is sharply angled, irregular or almost obliterated by secondary dentine.

b. Where the canal is obstructed by a fractured root canal instrument which cannot be retrieved or an imperfect root canal filling which cannot be removed.

c. Where the tooth has been crowned or supports a bridge retainer and where it is inappropriate either to drill through the restoration into the pulp chamber or remove it.

d. Where there is a continuous and copious drainage from a periapical cyst which would prevent effective sealing of the apical root canal. (In general it is preferable to root fill the tooth of origin by the orthograde route before removing a periapical cyst, though it may be wise to fill the root not more than 24 hours before the operation as sometimes an acute infection is precipitated following the root filling.)

Other indications for surgery include:

a. The presence of surgically accessible root perforations.

b. A fractured apex which can be removed to leave a sufficient length of undamaged root to support the tooth crown.

c. The removal of irritant root-canal filling material which has extended into the periapical tissues (*see* later).

d. Where for overriding social reasons a one stage procedure for treatment is required and orthograde root filling without periapical counter-drainage would be likely to fail.

e. Where for no obvious reason an apical granuloma fails to heal or where a small cyst fails to regress after orthograde root canal therapy.

It used to be taught that organisms in the apical delta of root canals or in the cell spaces of the apical cellular cementum were a cause of such failures but this is no longer believed to be the case. Drainage of a periapical abscess and the control of active infection by antibiotics should precede apicectomy. Drainage may be obtained through the root canal, or by an incision in the buccal sulcus, or both. Aspiration of periapical pus through the buccal mucosa with a syringe and wide bore needle after infiltration of the site with a local anaesthetic is an alternative to incision. While such measures may render the tooth symptomless they will not be sufficient to prevent recrudescence of the infection or, in some cases, cyst formation unless a proper apical seal is subsequently achieved.

APICECTOMY AND RETROGRADE APICAL SEAL

A common error in the performance of apical surgery is a failure to produce anaesthesia of a sufficient volume of tissue. As a consequence sensitive spots are encountered in the periapical bone or while enucleating a cyst and the insertion of sutures is painful. Buccolabially in the maxilla the alveolar process should be anaesthetized for the width of two teeth either side of the tooth or teeth to be operated upon. This will ensure the painless insertion of sutures. Also solution should be injected well above the sulcus to anaesthetize the superior dental neural arcade before it reaches the periapical lesion. Where a central incisor is to be operated upon either local anaesthetic solution should be introduced up the incisive canal or lignocaine urethral gel should be applied to either side of the nasal septum on ribbon gauze so as to anaesthetize the long sphenopalatine nerves. Both ends of a single strip of ribbon gauze should be used to prevent its displacement backwards into the inferior meatus.

A substantial degree of vasoconstriction is also desirable to ensure as far as possible a near bloodless field, particularly while the apical end of the root canal is identified and while the amalgam seal is placed. Contamination of the amalgam with blood is obviously detrimental to its properties. Therefore, although mandibular and lingual nerve blocks will readily provide a wide field of anaesthesia in the mandible, the infiltration of further solution buccally and lingually to the operation site is desirable. It will be seen that a total of 4 ml of local anaesthetic solution will be required for most cases. Even where a general anaesthetic is used the injection of an adequate amount of solution locally to produce vasoconstriction is necessary. Where it is feasible, the immediate preoperative placement of a root-canal filling will improve the prognosis perhaps by obliterating unidentifiable lateral canals which might lead to the failure of a solitary apical amalgam filling.

The operation may be performed through a broad based, three-sided, rhomboidal flap which includes the interdental papillae at either side of the tooth or teeth involved. This flap provides better access to and visualization of the operative field over and above the apex than the semilunar incision, and the ooze from the laterally placed margins is less likely to interfere with the operative procedure. The alternative semilunar incision carried out over the midpoint of the tooth root has the value of not disturbing the gingival margin related to a crowned tooth, but unless there is gingival pocketing, postoperative exposure of the edge of the crown can be overcome by the careful resuturing of a rhomboidal flap using vertical mattress sutures through the interdental papillae.

The mucoperiosteum is reflected well above the apex of the tooth, the position of which is estimated from any root convexity on the alveolar bone and by reference to the crown of the tooth and the relative root length in a radiograph. There may be a perforation in the cortical plate over the periapical bone defect, or exploration with the sharp pointed end of a Mitchell's trimmer may locate the cavity by penetrating the thin layer of bone over it. If the procedure is to be completed without excessive shortening of the root and with the accurate placement of a filling in the root canal, the undamaged apex must be uncovered first. An inverted semilunar cut is made with a No. 3 rose-head or narrow taper fissure bur over the estimated site of the apex and the labial cortex prised off. The cavity is gradually enlarged until the apex is exposed. There can be unexpected difficulty in the location of the apex of an upper lateral incisor which may lie at some depth, close to the palatal cortex. Once the apex has been uncovered a minimum amount of root tissue is shaved off at an angle of 45° to provide access to the apical canal. The canal can be identified by a probe. The top of the root must be seen clearly because it is possible to create an artefactual canal in the periodontal membrane between the root end and the bone.

A size one-half rose-head bur is carefully inserted into the apical opening to enlarge the end of the canal and to create an undercut cavity. It is possible to do this with a straight handpiece when operating on prominent, labially placed canines and central incisor roots by tilting the patient's head appropriately. However, a special right-angled handpiece with a miniature head makes both access and vision easier. A × 4 halo magnifier facilitates this stage of the operation. The apical areas should be curetted and irrigated free of debris and granulation tissue. The latter, which is essentially a non-infected reparative tissue, need not be meticulously removed. Indeed, the benefit is largely from the removal of a vascular tissue which may ooze during the next procedure.

The bony cavity is packed with ribbon gauze and the pack left in place for 5 minutes. The gauze may be moistened with a drop of 1 in 10000 adrenaline solution to aid local haemostasis. If there is still some ooze from the bone a small amount of Abseal (Ethicon Ltd) can be smeared on to the walls of the cavity with back of a spoon excavator. The apical canal is inspected to see that it is clean and dry and then filled with amalgam. Suitable miniature amalgam carriers can be made from spinal needles or 1 mm orthodontic tube and wire. The amalgam is condensed either with a ball ended plastic or the back of a spoon excavator. Any excess is scraped away and irrigated and sucked out of the cavity taking special care not to impregnate it into the cancellous bone. The seal is inspected by reflecting light onto the root end with a small mirror or polished retractor, then the wound closed with 3/0 black silk or resorbable sutures.

Accessible perforations may be treated in the same manner. A discharging sinus overlying the midpoint of the root of a tooth the subject of root-canal therapy is evidence of such a perforation and a reamer track directed towards the surface of the root may be demonstrable by obliquely taken periapical radiographs. However, both a chronic palatal periodontal abscess and an abscess related to a root with a longitudinal fracture may point on the labial aspect in this way. In both cases an elongated periradicular radiolucency will be seen in the radiograph. Where the cause is a deep palatal pocket, with care the reduced height of the palatal alveolar bone margin may be traced out in a good quality periapical radiograph and the presence of a deep pocket confirmed clinically, though not always is it easy to introduce a periodontal probe into it. A longitudinally fractured root is not amenable to treatment.

Where apical surgery is required to enucleate a cyst and where the canal has been root filled preoperatively it is not essential to perform an apicectomy. However, access to the cavity behind the root and detachment of the lining from this aspect of the periodontal membrane may prove difficult and an apicectomy may be carried out to improve access. The seal created by the root filling should be inspected as both gutta percha and silver points can be disturbed by the apicectomy and, if this is likely, a retrograde amalgam filling should be inserted.

Marked postoperative swelling lasting 4–5 days is not infrequently seen after an apicectomy and patients should be warned about this. One factor may be the vasoconstriction needed to ensure adequate visibility and a dry field for the placement of the amalgam seal. Reactionary hyperaemia and an ooze into the tissues may occur some time after closure of the wound. Swelling from this cause may be reduced by a pressure dressing over the lip where an anterior tooth has been treated. The preoperative administration of 10 mg of intramuscular or intravenous dexamethasone will reduce postoperative oedema where this is likely to cause concern. A course of antibiotics and appropriate analgesics should be prescribed and the first dose of the latter should be given before the patient leaves the surgery so that the drug is active before the local analgesia wears off.

Sometimes infection persists or recurs. A faulty apical seal or an unobliterated accessory canal in the unfilled canal below the amalgam filling may be the cause. It is possible that local resorption of the cut dentine can undermine the relatively shallow apical root filling and may follow from the lack of cementum repair over the root end. Re-treatment, perhaps in conjunction with simultaneous orthograde root filling, should be considered if the tooth is to be preserved.

Apicectomy with a retrograde seal may be carried out with care on most single-rooted teeth though it is doubtful if it is often justified on lower incisors. Access is not easy, the root ends are of such small diameter and a reduction in root length soon affects the long-term prognosis for the tooth. The position of the mental nerve and the curved course of the mandibular nerve as it approaches the mental foramen must be considered in the case of lower premolars.

The 2nd and 3rd lower molars are next to impossible to treat in this way. The overlying cortex is thick and the root apices some distance into the cancellous bone and access is poor. However, the lower 1st molar may be tackled by experienced operators.

As the upper 1st premolar usually has two apices a low resection of the buccal one may be necessary in order to reach and seal the palatal one. A transantral approach through a low alveolar extension of the antrum can be carried out but as it is rarely possible to keep the antral lining intact, great care must be taken not to lose bone debris, a root apex or amalgam fragments into the sinus cavity where they can cause chronic infection. With upper 1st molars the buccal roots are readily treated surgically, but the palatal one is usually impossible and is best root filled orthograde or excised and sealed at the level of the trifurcation, if necessary from the palatal side.

Other inaccessible molar roots may also be amputated and sealed close to the pulp chamber or the tooth hemisected to leave a single well supported root.

It is important, particularly where surgically difficult procedures are envisaged, to consider carefully the benefits and possible complications of what is proposed and to discuss these matters and the likely results in the long term with the patient. The patient must understand what will be involved and the chances of success or failure. Where the practitioner does not have the personal experience to undertake what is required there should be no hesitation in referring the patient to someone with the requisite special skill.

ENDODONTIC ENDOSSEOUS IMPLANTS

Endosseous implants may be used to stabilize teeth where attached root length has been lost either due to some pathological process or to excessive surgical enthusiasm. The technique has also been recommended to stabilize unsupported teeth following periodontitis. However, the prognosis in such a situation is poor unless there has been complete control of the periodontal bone loss and of active periodontal infection. The implant may be fabricated from Wiptam*: nickel chrome wire 1·3 mm or 1·5 mm in diameter. It must be of sufficient length to extend to the original position of the tooth apex and must also penetrate at least 5 mm into sound bone. At the coronal end sufficient wire will be required both for manipulation and also for the construction of a core to carry a crown. This may be done outside the mouth in the laboratory. Ready made endodontic implants together with appropriate bone drills are also available commercially.†

First the canal must be carefully and completely reamed to the implant diameter. The apical area is then exposed surgically, irrigated and dried with ribbon gauze and the canal also dried. The cement is then applied to the canal walls. This may be either EPA (epoxyorthobenzoic acid) or cold cure acrylic. The coronal half of the implant is also covered with cement and then the implant inserted into the canal and through the apex where it is carefully wiped with a sterile pledget of cotton wool prior to removing the ribbon gauze pack. The post may then be tapped firmly into the overlying bone and any excess cement carefully curetted and washed out of the bone wound. The closure is as described for an apicectomy.

---

* Wiptam clasp wire, Fried. Krupp, Essen, West Germany
† Dental Orotronic (UK) Ltd, 59 Queen Anne Street, London, W1M OHQ

Care must be taken in planning this procedure to ensure that the direction of the root is such that there will be apical bone to receive the implant. Occasionally with a Class 2, division II retroclined upper incisor where there is a concave alveolus the apex may be so superficial that an implant extends into the buccal soft tissues.

REMOVAL OF PERIAPICAL ENDODONTIC PASTE

Over-enthusiastic use of endodontic pastes may cause extrusion into the periapical bone. Usually this may be removed by a simple apicectomy. However, the introduction of a paraform containing paste into the inferior dental canal will give rise to impaired labial sensation which may persist. Transalveolar attempts to remove the paste from the molar region with or without extraction of the associated tooth often fail due to poor access and may damage the neurovascular bundle. Subsequent bone healing can even irreversibly obliterate the nerve canal.

The most rational means of removing such paste is by sagittally splitting off the outer cortex between two vertical cuts. The canal can often be exposed even without separation at the lower border, so that only an intraosseous wire is required for postoperative bony union. With a complete split intermaxillary fixation for 2–3 weeks is desirable.

SUGGESTED READING

Harty F. J. (1981) *Endodontics in Clinical Practice.* Bristol: Wright.
Monsour F. N. T. and Adkins K. F. (1985) Aberrations in pulpal histology and dentinogenesis in transplanted erupting teeth. *J. Maxillofac. Surg.* **43**, 8–11.
Nehammer C. F. (1985) Endodontics in practice: surgical endodontics. *Br. Dent. J.* **158**, 400–409.

CHAPTER 11

CYSTS OF THE JAWS

A cyst is an abnormal cavity lined by epithelium, fibrous tissue or occasionally by neoplastic tissue. Its contents may be fluid or semi-solid. Some cysts are believed to contain gas, but the only instances in which this is known for certain to be so are the gas filled cysts of the wall of the intestine and colon (pneumatosis cystoides intestinales).

While cyst contents may become infected so that pus is formed, cysts do not contain pus initially. Encapsulated chronic abscesses are not considered to be cysts although the pus may be described as 'encysted'.

Most forms of cysts in the jaws, floor of the mouth and neck are lined on the inner surface by a layer of epithelium. The connective tissue comprising the outer aspect of this sac forms a capsule and the whole forms a dissectable lining. Some types of cyst have no epithelial component to the sac, which in these cases is formed solely by a connective tissue membrane. This is often quite thin and may be intimately joined to the adjacent surrounding tissues so that it is not readily dissectable as in the ranula or the solitary bone cyst.

Cystic lesions of the jaws may be divided into three groups: odontogenic, fissural cysts and bone cysts. The odontogenic cysts arise from the epithelium concerned in tooth formation and comprise three main types: follicular (dentigerous), periodontal and keratocysts. There are also other cysts which are named on the basis of their clinical presentation, but which may not form a single entity and therefore are difficult to classify.

A simple classification of cysts of the jaws is as follows (*Fig.* 11.1):

Cysts of the Jaws
A. *Of odontogenic epithelium:*
   1. Derived from the dental lamina:
      a. Keratocysts:
         i. Solitary or primordial cysts
         ii. Pseudo-follicular or extra-follicular dentigerous cysts
      b. Calcifying odontogenic cysts.
   2. Derived from reduced enamel epithelium:
      a. Eruption cyst
      b. Follicular or dentigerous cysts:
         i. Pericoronal
         ii. Lateral
         iii. Residual.

3. Derived from epithelial debris of Malassez:
    a. Inflammatory periodontal (radicular):
        i. Apical
        ii. Lateral
        iii. Residual.
B. *Of non-odontogenic epithelium (Fissural):*
    1. Nasopalatine
    2. Nasolabial.
C. *Bone cysts:*
    1. Solitary bone cyst
    2. Aneurysmal bone cyst.

There are two phases to the growth of an epithelium lined cyst: initiation, which results in the first small cavity, and subsequent enlargement. The initiation is different for each group of cysts, but with variations the enlargement process is probably similar for all epithelium lined cysts. Nothing is known for certain about the origin of bone cysts and little about their mode of enlargement.

CYSTS OF ERUPTION AND FOLLICULAR OR DENTIGEROUS CYSTS

These form from the reduced enamel epithelium present on the surface of the tooth crown after it has become completely calcified. Normally this epithelium proliferates towards the surface of the alveolus where it meets and fuses with the downward proliferating basal cells of the alveolar epithelium. Lysis within this mass of cells forms an epithelium lined defect through which the tooth erupts (McHugh, 1961). Failure of the overlying alveolar epithelium to break down will give rise to an eruption cyst.

Cysts of eruption present as bluish, fluctuant swellings in the mucosa immediately over an erupting tooth. With few exceptions this is a primary molar but sometimes an incisor. Almost always the cyst ruptures spontaneously and the tooth erupts. Very occasionally the cyst remains intact and the child and parents suffer a succession of sleepless nights. If, under these circumstances, the cyst is incised a clear or yellowish fluid escapes from a cavity between the mucosa and the enamel of the tooth crown. If a segment of cyst wall is removed the cavity surface will be found to be incompletely lined by a thin, stratified, unkeratinized squamous epithelium. The histological appearance suggests that the follicular tissues have separated from the surface of the enamel, with patches of the reduced enamel epithelium adherent to their inner aspect.

Where eruption is impeded or delayed these cells may continue to proliferate around the crown of the tooth and then the mature inner layers undergo liquefaction degeneration leaving a pericoronal cyst. Occasionally the cyst is related to the lateral aspect of the crown or exceptionally may

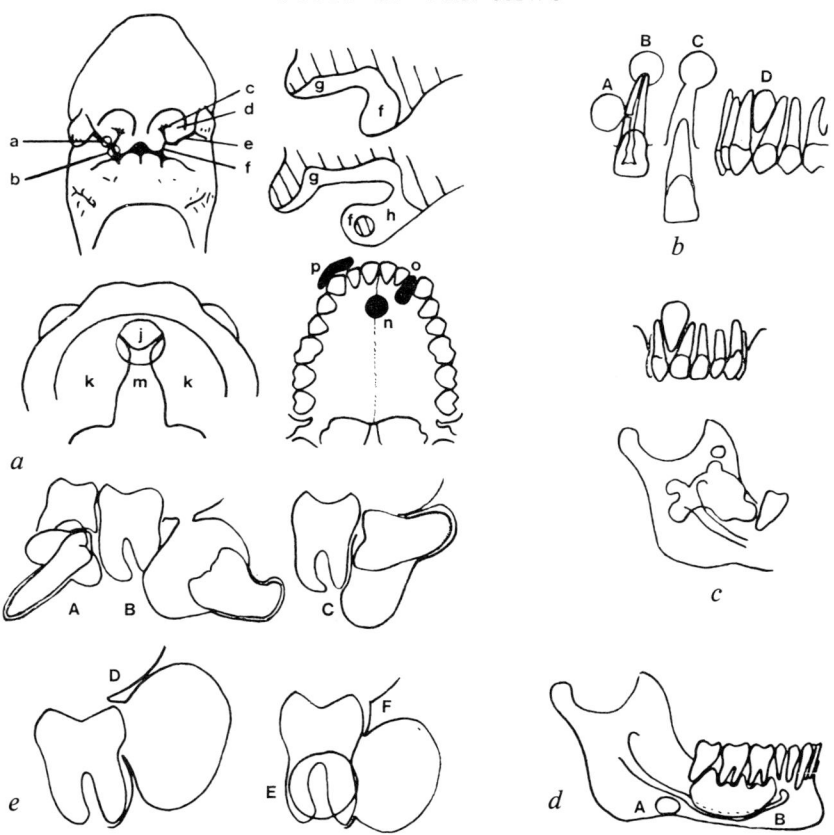

Fig. 11.1. Diagrams of cysts of the jaws.

a, Fissural cysts: *Top left.* Diagram of the face of a human embryo at 6 weeks. *Top right.* Diagram of sections through the developing nasal pit showing how the nasal fin is breached by maxillary and premaxillary mesoderm. a, Site at which nasolabial cyst develops. b, Site at which globulomaxillary cyst develops. c, Nasal pit. d, Lateral nasal process. e, Naso-optic or nasomaxillary groove. f, Nasal fin. g, Olfactory placode. h, Bucconasal membrane. *Bottom left.* Diagram of the developing palate. *Bottom right.* Sites of fissural or non-odontogenic developmental cysts. j, Primary palate or medial palatal process. k, Lateral palatine processes. m, Site of nasopalatine (incisive canal) cyst. n, Incisive canal cyst. o, Globulomaxillary cyst. p, Nasolabial cyst.

b, Periodontal cysts: A, Lateral. B, Apical. C, Residual. D, Residual (deciduous tooth).

c, Primordial cysts: *Top.* Replacing tooth. *Bottom.* Distal to 3rd molar.

d, Bone cysts: A, Stafne's idiopathic cavity. B, Solitary bone cyst.

e, Dentigerous and developmental periodontal cysts: Dentigerous cysts—A, circumferential; B, pericoronal; C and D, Lateral. Periodontal cysts—E, Lateral; F, Distal.

surround the neck or root of the tooth as it continues to erupt through it in which case it is described as being circumferential.

Where a lateral dentigerous cyst forms distal to a vertical or disto-angularly impacted 3rd molar a subsequent attack of acute pericoronitis may result in the rupture and regression of the cyst. Usually the cyst pulls away with the tooth if it is extracted but it has been known for the cyst sac to remain behind and to continue to enlarge as a residual cyst.

Dentigerous cysts (follicular cysts) form around the crown of an unerupted tooth. They involve teeth of the adult dentition or occasionally supernumerary teeth. The proliferation, liquefaction and separation process involving the reduced enamel epithelium which initiates cyst formation occurs at a time other than when eruption is briefly delayed. In some instances a cyst is discovered when only a short length of root has formed and long before the normal time of eruption. Where there is a deciduous predecessor even the process of root resorption may be far from complete. Other dentigerous cysts develop on teeth which are impacted or unerupted and where eruption is delayed. In some cases they develop in middle age when they can achieve a large size. The cyst sac is lined by a stratified squamous epithelium of variable thickness. Sometimes there are epithelial discontinuities and sometimes patches of mucus secreting goblet cells. The capsular connective tissue contains little or no inflammatory infiltrate.

The recognition of a dentigerous cyst radiographically in the early stages of development is not easy. As a tooth moves towards the alveolar crest when the time for eruption approaches the follicular space widens and the gubernacular opening enlarges. The bone is resorbed away from the crown producing a series of outlines like the opening of the petals of a flower. If the tooth is radiographed at the beginning of the eruptive stage the widened follicle may be mistaken for a cyst, particularly if the appearance of widening is enhanced by magnification due to projection over a distance on to the film.

Dentigerous cysts which develop around the crowns of 1st or 2nd molars may produce a bluish fluctuant swelling involving the overlying alveolar mucosa. However, unlike cysts of eruption, spontaneous rupture is uncommon and there is a substantial concavity in the underlying bone. Elsewhere the first indication of the presence of a dentigerous cyst is likely to be the failure of eruption of the involved tooth at the appropriate time. A radiograph will then reveal a rounded bone cavity surrounding the crown of the tooth. The tooth will be displaced by the expanding cyst away from the alveolar process, at first with its long axis radial to the cyst cavity but later as the root impinges on the inside of the cortex it is deflected to lie nearly tangential to the cyst.

Inflammatory Periodontal Cysts (Radicular Cysts)

The periodontal cyst arises from the cell rests of Malassez and usually forms at the apex of a tooth with a necrotic pulp where it appears to act as a lympho-epithelial barrier to the spread of pulpal infection into the surrounding tissues. If associated with an accessory pulp canal the cyst will develop in a lateral relationship to the root where it will be morphologically and radiologically indistinguishable from the lateral periodontal cyst associated with a vital tooth, which is presumed to be the result of cell rest proliferation brought about by bacterial provocation from the gingival crevice. Although periodontal cysts may regress spontaneously following root-canal therapy or extraction of the associated tooth, occasionally one may persist and is called a residual periodontal cyst.

Periodontal cyst epithelium is stratified squamous with rete pegs but varies in thickness and in some areas may be keratinized or even absent. The surrounding connected tissue capsule has a varying degree of inflammatory cell infiltrate often with dense foci of lymphocytes and monocytes. The infiltrate is usually more intense in the smaller and presumably younger cysts, than in the larger ones.

Keratocysts

Keratocysts arise from remnants of the dental lamina. Those which develop posterior to the 3rd molar, between standing teeth or, as occasionally happens, where a tooth of the permanent series is missing, are sometimes called primordial cysts. It has been suggested in the past, but without evidence, that primordial cysts arise by degeneration of the stellate reticulum in a tooth germ. This theory requires that there was a supernumerary tooth germ from which the cyst developed in cases where the adult dentition is complete, but many keratocysts arise in parts of the jaw where supernumeraries are uncommon. On the other hand, keratinizing cell rests of the dental lamina are particularly abundant in the submucosa of the retromolar regions, a part of the jaws where primordial cysts are frequently found, so that this more elaborate suggestion as to their origin is unnecessary.

Daughter cysts are sometimes seen developing from groups of epithelial cells in the capsule of a cyst wall removed at operation. The epithelial cells become orientated with the cuboidal basal cells on the outer, connective tissue aspect of the sphere, and the mature squamous ones towards the centre where they keratinize and are shed. Initially a keratin pearl is seen, but later, where the shed cells have degenerated, a cyst cavity forms.

Keratocysts may also develop from dental lamina rests immediately above a tooth in the gubernaculum between the follicle and the overlying mucosa (the epithelial 'glands' of Serres). Such cysts envelop the crown, displacing it and preventing its eruption. Clinically and radiographically these cysts resemble dentigerous cysts, but if they are opened the crown of the tooth is not seen protruding into the cavity. Histologically the cyst wall envelops the crown of the tooth which is separated from it by the tooth follicle, hence they are sometimes described as pseudo-follicular cysts or extra-follicular dentigerous cysts. The stimulus which initiates proliferation of the cell rests and hence the development of keratocysts is unknown. It may be genetic as seen in the basal cell naevus syndrome (*see below*).

The epithelium lining keratocysts is 6–8 cells thick and with a basal layer of cuboidal or low columnar cells with nuclei which may exhibit reversal of polarity. There is an abrupt transition between the stratum spinosum and a surface layer of para-keratinized cells. There are no rete pegs. The enucleated and fixed lining shrinks slightly with a tendency to separation of the epithelium from the underlying connective tissue. The contraction throws the keratin layer into small folds. The capsule is quite thin and normally free of inflammatory cells, but often contains strands of odontogenic epithelium resembling the dental lamina, cell nests, with central keratinization and daughter cysts. Sometimes the epithelial strands are connected to the basal layer of the lining epithelium as though developing from it.

The Basal Cell Naevus Syndrome
(Gorling and Goltz syndrome)

This could equally be called the multiple jaw cyst syndrome because it is usually through the appearance of jaw cysts that sufferers present. The condition follows a dominant mode of inheritance with high penetrance and variable expressivity but sporadic cases also occur.

The jaw cysts are keratocysts of both the solitary and the extra-follicular dentigerous (pseudo-follicular) varieties. These start to develop about the time of the eruption of the adult dentition. The skull is often brachicephalic with frontal and parietal bossing and ocular hypertelorism. Ocular abnormalities are apparent in childhood and a mild prognathism due to the short cranial base may be the cause of an orthodontic consultation.

During adolescence tiny whitish epidermal cysts or 'milia' appear in the skin around the eyes and tiny circular patches of epithelium may be shed from the thick skin of palms and soles to produce pitting. Epidermal cysts may develop under the skin in various parts of the body. Later, pinkish or white, circular skin plaques develop on the face, cheek and trunk which are basal cell naevi, some of which can progress to frank basal cell carcinomata. Ovarian cysts and rarely medulloblastoma formation can complicate the presentation.

A variety of skeletal abnormalities may be seen in radiographs including calcifications of the falx cerebri seen in postero-anterior skull radiographs, calcific bridging over the sella turcica on lateral skull radiography, fusion of cervical vertebrae or occult spina bifida in the cervical or thoracic regions and bifid ribs. Many other less common anomalies are described.

The Calcifying Odontogenic Cyst
(Calcifying and Keratinizing Odontogenic Cyst)

This rare lesion can occur in a unilocular and a multilocular form. The latter variant may develop a thick capsule into which strands of epithelium resembling the dental lamina proliferate, forming daughter cysts.

In both unilocular and multilocular forms dental tissues may be induced giving rise to multiple small odontomes. The variable presentation may account for its inclusion in the classifications of odontogenic tumours.

The most common site is the anterior part of the mandible with a peak incidence in the second decade.

Clinical and Histological Features

Mostly a single cavity lesion is discovered originating between standing teeth and displacing or resorbing their roots. Some appear to develop superficially with a substantial part producing a fluctuant subperiosteal swelling. Examples are sometimes found in the retromolar region entirely in the soft tissue and presumably developing from local dental lamina remnants. Tiny. highly radiopaque bodies may be spotted in the radiograph lying in a layer parallel to the inner surface of the bone cavity.

Histologically the odontogenic type lining epithelium is 6–8 cells thick and has a columnar or cuboidal basal layer of cells with their nuclei polarized away from the basement membrane. There can be a superficial resemblance to a keratocyst in a small biopsy. In patches the epithelium proliferates, the cells becoming swollen and then eosinophilic, due to a form of keratinization, but with persistence of pyknotic nuclei. These are called ghost cells. Later these cells fuse and tend to calcify. If pyknotic nuclei are included in the calcified mass it may resemble cellular cementum at first sight. It is the calcification in these epithelial cell masses which forms the opacities seen in radiographs.

Where the eosinophilic change involves the whole thickness of the epithelium it may be shed or incite granulation tissue to appear in the adjacent connective tissue capsule with giant cells phagacytosing some of the cells. Occasionally inductive changes are seen both under the ghost cell masses and the taller basal cells with the formation, first of an atubular dentinoid, and then tubular dentine. Unlike keratocysts, simple enucleation is never followed by recurrence.

NON-ODONTOGENIC FISSURAL CYSTS

These include the naso-palatine or incisive canal cysts and the nasolabial or nasoalveolar cysts. Globulo-maxillary, median mandibular, median alveolar and median palatine cysts are also described but their authenticity or even the actual existence of some of these entities is in doubt.

The Nasopalatine or Incisive Canal Cyst

Fusion between the primary palate and the two palatine processes of the maxilla is completed at the centre of a triradiate junction. Later the bony incisive canals are formed by the developing maxillary bones for the passage downwards of the terminal parts of the long sphenopalatine nerves and the passage upwards of the greater palatine vessels which will anastomose with the sphenopalatine vessels on the nasal septum. In the foetus, cords of epithelial cells which sometimes canalize, and which are referred to as the nasopalatine ducts, are found in relation to the incisive canals. Nasopalatine cysts are believed to develop from these structures.

Incisive canal cysts are nasopalatine cysts which produce a cavity in the bone. The majority develop within the incisive fossa and are covered only by palatal mucoperiosteum on the palatal aspect. They enlarge upwards and backwards towards the nose and palate but also forwards between the roots of the central incisors where a swelling in the labial sulcus may be produced.

A deep incisive fossa may be difficult to distinguish radiographically from a small cyst. As these cysts enlarge only slowly and do not cause problems until they reach around 1·5 cm diameter a policy of observation is the correct approach in doubtful cases. Indeed, in the absence of symptoms, only if the cyst is sizeable—and only rarely do they enlarge much beyond 2 cm diameter—is surgery necessary. Indications for treatment are encroachment on the central incisors, and attacks of infection, especially when a communication develops with the mouth and when a fluctuant palatal swelling appears, especially in the edentulous patient.

Particular care must be taken not to mistake an incisive canal cyst for an apical periodontal one arising from a central incisor because often the image of these cysts coincides with the apex of the incisors in periapical films. Examples involving just the incisive canals singly or bilaterally can be found.

Histological examination of these cysts reveals a lining which may be of stratified squamous epithelium or, less frequently, ciliated and pseudo-stratified columnar cells with mucous glands which secrete into the cyst.

Incisive Papilla Cysts

These develop entirely in the soft tissues of the incisive fossa and cause recurrent swellings just posterior to the incisive papilla. They produce no radiographic changes but frequently discharge a salty tasting fluid into the mouth. A tiny opening may be found lateral to the incisive papilla or longitudinal ruga.

Nasolabial Cysts

Nasolabial cysts are rare and arise above the buccal sulcus under the ala of the nose. They grow slowly, lifting up the nasolabial fold and bulging into both the inferior meatus of the nose and the labial sulcus. They lie outside the bone, but cause pressure resorption of the margin of the anterior bony aperture of the nose and the labial aspect of the base of the alveolar process.

A standard occlusal radiograph demonstrates the resorption of the inferior margin of the anterior bony aperture. Normally the two inferior nasal margins together with the buttress of the anterior nasal spine produce a 'bracket' shaped line in this view. A nasolabial cyst converts one half of this line into a concave rather than a convex shape.

The epithelium of the lining is usually pseudo-stratified columnar or cuboidal, or ciliated and with the goblet cells. Sometimes it is stratified squamous. The fluid is either straw-coloured or whitish with a mucoid consistency.

Several explanations have been advanced for their origin. Some believe that they are mucous cysts arising from epithelium lining the floor of the nose or a mucous gland in the labial sulcus. However, around 10% of cases are bilateral which supports the alternative explanation that they are developmental in origin, possibly fissural cysts. If so, sequestered epithelium from the depths of the groove between the maxillary and lateral nasal process would seem to be the most likely origin.

Other Types of Fissural Cyst

These have been described, notably the globulomaxillary cyst. At one time examples purporting to be globulomaxillary cysts were reported regularly, but when looked at critically most were apical periodontal cysts arising from pulpless lateral incisors. Since the canine erupts normally they must develop after this has happened.

The characteristic appearance of a globulomaxillary cyst is that it has a pear shape, occupies the interdental bone between the maxillary lateral incisor and canine roots, and pushes them apart. Radiographs of apical periodontal cysts on lateral incisors can be found which show how, in some cases, they enlarge progressively into the interdental bone rather than expand symmetrically about the tooth apex.

Cysts of the characteristic pear shaped appearance can be found where both the lateral incisor and canine have vital pulps but they are rare. It has been suggested that these may be residual apical periodontal cysts from teeth of the primary dentition, possibly a displaced lateral follicular cyst from the canine, or keratocysts (primordial cysts). Keratocysts are uncommon in the upper incision region and of course are readily recognized histologically.

If indeed globulomaxillary cysts exist as a rare developmental entity then they develop from sequestered epithelium from the nasal fin which is formed by fusion of the surface epithelia of the maxillary and medial nasal processes as they bulge forwards in contact with one another below the nasal pit. This epithelial sheet subsequently disappears and maxillary ectomesenchyme migrates medially.

The two palatine processes of the maxilla join first by fusion of the epithelium covering their edges and this subsequently fenestrates and breaks down to form keratin pearls and microcysts at the line of fusion. Epstein's pearls seen in many neonates in a diamond shape at the junction of the hard and soft palate are thought to derive from these epithelial remnants. However, no case of an inclusion cyst (median palatine cyst) developing in the midline of the palate posterior to the nasopalatine region has been reported in an unequivocal fashion and the existence of such cysts is doubted.

Some writers mention median alveolar cysts of the maxilla but the primary palate develops as a median structure which rules out such a possibility, and again no case which could not have been a nasopalatine cyst is described.

The mandibular mesenchyme from each side migrates medially and fuses beneath the epithelium to form the mandibular arch so that median mandibular fissural cysts should not exist. A number of authors have collected cases in which a cyst is present in the midline of the mandible between the divergent roots of vital central incisors. Such cysts could be residual apical periodontal cysts from the primary dentition, keratocysts which are common in the lower incisor region, or lateral periodontal cysts.

Median dermoid cysts of the floor of the mouth are seen from time to time, in the midline just behind the mandible, and of course the anterior two-thirds of the tongue develops from paired processes which develop on the back of the mandibular arch.

BONE CYSTS

The solitary or unicameral bone cyst is usually symptomless and detected as an incidental finding during a radiographic examination. If the cyst becomes large enough it may cause expansion of either the buccal or lingual cortex or both so that the patient complains of a swelling. They occur mostly in the premolar and molar region of the mandible above the inferior dental canal, but may be found also in the lower incisor region and the ramus. As they enlarge they push up into the interdental bone between the teeth to produce a characteristically scalloped outline to the upper margin.

Downward extension carries the cyst to the lower border, sometimes displacing the inferior dental bundle, but at other times progressing around it, so that the nerve and vessels are within the cavity. The cortex is usually thinned but expansion occurs late on and may first involve the lingual aspect below the mylohyoid ridge where it may be overlooked. The associated teeth are normally vital and the lamina dura persists around them for some time. The roots of related teeth may be displaced by the enlarging cyst and unerupted teeth, usually molars, are prevented from eruption. The inner aspect of the cavity is covered by a delicate vascular connective tissue, folds of which may contain neurovascular bundles to the apices of the teeth and enclose the inferior dental bundle. Clumps of granulation tissue containing masses of foamy macrophages may be encountered. The bony walls lack the smoothness of other jaw cysts and of course there is no dissectable lining composed of epithelium and a fibrous capsule. These lesions share features in common with the unicameral bone cysts of long bones and are found most often in the first, second and third decade but may be encountered in older individuals.

If the larger examples are aspirated with care a deep yellow coloured fluid may be obtained. This contains plasma proteins and will clot if left to stand. From smaller ones a heavily bloodstained fluid or fresh blood may be drawn off. If the bloodstained fluid is spun down, a yellow supernatant plasma will be recovered with, as in the case of the clear yellow fluid, a high content of bilirubin. It is quite easy to induce haemorrhage from the cyst wall so the aspiration of fresh blood is easily understood. The bilirubin is evidence of past haemorrhage and also a lack of drainage of the contents into the lymphatics. Some cysts are reported as 'empty' and it has been suggested that they contain gas such as nitrogen, oxygen and carbon dioxide.

Occasionally cysts diagnosed on radiographic grounds heal spontaneously. Others do so after aspiration which induces haemorrhage. Removing part of the bony wall and lightly curetting the lining membrane where no damage to neurovascular bundles will be caused usually provokes most bone cysts to heal. The wound is primarily closed after haemostasis. Recurrence tends to occur in the case of those operated upon before adolescence.

Histological examination of the wall of these cysts casts little light upon their origin. Outside a vascular connective tissue membrane, lamellar bone or sub-periosteal new bone is seen with either osteoclastic resorption or even bone deposition taking place on the inner aspect, but neither very actively.

Occasionally the cavity is associated with an area of fibrous dysplasia. Their origin is uncertain. A local abnormality of endosteal bone remodelling has been suggested with, from time to time, haemorrhage occurring into the cavity from the small vessels in the wall. There is no good evidence that they arise as a result of trauma.

The Aneurysmal Bone Cyst

This should not be confused with the solitary bone cyst. Indeed, the cavity in the bone is filled with a vascular sponge of soft tissue so it is not completely cystic. The name refers rather to the radiographic appearance of a blown out bone cavity outlined by subperiosteal new bone.

The lesion usually presents during adolescence as a large expansile lesion in the mandible or, more rarely, the maxilla. The radiographic features are an oval or spherical bone cavity showing substantial expansion and covered by sub-periosteal new bone but with internal ridges and incomplete septa giving a septate appearance. Occasional patches of fine bony trabeculation are seen in some examples.

Histologically the lesion is composed of sinusoidal vascular channels and cystic areas of varying size with connective tissue septa between. Woven bone may be deposited in these and aggregations of giant cells may be found. The histology of the solid component varies from that of a giant cell granuloma with spindle cells and multinucleate giant cells to tissue resembling an ossifying or cementifying fibroma, i.e. small trabeculae of osteoid, woven bone, or cementoid.

A persistent ooze impedes the operation of enucleation but once the soft tissue contents have been removed haemorrhage from the bony wall may be controlled by the application of Abseal (Ethicon Ltd), a putty-like mixture of fibrin and collagen. If necessary the cavity can be packed with ribbon gauze soaked in Whitehead's varnish. Recurrence occurs after incomplete removal and so large lesions may have to be resected as a benign tumour and reconstructed with an iliac crest bone graft.

OTHER CYSTIC ENTITIES
Gingival Cysts

Several types of small cyst may be found in the gingival mucosa. Bohn's nodules are tiny white keratin pearls seen on the crest of the ridge of neonates and probably represent superficial remnants of the dental lamina. In some negro children they may enlarge to 2–3 mm in diameter and take on a pale violet colour. After a few weeks they are shed spontaneously. Micro cysts and keratin pearls are sometimes found on histological examination of gingivectomy specimens and small cysts identified outside the alveolar bone in the buccal and labial mucosa. Some are small mucous cysts.

Developmental Lateral Periodontal Cysts

These are found lateral to the roots of the vital teeth. These cysts probably include more than one entity.

Cysts develop against the distal root surface of the lower 3rd molars which are clearly unrelated to the crown and are not lateral dentigerous in origin. They immediately destroy the lamina dura and adjacent bone whereas when a lateral dentigerous cyst enlarges downwards the lamina dura persists for some while. They probably arise from epithelial rests of Malassez proliferating as a result of bacterial provocation from organisms under the gum flap. Another entity develops in the bifurcation between the 3rd molar roots, either buccally or lingually but more often on the buccal side.

Hodson (1957) described a specimen which developed in continuity with a cord of epithelium arising from the reduced enamel epithelium. Crain (1976) demonstrated this relationship in a series of specimens and established an association with an enamel projection on the buccal aspect of the root bifurcation. He showed that the periodontal membrane was exterior to the cyst capsule, between it and the epithelial debris of Malassez which was inactive. He calls these cysts paradental cysts and believes chronic pericoronal infection initiates their growth.

Some of these cysts develop lingually in which case they soon perforate the lingual plate of the mandible below the mylohyoid ridge. Infection of such a cyst has been seen to produce a fulminating submandibular infection.

Another form of periodontal cyst involves the inter-radicular bone in the canine and premolar region. These may be residual cysts from carious primary molars as retained deciduous molar roots are found in the same location. They need to be distinguished from keratocysts which can develop at this site. Cysts found lateral to the canine and premolar roots which perforate the buccal wall of the socket may be gingival cysts which have enlarged inwards rather than cysts of periodontal origin.

CYST ENLARGEMENT

Once the initiation of cysts has been considered, their continued enlargement has to be explained. Any explanation for cyst enlargement has to account for:

a. An increase in the volume of the contents;

b. An increase in the surface area of the sac, and if this is lined by epithelium, this also has to increase in area; and

c. Displacement of the surrounding soft tissues or resorption of the surrounding bone where the cyst develops within bone.

If enlargement is prevented or delayed on one aspect by the consistency of the surrounding tissues, it will progress at other sites where the tissues are more easily displaced, stretched, resorbed or disrupted. Where there is an epithelial component, thickness of the epithelium depends upon the rate of multiplication of the basal cells, their speed of maturation and rate at which they are shed. The rate of mitotic division of the basal cells in a keratocyst is greater than in an apical periodontal cyst.

If proliferation of the epithelium leads to an increase in surface area which is closely related to the increase in volume, the inner surface of the sac remains smooth. If the increase in surface area exceeds the increase in volume of the contents, inwardly directed folds result to produce a papillary appearance on histological section.

In the case of some cysts like dermoid cysts, it is evident that desquamated epithelial cells, hair and secretions from sebaceous glands add to the volume of the contents. Where the lining is mucus secreting an accumulation of mucus explains the increase in volume. In the case of cysts of the jaws our understanding of cyst enlargement is incomplete, but the following stages are recognizable for the periapical inflammatory cysts.

Low-grade infection of a non-vital dental pulp stimulates the cell rests of Mallasez in the periapical periodontal membrane to proliferate to form arcades at the periphery of the periapical granuloma. They eventually form a confluent layer sealing off the apical foramen (Valdehaug, 1971) and the contained granulation tissue and round-cell infiltrate liquefies. Cyst epithelium does not appear capable of inducing an endogenous vascular connective tissue stroma in the same way as a solid epithelial tumour by releasing the so-called tumour angiogenesis factor, and so the cells are seen to proliferate in layers from the surface of the adjacent vascular connective tissue. This connective tissue becomes organized as the cyst capsule. In the periodontal cyst the epithelial–capsular interface usually forms rete pegs. The number of epithelial layers is presumably determined by the period of viability of each cell as it is separated from the basement membrane by the dividing basal layer and by the rate at which maturation and desquamation occurs. As these cells divide the cyst is able to enlarge within the rigid bony environment by the release of bone resorbing factors from the capsule which stimulate osteoclast function. These consist of prostanoids PGE_2 (Harris, 1978), PGI_2 (Harvey *et al.,* 1984) and leukotrienes (Makejka et al., 1985). Inflammatory cells which are commonly seen in the capsule also release cofactors. Lymphocytes release the lymphokine, osteoclast activating factor (OAF), and monocytes, interleukin I, which stimulates the fibroblasts to release the prostaglandins (Harvey *et al.,* 1984). This cyst enlargement is principally determined by the continued stimulation of epithelial proliferation which in turn activates the all-important capsule.

The osmotic theory of enlargement reviewed by Main (1970) and Harris and Toller (1975) is both popular and readily understood, but unfortunately the concept that epithelial cell breakdown products produce a hyper-osmolar cyst fluid which draws in fluid from the surrounding tissues is difficult to sustain as the principal mechanism of growth. The presence of large intracystic molecules such as globulins, fibrinogen and fibrin degradation products makes it impossible to consider the complex cyst wall as being a semi-permeable membrane. In fact the contents of periodontal cyst fluid suggests that transudation, exudation and haemorrhage all take place through the mural vessels. Furthermore, the apparent intracystic hydrostatic pressure measured by inserting a fine bore needle attached to a manometer (Toller, 1948) is more likely to result from a change in volume due to cyst wall contractility or swelling of the lining than from an outwardly acting force capable of inducing bone resorption.

Any process that leads to the involution of the cyst epithelium such as extraction of the necrotic tooth or endontic therapy, or its conversion to oral mucosa as with marsupialization, will cause the connective tissue capsule to regress and the cavity to be filled by bone or scar tissue. With marsupialization the cyst epithelium and capsule are replaced by oral mucoperiosteum. This may be incomplete with keratocysts where patches of cyst epithelium persist, potentially giving rise to superficial recurrent cyst formation. Where a cystic ameloblastoma is inadvertently marsupialized the cavity becomes filled with proliferating ameloblastoma epithelium.

CYSTS OF THE JAWS
CLINICAL PRESENTATION

Many cysts are discovered on routine radiographic examination, often before expansion of the jaw is noticed. However, a cyst should be suspected where there is a smooth, rounded expansion of either mandible or maxilla. Where resorption and deposition of subperiosteal new bone results in only a thin layer of overlying new bone the surface can be indented with the examining finger, fracturing the bone and producing the so called ping-pong ball effect. When only microscopic amounts of bone remain beneath the mucoperiosteum fluctuation can be elicited and the swelling may take on a dark bluish appearance. If two fluctuant swellings are present in the same jaw it may be possible to elicit fluctuation between them. This is a sign that there is only one cavity, if not then there may be two cysts, or the lesion may be multilocular. The fitting surface of a denture which has been made some years previously may also provide evidence for the length of time the swelling has been present.

Absence of a tooth from its place in the arch suggests the presence of a dentigerous cyst, particularly in the young. In the older patient, perhaps with a history that the tooth was extracted, a residual periapical cyst is more likely. Suitable radiographs will help to confirm or refute these deductions.

Dentigerous cysts tend to arise in relation to teeth subject to delayed eruption, i.e. 3rd molars, 2nd premolars and maxillary canines, and less often supernumerary teeth in the upper incisor region and the upper incisors themselves. Displacement of adjacent unerupted teeth in a child's jaw by a cyst may be deduced if their follicular spaces and gubernacular canals remain visible in radiographs.

A carious, discoloured, fractured or heavily filled tooth related to the swelling suggests an apical periodontal cyst. In a high percentage of cases a non-vital maxillary lateral incisor is involved because of caries, trauma or a cingulum invagination causing pulp necrosis. Tilting of the crowns of standing teeth indicates that their roots have been displaced by expansion of the cyst. Palatal inclination of the maxillary cheek teeth is common where a cyst expands to fill the antrum, whereas sideways displacement is seen where the cyst develops interdentally, notably with dentigerous cysts in children. Apical periodontal cysts arising from deciduous teeth are uncommon probably because they do not have sufficient time to develop before the tooth is shed, but when they do arise they often become quite large, displacing the succeeding teeth. Indeed any cyst will enlarge rapidly in the labile and responsive jaws of a child making prompt treatment essential.

Following the extraction of a tooth with a sizeable radicular cyst there may be an escape of cyst fluid. Provided it does not become infected the socket may still heal clinically leaving a residual cyst, but often a bony defect persists at the site of the socket which is visible radiographically and gives a clue to the source of the residual cyst.

Infected cysts present as painful, tender swellings which may already have developed a discharging sinus. Occasionally such cysts give rise to a cellulitis, but only rarely an osteomyelitis. Pathological fracture of the mandible in response to minor trauma is surprisingly unusual, mainly because there is more compensatory subperiosteal new bone on the buccal, lingual and inferior aspects than is readily apparent in the radiographs. Furthermore, the remaining bone has a tubular arrangement which gives it unexpected strength. However, social, sport or iatrogenic trauma may reveal such a lesion by producing a fracture.

Investigations

It is necessary to pulp test all teeth associated with a cystic lesion in order to help establish the diagnosis. If all the related teeth respond normally then a dentigerous cyst, keratocyst, solitary bone cyst or cystic ameloblastoma must be considered in the differential diagnosis, whereas the presence of a pulpless tooth at about the midpoint of the cyst suggests an apical periodontal cyst.

Radiology

A combination of rotational tomographic, periapical, occlusal and PA jaws radiographs will help to define the site, size and marginal outline of the cystic lesion. Good quality oblique lateral views of the mandible may add detail not evident in a rotational tomogram and can still have a place in difficult cases. Cysts arising in the premolar–molar region of the maxilla, and from the upper lateral incisor with its palatally placed apex, tend to enlarge upwards into the antrum and inferior meatus of the nose and therefore additional radiographs such as the lateral sinuses and occipitomental views are important.

Cysts developing in bone of uniform density take on a spherical shape, but otherwise tend to enlarge in the direction of least resistance. It is for this reason that maxillary cysts enlarge into the antrum and expand buccally before distending the tough, palatal mucoperiosteum. In the thickly corticated body of the mandible cysts push through medullary bone for a considerable distance to produce a sausage shaped cavity before penetrating the cortex at some point or points to produce a subperiosteal swelling. This behaviour is seen with all large benign cysts of the mandible and is not specifically characteristic of keratocysts. However, it also seems that some dentigerous cysts and periodontal cysts cease to enlarge after achieving a modest size.

Neurovascular bundles, particularly the inferior dental bundle, although displaced by cysts, retard enlargement, as they are displaced more slowly than the surrounding bone is resorbed, so they produce ridges on the cavity wall and indentations at the periphery.

As with periapical bone destruction an increase in radiolucency is the result of cortical bone destruction, not cancellous bone destruction, and is maximal when both plates are penetrated. Once there is complete perforation a map-like radiolucency with a distinct margin is seen which is obvious but which rarely coincides with the full extent of the lesion. An absence of linear trabecular images without a change of radiolucency marks the extent of medullary cavitation. The margin of the cavity within cancellous bone is therefore indicated by an abrupt return of trabeculation, but contrary to common opinion, rarely by a thin, peripheral, radiopaque line. Ridges inside the bone cavity and that part of the subperiosteal new bone which arises almost at right angles to the edge of cortical perforations externally will produce white linear images if the X-ray beam passes tangential to them. Both may give the false impression of a multilocular cavity, particularly if there is also uneven resorption of the cortex. The subperiosteal bone can give the appearance of a white linear margin; its image does not necessarily coincide with the periphery of the intrabony cavity.

Chronic infection of the sac can result in a noticeable zone of sclerosis around the cyst, a feature which is enhanced if there is a sinus present. Irregular resorption of the adjacent bone should arouse suspicion of a malignant change, although this is a rare occurrence. Where maxillary cysts extend into the antrum the margin of the intrusive opaque image forms part of a sphere and has a thin, dense or white linear outline, unlike the floppy shape, less dense margin of benign mucosal cyst of antral origin.

Sometimes difficulty arises in differentiating between a large antrum and a cyst. Often the problem is resolved by sinus views in which the opaque upper margin may be seen or by comparing the appearance seen in periapical views of both sides. There is usually a considerable degree of symmetry between the alveolar, palatal and tuberosity extensions of the right and left sinuses so a marked asymmetry is likely to be significant. Furthermore, the thin cortical bone of the antral wall normally forms a continuous linear white image which fuses with the lamina dura covering the tooth roots even if the antrum dips low between them. If the interdental bone lacks a white cortical line on the sinus aspect and ends as a cut off margin of cancellous bone the cavity is likely to be pathological and probably a cyst. Particularly is this so if the upper end of the interdental bone between several teeth ends in this way and the lamina dura is absent over the intervening tooth roots. Where doubt persists a wide bore needle can be introduced on a syringe through the anaesthetized cavity wall. Aspiration will produce air if it is the antrum and cyst fluid if it is a cyst. Provided the patient tips the head forward some sterile saline can be injected as a last resort. If the cavity is the antrum the saline will run out of the nose!

As periapical cysts tend to expand symmetrically, the apex of the tooth of origin is often centrally placed in relation to the margin of the cyst. Further evidence is the absence of the lamina dura over the apex and perhaps a root canal which is wider than in adjacent teeth, or even narrower due to the deposition of secondary dentine prior to pulp death, and of course incomplete formation of the root end where the pulp and dentine papilla have necrosed before development of the tooth was complete.

As cysts enlarge they displace adjacent tooth roots and if radiographs are examined critically in up to a third of such cases some resorption of the roots will also be seen. With large benign cysts the resorption can be substantial, although much resorption may arouse suspicion that the lesion is an ameloblastoma. While concurrent bilateral dentigerous cysts can occur, symmetrical cyst development around molar crowns suggests the presence of pseudo-dentigerous keratocysts.

Keratocysts in the retromolar region tend to expand with an amoeboid outline backwards into the ramus and up towards the coronoid process. Despite the increased rate of turnover of their epithelium keratocysts are relatively poor bone resorbers and are more readily confined to the medullary cavity, with comparatively late expansion of the cortical plates.

The point has been made already that irregular enlargement can produce a ridged cavity radiographically simulating a multilocular cyst. More keratocysts give the impression radiographically of being multilocular than are actually multilocular. However, an outpouching of the wall forming a significant part of a sphere suggests a daughter cyst and true multilocularity is certainly suggestive of a keratocyst. Whenever multilocular cysts are seen the differentiation between keratocyst and ameloblastoma becomes important and aspiration of the cyst contents may be helpful (*see below*).

The nasopalatine cyst presents as a central circular or occasionally heart-shaped radiolucency in the anterior palate. Nasolabial cysts as stated previously may resorb the thin margin of the inferior border of the nasal pyriform fossa, in which case the double curved 'bracket line' seen on the standard maxillary occlusal radiograph will be converted to a single backwards curve on the affected side. There will also be an increased radiolucency of the alveolar process over the lateral incisor and canine which occurs due to resorption of the overlying cortex. If appropriate to demonstrate the cyst's full extent, the contents may be aspirated and an aqueous radiopaque medium such as Triosil injected prior to further radiography.

Because cysts are the most common benign, intra-osseous lesions of the jaws, there is a tendency to describe any abnormal bone cavity seen in a radiograph as a cyst or 'cystic'. The features seen in several different views should always be studied, in particular an occlusal view which shows the lateral surface of the lesion where it is covered by subperiosteal new bone is of importance. If the margin is not entirely smooth the lesion is unlikely to be a simple cyst and may well be a solid, if benign, neoplasm. Loss of marginal definition implies a malignant tumour, especially a carcinomatous.

CYSTS OF THE JAWS

Aspiration

Where concern exists as to the nature of a lesion in the jaws, aspiration may be attempted using a wide bore needle and a 5 or 10 ml syringe after infiltrating a small amount of local analgesic solution into the overlying mucosa. It can facilitate aspiration if a narrow bore needle is also inserted close to the other to avoid the creation of a painful reduction of pressure in the cavity.

Dentigerous and periodontal cysts usually yield a clear pale straw-coloured fluid containing varying amounts of cholesterol crystals. These have a bright glistening appearance which can be seen if the syringe is held under a beam of light or if some fluid is expressed onto a dry swab. When haemorrhage into the cyst has recently taken place an opaque, dark brown fluid will be aspirated. Odontogenic keratocysts contain a creamy white, viscoid suspension of keratin.

Cyst fluid may be sent for electrophoresis, in which case dentigerous and periodontal cysts will reveal quantities of albumin and globulin resembling that found in serum with a total protein in excess of 4·0 g per 100 ml. Keratocyst contents tend to have much less protein on electrophoresis, most of which is albumin, but stained smears will show parakeratinized squames. This may be done by spreading a drop of cyst fluid thinly on to two cleaned slides, allowing them to dry and staining one with haemotoxylin and eosin and the other with the rhodamine B fluorescence method. The accurate diagnosis of a keratocyst may be achieved by a combination of the electrophoresis and smear techniques, although occasional false positives with other cysts and cystic neoplasms are possible.

The result of aspiration with an ameloblastoma depends upon the physical type. Some form a single large cyst from which liquid is readily aspirated, others are macroscopically multilocular, and if a largish cyst is penetrated fluid can be withdrawn. Yet others are clinically solid, though histologically have small cysts. In general the fluid does not contain cholesterol crystals, though considerable quantities may be formed if the ameloblastoma has been irradiated, as was the practice in some centres in the past.

A failure to aspirate liquid from the bone cavity usually means that a solid tumour is present, though this can happen if the needle is blocked by a fragment of solid debris or cyst lining. Fresh blood can be aspirated from vascular cyst walls, vascular solid tumours or from solitary bone cysts where bleeding from the wall is easily provoked. The ready aspiration of complete syringe-fulls of venous blood indicates the presence of an intramedullary cavernous haemangioma. Aspiration of bright red blood suggests an arterial or arteriovenous malformation, particularly if pulsation can be appreciated. Uncontrolled haemorrhage from the last two lesions is potentially life-threatening if full precautions are not taken. An angiogram must be performed where doubt exists.

Biopsy

Where there is any question as to the nature of the cyst it should be biopsied under local analgesia prior to surgery in order to clarify the diagnosis and surgical management. However, the site for biopsy needs to be chosen with care if a trustworthy report is to be hoped for and the material sent to a pathologist familiar with odontogenic lesions. Of course precautions should be taken to place the biopsy incision so that it can be excised with the lesion and to facilitate accurate closure so as to prevent infection which will delay treatment.

TREATMENT

General Considerations

Untreated cysts tend to increase in size and become infected. The presence of a large cyst within the mandible will weaken it. This makes it likely for a pathological fracture to occur as the result of an accidental blow on the jaw, or perhaps when a tooth is being extracted if the operator is unaware of the intra-osseous lesion.

Where possible functional teeth should be preserved. This will require the careful assessment of the vitality of all teeth related to the cyst. Pulpless teeth should be root filled within 24 hours prior to the operation provided the root canal can be maintained dry while the filling is placed and provided there has not been a recent acute infection involving the cyst. Root filling the tooth preoperatively shortens and simplifies the actual cyst operation. Where these conditions cannot be fulfilled an orthograde root filling may be placed during the operation and after enucleation of the cyst. To ensure a good apical seal a large gutta percha point may be condensed so as to protrude beyond the apex and trimmed flush with a hot plastic. Where this is not possible because of the presence of a crown or abnormally narrow root canal the tooth will require an apicectomy and a retrograde amalgam seal.

Contrary to popular belief vital teeth whose apices are adjacent to the cyst wall often retain their vitality if the cyst is enucleated with sufficient care, either because a thin layer of bone remains covering the apex or because in other cases gentle separation of the cyst sac may leave the apical neurovascular bundle intact, even though the apex is denuded of bone. If the root has accessory canals providing a substantial blood supply again the pulp may survive. In all cases it is important to monitor these teeth subsequent to the operation by clinical examination, periapical radiography and serial vitality tests until bone regeneration is complete and the vitality of the teeth confirmed.

Where there needs to be a delay before operating upon an infected cyst any acute episodes should be treated with antibiotics and drainage.

CYSTS OF THE JAWS

Operative Procedures

Epithelium lined cysts of the jaws may be treated in one of two ways:

　a. By marsupialization, which may be performed after removal of part of the lining or after enucleation of the whole cyst sac;
　b. By enucleation and primary closure.

It is the primary closure of the wound rather than the enucleation of the sac which distinguishes the second procedure from the first, which simply opens the cavity widely to the mouth or occasionally the maxillary sinus or nose.

MARSUPIALIZATION

Marsupialization opens the cavity widely to the mouth. The wider the opening, the shorter the time before undercuts and recesses are filled in as a result of regeneration of bone and the easier the irrigation and cleansing of the cavity. The cyst sac beneath the opening is removed so that the raw margin between lining and oral mucosa soon heals. In the case of dentigerous cysts the enclosed tooth starts to erupt towards the arch as the cavity fills in. Where the whole cyst lining is removed and the flap of oral mucosa is turned into the cavity it granulates, epithelializes and then reduces in size in the same way.

Marsupialization of odontogenic cysts is probably successful because of a variety of factors.

　a. Once the liquid contents are released, there appears to be an inherent tendency for the cyst lining to contract probably due to myofibroblasts in their walls. This allows endosteal bone formation to take place.
　b. As the cyst lining shrinks there is also a marginal ingrowth of normal mucoperiosteum which replaces the capsule with its resorptive potential. The ingrowing mucoperiosteum may provide additional bone regenerative factors.

Following marsupialization the patient has a cavity which needs to be irrigated free of stagnant food debris at regular intervals. It therefore requires a pack or bung to obturate the opening and prevent premature closure. If large and left uncovered it may alter the sound of the voice. Regular follow up visits are necessary to see that the cavity is filling up in a uniform fashion and to adjust the size of any bung or cyst plug. In a proportion of cases usually involving the maxilla, the cavity may not fill in completely and a supplementary procedure will be necessary to eliminate the residual cavity if it is an inconvenience. In general therefore marsupialization into the mouth is avoided wherever possible and primary closure of the oral wound is preferred.

However, marsupialization is still indicated under the following circumstances:

1. In a young person, for a dentigerous or pseudo-follicular keratocyst where marsupialization will permit the eruption of the enclosed tooth or any underlying developing teeth which have also been displaced.
2. Where a cyst other than a dentigerous cyst has enlarged between unerupted teeth and the oral cavity. In a child if development of the displaced teeth has not progressed very far enucleation will expose and damage the developing tooth germs.
3. Where a large cyst involves the apices of many adjacent erupted teeth and where enucleation could prejudice the support and vitality of these teeth or perhaps put at risk a major neurovascular bundle. As has been discussed above, with care enucleation may be possible without damage to the blood supply to the teeth even where radiographically it appears that their apices are incorporated in the cyst capsule.
4. If there is concern that enucleation and primary closure of a large cyst may lead to a pathological fracture. This is only true if marsupialization can be accomplished through a more limited bony opening than enucleation, and if the extraction of teeth, which might cause a fracture, can be avoided.
5. This method has a particular application in the very elderly or for patients who are unfit for a general anaesthetic because of advanced cardiac or respiratory disease or where there are other serious problems such as haemophilia. It may be feasible to make a modest opening under local anaesthesia with, if appropriate, simple sedation, where enucleation and primary closure would not be possible.

The Technique of Marsupialization

Where a substantial area of mucoperiosteum covered alveolar process is expanded a simple window may be made, removing an oval of mucosa, bone and underlying cyst wall. The opening must be made as large as possible compatible with the preservation of adjacent structures and the cavity packed. The specimen of cyst wall is submitted for histological examination. If the opening encroaches on the sulcus mucosa it will retract to expose a wide raw area but later it will contract, reducing the size of the opening.

In such circumstances a preferable technique is to create an inverted U-shaped flap based on the buccal sulcus which can be turned into the cyst cavity covering the margin (*Figs.* 11.2a and 11.3a). The incision is made around the anticipated outline of the surgical opening in the bone and cyst sac. It should leave at least 0·5 cm of continuous gingival margin around adjacent teeth or 1 cm between the incision and the crest of an edentulous ridge. The mucoperiosteum is reflected, starting in the lateral corners of the incision, over sound bone and working gently inwards over the central bulge. Through an initial opening in the bone the cyst lining is separated from the underside of the overlying bone (*Fig.* 11.2b) which is to be removed and the bone nibbled or cut away to form an adequate opening,

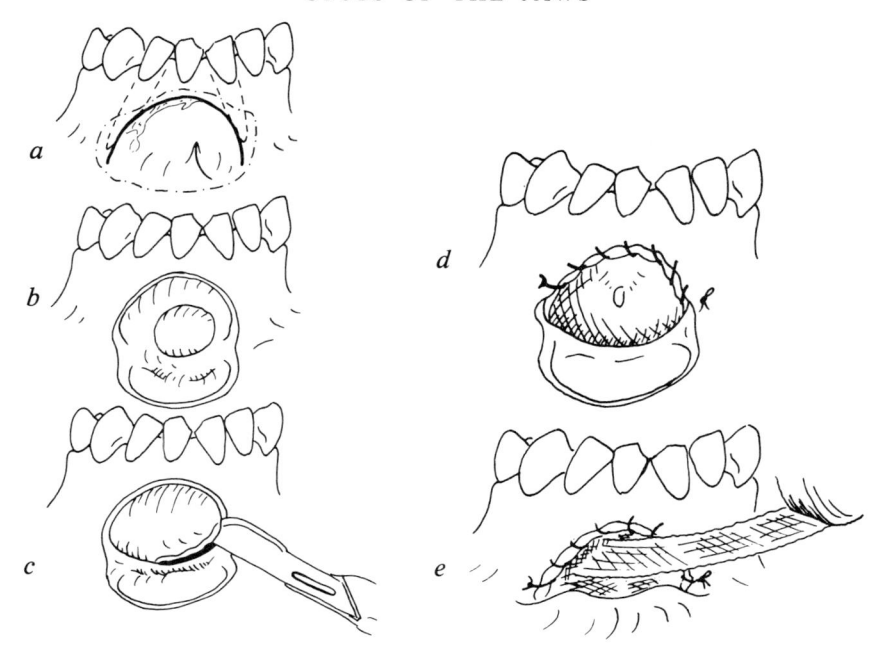

Fig. 11.2. Diagrams illustrating marsupialization of a cyst. *a,* A U-shaped incision over the margins of the future cyst opening. *b,* A mucoperiosteal flap reflected to reveal a perforation in the cortex. *c,* Bone removed to uncover the cyst lining which is incised from within outwards flush with the bone edge. *d,* The lining is sutured to the edge of the mucosa. Often the apex of the tooth of origin protrudes into the cavity and may be amputated flush with the lining. If un-rootfilled, a retrograde root filling can be inserted. *e,* The flap is turned into the cavity and packed into place with ribbon gauze soaked in Whitehead's varnish.

cutting the bone back to just underneath the still attached mucosa. A scalpel is stabbed through the lining against the bone edge and an opening made into the sac by cutting from inside the cavity out, against the bone margin (*Figs.* 11.2*c* and 11.3*b*). The specimen of lining is sent for histological examination, the flap is turned in and the cavity packed with half or one inch ribbon gauze soaked in Whitehead's varnish or bismuth iodoform paraffin paste (BIPP) (*Fig.* 11.2*d*). The latter is particularly effective in lubricating the pack and reducing infection but the taste is objectionable and occasionally produces a rash in those sensitive to iodine. All packs should be secured by sutures.

It does not matter if the flap overlaps the lining as the cyst epithelium will be destroyed. Surgical tidiness can be improved by running a continuous

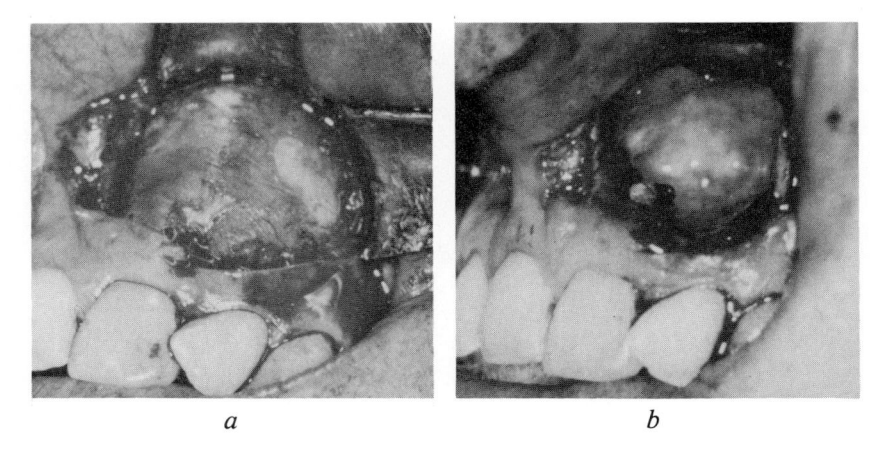

Fig. 11.3. *Left.* Marsupialization of a radicular (apical periodontal) cyst arising from pulpless |1. Note the dark coloured crown. The gum has been incised and a mucoperiosteal flap raised. Bone has been removed to uncover the cyst lining. *Right.* The apex of |1 enters the cavity and has been trimmed exposing the root filling. The displaced root of |2 is still covered by the cyst lining, the lateral half of which has been cut away.

catgut suture round uniting the oral mucosa and flap edge to the cut margin of the cyst before the pack is placed (*Fig.* 11.2*d*). Two weeks later the pack is removed. The patient irrigates the cavity regularly with a disposable syringe. Food may be kept out of the cavity and the opening prevented from contracting by a bung fashioned from black gutta percha or a soft acrylic, attached to a temporary plate.

Large cysts arising in the maxillary incisor region invariably perforate the bone on the palatal side and the capsule fuses with the underside of the mucoperiosteum. If such a cyst is marsupialized from the buccal aspect a deep, narrow slit-like cavity results as the lining fails to separate from the palatal mucosa. This may also prevent overlying teeth from erupting. In a child where enucleation would put at risk unerupted teeth a palatal opening may be made and kept patent by an extension on an acrylic palatal plate. This usually results in satisfactory cyst regression, eruption of the permanent anterior teeth and adequate regeneration of palatal bone.

About two-thirds of the cyst lining on average is left *in situ* by these techniques, which raises the possibility that more serious disease may be overlooked if the whole cyst sac is not submitted to the pathologist. Some ameloblastomas form a single large cyst with the more obvious tumour tissue in one or more nodules. However, although the whole lesion is an ameloblastoma, the thinner part of the lining epithelium is most likely to be mistaken for a keratocyst by an inexperienced pathologist. In all cases before the cyst is packed the cavity is irrigated and aspirated dry and the inner surface of the lining inspected for mural nodules. If one is seen it should be removed for section. A marsupialized ameloblastoma will heal in the same way as a benign cyst for a period of time, then fresh extension will occur and fleshy tumour tissue will appear in the cavity.

Carcinoma arising focally in odontogenic cyst linings is recognized as a very rare occurrence. It is most unlikely that malignant change would be so localized that some indication would not be seen in a reasonable segment of buccal cyst wall, nor indeed that the presence of a carcinoma would not soon be apparent within the opened cavity.

Contrary to popular belief keratocysts will respond satisfactorily to marsupialization and probably with a not much higher risk of recurrence than after enucleation. Indeed this may be the treatment of choice where enucleation would result in the loss of sound teeth or disturb erupting teeth in a child. Should a recurrence occur it will be superficially placed in the alveolus and may be spotted while still small if regular recall is practised, and it can be dealt with quite simply by enucleation.

ENUCLEATION AND PACKING

Where enucleation of the cyst lining is undertaken but previous infection in a large cyst suggests that primary closure of the wound would not be successful, a flap is turned in and the cavity packed. The cavity heals with granulation tissue until epithelialization is complete. Reduction in size takes place as after marsupialization with retention of the deeper part of the lining. Loose packing after enucleation is also used as a secondary measure where the wound breaks down after an attempt at primary closure.

ENUCLEATION AND PRIMARY CLOSURE

Where enucleation and primary closure is performed, once the flap has healed soundly the patient is often unaware of the healing cavity and regeneration of bone takes place from all its aspects. Also infrequent follow up appointments are required to monitor healing by radiography. Bone regeneration is often complete within six months for small cysts and one year for large ones. During this time also the vitality of adjacent teeth will be confirmed.

Keratocysts of course need subsequently to be reviewed annually for at least five years in order not to overlook recurrence. In general greater surgical skill is required for successful enucleation and primary closure, a greater volume of tissue will need to be anaesthetized if a local anaesthetic is used, or alternatively a general anaesthetic will be required.

Successful primary closure requires a different design of flap to that which is suitable for marsupialization so the decision as to the type of operation to be performed must be made before the surgeon starts. A short postoperative stage, less frequent follow up visits and a better contour to the

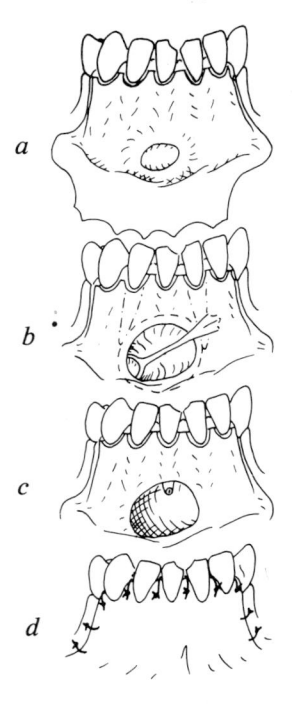

Fig. 11.4. Diagrams illustrating the enucleation of a cyst and primary wound closure. *a,* A three-sided flap is reflected. *b,* Bone is removed to uncover the cyst and the lining separated from the bony cavity. *c,* The lining removed. The apex of root-filled $\overline{1|}$ is seen. Note the broad zone of bone around the opening. *d,* The flap is sutured into place.

healed alveolar process all make this the preferred procedure where it is technically possible.

The operation can be performed under local or general anaesthesia, almost always operating intraorally (*Fig.* 11.4). Where general anaesthesia is available it is preferable for large cysts. If a general anaesthetic is used, infiltration of the operative site with 1 : 100000 adrenaline in saline will help to reduce haemorrhage and facilitate dissection. Buccal flaps are best designed with a gingival margin incision, preserving the interdental papillae. One or two relieving incisions extending as curved arcs into the buccal sulcus will be needed to provide adequate access and are made on sound bone. The gingival papillae facilitate replacement of the flap and provide tough tissue for suturing. Where the ridge is edentulous the incision is carried along the crest of the ridge.

In order to provide a broad zone of contact for the flap and a valve like closure of the wound the incision should be planned well wide of the

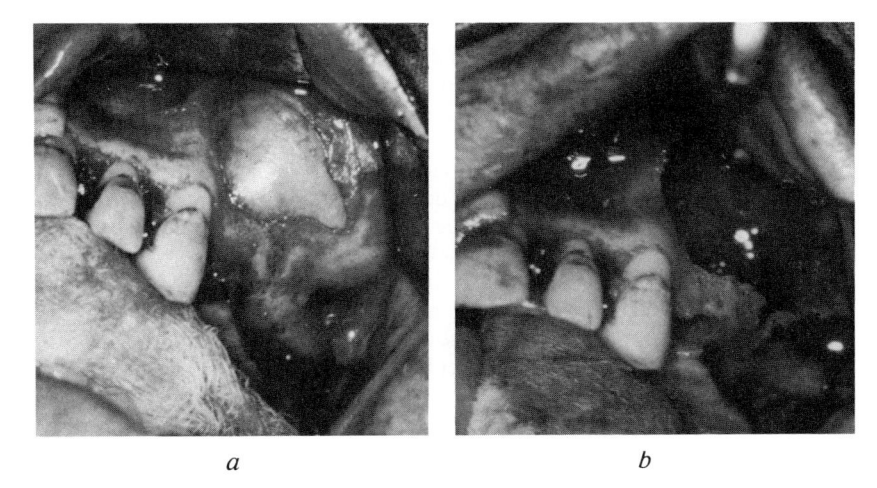

Fig. 11.5. *a,* A generous three-sided flap has been raised uncovering a perforation in the expanded bone and the cyst lining. *b,* The bone has been cut away to improve access and the cyst sac enucleated.

proposed opening in the bone. Reflection of the flap should commence firmly under the periosteum of the anterior buccal incision, working parallel to the gingival margin and undermining and detaching the papillae as the elevator is pushed distally. Where the cyst has eroded the overlying bone and become adherent to the underside of the flap, or at the site of a sinus or previous drainage incision difficulty may be encountered in separating the two layers. Patient pressure with the periosteal elevator close to the point of reflection from the cyst lining, perhaps with a layer of gauze swab around the periosteal elevator, will establish a plane of cleavage. Particularly adherent spots will require sharp dissection with scalpel or dissecting scissors.

Reflection should continue until sound bone has been reached all round the intended bony opening. Should the overlying bone be intact an opening should be made using chisels or a bur. A rose-head bur will cut out a disk of bone without puncturing the cyst lining which makes separation of the sac easier. The lining is separated with a Howarth's rougine from under the margin of the opening, which facilitates the removal of more bone with rongueurs until adequate access for enucleation of the sac has been created (*Fig.* 11.5).

Enucleation can be accomplished with a variety of instruments depending upon access. In large cysts a Howarth's rougine or a Ward's periosteal elevator are suitable. For smaller ones a Mitchell's trimmer or a large bi-angled spoon excavator, supplemented by curved Warwick James' elevators are better. The edge of the instrument slides over the surface of the bone, with the convex back towards the lining, lifting it off. A two-handed technique is particularly helpful peeling the capsule from the bone by using a blunt ended fine surgical sucker like the Kilner and retracting it with a periosteal elevator in the other hand. This ensures a bloodless field and a clear view of the site of dissection.

In general difficult and adherent areas, such as where the lining is fused to the nasal floor, are left to the last, if necessary emptying the sac to see the bottom of the cavity. Care should be taken with mandibular cysts which have resorbed the walls of the inferior dental canal. Separation of the lining from the neurovascular bundle is usually straightforward if it is peeled off along the length of the bundle, not across it. This also applies to large maxillary cysts where blind, forceful dissection may not only damage the infra orbital nerve, but produce an inconvenient and obscuring haemorrhage from its vessels.

Some difficulty may also be experienced where the lining is adherent to the periodontal membrane around the apices of teeth, hence the need to apicect non-vital teeth. Teeth that prior to the operation respond to vitality tests may remain vital if the lining is peeled off the apices along their length without scraping either root or bone. If possible the sac is removed in one piece as this ensures none is left behind. The bony cavity is irrigated and inspected for any retained fragments of lining, then packed with saline moistened ribbon gauze. This is removed after 5 minutes and the wound checked for haemostasis. Any oozing patches are treated with Abseal.* This way it is hoped the clot will be confined to the cyst cavity and the flap will adhere firmly to the surrounding bone. The wound is closed with care.

Where a maxillary cyst has produced a palatal swelling rather than a buccal one a palatal flap may be raised from the gingival margin, an opening made in the bone and the cyst lining enucleated from this aspect with less risk of damage to the standing teeth. After the flap has been sutured back in place a small piece of soft black gutta percha is applied to the fitting surface of a previously made acrylic plate and pressed into place. The gutta percha corrects the contour of the palate and the plate holds the mucosa close to the bone around the margins (*Fig.* 11.6).

Large cysts of the maxilla invaginate the maxillary antrum and are covered by a thin shell of subperiosteal new bone, between the cyst capsule and the antral lining. When the cyst occupies most of one side of the maxilla the antrum is reduced to a narrow slit above and behind the cyst from which the drainage of secretions is impaired. The stagnant secretions are likely to become infected from time to time. If a simple enucleation and primary closure is performed remodelling will be prolonged. It is better to remove the partition between the cyst and the residual antral cavity.

---

*Ethicon Ltd., P.O. Box 408, Bankhead Ave, Edinburgh EH11 4HE.

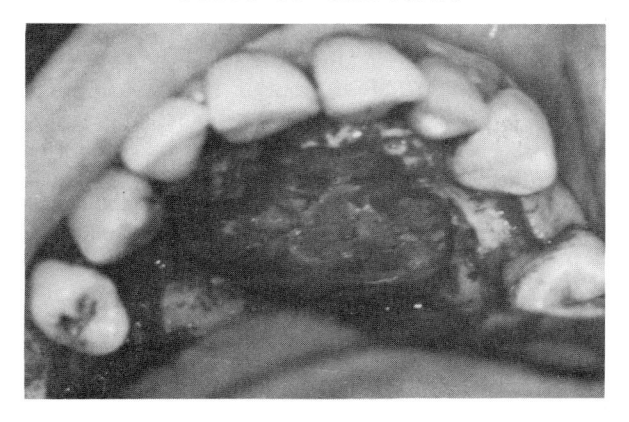

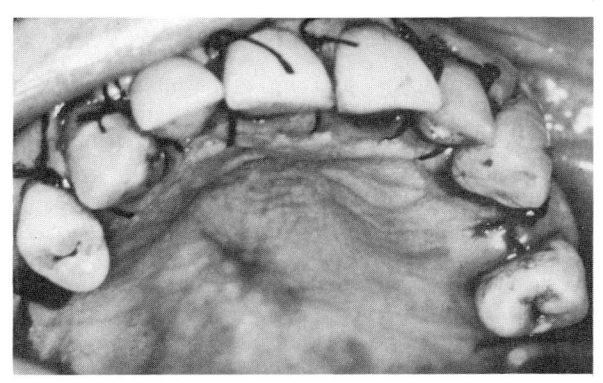

Fig. 11.6. *Top.* An apical, periodontal cyst from pulpless ⌊2 is expanding palatally. ⌊2 has been root-filled preoperatively. The palatal mucosa has been reflected and bone removed to uncover the cyst. *Bottom.* The cyst has been enucleated and the flap sutured back into place. Palatal contour has been restored and will be maintained by a gutta percha lined acrylic plate.

After enucleation of the cyst lining the partition is penetrated outwards towards the zygomatic extension of the antrum. A Howarth's rougine is slipped into the antral cavity and the thin partition fractured away. The antral lining which previously covered the partition should be left attached by one margin, but the thin bone nibbled back flush with the wall. Then the flap of antral lining can be pressed into contact with the bare bone of the cyst cavity. A trochar and cannula or curved Spencer Wells forceps is passed through the nostril, under the inferior turbinate and into the cyst cavity to create an intranasal antrostomy for drainage and a length of Yeats drain pulled through into the nose. It is secured by a stitch to the ala of the nose.

The oral wound is carefully closed. This technique prevents the accumulation of haematoma and ensures subsequent drainage from the new antral cavity. The drain is removed after about 48 hours—it is easier and more comfortable for the patient to draw out a soft plastic drain than the gauze pack which is sometimes used.

If large cyst cavities are not partly decompressed after enucleation they become overfilled by haematoma, creating tension on the suture line which breaks down. Large mandibular cysts, i.e. those greater than 5 cm in the long axis, should be drained. The size of the dead space in the cyst cavity should be reduced by removing as much as possible of the thinner and more expanded wall, which is usually the buccal one, and a vacuum drain is inserted, passing it down and out through the submandibular skin. The intraoral wound must be closed with special care to evert the wound margins and produce maximum contact between the raw flap surfaces. Either interrupted vertical mattress sutures or a continuous horizontal mattress, oversewn with a continuous plain stitch, will achieve a hermetic seal. The drain should be left for at least 24 hours. If the cyst is in the ramus the vacuum will pull the deeper part of the masseter into the cavity further reducing the dead space.

A special comment is required for the keratocyst. Recurrences variously reported as occurring following 10–62 per cent of operations are due to a variety of causes. Because the cyst lining is thin and easily torn small amounts of cyst lining may be left inadvertently in the bony cavity. Patience and gentleness will help to reduce the chance of this and careful inspection after irrigation should enable the operator to remove any remaining fragments. The bimanual sucker and periosteal elevator technique aids precise dissection. Not infrequently large cysts extend up the ascending ramus into the coronoid process and become inaccessible. Stripping off the temporalis tendon and performing a coronoidectomy with a fissure bur will open the cavity to direct vision. All cyst linings are difficult to separate from the periosteum where the bony wall is perforated. The thin keratocyst lining is particularly adherent and careful, sharp dissection may be required.

It is possible that the microscopic daughter cysts which can be found in the capsule may extend into the cancellous bone and be left behind when the lining is enucleated. It is possible that the incidence of this type of recurrence can be reduced by skimming off a shallow layer of bone from the cancellous component of the cavity wall. This is accomplished with a large round bur, using minimal pressure and cutting under a generous water spray. Care must be taken not to damage adjacent structures, particularly adjacent nerves, or to implant living cells into the freshly opened cancellous spaces. The necrosis of an uncertain zone of wall with caustic chemicals or cryosurgery is not in keeping with good surgical practice, particularly as in a substantial percentage of cases no recurrence will occur even without such treatment. Such imprecise methods may unnecessarily damage adjacent structures.

A small proportion of keratocysts are multilocular and develop multicentrically from a zone of dental lamina. Provided that there are only a modest number of cavities and that care is taken to enucleate all the cysts, many will heal without further trouble. It should not be forgotten that new cysts may arise in adjacent unstable dental lamina, but recurrence from this cause will not be prevented by the drastic measures mentioned above. In patients with the multiple cyst syndrome further cysts may arise anywhere in the dental lamina and new cysts appear at any age though the maximum incidence is during the second decade. Only careful long-term follow up will permit these to be dealt with when small. They are not preventable.

Attention has been drawn to dental lamina residues in the mandibular retromolar mucosa. In the case of ramus cysts this mucosa can be excised before the wound is closed, but recurrences rarely arise superficially at this site. The notorious reputation for the keratocyst to recur has also encouraged some surgeons to excise the mandible where there is a large lesion. This may be justified where there is a multitude of cysts which would defy individual enucleation, but many large keratocysts are unilocular despite their appearance in radiographs due to ridges on the wall.

Large cysts can be enucleated by gentle, diligent surgery, so that such radical treatment for a non-malignant condition is generally unnecessary. Careful follow up enables any small recurrences to be detected early and removed, and the overall morbidity for the patient is considerably reduced. Indeed in some cases where subperiosteal resection with bone grafting of the defect has been carried out, recurrence within the graft has been reported.

Where the cyst has penetrated out to the periosteum it is just as difficult to separate the periosteum from the lining while resecting the mandible as during enucleation of the lining from within the bony cavity. If patches of lining are left on the periosteum then recurrence in the graft is virtually certain to occur so that the more radical approach does not necessarily have a therapeutic advantage.

Some recurrences have occurred down in the neck suggesting implantation of free fragments as a cause. Careful and copious irrigation of the wound before closure and care to avoid soiling the wound with cyst contents and fragments of lining should help to prevent this type of complication.

ENUCLEATION AND PRIMARY CLOSURE WITH BONE GRAFTING

The highly vascular periosteum and endosteum of the jaws have remarkable powers of bone regeneration so that large cavities are filled with little evidence of the original defect except for a delicate radial pattern to the bone trabeculae. This makes the grafting of these cavities with autogenous cancellous bone chips largely unnecessary. The use of other materials such as absorbable haemostatic materials or processed stored bone of various types as cavity fillers is contraindicated as they interfere with normal healing. Just occasionally following enucleation there is a local loss of ridge contour which will impair the success of a subsequent prosthesis, and under such circumstances chip bone grafts may be justified, but there is always a risk of wound breakdown and of their loss through infection.

PATHOLOGICAL FRACTURES

Intra- or postoperative fracture of the mandible following the removal of a large cyst is uncommon because compensatory subperiosteal bone deposition keeps pace with the expansion of such slow growing benign lesions. Thus despite a dramatic, large, radiolucent cavity to be seen on a rotational tomographic radiograph, there is invariably substantial amounts of bone buccally, lingually and inferiorly to maintain continuity.

However, where the mandible is generally thin and fragile, splints or arch bars should be prepared preoperatively and the patient warned of the risks to be faced. Should a fracture take place, the cavity should be packed with Whitehead's varnish impregnated ribbon gauze and the mandible immobilized.

Occasionally a pathological fracture occurs postoperatively, usually when the oedema and discomfort have subsided and the patient chews more adventurously, or is accidentally struck. Where there is no displacement, satisfactory healing will often take place merely with a regime of soft diet and reassurance. Otherwise apply intermaxillary fixation, open up the operation site, reduce the fracture and pack the cavity to splint the fragments in alignment.

NASOPALATINE CYSTS

These cysts are enucleated after the reflection of a palatal flap, incising around the gingival sulci of any standing teeth. Avulsion of the vessels entering the incisive fossa from the flap as it is raised usually leads to retraction of their walls and spontaneous cessation of bleeding. If this is delayed the vessels may be crushed with a mosquito artery forceps. The cyst is then peeled from the cavity with a narrow periosteal elevator or the curette end of a Mitchell's trimmer. The terminal fibres of the long sphenopalatine nerves are usually spread over the surface of the capsule. These have to be divided to free the cyst sac and this can be painful under a local anaesthetic. A few drops of solution injected in the top of the sac a few minutes before this is done will help.

It is worth remembering that small 'cysts' (i.e. less than 7 mm) seen in radiographs often prove to be deep incisive fossae. In the absence of swelling or symptoms, radiographic review is preferred to surgery. The palatal flap may be sutured back with sutures between the palatal and buccal gingival papillae. Some operators prepare an acrylic plate retained with cribs to prevent haematoma formation. If this has been omitted a small stab incision made in the midline of the flap over the bony cavity will help to prevent excessive distention of the flap.

SOLITARY BONE CYSTS

Surgical exploration should be carried out as described for enucleation in order to confirm the diagnosis. It is wise to submit the segment of bone removed to gain access to the cavity for histological examination. Occasionally this has a structure resembling fibrous dysplasia. Currettage of the bony walls leads to haemorrhage and disrupts the thin connective tissue covering. Closure of the wound usually produces rapid healing. However, these patients should be kept under review as occasionally a recurrence takes place. Recurrence is not uncommon where the patient is a child, but is unusual after skeletal growth is complete.

FISSURAL CYSTS

These rare cysts are best enucleated and of course submitted for histological examination.

POSTOPERATIVE FOLLOW-UP

This will be required for:

1. Keratocysts in order to detect early and deal with any recurrence;
2. Associated teeth in order to ensure that latent loss of vitality does not lead to an abscess or further cyst formation;
3. Unerupted teeth which may require exposure and orthodontic treatment if their eruption has been disturbed.

SUGGESTED READING

Craig G. J. (1976) The paradental cyst: a specific inflammatory odontogenic cyst. *Br. Dent. J.* **141**, 9–14.

Harris M. (1978) Odontogenic cyst growth and prostaglandin-induced bone resorption. *Ann. R. Coll. Surg.* **60**, 85–91.

Harris M. and Toller P. (1975) Pathogenesis of dental cysts. *Br. Med. Bull.* **31**, 2, 159–163.

Harvey W., Cuat Chen F., Gordon D. et al. (1984) Evidence for fibroblasts as the major source of prostacyclin and prostaglandin synthesis in dental cysts. *Arch. Oral Biol.* **29**, 223–229.

Hodson J. J. (1957) Observations on the origin and nature of the adamantinoma with special reference to certain muco-epidermoid variations. *Br. J. Plast. Surg.* **10**, 38–59.

Killey H. C., Kay L. W. and Seward G. R. (1977) *Benign Cystic Lesions of the Jaws, their Diagnosis and Treatment,* 3rd ed. Edinburgh, London and New York: Churchill-Livingstone.

Main D. M. G. (1970) Epithelial jaw cysts, a clinico-pathological reappraisal. *Br. J. Oral Surg.* **8,** 114–125.

Matejka M., Porteder H., Ulrich W. et al. (1984) Prostaglandin synthesis in dental cysts. *J. Maxillofac. Surg.* **23,** 190–194.

McHugh W. D. 91961) The development of the gingival epithelium in the monkey. *Dent. Practit.* **11,** 314–324.

Pindborg J. J. and Kramer I. R. H. (1971) *Histological Typing of Odontogenic Tumours, Jaw Cysts and Allied Lesions.* World Health Organization.

Rule D. C. (1976) Dermoid cyst of the lower lip. *Br. Dent. J.* **141,** 116–119.

Shear M. (1983) *Cysts of the Oral Regions,* 2nd ed. Bristol: Wright.

Toller P. A. (1948) Experimental investigation into factors concerning the growth of cysts of the jaws. *Proc. R. Soc. Med.* **41,** 681–688.

Tonge C. H. and Luke D. A. (1976) Dental anatomy—cleft palate. *Dental Update* (May/June). 138–143.

Valdehaug J. (1972) A histologic study of experimentally induced radicular cysts. *Int. J. Oral Surg.* **1,** 137–147.

CHAPTER 12

SOFT-TISSUE SWELLINGS OF THE ORAL MUCOSA

SWELLINGS OF THE ORAL MUCOSA

A variety of superficial swellings can be found arising from and beneath the oral mucosa most of which are inflammatory hyperplasias and granulomas. A completely logical classification of the tumours on aetiological grounds is not possible for reasons which will become apparent. A practical grouping, however, can be made partly based on the site of origin of the lesion and partly on the basis of aetiology and histological appearance.

As an initial step they can be divided into those which arise from the mucosa covering the alveolar processes and those which arise elsewhere in the oral cavity (*see below*). Some of those which arise from the alveolar process mucosa have the word 'epulis' as part of their name, but others do not. An epulis is a lump arising from the gingiva. Those which arise from the masticatory mucosa on the alveolar process clearly fall into this group, but those which arise from the masticatory mucosa of the palate are not classified as epulides. Some lumps have different histological appearances at various stages in their evolution so that a histological grouping can contain several entities.

Despite their apparently benign character it is essential that all masses which are excised should be sent for histological examination.

a. *Swellings of the gingiva*
   i. *Discrete (epulides)*
      Fibrous epulis
      Denture-induced granuloma (denture hyperplasia)
      Pyogenic granuloma
      Pregnancy tumour
      Giant cell epulis
      Haemangioma
      Neurofibroma
   ii. *Diffuse enlargement*
      Drug-induced
      —diphenylhydantoin
      —cyclosporin A
      Fibromatosis gingivae
      Fibromatous enlargement of the tuberosities
      Sarcoid
      Chrohn's disease
      Wegener's granuloma

b. *Swellings of the buccal and palatal mucosa*
   Fibro-epithelial polyp
   Fibroma
   Papilloma
   Neurofibroma
   Lipoma
   Crohn's Disease
c. *Swellings of the tongue*
   Pyogenic granuloma
   Fibro-epithelial polyp
   Median rhomboid glossitis
   Lymphoid nodules
   Lymphangioma
   Haemangioma
   Granular cell myoblastoma
   Amyloid

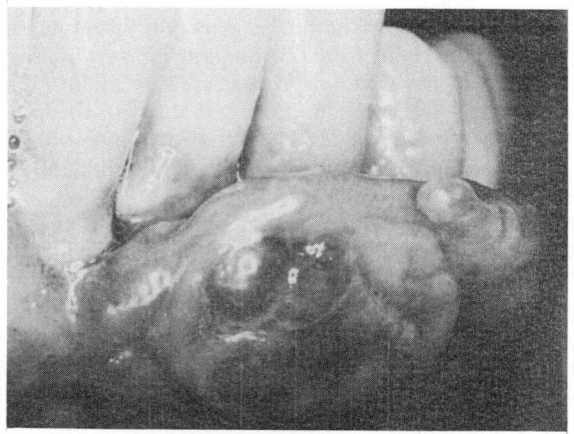

Fig. 12.1. A fibrous epulis arising in relation to periodontally involved $\overline{123}$.

SWELLINGS OF THE GINGIVA
Fibrous Epulis

Most fibrous epulides arise from an interdental papilla. They arise as a hyperplastic response to chronic irritation or trauma, usually where there is poor oral hygiene. The irritant factor may be the sharp edge of a carious cavity, or of an inadequately contoured restoration, or calculus, particularly subgingival calculus, and plaque. As the inflammatory mass enlarges it bulges out on either the buccolabial or palatolingual side and overlaps the adjacent teeth and alveolar process (*Fig.* 12.1). Where there is a large approximal, carious cavity in a posterior tooth the mass may enlarge to fill the cavity. It is then described as a gum polyp, in contrast to a pulp polyp which develops from a widely exposed pulp.

Initially the inflamed hyperplastic papilla is soft and red and bleeds easily. Even when the enlargement has become too great to be regarded merely as a hyperplastic papilla the lump is still soft and vascular and composed of immature, cellular, fibrous tissue supplied by many dilated capillary blood vessels and infiltrated by mixed inflammatory cells. Histologically at this stage it is indistinguishable from a pyogenic granuloma. In the course of time the mass becomes larger, up to 1·5–2 cm in diameter, but rarely more than 2 cm, pale pink in colour and firm.

Some fibrous epulides are sessile at first sight, but a blunt, periodontal probe can be passed underneath the lump from various angles to define the narrow point of attachment. Mature fibrous epulides become less vascular, are covered with stratified squamous epithelium and are composed of a mature collagenous fibrous tissue. Inflammatory cells are seen only in relation to sites of irritation or ulceration.

From time to time fibrous epulides are abraded during mastication and develop an ulcerated surface which may be sore enough to encourage the patient to seek professional help. Sometimes the ulcerated and inflamed mass resembles a malignant neoplasm at first sight. Woven bone develops in the centre of long standing fibrous epulides and may increase in amount until only a small zone at the periphery remains unossified.

Treatment

Simple conservative local excision is sufficient to remove the epulis. Where it is attached by a narrow peduncle this is sectioned parallel with the adjacent surface. Those attached by a broad peduncle or which are sessile and involve the interdental tissues require incision down to bone immediately around the attachment, and the mass with enlarged papilla removed together.

The important aspect of treatment is to identify and remedy the source of chronic irritation. This is usually obvious once the epulis is removed, if not before. Failure to do this and to establish adequate regular cleansing of the now open interdental space will result in recurrence. A periodontal pack is usually needed to control ooze from the raw surface and to protect it until it has healed.

Denture Induced Granuloma (Denture Hyperplasia)

A denture induced granuloma occurs as a hyperplastic response of the underlying tissues to the flanges of a mobile, ill-fitting denture. The hyperplastic mass may develop opposite just one part of the denture, such as the lower labial flanges or in relation to the entire periphery. Mostly the flanges dig into and irritate the sulcus tissues as a result of shrinkage of the alveolar ridge. Occasionally a local expanding intra-bony lesion such as a

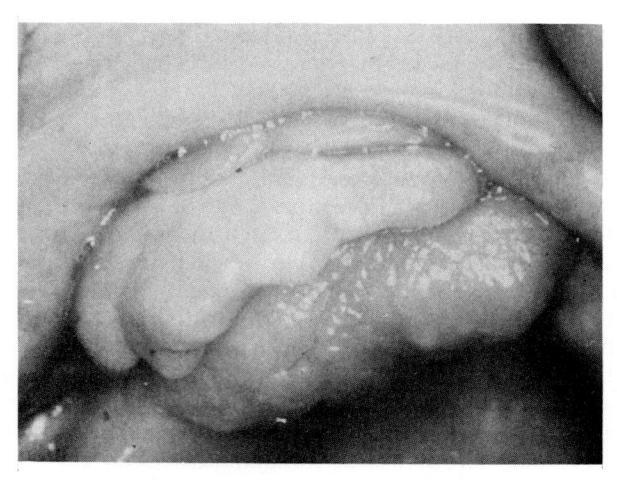

Fig. 12.2. A denture induced granuloma 4–1| region. The denture flange fits in the groove between the two components. The inner one fills the space between the denture flange and the resorbed ridge. It is red, granular and infected with candida. There is a large and small component to the outer part which fits over the denture flange.

cyst, or even more rarely a carcinoma from the antrum, causes the denture to rub and produce a hyperplastic mass which disguises the primary lesion.

Where there has been ridge resorption the hyperplasia develops as two adjacent and parallel masses with a groove in between in which the denture flange fits. One mass occupies the space beneath the denture and the other arises at the outer margin of the flange and overlaps it (*Fig.* 12.2). Sometimes in the lower anterior region there are successive rows of hyperplastic tissue extending from the ridge out into the sulcus and even onto the inside of the lip. Each layer of tissue is pale pink in colour and firm, sometimes with a granular surface. It is thicker in the centre but tapers towards the ends and is attached at one edge to the sulcus mucosa by a long, narrow, linear peduncle.

Similar lesions may develop across the palate at the posterior border of a full upper denture and on the mucosa overlying a resorbed anterior maxillary ridge which has been the subject of chronic trauma from lower standing natural teeth.

The leaf like pedunculated fibro-epithelial polyps of the palate always develop under a denture so can be looked upon as a form of denture induced granuloma. They are attached by a small peduncle and presumably would be spherical or pear-shaped were they not flattened by the palate of the denture. When the plate is removed they are seen to lie in an indentation in the palatal mucosa.

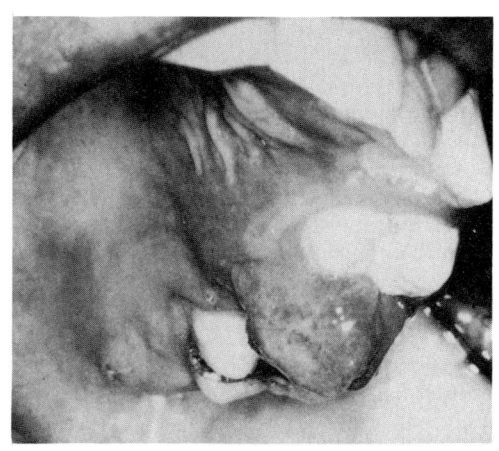

Fig. 12.3. A pyogenic granuloma arising in relation to a recently erupted $\underline{4|}$.

These lesions are primarily inflammatory in origin, perhaps developing at the margin of sites of repeated ulceration, and the vast majority remain quite benign. Occasionally areas of white or speckled leukoplakia develop on a hyperplastic lesion which may be infected by *Candida albicans*.
Treatment is dealt with in Chapter 4.

Pyogenic Granuloma

Like the fibrous epulis this lesion arises in response to chronic irritation and non-specific infection. Calculus, plaque, overhanging cervical margins of restorations, food impaction in interdental embrasures and periodontal pockets are common causes. They also arise where a deciduous molar has recently been shed, but has left behind a sharp fragment of dentine and enamel or a root. The deep crevice between the gingival margin and the crown of an incompletely erupted tooth, if infected, can also give rise to a pyogenic granuloma (*Fig.* 12.3).

Most lesions present as a sessile or pedunculated vascular mass with an ulcerated surface. They are purplish-red in colour, painless and soft, enlarge quite rapidly, but only occasionally exceed 1 cm in diameter (except during pregnancy—*see below*). Histologically they are composed of immature and very vascular fibrous tissue infiltrated with mixed acute and chronic inflammatory cells. Typical lesions most often appear in children and young adolescents where they are seen in circumstances similar to those which produce fibrous epulides in older adolescents and adults.

Young, immature fibrous epulides, it will be remembered, are very similar in clinical features and histological appearance but the typical pyogenic granuloma will retain these features over a long period of time while achieving a size similar to the mature fibrous epulis. The justification for describing this lesion as a separate entity is that some can retain their vascularity and softness over several years, including examples seen in men and non-pregnant women. On the other hand, it is also probable that some of the lesions which start in childhood as pyogenic granulomas, subsequently mature as fibrous epulides as the patient gets older.

Occasionally a vascular antral polyp may prolapse through an oroantral fistula created by the extraction of an upper molar and may be confused with a pyogenic granuloma. However, this lesion is initially very soft and may be displaced upwards into the antrum again with a blunt probe. It is important to remember that exuberant granulation tissue is seen over infected sequestra and foreign bodies or at the entrance to discharging sinuses which may be overlooked. These lesions rapidly regress if the infected body is removed or if drainage from the sinus ceases.

Pyogenic granulomas can be looked upon as a form of exuberant granulation tissue which proliferates to form a substantial mass, is covered by stratified squamous epithelium and persists over a considerable period of time.

A preoperative radiograph will confirm the presence or absence of a retained root, a tooth fragment or an erupting tooth.

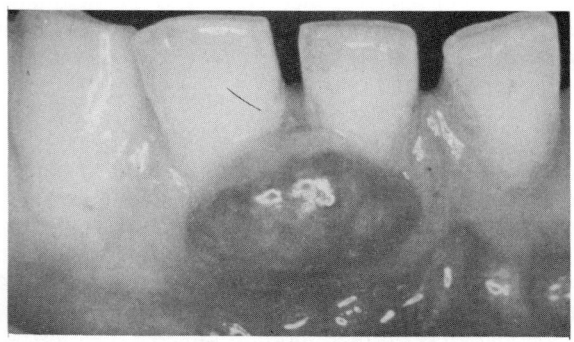

Fig. 12.4. A pregnancy tumour (epulis) in the lower incisor region. The mouth is generally clean and the gingival margins healthy, but calculus has accumulated on the teeth adjacent to the epulis and the local gingival margins are inflamed.

Treatment

The lesion is infiltrated with local anaesthetic and excised, curetting away any remaining fragments at the base. The resultant wound is dressed with a periodontal pack. As with fibrous epulis the underlying irritant factors must be dealt with and poor local oral hygiene corrected.

Some lesions in the premolar region in children tend to recur. This usually ceases once the adult teeth have fully erupted. If the causative factor is removed or corrected, but the epulis is not removed, both the pyogenic granuloma and the fibrous epulis tend to shrink, but rarely disappear completely.

Pregnancy Epulis (Pregnancy 'Tumour' or Granuloma)

This lesion is a variant of the pyogenic granuloma which arises in pregnancy and has similar clinical and histological appearances (*Fig.* 12.4). There is an exaggerated inflammatory response to plaque in some pregnant women which results in pregnancy gingivitis and which is thought to be due to increased levels of circulating progesterone.

Pregnancy tumours tend to arise from the third month of pregnancy onwards, but are most often seen in the last trimester. They may develop in a patient who has a generalized pregnancy gingivitis or even where the oral hygiene is good, but where there is some local irritative factor.

Patients with pregnancy gingivitis tend to abandon oral hygiene measures as tooth brushing makes the gums bleed and is painful. A pregnancy tumour also is vascular, ulcerates readily and bleeds in response to minor trauma, so plaque and calculus soon accumulate locally, adding to the irritation.

Occasionally the pregnancy granuloma may develop into a sizeable mass; however, even if untreated these florid lesions regress to a relatively avascular fibrous epulis after delivery. Smaller lesions may disappear completely.

Treatment

A professional scale and polish, the re-establishment of tooth cleaning with a soft toothbrush and floss and plaque control with chlorhexidine dental gel are the first measures in treatment. Irritant factors local to the pregnancy tumour should be sought and removed.

Large and haemorrhagic granulomas which are a nuisance to the patient should be excised under local anaesthesia. A unipolar cutting electrode as used for gingival surgery is ideal and reduces haemorrhage which otherwise can be quite brisk and on occasions profuse. A firm gingivectomy pack both covers the raw wound and controls postoperative ooze. Any recurrence is best left untreated until after delivery.

The Giant Cell Epulis

The term giant cell reparative granuloma was used to distinguish the intraosseous giant cell jaw lesion from the osteoclastoma of long bones. Histologically the epulis is remarkably similar to the intraosseous lesion and has therefore been referred to as the peripheral giant cell granuloma.

This epulis is much less common than the fibrous epulis or the pyogenic granuloma but also seems to arise in relation to local sources of gingival irritation. They present as a pedunculated lesion, but usually with a broad peduncle, and vary from a firm pink fibrous-looking lesion to a red, haemorrhagic, or mottled purplish colour (*Fig.* 12.5). They are firmer than a pyogenic granuloma but softer than a mature fibrous epulis, can enlarge

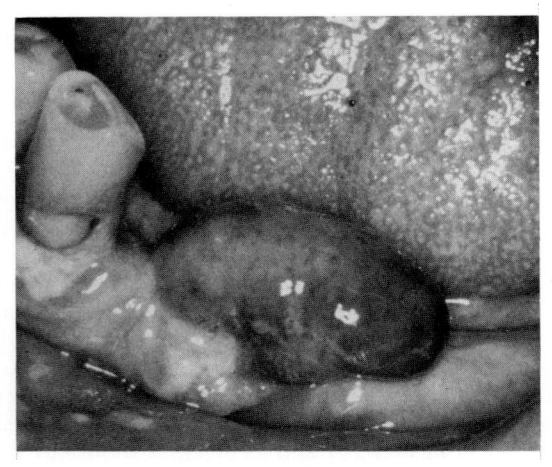

Fig. 12.5. A giant cell epulis related to a retained root. It is dusky purple in colour.

rapidly, but rarely exceed 3 cm in diameter, and are more common in females then males.

Radiologically there may be a localized shallow resorption of the surface of the underlying bone. The lesion must be distinguished from the subperiosteal form of the central giant cell granuloma, which is more often seen in the canine premolar region in children and young adolescents at puberty. The subperiosteal giant cell granuloma presents as a bulky submucosal swelling which overlies a laterally spreading, intrabony lesion which often involves the developing teeth. As the bone on just one aspect of the alveolar process is destroyed the extent of the involvement may not be obvious in radiographs. By comparison the epulis involves only the gingival mucosa.

Histologically groups of osteoclast-like multinucleate giant cells are seen in a spindle cell stroma which contains many thin walled vessels and macrophages. Haemorrhage into the tissues as a result of minor trauma is common. The lesional tissue is not encapsulated but demarcated by a narrow zone of subepithelial connective tissue. At the base the lesional tissue is usually in contact with the underlying, interdental bone. Small amounts of woven bone may develop in the deeper and more mature parts.

Giant cell epulides are occasionally a feature of hyperparathyroidism in the same way as intrabony 'brown tumours' and so fasting serum calcium, phosphorus, alkaline phosphatase and an immunoparathyroid hormone assay, together with a 24-hour urinary calcium and hydroxyproline estimation, are necessary to exclude this disorder.

Treatment

Local excision, light curettage of the underlying bone and the application of a surgical pack is adequate treatment, with of course removal of any irritant factor.

Congenital Epulis

The congenital epulis is present in the neonate from birth as a pedunculated mass which is large in proportion to the size of the mouth and attached to one of the gum pads. The base of the peduncle is usually broad, but some mucosa can be conserved from its margins to close the defect resulting from its excision.

The histology shows large closely packed cells containing fine acidophilic granules. The nature of the lesion is controversial and has been looked upon as a form of granular cell myoblastoma, a fibroblastoma, or a dental hamartoma (a malformation resembling a neoplasm caused by defective tissue combination or maturation). A connection has been described with the enamel organ of an underlying developing tooth. A rare type of ameloblastoma features similar granular cells so this may be an analogous change in cells of odontogenic epithelium origin.

Treatment

It is easily excised without risk of recurrence.

Haemangiomas

These occasionally present as a small localized sessile or pedunculated hamartomatous gingival swelling. They may be excised for histological examination, but if they recur can be treated by cryosurgery. They can be distinguished from a pyogenic granuloma which they resemble by the way that they can be emptied of blood with pressure. Incidently, gingival pyogenic granulomas are sufficiently vascular that they may be reported as a capillary haemangioma by a general pathologist unfamiliar with oral lesions.

Diffuse Gingival Enlargements

Drug-induced Gingival Hyperplasia

A diffuse, firm hyperplasia of the gingiva may occur as a result of anticonvulsant therapy with diphenylhydantoin (Epanutin, Dilantin sodium). The incidence appears to vary from group to group and may be as high as 50 per cent. The swelling, which starts with the interdental papillae, is confined to the gingival margins of erupted teeth and tends to be pink and firm and non-haemorrhagic, but occasionally bleeding and ulceration do occur. The enlargement may become so gross as to cover the surfaces of the teeth. The gingival mucosa is enlarged as a result of a substantial proliferation of collagen fibres. The overlying epithelium features downgrowths of the rete pegs into the underlying corium. In approximately 12 per cent of patients root deformities such as apical resorption or spindly narrowing are also seen as a result of the drug interfering with tooth formation.

Treatment consists of surgical removal by gingivectomy to eradicate the soft tissue mass which can be prevented from recurring by meticulous plaque control. Unfortunately this may not be feasible with severely affected epileptic patients incapable of personal oral hygiene. With the use of alternative anticonvulsant drugs this unexplained phenomenon may be avoided.

A similar gingival hyperplasia is induced by the use of cyclosporin A for immunosuppression. This drug is often used in renal, bone marrow, liver and heart transplantation, and some 25–30 per cent of kidney transplant and 2 per cent of bone marrow transplant patients develop the gingival enlargement. Once it commences it develops quite rapidly and is softer than that seen in Epanutin hyperplasia where the hyperplasia evolves slowly. Stringent oral hygiene measures effect only marginal control and substantial haemorrhage can accompany gingivectomy. Interestingly, hypertrichosis may also occur with the use of this drug.

Fibromatosis Gingivae (Hereditary Gingival Fibromatosis)

This is a rare condition in which there is a diffuse fibrous overgrowth of the gingiva which may be limited to the posterior segments or involve the whole gingival margin. The mode of transmission is usually a dominant trait, although sporadic cases present. It may also be associated with hypertrichosis and mental retardation. The condition is rarely present at birth and most commonly becomes apparent with the eruption of the permanent dentition. The condition may be related to other benign but troublesome fibromatoses occuring in childhood and adolescence elsewhere in the body.

Treatment is by gingivectomy which in adult patients may be permanently successful. In other cases the hyperplastic tissue recurs and may even produce a thickening on the edentulous ridge after all the teeth have been extracted.

Fibromatous Enlargement of the Maxillary Tuberosities

The enlargement affects the mucoperiosteum on the palatal and distal aspects of the 2nd and 3rd molars more than the buccal tissues. It can produce substantial, bilateral, hard, rounded fibrous masses which create false pockets against the crowns of the adjacent molars. Similar, but less bulky hyperplasia may affect the lower retromolar pad and the lingual gingival tissues adjacent to the lower molars. While there is some similarity to gingival fibromatosis there appears to be no connection with the genetically determined generalized enlargement. The tuberosity masses, if large may interfere with speech and swallowing and prevent the fitting of dentures. In time true pocketing may develop as a result of food impaction between the enlarged gum and the molar teeth and accumulation of plaque. For treatment *see* Chapter 4.

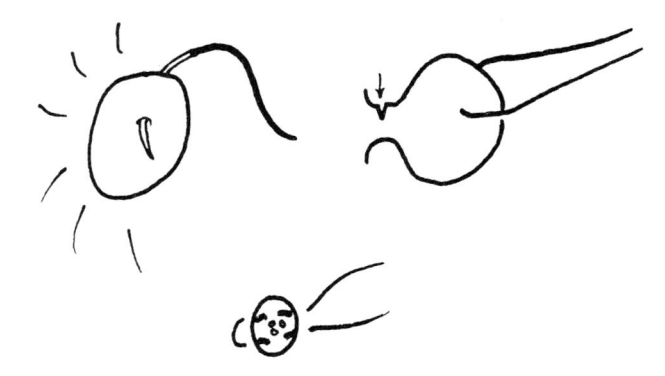

Fig. 12.6. A diagram illustrating the removal of a fibro-epithelial polyp from the inner aspect of the cheek. A stitch is inserted into the polyp which is drawn gently away to expose the pedicle. The pedicle is divided close to the lump and a mattress suture inserted which deliberately picks up the tissues either side of the vascular supply to the polyp so as to effect haemostasis.

SWELLINGS OF THE BUCCAL AND PALATAL MUCOSA

Fibro-epithelial Polyps

Pedunculated fibrous hyperplastic lumps arising from the mucous membrane lining the oral cavity are relatively common, but true fibromas are rare tumours in the mouth.

The cheek lesions often develop on the buccal mucosa opposite a space in the dentition into which they are sucked during deglutition. Some on the lips and cheek appear to develop initially as a round, flat, fibrous, submucosal scar where sharp opposing teeth traumatize the cheek. Again the suction of deglutition or a chewing habit may raise the initial flat lesion into a pedunculated swelling. Similar lumps develop on the tip of the tongue opposite sharp incisal edges or a diastema but arise from a tiny peduncle. The pedunculated, fibro-epithelial polyps of the hard palate have already been described under denture induced granuloma. They tend to be pale pink in colour. Some are quite soft, while others are firm.

Histologically they possess a normal stratified squamous epithelium which may be hyperplastic or ulcerated in response to trauma. The bulk of the lesion is composed of a vascular and cellular fibrous connective tissue with varying degrees of inflammation. True fibromas are reputed to be less vascular and to possess a distinct capsule.

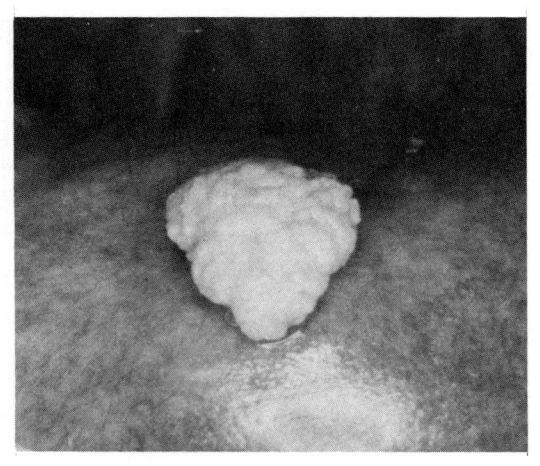

Fig. 12.7. A papilloma on the inner aspect of the lower lip.

Treatment
They are readily excised. A suture is passed through the lump and acts as a handle to control it. Too much tension should not be applied as this pulls the adjacent tissues out into the peduncle. An elliptical incison is made around the peduncle close to the base to remove it, and the defect sutured with one or more interrupted resorbable sutures. Sometimes a horizontal mattress is needed to pick up and control the divided blood supply to the polyp (*Fig.* 12.6).

Papilloma
Papillomas are uncommon benign tumours of the oral mucosa, but probably occur with equal frequency on the cheek, soft palate, fauces and tongue. They tend to occur in children and young adults and may be viral in origin. Papillomas are usually white or pinkish and pedunculated, consisting of a delicate polypoid mass of keratinized epithelium on a connective tissue base (*Fig.* 12.7). Occasionally several may arise in different parts of the mouth. An important differential diagnosis in an older patient is a verrucous carcinoma.

Treatment
The lesion is excised at its base with a narrow margin of normal mucosa. Haemorrhage can be controlled by a mattress-suture bringing the undermined edges of the mucosa together. Alternatively, electrocautery may be used and the wound allowed to granulate.

SOFT-TISSUE SWELLINGS OF THE ORAL MUCOSA

Neurofibroma

Neurofibromas are uncommon in the mouth and present as soft pedunculated swellings of the cheek, tongue or palate, or as sessile masses on the gingiva. Deeper lesions produce a fusiform swelling often soft and lobulated in the substance of the cheek, tongue or palate, and may be mistaken for a lipoma. It is important to examine the skin for other swellings and for brown (café-au-lait) patches which make up von Recklinghausen's neurofibromatosis. Lesions arising from the inferior dental nerve will enlarge the bony canal or even create a significant intra-osseous radiolucency. There is no associated neurological defect.

Plexiform neurofibromatosis may affect the head and neck region. In these unfortunate patients, a whole plexus of nerves is thickened producing a marked deformity due to the soft redundant mass within the facial tissues. The effect is that of a hemifacial hypertrophy.

Histologically there is a proliferation of the Schwann cells of the nerve sheath producing 'schwannomas' or 'neurilemmomas' or 'neurinomas'.

Occasionally the nerve is displaced and the tumour can be shelled out but in many cases there is no separation between the connective tissue mass and the nerve fibres.

Neurofibrosarcomas are rare.

Treatment

Treatment is excision where necessary but the involvement of related nerves presents obvious technical problems and a likelihood of nerve damage. Incomplete removal, as for instance with plexiform neurofibromatosis, will lead to a recurrence.

Lipoma

Lipomas are rare in the mouth, usually arising in the cheek from the buccal fat pad or in the floor of the mouth. They are soft and fluctuant, and may appear yellowish through the mucosa.

Treatment

Extracapsular excision.

SWELLINGS OF THE TONGUE

Fibro-Epithelial Polyp and Pyogenic Granuloma

Fibro-epithelial hyperplasias (fibro-epithelial polyps) may arise on the tongue, usually on the lateral border, whereas pyogenic granulomas may occur on the dorsum and contain food particles. Similarly, the less common lesions such as neurofibromas, fibromas and even lipomas may be found. However, the most characteristic swellings are median rhomboid glossitis, lingual lymphoid tissue, lymphangiomas and haemangiomas and the granular-cell myoblastoma.

Median Rhomboid Glossitis

This presents as a smooth or nodular oval mass on the mid-dorsum of the tongue just anterior to the junction of the anterior two-thirds and posterior third. It is devoid of papillae and tends to have a purple-pink hue.

Although considered, for many years, to be a developmental defect due to the failure of the lateral lingual swellings to fuse over the tuberculum impar, this explanation has been questioned. It is now thought to be a form of chronic hyperplastic candidiasis. However, the infection with candida may be secondary to the presence of an abnormal mucosa. Treatment of the candidiasis does not result in the disappearance of the nodular, non-papillated lesion. It is painless and treatment is usually unnecessary, although in some cases patients develop a cancerophobia, especially if examined by a non-dentally qualified clinician.

A simple V resection may be used to eliminate bulky lesions. Before excising a lesion be sure it lies anterior to the foramen caecum. Lingual thyroids present at and behind the foramen caecum and may be the patient's only thyroid tissue.

Lingual Lymphoid Tissue

This may be found where the lateral border of the tongue fuses with the faucial pillars. The smooth lobulated red and occasionally vascular tissue is both normal and desirable. However, it may also give rise to cancerophobia in a neurotic or hypochondriacal patient especially when a psychogenic pain has drawn attention to the area.

Firm reassurance that this is normal tissue is essential. Sometimes the foliate papillae, found at the same site, become inflamed and tender. Topical gentian violet 1 per cent solution for a few days usually brings about resolution.

Lymphangioma and Haemangioma

Lymphangiomas present as fine nodular semi-translucent lesions which tend to persist with growth of the normal tongue. Excision of circumscribed lesions usually presents no problems. Some are ideally removed with a cutting laser. Others require wedge resection correcting at the same time the macroglossia which the lesion causes. Significant postoperative swelling must be expected, but subsides within 2 weeks.

Cavernous haemangiomas may be solitary or part of a widespread orofacial vascular malformation. The tongue has an irregular bluish enlargement. Rarely this may be found to contain the concentric opacities of phleboliths when radiographed. If discrete and troublesome, excision under general anaesthetic with careful haemostasis using diathermy and deep sutures is advisable. Where a large volume of the tongue is involved by a cavernous malformation, demarcation with selective angiography and embolization with particles of polyvinyl alcohol (Ivalon) is the treatment of choice.

SOFT-TISSUE SWELLINGS OF THE ORAL MUCOSA

Amyloid

Diffuse firm enlargement of the tongue is produced by amyloid infiltration. This is often a manifestation of latent or known myelomatosis. Histologically the tongue is infiltrated with eosinophilic hyalinised material especially around blood vessels. This is a complex glycoprotein which gives a green birefringence on light microscopy when stained with congo red.

Myeloma paraproteins should be detectable in the plasma and urine and a radiological skeletal survey may reveal widespread punched out radiolucencies.

Granular-cell Tumour (Myoblastoma)

This rare lesion may present as a smooth symptomless swelling in the dorsum of the tongue. It is usually pale, firm and non-tender. The origin of the lesion is considered to be the Schwann cell and local excision is invariably successful. The histological appearance is of large polyhedral cells with small central nuclei and eosinophilic granular cytoplasm. The overlying epithelium shows pseudoepitheliomatous hyperplasia which in a superficial biopsy can lead to a mistaken diagnosis of carcinoma.

OTHER CONDITIONS PRODUCING SOFT-TISSUE SWELLING

Sarcoid

Sarcoid may produce a localized swelling or a diffuse, tender hyperplasia of the gingiva. Biopsy will reveal a tuberculous-like non-caseating epitheloid and giant cell granuloma. The condition occurs in young people, often negroes, and involves the eyes, skin, lymphoid tissue and cranial nerves. The cause is unknown.

Orofacial manifestations include lymph node enlargement which may be firm, non-tender and occasionally considerable in size, swollen salivary and lacrimal glands and uveitis. A chest X-ray will reveal enlarged hilar lymph nodes, the Kveim skin test is usually positive, and the serum angiotensin converting enzyme is raised.

A biopsy of the mucosa of the hard palate or gum is also said to be diagnostic in about 40 per cent of cases.

Treatment

The sensitive gingival lesions can be treated with topical steroid gel (0·1 per cent triamcinolone in Orabase). Grossly enlarged lymph nodes are easily removed for aesthetic reasons. Uveitis and extensive pulmonary disease require systemic corticosteroids.

Crohn's Disease

This is an uncommon, idiopathic, granulomatous condition of the alimentary canal which occasionally affects the mouth. Lesions are often red granulomatous areas on the gingiva or irregular 'cobblestone' patches on the buccal mucosa. The lip may swell suggesting angio-oedema except that the swelling is persistent and does not respond to antihistamines. Crohn's disease may not be suspected unless there is a history of lesions elsewhere in the gut. A biopsy will reveal granulomatous areas consisting of macrophages, lymphocytes and multinucleate giant cells, resembling a foreign body reaction or sarcoid.

No specific treatment is required for the oral lesions although topical steroids may be useful. An unsightly persistent swollen lip may require local steroid injections or even systemic steroids.

Note: The Melkersson–Rosenthal syndrome is usually considered to be a combination of swollen lips (cheilitis grandularis apostomatosa, or cheilitis granulomatosa), scrotal tongue and facial palsy. It is often difficult to establish the diagnosis if all the features are not present. When it occurs with facial palsy the condition is probably sarcoid, but without the cranial neuropathy, cases may be Crohn's disease or merely angio-oedema.

Malignant Granuloma (Wegener's Granulomatosis)

This may present as a haemorrhagic hyperplastic pale granular gingival overgrowth which is usually localized or occasionally diffuse or multifocal within the mouth. This diagnosis should be suspected if there is substantial destruction of the underlying bone and in particular the presence of lesions on the nasal mucosa or within the antrum. It is important to establish whether the condition is the localized destructive granuloma (Stewart's) or the generalized Wegener's variety which will lead to fatal renal failure if not treated early.

Histologically the dense infiltration of lymphocytes and plasma cells associated with necrosis may be difficult to diagnose unless the characteristic vasculitis is evident. Apart from a raised ESR there may be no other specific features and a careful search for lesions elsewhere must be made.

Treatment

Local lesions may be arrested with radiotherapy but this is not invariable, and progressive destruction of the face may lead to death through aspiration pneumonia. The systemic disease is treated with corticosteroids and azathioprine.

SUGGESTED READING

Barker B. S. and Lucas R. B. (1967) Localised fibrous overgrowths of the oral mucosa. *Br. J. Oral Surg.* **5**, 86–92.

Lee K. W. (1985) *Colour Atlas of Oral Pathology.* Philadelphia, Lea & Febiger.

Rateitschak-Pluss E. M., Hofti A. and Rateitschak K. N. (1983) Gingival-hyperplasie bei Cyclorsporing A Medikation. *Acta Paradontoligica* **93**, 57–65.

Sunderland E. P., Sunderland R. and Smith C. J. (1983) Granular cells associated with the enamel organ of a developing tooth. *J. Oral Path.* **12**, 1–6.

Tyldesley W. R. and Potter E. (1984) Gingival hyperplasia induced by cyclosporin A. *Br. Dent. J.* **157**, 305–309.

CHAPTER 13

THE DIAGNOSIS AND MANAGEMENT OF OROFACIAL PAIN

Pain is an unpleasant emotional experience due to either physical or psychological trauma. Most cases of facial pain are easily recognized as being toothache, sinusitis, trigeminal neuralgia, or even the more rare conditions such as facial migrainous neuralgia. However, the greatest difficulty in the management of facial pain is the failure to appreciate the common occurrence of psychogenic pains and the means of diagnosing and treating them.

THE HISTORY

The patient's account of the pain is of the utmost importance. Indeed where there are no other associated symptoms and no detectable physical signs the patient's history is the only evidence upon which the clinician can base a diagnosis.

Dentists, like other practically inclined and surgically trained clinicians, tend to spend too little time taking a history and may even feel uncomfortable if they do not promptly offer practical help to the patient. Where the diagnosis is straightforward, treatment can be prescribed immediately. For many patients who present with pain the clinician may not be certain of the diagnosis after the first consultation and inappropriate, empirical treatment may hinder and complicate the diagnostic process.

It often takes time to persuade the patient to tell all of his or her story, to sort out the details in chronological order, establish valid relationships and separate out the accumulation of beliefs and assertions of the patient's relatives, friends and professional advisors.

At the first visit patient and clinician meet as strangers and it may not be until a subsequent consultation that enough rapport is developed for important details to be revealed. Sometimes a female patient may confide the essential clue to the surgery assistant. Not infrequently patients censor certain pieces of information on the grounds that they are not the business of a dentist!

Pains due to local disease processes have a recognizable pattern, but more importantly there are usually other associated symptoms and physical signs to be uncovered by appropriate investigations. Also, as the disease progresses the clinical picture evolves accordingly. Patients who have a remittent or continuous pain, unchanged in character over many months or years and without the appearance of new symptoms or signs, are most unlikely to have either an occult infection or a malignant neoplasm and, at least, can be reassured on that point at the first visit. There are, however, pains which follow a similar pattern and are probably due to an ill-understood physical disease process, even though there is little in the way of physical signs. Examples of such pains are migraine and trigeminal neuralgia. Finally there are the psychogenic pains which are difficult to recognize without experience, and whose underlying mechanisms are still a matter of speculation.

The site of origin of a pain from a superficially placed disease process is usually accurately located by the patient, often with one finger, except when the pain is referred from a site innervated by an adjacent branch of the same nerve. In the latter case the site of complaint is non-tender. Such pains are often sharp and intense, but a dull, burning pain subsequently spreads out from the original focus, involving eventually a wide area. It is important therefore to determine where the pain started. If on physical examination a cause is found consistent with the patient's history 'the causal relationship' is assumed, but it is helpful, and indeed may be important, to find confirmatory evidence of current activity of the disease which would account for the complaint of pain. Some psychogenic pains may be experienced at a particular site to which consistently the patient points. The finding of a heavily filled tooth, unresponsive to vitality tests but without evidence of active infection, is not conclusive. Similarly many innocent impacted wisdom teeth or retained roots are wrongly incriminated. The clinician should reserve judgement that this is the sole cause, or even the likely cause, of the complaint, unless the symptoms match the signs.

Pains which arise from a focus of disease in the depths of the tissues are less well localized. If the pain is due to nerve involvement then the pattern of neurological signs may give a clue to the anatomical site of the lesion. If there are sensory changes involving more than one branch of the trigeminal nerve the appropriate division is likely to be involved. If more than one division is affected the lesion is at or inside the base of the skull. Lesions just outside or inside the skull may also involve other cranial nerves. Long tract signs usually mean a lesion within the brain or several disseminated lesions.

Important management problems relate to the further investigation of the patient and the use of empirical treatment as a therapeutic test. It is necessary to investigate a patient with sufficient thoroughness to avoid overlooking a detectable and treatable cause. On the other hand the indiscriminate use of investigations subjects the patient to avoidable discomfort, inconvenience and perhaps even complications. Indeed some investigations are not only hazardous, but expensive and the thoughtless use of diagnostic resources adds to the cost of health care and can even delay the investigation of more urgent cases.

Trying the effect of treatment where a plausible cause of the pain has been found may well be justified, but in the absence of certainty as to the diagnosis may increase the patient's symptoms and impede progress towards a correct understanding of the case. Both inappropriate investigation and inappropriate treatment may confirm in the mind of a patient with psychogenic pain the presence of serious physical disease which the clinician has not found or is concealing from the patient. Examples of these problems will be given when discussing specific entities.

In order to diagnose any pain and in particular distinguish between organic and psychogenic pain it is essential to take a history which includes the following information.

1. The character of the pain—is it sharp, dull, throbbing, burning or stabbing?

2. The site at which it is felt and any radiation. This should be recorded as a line drawing.

3. The timing—when the very first attack occurred and the frequency and duration of subsequent attacks. It is important to consider the timing of attacks during the day, whether the pain is worse in the morning, afternoon, evening or night, and if it prevents or disturbs sleep.

4. Provoking factors—these may include hot, cold, sweet and sour food and drinking, biting, chewing, yawning or talking, and bruxism—nocturnal or diurnal. But also establish the effect of anger, anxiety or alcohol.

5. The relieving factors—is it controlled by analgesics, alcohol, the application of heat, or does the pain disappear spontaneously?

6. What are the associated clinical features—swelling, unpleasant taste, trismus, nasal obstruction, loss of facial sensation, epiphora, anxiety or depression?

7. It is necessary to establish whether the patient suffers from pain or discomfort elsewhere in the body, such as headaches, migraine, neck or back pain, chest, abdominal or pelvic pain and pruritus. The timing, duration and management of these pains should be recorded. In this way it can be seen whether or not the facial pain belongs to a whole body syndrome.

8. The current and past general medical history, including drug therapy.

9. It is important to establish the patient's emotional history and determine whether the patient has suffered periods of anxiety or depression.

10. A standard family history, including the ill health or death of parents, brothers and sisters, spouse and children, is of crucial importance and often forgotten.

CLINICAL PRESENTATION
The Teeth—Odontalgia

Pulpal pain—irritation or inflammation of the dental pulp—arises from caries, loose or lost restorations and the latent split tooth. A transient sharp pain as a response to acid, sweet and thermal changes is a feature of uninsulated dentinal tubules. However, once the pulp becomes inflamed, the sharp pain becomes more severe and lasts for perhaps 10 or 20 minutes following contact of the tooth with cold or sweet food. Spontaneous episodes of sharp pain herald the onset of a persistent throbbing pain which is characteristically worse following stimulation and when lying down at night. It may be well localized, particularly on biting and chewing, but occasionally the pain becomes diffuse or is referred to the opposite jaw and may also be obscured by painful ipsilateral reflex muscle spasm.

All teeth must be carefully examined with a mirror and probe and percussed for sensitivity. Electrical and thermal pulp testing may also prove valuable in localizing a hypersensitive or non-vital tooth. Additional help may be obtained by injecting a local anaesthetic solution at the considered source of the pain. If the pain persists despite good analgesia alternative teeth should be re-examined.

The diagnosis of the split tooth can be difficult but the possibility should be considered, especially with heavily filled upper premolars or lower 1st molars. Sharp pain may only be provoked by getting the patient to bite firmly on a wool roll placed buccolingually over the tooth. A small fibreoptic light source is invaluable and removal of the restoration usually reveals a crack through the base of the cavity.

Toothache in the absence of appropriate physical and radiological signs—atypical odontalgia—is a psychogenic vascular pain which may mimic common dental pain and is discussed in detail later in this chapter.

Radiographs should include bitewing and periapical films of the suspected teeth. Where there is difficulty in establishing a diagnosis, especially with root-filled teeth, two long cone periapical projections taken obliquely in the horizontal plane to reveal the individual apices of multirooted teeth are invaluable. For pain arising in the upper dentition, an occipitomental view of the antrum is essential, to eliminate the possibility of sinusitis or, occasionally, a carcinoma.

Periodontitis

Pain from the inflamed periodontal membrane is invariably dull and continuous, and initially relieved by clenching the teeth, but later on is aggravated by this action. Periodontitis may be as a result of primary infection of a pocket due to food impaction, or secondary to an apical pulpal infection, or occasionally due to a longitudinally split root.

The treatment will depend on the cause. If a primary acute periodontal abscess is present, drainage of exudate and irrigation of the pocket with an antiseptic such as povidone-iodine or alcoholic tincture of iodine has a soothing effect which may be assisted by grinding the tooth out of occlusion. Unless periodontal surgery is carried out, the condition will recur. A secondary periodontitis can be treated only by removal of the infected pulp or tooth.

Bone Pain

The principal causes are alveolar osteitis (dry socket), infected cysts, fractures, osteomyelitis, and primary or secondary malignant tumours. (These are dealt with in detail in the appropriate sections.)

The pain varies from a dull, continuous ache to a severe throbbing which is relieved by antibiotics and analgesics. Inflammation producing thrombosis in the vasa nervorum or the infiltration of the inferior dental neurovascular bundle by a malignant tumour will give rise to mental analgesia. A rare cause of mandibular pain with mental anaesthesia is a sickle cell crisis.

Radiographs taken in either two or three planes will help to determine the exact site and extent of the disease.

As metastatic carcinoma may mimic an area of inflammatory bone destruction, where there is any doubt about the diagnosis, the lesion should be explored and a specimen taken for biopsy.

PRIMARY ORGANIC JOINT DISEASE

Traumatic Temporomandibular Joint Arthritis

This follows damage to the capsule and meniscus due to direct trauma and may follow a blow on the mandible or subluxation. The pain may be moderate to severe, is well localized and aggravated by movements of the mandible which are restricted. The mandible will deviate towards the painful side on attempted opening and a tender joint effusion may be visible and palpable.

Radiographs should include a rotational tomogram which can give the clearest picture of the condylar head and fossa. In addition, the transpharyngeal view is valuable, particularly if the mandible can be opened. The traditional superior oblique transcranial radiograph is difficult to interpret and gives a distorted view of the joint surfaces. Where an unreduced anterior dislocation of the meniscus is suspected to be the cause of the problem, an arthrogram will visualize the displaced meniscus.

Treatment consists of resting the joint and relieving pain with adequate analgesia such as aspirin 1 g, or ibuprofen 400 mg, t.d.s., 4–6-hourly. Persistent pain despite conservative therapy will be discussed under chronic dysfunction.

Acute arthritis of a non-traumatic aetiology is rare. Children may suffer juvenile rheumatoid arthritis (Still's disease) or an arthritic reaction to rubella immunization. In adults, acute rheumatoid arthritis is part of a systemic disease and is usually readily diagnosed. Rarer causes include psoriasis, gout and infective arthritis.

Investigations will include serological tests for rheumatoid arthritis, serum uric acid for gout and aspiration of any effusion for microscopic and microbiological investigation. Treatment will be determined by the underlying cause.

Osteoarthritis of the Temporomandibular Joint

This is a degenerative condition of the joint which occurs commonly without symptoms in the elderly, but has been observed clinically and radiographically in younger patients when it may follow long-standing untreated facial arthromyalgia. Immediately this creates the problem of diagnosis where it appears that a functional psychosomatic disorder may give rise to a structural organic lesion. Even in older patients where degenerative joint changes occur together with repetitive chronic mechanical insult (such as may follow using inadequate dentures), emotional tension can be an important predisposing factor and result in painful symptoms.

Since the degenerative changes in the joint cannot be reversed, attention must be diverted to correctable factors. Prolonged vigorous movements as may accompany singing or the use of old, ill-fitting dentures, particularly if they are worn continuously day and night, may be contributory factors. Lack of adequate occlusal support from the posterior teeth may transfer chewing stresses to the anterior ones with increased leverage on the joint tissues.

The pain is well localized to the affected joint and is provoked by chewing and other jaw movements. On examination, there is tenderness and both palpable and sometimes audible crepitus in the joints. When acutely inflamed, an effusion with periarticular swelling may be seen. If the pain is sharp and severe in an elderly patient, the differentiation from a paroxysmal trigeminal neuralgia can be difficult. Furthermore, it would appear that temporomandibular joint osteoarthritis can be a trigger for a true paroxysmal neuralgia in some patients.

The radiographic changes are best seen on the transpharyngeal and rotational tomographic views of the joint and include a loss of cortical definition, erosions and subarticular cysts together with calcific or osseous metaplasia at the insertion of the lateral pterygoid tendon, which together produce flattening and an angular beak-like remodelling of the condylar head.

Treatment

1. Correction of the occlusion with adequate dentures is of primary importance.
2. A course of an anti-inflammatory analgesic, such as ibuprofen 400 mg, 3 times a day with meals, or naproxen 250–500 mg once or twice a day, is useful, especially where there is an acute painful effusion.
3. Where an element of tension or depression is provoking bruxism an anxiolytic antidepressant drug such as 25–50 mg of dothiepin is of great

value. The tricyclic antidepressant drugs also have a synergistic effect on analgesics for pain relief.

4. Persistent pain may respond to one or two intra-articular injections of an anti-inflammatory steroid, such as 1 ml of triamcinolone (40 mg) or dexamethasone 1 ml (4 mg). Unfortunately, it is impossible to be certain whether intra-articular steroids have any long-term beneficial effects over that of the oral non-steroidal analgesic. Repeated intra-articular injections of steroids can induce resorption of the condylar head so, if there is no benefit from one or two injections, further doses are not advisable.

5. Smoothing of the condylar head by open surgery. The high condylar shave is advocated by some authors for cases with persistent, intractable pain. However, although immediate relief is achieved in some patients, the long-term value is uncertain. Simple smoothing of discrete osteophytes is preferred. The benefit of meniscectomy is short lived and further severe degenerative changes in the condylar head follow. Where there is gross degeneration of the meniscus, or in cases that have undergone previous surgery, a conservative smoothing operation with the insertion of a 2 mm silicone elastomer membrane suspended from the condylar fossa and overlying the eminence is the treatment of choice, in combination with the analgesic regime.

FUNCTIONAL TEMPOROMANDIBULAR JOINT DISORDERS

Because the mandible is bent into a U shape with the joints at either end in the same plane both must move together and in harmony with one another. Any abnormality in the movement of one TM joint imposes an abnormal movement on the other. Thus a patient may complain of pain and perhaps clicking in one joint in which the condyle is found to be moving forwards to the point of subluxation when the jaw is opened while the opposite condyle merely rotates and does not translate, hence the excessive movement of the other.

Movement of the condyles must also be guided by the muscles so that when the teeth articulate and move against one another in function they do so without discomfort. This must be managed despite the fact that few dentitions permit unimpeded movements of the jaw. Indeed some joints may act at a distinct mechanical disadvantage because of abnormal occlusal relationships. For example, where there is marked mandibular retrognathism the mandible must be protruded to incise food so that a closing force is exerted with the condyle held far forward on the articular eminence.

Such factors alone do not usually cause symptoms, but predispose the joint to disturbed function, pain, clicking and limitation of movement if other insults are added such as prolonged active opening during dental treatment. When the new factor can be reversed, or one of the predisposing

THE DIAGNOSIS AND MANAGEMENT OF OROFACIAL PAIN

factors eliminated, symptomless function may be restored. In some cases the underlying or precipitating factors are psychogenic in origin and the failure to recognize or treat such a problem may lead to chronicity.

PSYCHOGENIC PAIN

Psychosomatic disturbances are now recognized as being a common category of illness. When emotional strain gives rise to disturbances in the cardiovascular system, gastrointestinal tract or skin, the identifiable physical changes, such as increased blood pressure, tachycardia, peptic erosion or eczema, make the diagnosis respectable to the clinician and acceptable to the patient. Unfortunately, if the clinical presentation is simply pain, then there is often a failure to appreciate on both sides that real pain may arise in peripheral organs as a result of a central emotional disturbance. The pain usually arises in tense muscles or dilated blood vessels and is rarely the peripheral referral of a central disturbance, i.e. a conversion symptom, or an hallucination.

Psychogenic pain may arise in a variety of situations:

1. As a result of a stressful life event in a previously normal individual.
2. As a manifestation of transient emotional illness such as anxiety, neurosis or depression.
3. As an abnormal personality trait which will persist throughout life. This may be hypochondriacal or hysterical in character.
4. As the manifestation of psychosis.

The first two groups are by far the most common and most amenable to treatment.

As with all pain problems the history is the key to the diagnosis, and the following areas should be explored:

a. General pain symptoms. Symptoms of other psychosomatic conditions which occur simultaneously or sequentially with orofacial pain, e.g. migraine, tension headaches, neck and back ache, pelvic pain, especially dysmenorrhoea often associated with menorrhagia, irritable (spastic) colon, pruritus and non-allergic vasomotor rhinitis. By establishing the positive relationship of these conditions with orofacial pain, not only is the diagnosis clarified, but the patient is reassured that unexplained pain or continuous illness that has been a trouble for years with fruitless investigations and operative procedures can be explained in a more rational way.

b. Family history. As stated, a detailed family history is often a crucial key to diagnosis. Features of importance include a history of emotional disturbance in the parents or siblings, bereavement immediately prior to the onset of the condition or the occurrence of a congenital deformity or chronic illness often in a child or spouse. Weddings and pregnancies in the family which normally are a source of joy are sometimes the cause of distress or anxiety.

    c. Social history. Psychosomatic pain can arise in the first decade in children who adapt poorly to school, or who have difficulty tolerating sibling rivalry. In older children the pressure of examinations can be a cause. Vocational pressures in adults including unemployment and marital problems such as alcoholism or sexual maladjustment are important. Later still, social isolation or responsibility for a chronic invalid produce psychosomatic illness.

    In summary, the dental clinician has no difficulty in establishing the patient's general medical history, but is often reluctant to ask if the patient suffers from 'worry or depression' or has been treated for these conditions, and often overlooks the need to explore the family medical history and social history.

Clinical presentations of psychogenic pain include:
—Facial arthromyalgia (TMJ dysfunction, myofascial pain dysfunction syndromes).
—Atypical facial pain (atypical facial neuralgia).
—Atypical odontalgia.
—Oral dysaesthesia.
—Factitious ulceration.

Facial Arthromyalgia
(The Temporomandibular Joint Dysfunction Syndrome)
(The Myofascial Pain Dysfunction Syndrome)

After toothache the most common facial pain arises in the temporomandibular joints and facial muscles. There is still reservation amongst some clinicians as to the principal cause of temporomandibular joint pain. The overwhelming evidence is that this joint and its associated musculature are commonly the sites of psychogenic dysfunctional pain and that pure organic causes are considerably less frequent. (*See* Primary organic joint pain *above.*)

Clinical Presentation

The condition may vary from clicking and sticking of the jaw joint on chewing, talking and yawning to a severe, continuous dull ache in one or both temporomandibular joints associated with trismus. Although the onset may be acute, the pain commonly radiates up into the temporal region, down to the angle of the mandible and is often associated with occipital, sternomastoid and cervical pain.

    The patient can describe the pain as being an earache and may suffer from a stuffy sensation or popping noises within the ears and tinnitus. Questioning will usually reveal a history of headaches, migraine, cervical and back pain, in addition to abdominal and pelvic pain and pruritic skin. Thus the patient will have been treated for what is often diagnosed as a slipped disc, irritable colon, dysmenorrhoea and eczema.

Although referral is often due to a recent exacerbation, it is important to determine previous episodes of pain which may have occurred intermittently over many years.

The pain may be present on waking together with trismus and tend to improve during the day, in which case there may be a history of nocturnal bruxism or jaw clenching. Other patients tend to develop the pain during the course of the day, especially when tired and stress is discernible as a related factor. Bruxism and comparable oral habits such as nail, pencil or pipe biting and cheek or lip chewing are frequently associated features.

After establishing whether the patient is aware of bruxism or facial tension, it is important to ask whether they suffer from anxiety of depression. Many patients will be reluctant to reveal a previous psychiatric history, at least at the first interview. Other important factors which often arise in the absence of any emotional disturbance are adverse life events. These include, in children, difficulties with school examinations or sibling rivalry, a history of bereavement or family illness which may include congenital malformation in a child, or alcoholism in a husband, marital disharmony, and professional stress. These factors can only be elicited by taking a detailed family history.

On clinical examination, there is usually tenderness in one or both joints and also in a variety of facial muscular sites, including the temporalis and masseter muscles. Trismus may be present and there is usually deviation of the mandible on opening towards the most painful side. Intraorally, ridging of the buccal mucosa and tongue margins is pathognomonic of a persistent clenching habit and bruxism may also be seen in the worn facets of the anterior teeth. It is, of course, important to examine the dentition for carious lesions, pulpitic teeth and gross occlusal defects.

The pain appears to be a combination of a traumatic arthrosis due to bruxism and painful muscular vasodilatation. The poor response to analgesics and effective control by tricyclic antidepressant drug therapy suggest that the intensity and persistence of the painful symptoms may also be due to failure in a central amine pain suppressor mechanism.

Much emphasis has been placed on malocclusion as the prime aetiology of this condition, despite the fact that no clinical trial has been able to establish malocclusion as the cause or occlusal equilibrium as a consistent cure of the condition. Acute or subacute forms may be provoked by an inflamed tooth, or gross occlusal disturbance such as a recent badly contoured dental restoration or a sudden loss of posterior occlusal support. However, most cases do not display any gross malocclusion and in some the dental disorder appears to trigger off, or localize, a chronic pain problem.

Some 60 per cent of patients appear to be suffering from either a neurotic or depressive illness, while the remaining 40 per cent, although psychiatrically normal, often give a history of stressful life events. Although the patients who attend for treatment are predominantly adult married females, there is a wide age range extending from the first decade upwards, and it would appear that many men suffer a mild form of the condition but do not attend for treatment. In children the condition is misdiagnosed as earache.

The pain is best considered to be part of a whole body psychosomatic syndrome in patients who are often competent individuals with obsessional perfectionist traits, particularly those who hold responsible positions.

Treatment

1. All dental disease must be eliminated, including carious cavities, periapical abscesses and pericoronitis. There is no evidence that minor occlusal disharmony or partially and unerupted wisdom teeth are responsible for the condition. Major restorative dental procedures aimed at modifying the occlusion can make the patient worse, producing severe intractable pain so that there is difficulty in separating the original problem from the secondary somatopsychic disturbance.

2. An appreciation of the underlying stress is important to the patient who responds well to the reassuring explanation that emotional tension expressed as bruxism can create joint pain and with painful dilated blood vessels, muscle spasm. It is important to emphasize to the patient that the pain is a 'real pain—comparable to migraine' and is not imaginary.

3. Tricyclic antidepressants such as nortriptyline, starting with 10 mg at night and increasing to 30 mg at seven days and then maintaining this regime for three weeks will produce marked relief of both local and general symptoms. Where pain persists the patient should be encouraged gradually to increase the dosage to a maximum tolerated level which may be 100 mg. Side effects such as drowsiness and a dry mouth soon wear off especially as the drug is taken at night before retiring. Where there is no remission small doses of a phenothiazine appear to be beneficial and are used as a combined medication with the tricyclic, e.g. trifluoperazine, 2–4 mg in the morning. A useful and well tolerated drug combination is Motival (fluphenazine 0·5 mg and nortriptyline 10 mg), one to two at night. Again this dose should be increased gradually as required. Flupenthixol 0·5–1·5 mg twice daily is also a useful alternative regime where a tricyclic drug fails.

It may be necessary in severe, persistent cases to use a monoamine oxidase inhibitor such as Parstelin (tranylcypromine 10 mg and trifluoperazine 1 mg) 1 t.d.s. at 8, 12 and 4 p.m. with 2–5 mg diazepam at night to prevent insomnia.

It is important to stress that the medication is being used for its centrally acting muscle relaxant analgesic effect and not as an antidepressant.

4. A bite-guard may be used either at night or during the day, between meals, to discourage bruxism and may be effective in a number of cases.

However, many patients quickly cease to use or even lose the bite-guard and its value appears to be a placebo effect and is therefore best used in young patients and those who are reluctant to take psychotropic drugs.

5. Severely disturbed and intractible cases invariably benefit from a psychiatric consultation and if necessary, treatment. Unfortunately, many patients are reluctant to be referred to a department of psychological medicine and not all psychiatrists show interest in psychosomatic facial pain.

6. The role of surgery is controversial. Although a blind condylotomy has been shown in one retrospective series to be of value, many patients have gradually relapsed. The diagnosis of internal derangement of the joint with anterior dislocation of the meniscus has become fashionable since the increased use and understanding of temporomandibular joint arthrography. Anterior dislocation of the meniscus without reduction can produce both chronic pain, erosion of the anterior surface of the condylar head and even condylar remodelling with loss of ramus height and an anterior open bite. However, many of these cases respond to conservative therapy, that is reassurance, analgesic and antidepressant drugs. Even so, an increasing number of patients are being subjected to a high condylotomy and posterior re-attachment of the meniscus as an open procedure. There is no controlled published work to establish the degree of success of this surgical procedure, and many cases can be seen in time to become either worse or develop marked degenerative changes with osteophyte formation of the condylar head.

In summary, the authors do not support the need for surgery except in extreme cases, which may be determined by the following criteria:

a. Where the patient has had longstanding pain and trismus unrelieved by conservative drug therapy for a minimum of 12 weeks.

b. Where an arthrogram or computerized tomogram or arthroscopy confirms anterio-medial or posterior dislocation of the meniscus, adhesions or gross osteophytes of the condylar head.

At surgery the joint space is opened up by a Juniper joint distractor. If a displaced disk can be freed and repositioned it is sutured to the posterior capsule. Grossly adherent and torn menisci are probably best removed and replaced by a 2 mm Dow Corning disk prosthesis suspended from the fossa by fine wire ligatures. Adhesions may be divided by arthroscopy without open surgery.

It is important to remember that following longstanding trismus a temporalis contracture may develop which will give rise to an extra-articular ankylosis and prevent opening under a general anaesthetic. This can only be treated by bilateral temporalis myotomies or coronoidectomies. Vigorous postoperative exercises are essential.

Finally, one important feature of all psychosomatic conditions is that the vulnerability of the patient persists throughout life, predisposing to relapse and recurrence. The patient should be made aware of this and given instructions as to how they can cope, for instance, by returning to their former course of medication. It has also been shown that medication is required for at least a year for many patients with longstanding joint and facial pain. Shorter periods of treatment lead to relapse often within 3–4 weeks. (*See also* sections on Atypical facial neuralgia and Atypical odontalgia *below*.)

Atypical Facial Pain
(Atypical Facial Neuralgia)

Although this painful condition may occur alone, it frequently presents sequentially or even simultaneously with facial arthromyalgia and would appear to be a non-muscular, non-joint variant of the facial psychogenic pains.

This is a common form of facial pain, often described as a continuous dull ache with intermittent excruciating throbbing episodes. It is characteristically localized to non-muscular, non-joint areas, such as the facial bones, alveolus and teeth, where the localized variant, atypical odontalgia, will be discussed separately. It may be bilateral and is not provoked by any identifiable factors such as temperature changes or jaw movements and is not relieved by analgesics. Like facial arthromyalgia it is associated with pains elsewhere in the body. A common feature is a sensation of nasal stuffiness or obstruction. This is a non-allergic vasomotor rhinitis and is usually firmly described as a history of chronic sinusitis.

The pain episodes may be intermittent or continuous over a period of many years. Quite often there is a history of a placebo response to antibiotics which, as a result, may be prescribed frequently but without obvious reason. Dental treatment also can provoke or potentiate the pain. A frequent additional complaint is of swelling and redness of the face, or redness of the oral mucosa. There may indeed be slight oedema and redness of part of the face or minimal hyperaemia of the oral mucosa. Such appearances may form the basis for the use of antibiotics but without regression of the swelling.

Infiltration of the painful site with local anaesthetic may give temporary relief, but has no diagnostic value. The association with migraine and vasomotor rhinitis suggests that the pain mechanism is vascular with intermittent or perhaps persistent vasodilation giving rise to the release of local pain producing substances. Although the absence of physical signs and the difficult history may tempt the clinician to assume the problem is imaginary, this is unhelpful and will obscure the true nature of the condition and impair management.

Another difficult feature of many patients is their extreme reluctance to accept a diagnosis of psychogenic pain, even when it is sympathetically and emphatically explained that the pain is nevertheless a real and distressing one. These patients will often insist in an obsessional way that there is a physical cause giving details of the supposed anatomical disturbance and demand surgical treatment. This should be completely resisted as the extraction of teeth and exploratory operations complicate the picture. While surgery often produces short-lived relief, it is usually followed by an exacerbation of the problem. Such treatment adds an additional failure of clinical expertise to some patients' log book, indeed some hypochondriacal patients give the impression of competing with the clinician. This has been described as the pain game, and unfortunately, the tendency to manipulate and dominate may, in aggressive and paranoid patients, become a basis for medicolegal attack. However, if the patient is treated firmly with repeated assurance that surgery is both unnecessary and harmful, and that only medical drug therapy is suitable, the majority of patient's problems can be controlled. In a few cases, however, the pain persists. Severe and persistent pain, or a marked emotional disturbance, are indications for referral to a psychiatrist.

There are good reasons for maintaining these patients under continuous review, which should include regular careful neurological examination. While with experience and care the clinician may have confidence in the diagnosis, continuing observations will ensure that the first clinical manifestations of physical disease will not be missed. Any suggestion of sensory change indicates the need for a CT scan. In any case the patients benefit from a regular supportive interview with someone they have come to trust, and finally it avoids the beginnings of a new disease being overlooked because the symptoms are looked upon as new manifestations of the old complaint.

The treatment is the same as facial arthromyalgia.

Atypical Odontalgia
(Idiopathic Periodontalgia)

Pulpitis and periodontitis are common recognized causes of orofacial pain. However, an atypical odontalgia with identical features consisting of persistent or throbbing pain provoked by biting, chewing and thermal changes can arise without any detectable structural lesion. The condition becomes more readily recognizable if teeth in more than one quadrant are affected. However, should a single, heavily filled tooth become painful, there is a strong temptation to remove first the filling, then the pulp, and then after root filling and apicectomy, extract the tooth, even without any clear clinical indication. An additional complicating factor is that atypical odontalgia is commonly precipitated by a dental procedure such as the fitting of a crown or bridge or an extraction and is made worse by further active treatment.

The important differential diagnosis in these cases is the latent split tooth. The history is therefore one of pain in the teeth followed by repeated dental procedures, including pulp extirpations and extractions, followed by a 'dry socket' from a mouth where certain of the residual teeth, although sound and vital, are still tender to percussion and hyper-responsive to other stimuli.

In other cases the patient complains of pain in a completely sound tooth. Extraction of the tooth relieves the pain, but several months later the patient returns with a similar complaint about a further blemish-free tooth. This cycle can be repeated until four or five normal teeth have been removed and the clinician's suspicions aroused.

Like atypical facial neuralgia, the pain appears to be vascular in origin and is related to other pains of a similar nature. Although many patients reveal significant emotional problems, some do not, and attempts to force a psychiatric diagnosis on these patients are of no therapeutic advantage. However, it is important to stress to the patient that the pain is a real pain and is best considered to be a 'dental migraine' which will respond to drug therapy. Apicectomies, refilling or extracting teeth where there is no clinical indication of the need for such treatment should be avoided at all costs.

The treatment is that of facial arthromyalgia and atypical facial neuralgia.

Oral Dysaesthesia

This group of conditions tends to be non-painful and more commonly occur in the elderly with latent or overt problems of bereavement and loneliness. In some cases there may be evidence of an organic psychosis due to cerebral ischaemic changes. The most common presentations are:

1. Burning tongue—glossodynia or glossopyrosis.
2. Dry mouth in the presence of saliva 'salivary sand'.
3. Denture intolerance.
4. Phantom bite syndrome.
5. Abnormalities of taste, including the obesssional fear of halitosis or a conviction of a 'discharge' from a particular corner of the mouth.

1. The burning tongue, glossopyrosis or glossodynia, is probably the most common and may also extend to involve the gingiva, lips and palate. The patient is often middle-aged and female, but can be of any age or sex. The discomfort is not present on waking, but gradually increases during the course of the day, until, towards the evening, it becomes intolerable. Nevertheless, it never prevents or disturbs sleep. An important diagnostic feature is that it is usually, but not invariably, relieved by eating and drinking, which distinguishes this from organic disturbances, such as vitamin B_{12} or iron deficiency, or benign or malignant ulceration. Although the condition is often attributed to a fungal infection, there is rarely any evidence of this. A secondary problem is cancerophobia, which is often confirmed in the patient's mind by a bright red tongue, with scalloped margins. This appearance is due to compression of the tongue against clenched teeth.

2. The problems of a dry mouth sensation or 'sand in the saliva' occur despite adequate salivary flow, and investigations of salivary gland function, including tests for Sjögren's disease, prove to be negative.

3. In the same way, some patients have prosthodontic problems which appear to have no physical justification in that there are good ridges as a foundation for dentures. The suspicion is borne out by the large bag of dentures, each made by one of a number of competent clinicians, and which the patient usually carries with her. The underlying complaint is usually of oral mucosal hypersensitivity such that even pressure with a finger, let alone the dentures, is not tolerable.

4. The phantom bite syndrome is the situation where a patient cannot find a position of comfort despite having worn dentures for many years. The disturbance is invariably precipitated by the provision of new dentures to correct the loss of fit and occlusal height in the old set! Here a neurotic or even psychotic reaction is triggered off by a disturbance in orofacial posture. In addition the patient may develop an obsessional concern for some single feature, be it the shape of the teeth or the appearance of the tongue or the colour of a crown. These conditions are best described as a mono-symptomatic hypochondriacal neurosis. If the symptoms become more bizarre and obsessional in character, then it is a hypochondriacal psychosis. The phantom bite syndrome may also occur in the dentate patient following occlusal rehabilitation.

5. A variant form of mono-symptomatic hypochondriacal neurosis is the complaint of perversion of taste, i.e. cachageusia. The patient may describe a constant acid or foul taste or be obsessed with having halitosis. Clinically, there is no evident cause and in most cases fruitless investigations of the sinuses, chest and stomach have usually been carried out. Treatment should be strong reassurance, simple instructions on oral hygiene including cleaning the dorsum of the tongue with a soft wet toothbrush, supplemented by the following medication. These patients respond better to a phenothiazine and related drugs than the tricyclic antidepressants. Flupenthixol, commencing with 0·5 mg bd, and increasing the dose as required to 3 mg a day. An alternative is trifluoperazine 2–4 mg as slow release spansule twice a day.

Factitious Ulceration

Painful factitious (self-inflicted) ulceration may be difficult to recognize, particularly if the lesion resembles an aphthous ulcer or a stomatitis. The mucosa may be abraded with either finger nails or the application of a corrosive substance such as aspirin. Patients invariably deny causing the lesion and the diagnosis has to be made on the basis that the site and presentation do not fit a recognizable, pathological entity. In addition, there is usually a history of emotional disturbance. Conversely, where lesions appear to be bizarre or resemble some rare disease, a diagnosis which is not borne out by the microbiological or histological evidence, a self-inflicted lesion should always be considered.

As these lesions appear to be an unconscious manifestation of stress, a phenothiazine, e.g. trifluoperazine 2–4 mg a day can be tried with a psychiatric assessment or treatment as necessary.

OTHER SITES OF PAIN

The Tongue

Lingual pain may be sharp or burning and can be referred to the ear. When the cause is an organic lesion, it is provoked by spiced or hot food or drink, and by swallowing.

The benign mucosal causes include aphthous and viral ulceration, erosive lichen planus, bullous lesions, and the atrophic glossitis of iron deficiency or vitamin B_{12} deficiency. Occasionally, the enigmatic geographical tongue will give rise to discomfort.

The possibility that an ulcer may be malignant is an important consideration. Carcinomas which arise at the posterior end of the lateral border, in the vallecula and on the posterior third of the tongue may cause pain as the first symptoms and can be particularly difficult to detect while still small. In all cases, the tongue should be examined carefully by drawing it forward and holding it with a dry gauze swab. Some skill in using a laryngeal mirror is necessary to see down as far as the epiglottis. If any doubt persists in the clinician's mind an examination under anaesthesia with biopsy should be arranged.

The most common cause of lingual discomfort is the burning tongue of glossodynia or glossopyrosis. This has been discussed in detail above—*see* p. 327. Investigations will include biopsy, easily done under local anaesthetic, serum iron and iron binding capacity, serum B_{12} and folate.

Each condition will require specific therapy. However, persistent pain due to an inoperable carcinoma of the posterior third of the tongue may be relieved by the division of the glossopharyngeal nerve in the tonsillar fossa.

Salivary Glands

Pain is variable in character, often intermittent and dull, but well localized and associated with a swollen gland which usually enlarges whilst eating. With infection, pus can be expressed from the opening of the secretory duct, the mouth of which will be seen to be inflamed. Intermittent swelling due to obstruction can be provoked clinically by lemon juice.

The important differential diagnosis is mumps where the swelling usually becomes bilateral and the patient is febrile and ill and may develop inflammation at other glandular sites such as the testes, pancreas or breast. With mumps the serum should be screened for S and V antibodies when the patient is first seen and again ten days later.

THE DIAGNOSIS AND MANAGEMENT OF OROFACIAL PAIN

Obstructive causes for sialoadenitis include calculi, which are usually seen in the submandibular gland and occasionally in the parotid. Calculi can be diagnosed by plain radiography or may need to be confirmed by sialography which should be done after an acute inflammatory phase has been brought under control with antibiotics. Occasionally, the cause of obstruction may not be seen, especially in the parotid, and is attributed to a mucous plug, buccinator spasm or stricture of the duct. Just occasionally, salivary gland tumours produce obstruction.

The persistent tender nodule in the parotid may be an adenoid cystic carcinoma.

Many patients complain of persistent or intermittent pain and swelling of the parotid area, occasionally strongly supported by the evidence of family or friends which after careful consideration and investigation proves to be psychogenic joint pain—facial arthromyalgia. The history is usually of several months duration with pain provoked by eating and not drinking and no actual swelling of the gland is seen despite repeated examination.

The Maxillary Antrum

Acute sinusitis presents as a dull and often severe maxillary pain, either unilaterally or bilaterally, which is characteristically worse on bending. Unfortunately, the diagnosis may be obscured by sensitivity in one or more of the premolar and molar teeth which can be exquisitely painful on percussion, giving the impression of a pulpitis. However, the patient has usually suffered a recent upper respiratory tract infection with nasal obstruction and an anterior and posterior nasal discharge. The cheek is tender to pressure and occipitomental radiographs will show an opaque sinus often with a fluid level.

Chronic sinusitis consisting of intermittent nasal obstruction with radiographic changes showing mucosal thickening and polyp formation rarely gives rise to facial or dental pain. The condition may require active treatment, or the persistent mucosal changes justify biopsy in case they represent a carcinoma. An ENT surgeon will advise if this is so. In the absence of clinical evidence of active disease the changes may be no more than residual fibrosis of the mucosal thickening.

Where the patient is in fact suffering from persistent psychogenic pain repeated medical and surgical treatment on the basis of such radiographic appearances alone may be harmful rather than beneficial.

Carcinoma of the antrum tends to remain painless until late in its development and patients are more likely to present with nasal obstruction with epistaxis, facial enlargement, loose teeth, epiphora and elevation of the eye. Pain is usually due to invasion of the nerves in the wall of the sinus so is often associated with impaired sensation in the distribution of the maxillary nerve.

All patients with otherwise unexplained maxillary pain should have an occipitomental radiograph as part of their investigation to exclude carcinoma, particularly as a rotational tomograph may not reveal such a lesion if it lies in part of the antrum outside the sharp plane of the tomogram. An opaque soft tissue mass associated with bony erosion is the characteristic radiological appearance.

The Ears

A painful otitis externa due to a furuncle, impacted wax or a fungal infection may occasionally be referred to the mandibular area. The pain, however, can be elicited by rotating the pinna and examination with an auroscope will reveal the site of inflammation. Treatment by the GP or ENT surgeon is directed towards the cause. Middle ear infection is associated with an inflamed or ruptured tympanic membrane and requires urgent specialist care.

Tonsils

The peritonsillar abscess (quinsy) occasionally presents as pain in the maxilla with trismus, which the patient misinterprets as toothache. However, on examination the palate is seen to be swollen between the uvula and tonsillar fossa.

Treatment is with antibiotics, incision and drainage of the abscess. This may be done in suitable patients in the upright position, anaesthetizing the swelling first with topical, then with a submucosal injection of a local analgesic. The alternative is to use a short-acting intravenous anaesthetic with the head of the patient well extended in the supine position and a good sucker to prevent inhalation of the pus.

The Elongated Styloid Process (Eagle's Syndrome)

Painful dysphagia may follow fracture of the styloid process. Eagle's syndrome is pain arising from an elongated styloid process where a diagnostic feature is said to be tenderness on palpation in the tonsillar fossa. Whether an elongated styloid process is really the cause of such pain is questionable. Radiographs reveal elongated styloid processes in many middle-aged and elderly patients and pain of an acute nature in the pharyngeal area should be considered to be a glossopharyngeal neuralgia, a nasopharyngeal tumour or possibly psychogenic atypical facial neuralgia in the first instance.

Pain in the Region of the Eyes

Acute glaucoma has been described as presenting with an ill-defined, acute facial pain. However, the association of blurred vision and a palpably hard eye should establish the diagnosis. A patient considered to have acute glaucoma should be referred as an emergency to an ophthalmic surgeon. Treatment consists of pilocarpine and surgery.

THE DIAGNOSIS AND MANAGEMENT OF OROFACIAL PAIN

Angina Pectoris

Occasionally, a manifestation of ischaemic heart disease is angina pectoris referred to the angle of the left mandible or even the premolar region via their common autonomic sensory innervation. The pain is provoked on effort and will be associated with ischaemic changes on an electrocardiogram. Instances are known, however, where patients with a cardiac infarct have presented with continuous severe pain in the left mandible which they have attributed to a bad tooth. An extraction under these circumstances would clearly have serious consequences.

PRIMARY NEURALGIAS

The most common paroxysmal neuralgia arises in the trigeminal nerve. Occasionally, the condition also affects the glossopharyngeal nerve or superior laryngeal branch of the vagus nerve. The aetiology of this pain is unclear and has been attributed to viral damage within the ganglion, demyelination of intracranial nerve roots due to nerve compression by small vascular loops, by dural bands or by narrowing of the nerve foramina, and even to ill-defined foci of chronic osteitis within the jaws.

Paroxysmal Trigeminal Neuralgia (Tic Douloureux)

Usually affecting the middle aged and elderly. The patient presents with a sharp, often severe stabbing pain lasting seconds which is provoked by talking, chewing, swallowing or by touching a specific area called the trigger zone. However, rapidly repeated attacks at intervals throughout the day may lead the patient to describe the pain as continuous. Women are more often affected than men. The most common sites involved are the mandibular mental and maxillary canine areas. The ophthalmic distribution of the trigeminal nerve is rarely affected.

Attacks do not occur during the night except when the patient suffers from insomnia. Although periods of remission are well recognized, the condition tends to recur or persist throughout the patient's remaining life without any objective neurological signs appearing. The diagnosis may be complicated by the fact that the pain can be provoked by an osteoarthritic temporomandibular joint. The patient justifiably becomes depressed and in between episodes of trigeminal pain may present with a persistent ache or burning sensation which is usually an atypical facial neuralgia.

The pain can also be an early manifestation of disseminated sclerosis, or of an intracranial neoplasm (*see* later under secondary neuralgias). The development of fresh symptoms or detectable neurological signs therefore calls for prompt further investigation.

Treatment

The anticonvulsant carbamazepine (Tegretol) 100–400 mg taken immediately on waking and 5–6-hourly, i.e. three times a day in all, controls the condition in most cases. It is important to introduce the drug gradually to avoid nausea, drowsiness and ataxia. With time, these symptoms tend to decrease, although in some patients the onset of an allergic dermatitis may necessitate its withdrawal. Unfortunately, there is no equally potent alternative drug, although phenytoin 200–400 mg twice a day may be useful. Clobezam 10 mg three times a day may also be of value as a supplement to carbamazepine or phenytoin. Contrary to earlier reports, agranulocytosis, due to carbamazepine, is very uncommon.

Where drug therapy is inadequate, or immediate relief is essential, good control can be achieved by injecting 1 ml of 60 per cent or 90 per cent alcohol into the mental or infraorbital foramina, taking care to avoid entering a blood vessel by aspirating before the injection. The alcohol can also be infiltrated in the region of the mandibular foramen at the lingula. In all cases, 2 ml of 2 per cent lignocaine should be given five minutes before the injection to avoid unnecessary pain. The immediate relief is valuable in distressed patients and may last for 6–12 months, although as with all peripheral blockades recurrence in adjacent areas, that is displacement, often arises sometimes within a matter of a few days. Peripheral neurectomy and cryotherapy at these sites have comparable results. With cryotherapy, an early return of sensation before recurrence of the pain is said to be an advantage.

Intraganglionic alcohol injection or radiofrequency thermocoagulation performed through the foramen ovale under radiographic control is necessary when medical or peripheral measures fail. The advantage of thermocoagulation is that the destruction of the nerve fibres may be modulated to include principally the unmedullated pain fibres, preserving some sensation and reducing paraesthesia.

Finally, an intracranial preganglionic section of the mandibular or maxillary nerve trunk or division of the mandibular and maxillary nerve fibres in the nerve root may be required where all other measures fail.

Intracranial vascular loops that compress the trigeminal nerve may be divided and this may relieve the pain.

Glossopharyngeal Neuralgia

Glossopharyngeal neuralgia is brought on by swallowing and the pain shoots both down into the throat and into the ear. The treatment is analagous to that of trigeminal neuralgia above.

SECONDARY NEURALGIAS

Secondary neuralgias arise from irritation of the trigeminal ganglion or nerves by some identifiable lesion and may either mimic exactly the primary paroxysmal pain, or present as a less specific disturbance.

Important differentiating features are the associated local sensory, reflex or motor impairment which may or may not be present when the patient first presents. The lesion causing the disturbance can arise either extracranially, within the cranial base, or intracranially.

Extracranial Lesions

Two mental nerve syndromes may give rise to neuralgia, commonly in elderly patients. The more common arises from the pressure of a lower denture flange which compresses a mental nerve which has become superficial as a result of alveolar bone resorption. The pain may be elicited by digital compression at the appropriate site and radiographically the mental foramen is seen to be at the alveolar crest. Treatment in the first instance may consist of relieving the denture over the origin of the nerve or inserting a soft lining. However, in many cases, the nerve will have to be set down surgically below the buccal surface of the residual alveolar process.

A less common mental nerve neuralgia is due to entrapment arising from narrowing of the mental foramen itself and this may give rise to a paroxysmal pain indistinguishable from a true tic douloureux. The diagnosis is made easier if the patient is not a denture wearer and the alveolar process is well preserved, in which case radiologically there is evidence of a narrow foramen. Treatment consists of decompression of the mental nerve by the careful removal of a ring of bone around the margin of the foramen.

Causalgia

Causalgia is pain arising at the site of a nerve injury. Despite extractions and frequent operative procedures to the mandible and maxilla, true causalgia appears to be very rare. Its presentation may be a well localized persistent burning or throbbing pain at the site of a traumatic surgical procedure. This is commonly the upper lateral incisor or the lower 3rd molar and relief can only be obtained by a complete local analgesic blockade of all sensory pathways from the relevant jaw.

Some causalgias have been attributed to traumatic neuromas but, unfortunately, excision of these discrete painful areas of mucosa has only provided relief of pain in 50 per cent of patients. It is important to consider the alternative diagnosis of atypical facial neuralgia which is probably a vascular pain precipitated by an emotional disturbance.

Some cases of causalgia appear to arise following repeated irrelevant surgery for the treatment of atypical facial neuralgia, and it may be possible to convert the psychogenic vascular pain into an intractable causalgia in this way. It is typical of causalgia that exploration of the injured site and excision of scar tissue results in relief of the pain, but the pain returns as healing is completed and new scar tissue forms.

TREATMENT

In the first instance the case is best considered to be an atypical facial neuralgia, exploring the patient's history and using an appropriate antidepressant drug therapy. With a true causalgia, nerve blocks will provide immediate, reproducible and long-term relief. However, with atypical facial neuralgia, if relief is achieved it is invariably of a short duration—often no more than 10–20 days—and the pain will recur despite persistent loss of sensation. For this reason, nerve section or ganglion blocks should be withheld until the diagnosis appears to be certain.

In order to avoid irreversible nerve damage, cryotherapy to the appropriate nerve, which is usually the inferior dental, will enable the pain to be abolished without irreversible sensory loss. It may be repeated, or if necessary the nerve itself avulsed.

Avulsion of the inferior dental neurovascular bundle is best done under a general anaesthetic when it is identified at the lingula. The lingula should then be removed using a chisel or an osteotome parallel to the lingual cortex. This enables a satisfactory length of bundle to be grasped. Two resorbable ligatures are best passed around the entire bundle and tied before the bundle is divided. The nerve is then exposed at the mental foramen and sectioned and avulsed by applying traction to the proximal end.

Intracranial root sections must be avoided in these patients as the recurrence of pain and hence uncertainty about the diagnosis is high. Therefore, rather than expose the patient to unnecessary surgical morbidity, a better alternative is to prescribe a continuous course of appropriate analgesics such as diflunisal or pentazocine.

Frey's Auriculotemporal Syndrome

This condition arises following parotid or rarely temporomandibular joint surgery or trauma. Occasionally it may arise spontaneously in cases of diabetic neuropathy or following cervical sympathectomy.

The patient may complain of a burning sensation in the temporal or facial region associated with flushing and profuse sweating on eating. Occasionally there is persistent hyperalgesia between attacks. Cases have also been reported provoked by certain foods, including cheese.

The syndrome is attributed to parasympathetic secretomotor fibre reinnervation of the cut ends of sympathetic vaso and sudomotor nerves. However, recovery in the post-surgical group and spontaneous onset in those cases that arise following diabetic neuropathy suggest that the cause may be a lack of inhibitory sympathetic tone. In some cases, the symptoms appear to remit spontaneously after one or two years, although paradoxically many cases also arise suddenly a long interval after surgery.

Conservative therapy with parasympathomimetic blockade using poldine methyl sulphate 2–4 mg 3 times a day has varying degrees of success but may produce an uncomfortable dry mouth and constipation. Nerve avulsion including the auricular temporal nerve or intracranial section of Jacobsen's nerve is usually unhelpful. The topical application of an anticholinergic such as 2 per cent glycopyrrolate or hyoscine cream may produce relief lasting up to 48 hours, and therefore can be repeated on a daily basis.

Herpes Zoster

The pain in this condition invariably precedes the vesicular eruption which may affect any peripheral nerve. However, in the head and neck region, the ophthalmic division is commonly involved. The infection is thought to arise due to activation of the varicella virus resident in the nerve ganglia, which can occur at any age but is more common in the elderly and following some debilitating disease, radiotherapy or steroid therapy. Where the virus has also involved the geniculate ganglion the patient will have a facial palsy, the so called Ramsay Hunt syndrome. Unfortunately, if the pain is initially localized to a tooth, this may be extracted unnecessarily.

The vesicular eruption is best treated with the topical application of 0·1 per cent aqueous idoxuridine to oral mucosal lesions and a 5 per cent suspension of idoxuridine in dimethylsulphoxide to the cutaneous lesions. This must be done four times a day for four days, but needs to be applied early in the course of the eruption to be beneficial. Acyclovir, which can be given as tablets systemically as well as applied topically to the lesions, may prove to be more effective.

Post-herpetic Neuralgia

This unfortunate complication may arise following untreated herpes zoster and presents as a persistent burning pain in an area of diminished sensation, hence the term 'anaesthesia dolorosa'. It is attributed to the destruction of the large myelinated sensory fibres by the zoster virus which abolishes their modulating inhibitory effect at the posterior horn substantia gelatinosa gate mechanism. The pain usually diminishes in six months to two years.

Treatment consists of analgesics such as ibuprofen 400 mg, 4–6-hourly, which may be supplemented with a tricyclic antidepressant drug such as nortriptyline 10–100 mg. Occasionally, stronger analgesics such as pentazocine will be necessary. Entonox, 50 per cent oxygen and nitrous oxide, is useful during the acute attacks. The condition is not amenable to nerve block, cryotherapy or surgery.

Nasopharyngeal Carcinoma (Trotter's Syndrome)

Nasopharyngeal carcinoma is more common in South-East Asia, affecting principally the Chinese, but it also appears to be a common lesion in Alaskan Eskimos. It may arise in young people and is thought to be related to the oncogenic Epstein–Barr virus.

The classical lesion arises in the fossa of Rosenmüller behind the opening of the eustachian tube and obstructs its aperture producing conductive deafness. As the tumour infiltrates laterally, the mandibular and maxillary divisions of the trigeminal nerve are involved giving rise to a combination of facial pain, cutaneous analgesia and wasting of the masseter muscle. Direct invasion of the soft palate and the medial pterygoid muscle produces ipsilateral elevation of the uvula, dysphagia and trismus. Extension towards the base of the skull will eventually involve other cranial nerves.

The lesion may be detected by mirror inspection of the nasopharynx, particularly under anaesthesia, and by lateral pharyngeal soft tissue radiographs, but computerized tomography provides the best means of visualization.

Treatment is by radiotherapy and cytotoxic drugs.

Cranial Base Lesions

Petrous Temporal Osteitis (Gradenigo's Syndrome)

Very rarely, infection of the middle ear may spread through the petrous temporal bone so that the osteitis reaches the meninges and involves cranial nerves such as the abducen nerve and trigeminal ganglion. This produces a lateral rectus palsy and facial pain usually with cutaneous analgesia. This rare presentation is usually an extension of the so-called malignant otitis externa in which an ischaemic necrosis arises in cases of diabetic vasculopathy.

Treatment consists of careful debridement of the infected bone, a course of metronidazole and vascularization of the dead space with a temporalis muscle flap.

Cholesteatoma

A cholesteatoma may present with chronic facial pain and hypoaesthesia. This is a slow growing lesion within the petrous temporal bone. The diagnosis is made by computerized tomography, and the treatment is surgical removal.

Other Cranial Base Lesions

Other cranial base lesions involving the cranial nerves include fractures, paragangliomas nasopharyngeal tumours extending upwards, intracranial lesions extending downwards and metastatic lesions from remote areas. Rarely, Paget's disease may lead to platybasia, compressing nerves in their foramina. However, these conditions usually give rise to important physical signs in other parts of the body.

Intracranial Lesions

Tumours of the Posterior Cranial Fossa

The classical example is the schwannoma (acoustic neurinoma) arising on the VIII cranial nerve in the cerebellopontine angle. The trigeminal, facial and vestibulo-acoustic cranial nerves are enclosed in the narrow triangular space between the pons, cerebellum and medial surface of the petrous bone. Thus the enlarging neuroma produces trigeminal pain and sensory loss, deafness and ataxia. These together with nystagmus and a reduced corneal reflex may be observed clinically. Further investigations should include radiography of the internal auditory canal and computerized tomography (CT). Although this is a benign lesion, early removal is essential to reduce operative and postoperative complications.

Middle Cranial Fossa Lesions

These include pituitary tumours and aneurysms of the internal carotid artery. The latter enlarges within the cavernous sinus. Both ultimately exert pressure on the optic chiasma and the nerves contained in the cavernous sinus which include the ophthalmic division of the V and the III, IV and VI cranial nerves. Thus tumours in this region produce facial pain, cutaneous analgesia together with disturbances in vision and in extra-ocular movements. Investigations will include plain skull radiographs, angiography and a CT scan.

Multiple Sclerosis (Disseminated Sclerosis)

This condition can occasionally present as a tic douloureux which is indistinguishable from the idiopathic form. However, most cases have accompanying neurological disturbances, such as loss of taste, disturbance in facial sensation and neurological deficits of a sensory, reflex or motor character elsewhere. These symptoms may remit or change, giving rise to the characteristic dissemination in time and space, that is the pathological features come and go in varied anatomical sites.

The condition should be suspected when a paroxysmal neuralgia occurs in a young person. However, there may be a latency of many years before the spread of the demyelinating disease becomes apparent.

The treatment is as described for the primary neuralgia. In the absence of specific treatment for multiple sclerosis, a failure to make the diagnosis during the patient's first presentation is not detrimental and does not affect the prognosis.

VASCULAR PAINS

Migraine

This is a recurrent unilateral throbbing headache associated with visual disturbances, nausea and ataxia. The pain is intensified by sneezing, coughing and movements of the head. It appears to be due to painful pulsatile extracranial vasodilatation associated with intracranial vasoconstriction. There are a multitude of precipitating factors which include hormonal and emotional disturbances, hypoglycaemia, alcohol and foods containing vasoactive amines such as cheese (tyramine) and chocolate (beta-phenylethylamine). Migraine may also be associated with tension headaches, facial arthromyalgia and atypical facial neuralgia.

Many patients achieve relief with simple analgesics which include aspirin 600–1200 mg, paracetamol 0·5–1·0 g, and mefenamic acid 500 mg. A continuous course of a sedative tricyclic antidepressant such as fluphenazine

0·5 mg with nortriptyline 10 mg (Motival, Squibb) can be highly effective in preventing frequent attacks.

The vasoconstrictor ergotamine tartrate is widely used, either 2 mg sublingually, 0·36–0·72 mg by inhaler or 0·25 mg intramuscularly or subcutaneously. However, ergot preparations have to be given as early as possible in the attack for satisfactory relief, and can add to the malaise and nausea of the attack if repeated too frequently. The drug should be avoided in pregnancy and in patients with vascular disease, for whom simple analgesics and prochlorperazine 5 mg are recommended.

Pizotifen is an antihistamine and anti-serotonergic drug related to the tricylics and may also be used prophylactically. Dose is 0·5–3 mg nocte, increased slowly to avoid drowsiness and anticholinergic effects.

Facial Migrainous Neuralgia (Also known as Horten's Syndrome, Sluder's Syndrome, Cluster Headaches, Histamine Cephalgia, Spenopalatine Neuralgia, Vidian Nerve Neuralgia, Alarm Clock Headache, etc.)

The many names for this condition reflect the problems associated with its diagnosis and treatment. As with other types of migraine, the pain is attributed to spastic dilatation of blood vessels, which in this condition are the maxillary branches of the external carotid artery. It affects principally men and classically occurs at night, waking the patient in the early hours, hence the name 'alarm clock headache'. It is an intense, throbbing pain, usually lasting about half an hour, and the patient may notice that his eye is red and his nose feels congested on that side. The attacks occur at regular intervals and are sometimes repeated as a series over a week or more before they subside. Occasionally alcohol or coffee are precipitating factors.

The attacks may be prevented with ergotamine suppositories used nightly before going to sleep until a phase of remission occurs. As with simple migraine tricyclic antidepressant drugs are a valuable prophylactic.

However, there appears to be a strong clinical association between facial arthromyalgia, migraine, facial migrainous neuralgia and atypical facial neuralgia, suggesting that they all represent related vascular pain mechanisms. Thus when conventional migraine therapy has been ineffective or where there is a history of anxiety or depression the therapeutic regime for atypical facial neuralgia is often successful.

Giant-cell Arteritis (Temporal Arteritis)

Arteritis of the superficial temporal artery presents as a headache or local pain. However, the condition can affect other branches of the external carotid with varying sites of pain. When the maxillary artery is involved, the pain may present as intermittent claudication in the masticatory muscles on chewing. If the lingual artery is involved ulceration and necrosis of the tongue can occur. The great danger is involvement of the ophthalmic artery with retinal infarction and blindness.

Occasionally the arteritis is associated with polymyalgia rheumatica in which the patient complains of widespread stiffness and joint pain. The patient is usually elderly, and may also suffer from diabetes mellitus. The erythrocyte sedimentation rate may be high and rheumatoid serological tests positive.

If a superficial artery, such as the superficial temporal or facial, is accessible for biopsy, the diagnosis may be confirmed by histology.

Where the condition is suspected, systemic steroids beginning with prednisone 60 mg or dexamethasone 10 mg a day should be commenced immediately to prevent blindness. The doses will be maintained for ten days and then reduced until the condition is under control.

SUGGESTED READING

Blau J. N. (1982) How to take a history of head or facial pain. *Br. Med. J.* **285**, 1249–1251.

Fienmann C., Harris M. and Cowley R. (1984) Psychogenic facial pain, presentation and treatment. *Br. Med. J.* **288**, 436–438.

Fisher F. J. (1982) Toothache and the cracked cusp. *Br. Dent. J.* **153**, 298–300.

Griffiths R. H. (1983) Report of the President's Conference on the examination, diagnosis and management of temporomandibular disorders. *J. Am. Dent. Assoc.* **106**, 775–777.

Guralnick W. (1984) The temporomandibular joint. *Br. Dent. J.* **156**, 353–355.

Rosen H. (1982) Cracked tooth syndrome. *J. Prosthet. Dent.* **47**, 36–43.

Seldin E. B. (1983) The emperor's new meniscus. *J. Am. Dent. Assoc.* **106**, 615–616.

Speculand B., Hughes A. D. and Goss A. N. (1984) Role of recent stressful life events experience in the onset of TMJ dysfunction pain. *Community Dent. Oral Epidemiol.* **12**, 197–202.

Sutton R. B. O. (1982) The problem of obscure facial pain. *Dent. Update* **9**, 159–164.

CHAPTER 14

DRUGS AND ORAL SURGERY

When a patient attends the practice for the first time the dentist will usually take a full history, recording the details in the patient's records. Such details as:

    a. The present state of the patient's general health;
    b. Past illnesses and accidents;
    c. Current and, where appropriate, past medication, particularly therapeutic drugs received during the past twelve months; and
    d. Allergies to drugs, dressings and other substances,

will all be included. Some of these factors may modify the patient's dental management and will be discussed in this chapter. Where the patient is allergic to certain drugs or dressings or is taking drugs which are likely to interact with those the dentist may administer or prescribe, or suffers from a chronic disease relevant to the conduct of dental treatment, the fact should be noted in a special, prominent location at the front of the notes or record card.

Not infrequently patients do not know the names of drugs which they have obtained from their medical practitioner. They may also claim allergy when in fact the untoward reaction was either a manifestation of the actual illness or an idiosyncrasy, i.e. the drug's normal side-effects occurring at a much lower dose than usual, or even a placebo reaction. Placebo responses are those endogenous changes stimulated by the act of taking a drug, by the clinician's attitude and management, and by the environment. This response may be positive—as will be discussed in pain control—or even negative. A patient experiencing side-effects such as drowsiness and dizziness when unknowingly given an inert tablet is a form of placebo response. It is because of these complex and often unpredictable reactions that the therapeutic value of any drug treatment can only be established by a controlled trial.

Before each new course of treatment enquiries should be made about any change in the state of the patient's health, current medication, or any new allergies, and fresh entries made on the front of the records if appropriate. If during the course of treatment drugs are to be prescribed a further brief question about allergies is an additional safeguard.

There will be a basic range of drugs which the practitioner will use frequently and with which he or she will be thoroughly familiar. In the case of all other drugs it is worthwhile referring to a formulary to check dosage, the size of tablets or the concentration of solutions, etc., available from the pharmacist, and the usual total quantities prescribed. Formularies, like the *British National Formulary* and the *ABPI Data Sheet* compendium will also have a paragraph about special precautions, drug interactions and side-effects under each entry.

PAIN CONTROL

This important area provides the best examples of the complexity of drug usage (*see* review by Seymour and Walton 1982). For instance, the placebo response in pain control, which explains the great variations in pain response to surgery, appears to be dependent on the release of endogenous analgesic substances in the central nervous system. These so called endogenous opioids include the enkephalins and endorphin. This system provides an important protection against pain and, although readily activated in acute situations such as war and sports injuries, clinically it can only be stimulated by careful patient control. Therefore a basic formula for pain control is a combination of confident and reassuring management enhanced by the use of sedation and a rational use of analgesics.

If pain does not respond to analgesia ensure that:

a. The patient is receiving an adequate dose at appropriate intervals. For example, for optimum analgesia opiate analgesics should be used in moderate amounts at short intervals or on demand, whereas aspirin needs to be prescribed in large doses at less frequent intervals.

b. The underlying disease has been appropriately dealt with, i.e. pus has been drained, infected roots removed, all fractures detected and immobilized, and exposed soft or hard tissues dressed.

c. The pain is not psychogenic in origin. Psychogenic pain will not respond well to analgesics and requires antidepressant drug therapy, e.g. dothiepin hydrochloride (Prothiaden) 25–150 mg nocte. Tricyclic antidepressant drugs also appear to have a centrally acting analgesic effect which potentiates simple analgesics and opiates.

d. The pain is not a paroxysmal neuralgia such as trigeminal neuralgia which responds only to an anticonvulsant type of drug such as carbamazepine (Tegretol) 100–200 mg 3 or 4 times a day.

Non-steroidal Anti-inflammatory Analgesics

This group of drugs which includes aspirin act by the inhibition of prostaglandin synthesis in damaged and inflamed tissues. The prostaglandins amplify the local effects of pain mediators. Therefore analgesics should be used where possible prophylactically, commencing therapy before the onset of anticipated pain and continuing it at regular intervals to prevent pain becoming established. Simple analgesics used in this way are highly effective following most surgical procedures and only cease to be useful when too little is taken too late.

Aspirin (Acetylsalicylic Acid)

Aspirin remains the most important analgesic and possesses antipyretic and anti-inflammatory effects.

PREPARATIONS AND DOSAGE

The optimum analgesic dose is 600–900 mg aspirin for an adult, every 4–6 hours if necessary. It may be prescribed as soluble tablets or enteric coated tablets each of 300 mg, or as aspirin 400 mg and codeine phosphate 8 mg which is available as soluble tablets and taken dissolved in water up to 4 hourly if necessary.

Because there is evidence that aspirin may be a contributory factor in the causation of Reye's syndrome (an acute encephalopathy with fatty changes in the liver following a viral infection) aspirin should *not* be given to children under the age of 12 years. (Committee on Safety of Medicines, letter MF 490/140 dated 10 June 1986.)

Adverse reactions include nausea, abdominal discomfort or gastric erosion and bleeding, and therefore the drug must be avoided in any patient who has peptic ulceration. All anti-inflammatory analgesics are best taken after meals. Allergy may produce asthma, angioedema, urticaria and rashes. By inhibiting platelet thromboxane synthesis aspirin can interfere with platelet aggregation and produce haemorrhage and is therefore contraindicated in any patient with a bleeding disorder or on anticoagulants. Also its protein-binding effect displaces inactive albumin-bound anticoagulant, therefore amplifying the anticoagulant effect. Tinnitus is not uncommon with the continuous use of high doses. Aspirin should be avoided in patients with renal damage, which may be increased by the drug, especially if excretion is impaired.

Tablets containing mixtures of aspirin, paracetamol and codeine probably offer more analgesic effect with reduced individual side-effects, e.g. aspirin and codeine or aspirin, paracetamol and codeine. Where a codeine-containing preparation is used, constipation may be produced.

Paracetamol

Taken 500 mg–1 g, 4–6-hourly, paracetamol is probably less potent an analgesic than aspirin with less anti-inflammatory effect, and where inflammation is the underlying cause of pain, aspirin may be preferable. Severe liver damage may result from taking 10 g (20 tablets) at once. However, the drug is useful in patients with peptic ulceration or bleeding disorders and is suitable for infants.

Paracetamol is also available in combination forms, paracetamol 325 mg and dextropropoxyphene 32·5 mg (a soluble preparation is available), or paracetamol 500 mg with codeine phosphate 8 mg, 2 tablets 3 or 4 times a day. In both cases the adult maximum dose of 8 tablets in 24 hours must not be exceeded.

DRUGS AND ORAL SURGERY

Propionic Acid Derivatives

This large group of drugs are analgesic with mild to moderate anti-inflammatory reactions but with less adverse effects than aspirin, hence they are used where chronic medication is required such as musculoskeletal disorders as well as for short-term pain control.

Mefenamic Acid

Taken 500 mg t.d.s. after meals, mefenamic acid may produce diarrhoea and rarely haemolytic anaemia but gut blood loss is low. The drug will increase anticoagulant effects.

Ibuprofen

Taken 200–400 mg, 6-hourly, ibuprofen does not appear to displace and potentiate anticoagulants. Available as a suspension 100 mg/5 ml.

Narcotic Analgesics

This group, sometimes termed major analgesics, are centrally acting and in most cases produce dependency when used for prolonged periods of time. However, for short-term management of surgical patients this is no disadvantage compared with their important analgesic effect. A more immediate problem is their emetic effect and it is therefore advisable to combine the analgesic with an anti-emetic such as perfenazinel 4 mg by mouth or 5 mg by injection, or metoclopromide 10 mg i.m. or i.v.

Codeine (Methyl Morphine)

Codeine may be injected as the phosphate 30 mg up to 4-hourly, to a maximum of 200 mg in 24 hours. Although not as potent as morphine, it is a useful mild postoperative analgesic in cases where head injury or surgery may predispose to a latent intracranial bleed as it does not interfere with pupillary reflexes and produce meiosis.

Pethidine

Dosage is orally 50–100 mg, intramuscularly 25–100 mg, intravenously 25–50 mg, lasting 3–4 hours. Pethidine is more potent than codeine but less so than morphine. It also has a shorter effective analgesic duration but little hypnotic effect. The pupils are not constricted and it does not tend to cause constipation. However, it may cause vomiting and has an atropine-like effect producing dry mouth.

Pentazocine

Adult doses are orally 25–100 mg, 3–4-hourly after food, i.m. or i.v. 30–60 mg, every 3–4 hours. It is a potent analgesic when injected but less so when taken by mouth, with a lower tendency than other narcotics for producing dependency. In addition to the common adverse effects of nausea, vomiting, dizziness and sweating, it may produce hallucinations or unpleasant dreams in some patients. Despite this, the drug has considerable value in the management of benign, intractable facial pain with apparently minimum side effects, for which up to 500 mg a day may be required in divided doses.

Morphine

Dosage of 10–20 mg subcutaneously, intramuscularly or intravenously produces potent analgesia and euphoria and is valuable in the control of severe pain. However, in addition to its depression of the cough reflex, it depresses respiration, stimulates vomiting, produces miosis, bronchospasm especially in the asthmatic, and spasm of the gut muscle. An important postoperative effect of morphine may be delayed micturition due to spasm of the bladder sphincter. In some patients this may lead to severe urinary retention requiring catheterization.

Papaveretum (Omnopon)

This is a reconstituted mixture of purified opium alkaloids which probably does not differ substantially from the effects of morphine.

Buprenorphine (Temgesic)

Dosage is 0·3–0·6 mg intramuscularly or by slow infusion intravenously, 6-or 8-hourly. It can also be taken sublingually 0·2–0·4 mg 6–8-hourly. This is a new potent synthetic analgesic with rapid onset and prolonged duration and little disturbance of respiration, cardiovascular function and minimal dependency. However, in all other respects it resembles the opiates and may have a potent emetic effect with some patients.

Remember that prolonged opioid analgesia after major surgery, especially where the patient is confined to bed, may produce constipation leading to faecal impaction and inflamed haemorrhoids. This may be avoided by giving liquid paraffin and magnesium hydroxide mixture in small doses or dioctyl sodium sulphosuccinate starting 24 hours before the operation. For established constipation give a suitable laxative such as bisacodyl (Dulcolax) given orally 5–10 mg or as a suppository in the morning.

Special Analgesic Considerations

Diamorphine (Heroin)

This is a potent opiate producing a high degree of dependency and is therefore reserved for terminal cancer patients. Its value is analgesia and euphoria when administered by mouth, commencing at 5–10 mg as heroin hydrochloride in various mixtures, e.g. Brompton or Saunders mixtures, and is used for comforting the dying. In these cases the analgesic should be given frequently and adjusted to the patient's needs, e.g. 3–4 hourly, preventing rather than suppressing pain. The addition of a tranquillizer or antidepressant and anti-emetic is preferred to cocaine as in the traditional mixtures and helps with the control of the emotional aspects of pain.

The dying require a sense of security and companionship which may best be provided at home but when necessary the essential symptomatic treatment and medical nursing will have to be arranged in an appropriate hospice. It is important also to remember that relatives also require support and even antidepressant therapy.

Fentanyl

This is a synthetic opiate which is more potent but shorter acting than morphine. It is used as an adjuvant agent intravenously or together with droperiodol, a major tranquillizer, for so called neuroleptanalgesia. This combination enables the patient to be sedated and analgesed rapidly but remain cooperative. However, respiratory depression readily occurs and administration should be slow and well controlled with spontaneous respiration.

Dosage is 50–200 μg then 50 μg every 20–30 minutes as required; children 3–μg/kg. With assisted respiration doses of up to 600 μg may be given to adults and 10–15 μg/kg to children.

Phenoperidine

This an alternative choice to fentanyl. Adult dose is 0·5–5 mg i.v.

PREMEDICATION AND SEDATION

Premedication is intended to produce sedation, amnesia and analgesia and, where appropriate, inhibition of parasympathetic activity, such as reduced salivation, bronchial secretion and vagal inhibition. In an anxious patient sedation may be required days before the procedure. In ambulant patients diazepam 2–5 mg nocte with a further dose an hour before entering hospital for out-patient surgery is very useful. Children may be given 2 mg as a small pill or syrup, or alternatively trimeprazine forte syrup 1–2 mg per kilogram body weight.

Diazepam used as intravenous sedation has proved to be both safe and effective. Slow intravenous administration of up to 10 mg is adequate for most patients. The use of higher doses such as 2 mg per stone body weight produces the onset of ptosis, the Verril sign, and is often close to a hypnotic level with loss of patient control. As diazepam is slowly excreted, even though the patient is conscious and appears co-operative, he or she should always be accompanied home. A common problem is thrombophlebitis at the site of the injection which may now be avoided by using a diazepam emulsion (Diazemuls—Kabi Vitrum).

Like diazepam, midazolam (Hypnovel-Roche) can be used to produce sedation for the ambulant patient by intravenous injection. It has the advantage that it is water soluble and hence less likely to cause thrombophlebitis. Both the onset of sedation and initial recovery are rapid, but like diazepam residual effects may last for 8 or more hours and patients should not drive cars or handle machinery until the next day. It is supplied in 5 ml ampoules, each containing 10 mg midazolam; 1·75 ml of the solution containing 3·5 m of midazolam is given initially, then after a pause of 2 minutes further increments of 0·25 ml (0·5 mg) can be given with appropriate pauses to assess if sedation has been achieved. Adult dose is usually between 2·5 mg and 7·5 mg.

The control of secretions and the prevention of vasovagal effects are achieved with atropine 6 mg or hyoscine 4 mg subcutaneously or intravenously one hour before the operation. Promethazine hydrochloride (Phenergan) 25 mg is also used because of its sedative anti-emetic and atropine like qualities.

The inhalation of 30 per cent to 50 per cent nitrous oxide with oxygen, the proportion of nitrous oxide carefully graduated to need, is also useful as a sedative-analgesic.

POSTOPERATIVE MEDICATION

As stated, postoperative analgesics such as pethidine or morphine should be given in adequate doses at frequent intervals if pain demands it. The combined emetic effect of the anaesthetic, the accumulation of blood and gastric secretions within the stomach, as well as the action of opiate analgesics, can be controlled by anti-emetics such as metoclopramide (Maxolon) 10 mg i.m. or perphenazine (Fentazin) 10 mg. Both drugs may produce extrapyramidal symptoms such as distonia with facial spasm or torticollis, although the adverse effect occurs in only about 1 per cent of cases. In high dosage tardive dyskinesia may occur.

NIGHT SEDATION

The following drugs help the many patients who have difficulty in sleeping in hospital, especially the night before an operation.

Dichloralphenazone (Weldorm—S & N Pharm.)

Available in 650 mg tablets the dose is 2–3 tablets taken with water nocte. Also available as a syrup 225 mg in 5 ml which should be taken well diluted with water.

Nitrazepam

Dosage is 5–10 mg and may produce hangover with drowsiness during the following day.

DRUGS AND ORAL SURGERY

Chlormethiazole Edisylate (Heminevrin—Astra)
Available in 192 mg capsules, the dose is 2 capsules nocte. This drug produces less hangover and is less cumulative than nitrazepam.

DIABETES MELLITUS

The principal problem of the diabetic is control of the carbohydrate metabolism, but a sufferer is also at risk because of vascular disease affecting the heart, kidneys and lower limbs, and neuropathies which may impair cardiorespiratory reflexes. Hence, apart from minor procedures, the diabetic patient requires preoperative medical assessment.

Overweight, middle aged and elderly diabetics are normally treated by diet alone in the first instance. Oral hypoglycaemic agents may be prescribed if control is not established, despite adequate weight loss and an appropriate dietary regime. Children and young adults and underweight diabetics usually need injections of insulin to achieve control and permit normal development.

Hypoglycaemic coma develops if the normal dose of hypoglycaemic agent is taken, but a meal is missed. Sometimes hypoglycaemia follows the rapid absorption of an injection of insulin, an error in the dose administered by the patient or substantial unexpected exercise. Most patients recognize the premonitary symptoms and will have learnt to take some sugar. These symptoms may be mistaken by an observer for apprehension or even the effects of alcohol. Once unconscious the patient will be cold and wet with perspiration. Initially the hypoglycaemia could be easily confused with a faint, but the patient does not respond rapidly to being put flat. The hypoglycaemic state should not be allowed to persist in case permanent brain damage results. When the premonitory symptoms are experienced or observed 3–4 lumps of sugar dissolved in a squash drink can be given by mouth. Once consciousness has been lost up to 50 ml of 50 per cent glucose for injection is given intravenously. It should be given slowly into a large vein.

The patient will usually recover consciousness during the injection. Sterile saline 5–10 ml for injection should be given through the same needle to prevent the concentrated sugar damaging the vein wall and causing thrombosis. Where venepuncture proves difficult an injection of glucagon can be given and can be particularly useful in children, 0·5–1 unit (0·5–1 mg) being given by the intravenous, intramuscular or subcutaneous route.

Glucagon is normally produced by the cells of the islets of Langerhans and mobilizes liver glycogen, raising the plasma glucose level. Either a 5 per cent dextrose intravenous infusion should be started or sugar should be given orally as soon as the patient recovers consciousness until a stable blood sugar is achieved. Blood sugar levels can be determined by doing a

Dextrostrip blood sugar on a capillary blood sample and reading it with an Ames Glucometer. Diabetic patients who have been unable to eat normally because of a painful and tender tooth are at risk of hypoglycaemia if they have taken their normal insulin. So also are those who arrive as an emergency expecting a general anaesthetic and who have starved themselves in anticipation.

Minor surgical procedures under local anaesthesia should not interfere with meal times and require no change in the patient's insulin or drug regime. It is important to confirm that diabetic patients have had sufficient food with their insulin and if not to provide a glucose drink before commencing surgery. It is also important to stress that normal food or the equivalent in replacement carbohydrate should be taken postoperatively, later in the day.

Diabetic coma comes on gradually and insidiously and will not present as a sudden emergency. However, infection increases the requirement for insulin and a patient with an acute dental infection may be out of control with incipient ketosis. Patients admitted as a casualty or trauma case may also present with this complication. There is an obvious risk to administering a general anaesthetic in such a situation. In general dental practice if it is suspected that the patient is hyperglycaemic or ketotic the general medical practitioner should be contacted urgently, or failing this the patient taken to the casualty department of the local hospital.

For all routine dental treatment (except when a general anaesthetic or a substantial period of sedation is involved) diabetic patients can be treated in the same way as other patients. They should of course conform to their normal dietary habits and treatment regime. An injection of a local anaesthetic solution containing adrenaline may result in the transient release of glucose from liver glycogen into the blood stream, but as this does not lead to ketosis, it is of no importance.

Diabetics are more prone to infection than other patients so that any infections should be treated vigorously and special care taken to avoid postoperative infection.

There are two problems associated with the administration of general anaesthetics to diabetics. The obvious one is the problem of maintaining control of the diabetes when, as a result of the surgery, the demand for insulin may vary, and of course, the supply of sufficient carbohydrate to avoid hypoglycaemia. Hypoglycaemia is a particular hazard in the already unconscious patient where pallor and sweating may be the only clinical indication of its onset. The other problem relates to the proneness of diabetics to cardiovascular disease and special attention should be given to the patient's status in this respect.

Procedures under General Anaesthesia

For short anaesthetics on an out-patient basis patients on oral hypolycaemic agents simply omit the drug on the morning of the operation. Patients on insulin may do likewise, subsequently injecting a suitable proportion of the daily requirement as soon as they are able to eat after the anaesthetic. Alternatively, where just a single extraction is required the patient may have the normal insulin and breakfast, then receive the anaesthetic a short period before the next meal is due. The calorie equivalent of the next meal must be consumed as soon as possible after recovery from the anaesthetic.

As a general rule diabetic in-patients are better admitted to hospital at least 24 hours prior to the anaesthetic, and put on a routine 3-hourly diabetic observation chart which includes fasting and postprandial blood sugars. With unstable diabetics admission 2–3 days prior to surgery is essential to put the patient on a soluble insulin regime 3 times a day, and stabilize their blood and urinary sugar.

Where possible diabetics should be operated on in the morning, and a fasting blood sugar (a venous blood laboratory test if possible) should be done in the ward preoperatively.

Preoperative Management

All patients are starved overnight. No hypoglycaemic agents are given on the morning of the operation and a fasting blood sugar done. If the blood glucose level is more than 5 mmol/l the premedication is given and the patient sent to the operating theatre.

If the blood sugar is less than 5 mmol/l an intravenous infusion of 5 per cent dextrose is started before the premedication is given.

Intraoperative

In the operating theatre all insulin-dependent diabetics have an intravenous drip of 5 per cent dextrose.

During the operation the blood glucose level is monitored every hour using the glucometer and insulin or glucose given as necessary. If the blood sugar is more than 10 mmol/l, 10 units of a rapidly acting neutral insulin such as Actrapid insulin is given i.v., and if less than 3 mmol/l, 50 ml of 50 per cent dextrose is given i.v. It is advisable to maintain the blood sugar around 8–10 mmol/l during the operative and postoperative periods.

When close monitoring of the patient is possible before, during and after the operation an intravenous infusion of soluble insulin may be given at a rate of 1 to 2 units per hour and balanced by 5 per cent glucose and 4 per cent glucose–saline infusions. Potassium supplements may be needed. The amounts of insulin given are monitored by frequent blood sugar estimations.

Postoperative

It is essential to avoid hypoglycaemia during this period and therefore insulin is avoided until the blood sugar level is above 10–12 mmol/l. It would be prudent to maintain an intravenous drip of 5 per cent dextrose for 24 hours after the operation in all labile and insulin dependent diabetics.

During this period the blood sugar is checked 3-hourly, and a regime of soluble insulin, 2 units per mmol blood sugar, is continued 6-hourly until the patient is fit enough for his normal regime, and can be fed by mouth.

For afternoon surgery a light breakfast may be given and treatment is then as before.

Operative stress and infection in diabetics will increase their insulin requirements hence antibiotic cover to eliminate and prevent infection is essential.

All confused and unconscious patients admitted with maxillofacial injuries should have a urinalysis for glucose and ketones and a blood sugar estimation. Rarely a hyperglycaemic state may predispose to an accident and may be confused with excess alcohol consumption. Blood should then be taken for an accurate estimation of glucose, electrolytes and pH and the patient is rapidly rehydrated with saline. Insulin should be given 20 units intramuscularly immediately and then 6 units/hour as an intravenous infusion. Potassium loss requires correction in these patients and medical advice should be sought.

Where emergency surgery is necessary the blood sugar should be maintained between 8·5 and 10 mmol/l (150–180 mg/100 ml).

CORTICOSTEROIDS

Following an injury, either accidental or planned in the form of surgery, a serious infection, or during a general anaesthetic, the adrenals are stimulated by ACTH to secrete a greatly increased amount of the adrenal glucocorticoids, cortisone and hydrocortisone (cortisol). Failure of this response results in a fall in blood pressure and blood volume. There are two circumstances in which this may occur: on the one hand where there is damage to the hypothalamus or a lack of functioning adrenal or pituitary tissue, and on the other where secretion has been suppressed as a result of the therapeutic administration of corticosteroids.

The adrenals may be destroyed as a result of a vascular catastrophy, by an autoimmune mechanism as is often the case in Addison's disease, or by diseases such as tuberculosis or amyloidosis. Therapeutic bilateral adrenalectomy is an important cause and hypophysectomy has a similar effect by removing the stimulation of the adrenal cortex by ACTH. Diseases involving the hypothalamus or anterior pituitary also interfere with the hypothalamic–pituitary–adrenal axis. Aminoglutethimide is given to post-menopausal women with metastatic carcinoma of the breast because of its ability to inhibit the conversion of androgens to oestrogens in the peripheral tissues. However, it also inhibits adrenal steroid production.

In all these circumstances the patients will be receiving maintenance doses of corticosteroids, and following an accident, or surgery, or a severe infection with toxicity, additional corticosteroids will be needed to simulate the normal response to such stress-producing experiences. A suitable regime for such patients is 100 mg of hydrocortisone sodium succinate given intravenously 6-hourly, starting 1 hour preoperatively, and with the amount halved daily until the normal oral maintenance dose is once more achieved. Although the doses involved are large they are given for short periods of time only and consequently the anti-inflammatory and immunosuppressive activity of the steroids can be ignored.

Where major surgery has been undertaken involving many hours under a general anaesthetic it may be necessary to maintain the administration of 100 mg hydrocortisone sodium succinate 6-hourly, at first intravenously and then intramuscularly, for up to 72 hours from the time of premedication. This high dose again given i.m. will be maintained even longer if complications like serious infections supervene, particularly if the patient is unable to take or retain oral preparations.

For routine oral surgery procedures lasting, say, up to two hours under a general anaesthetic 100 mg hydrocortisone sodium succinate given 8-hourly intramuscularly starting with the premedication and then for the first 24 hours is likely to be sufficient. The normal oral maintenance dose is continued thereafter.

For minor surgical procedures under a local anaesthetic as an out-patient a single dose of 100 mg hydrocortisone sodium succinate intramuscularly given 1 hour preoperatively is usually adequate, or alternatively twice the normal oral dose for 36 hours followed of course by the normal oral maintenance dose.

All operative procedures for these patients are best scheduled for first thing in the morning so that the initial postoperative observations are made while the full day staff are still on duty. The blood pressure should be measured every 15 minutes during the initial postoperative period, until the patient's condition is considered stable, then hourly up to 12 hours in the case of routine cases and 2–3-hourly for the remainder of the period when the maximum dose is judged appropriate for major cases. (However, a balance must always be achieved between adequate, safe levels of observation, the consequent disturbance of the patient's much needed rest and the demands made upon nursing and resident staff.)

Patients who have had exodontia or minor oral surgery under local anaesthesia as out-patients should be kept under observation for several hours before they return home. They and their relatives should be warned to report promptly to a practitioner in the event of any nausea, vomiting, feeling of faintness, etc.

The other group of patients at risk in this category are those with partial or complete suppression of adrenal cortical activity as a result of the therapeutic administration of steroids. The drugs are given for their ability to suppress the manifestations of various inflammatory and hypersensitivity reactions. If circulating concentrations of glucocorticoids at or above physiological levels are achieved corticotrophin releasing factor is not produced by the hypothalamus to stimulate secretion of ACTH by the anterior pituitary. As a result either partial or complete atrophy of the adrenal cortex occurs. Where relatively small doses are involved atrophy can be minimized by giving them on alternate days and to coincide with the early morning circadian peak of normal steroid secretion.

Supplementary hydrocortisone sodium succinate should be given whenever a therapeutic regime has been continued for a week or longer. Mostly topically applied preparations and inhaled aerosol spray do not result in a sufficient systemic effect to warrant supplementation. However, high doses of aerosol spray and potent preparations applied topically under occlusive dressings may produce a negative feedback effect on the pituitary. Where substantial doses are involved similar regimes to those given above are required. Where small doses are involved and only partial atrophy is likely a single intramuscular dose of 50–100 mg of hydrocortisone sodium succinate for out-patients, and a similar dose 8-hourly for 24 hours for in-patients, should be sufficient.

It must be remembered in such cases that the manifestations of the underlying disease are merely suppressed by the steroids not cured, and potential complications of the disease itself in the face of surgery should be given due weight.

Withdrawal of the steroid is usually effected once spontaneous remission of the underlying disease seems likely. This is done in stages over a substantial period of time. Even so it takes months for full recovery of the adrenal cortex to occur. A single dose of 100 mg of hydrocortisone sodium succinate should be given within 6 months of a prolonged course of treatment or 3 months of a short course.

Postoperative patients who suffer an unexplained, rapid fall in blood pressure should be treated with a further intravenous injection of hydrocortisone sodium succinate as a matter of urgency. However, once this has been done other causes of shock such as a cardiac infarct, concealed haemorrhage, or a septicaemic infection should be excluded. Indeed serious infections may occur without the normal obvious physical signs. Patients who have been on prolonged therapeutic regimes may not gain wound strength at the normal rate, bone healing may be delayed and they are susceptible to postoperative infections. These factors must be taken into account in planning the surgery.

All patients who are receiving corticosteroids should carry a steroid card. This will record who has prescribed the drug and the dosage and advises patients to show the card to the dentist. It also warns that the treatment should not be stopped without medical advice and that additional steroid may be appropriate in case of infection, accident or operations. It is both helpful and courteous to discuss the proposed steroid supplementation with the doctor prescribing the steroids.

The synthetic anti-flammatory steroids dexamethasone and betamethasone have been shown to reduce significantly postoperative swelling under controlled conditions without any evidence of delayed healing, infection or other morbidity. Dexamethasone 4 mg given intravenously with the anaesthetic induction agent and repeated the following day, orally or intramuscularly, has no detectable effect on plasma cortisol or electrolytes, but only reduces the swelling to about 85 per cent of the controls and does not affect trismus. Dexamethasone 10 mg used in this way will produce a detectable plasma cortisol depression to the lower limit of the normal range, gradually recovering over 3–5 days. However, there is a significant reduction in swelling ranging from 66 per cent on day 1 through to 15 per cent of controls on day 7. This dose also reduces postoperative trismus. Wound infection and healing were unaffected. Therefore some clinicians use for minor oral surgery 10 mg i.m. with the premedication (or i.v. with the anaesthetic) and 10 mg i.m. or orally 24 hours later. For maxillofacial procedures dosage is as follows:

Day 1	10 mg Dexamethasone with premedication
Day 2	10 mg Dexamethasone 12-hourly
Day 3	5 mg Dexamethasone 12-hourly
Day 4	5 mg Dexamethasone mane

Used with discretion, these regimes are valuable. However, it must be emphasized that the routine administration of these steroids should not be necessary if tissues are handled gently, haemostasis is obtained before wounds are sutured and vacuum drains placed in all major wounds, particularly where there is a potential dead space. If gross swelling results as a routine the operator's surgical technique should be reviewed.

ORAL ANTICOAGULANTS

Immediate and short-term anticoagulation is produced by intravenous heparin and withdrawal of the drug is usually sufficient in the event of unwanted bleeding. Phenindione (dindevan) and coumarins, particularly warfarin, are used for sustained or long-term anticoagulation. These drugs are given orally and antagonize the effects of vitamin K by substrate competition. Warfarin is currently the most popular drug.

Anticoagulants are prescribed to prevent intravascular clotting, propagation of thrombus and embolism. They are prescribed for deep vein thrombosis, patients with prosthetic heart valves and those with poorly controlled atrial fibrillation. There is a long period of 36–48 hours before warfarin is fully effective and it is during this period that heparin is given if immediate anticoagulation is required. Because of the serious nature of the complications which anticoagulation seeks to prevent, stopping the treatment completely is usually avoided. Further sudden stoppage may lead to a rise in factor VIII levels to above normal. Patients are usually maintained with a prothrombin time between 2·0 and 4·0, British Comparative Ratio (BCR), at which level spontaneous haemorrhage is usually avoided. The equivalent thrombotest level is 5–15 per cent prothrombin activity.

If oral surgery is necessary for a patient taking oral anticoagulants the patient's physician is contacted, a full medical summary obtained and a suitable regime agreed. Patients on anticoagulants should carry an anticoagulant treatment card which records the dose of warfarin and the BCR each time tests are done. This will give an indication of the level of anticoagulation normally achieved.

The current prothrombin time is determined. At a BCR of 2·0 it is normally safe to perform routine extractions, a few at a time, or limited minor oral surgery. If the BCR is greater than 2·0 a dose or doses of warfarin are omitted to let the prothrombin time reach a safe level. Because of the delay before warfarin is fully effective a normal dose should be taken immediately after the operation.

Where a more rapid return to the anticoagulated state is desirable 5000 units of sodium heparin may be injected subcutaneously starting as soon as stable haemostasis is ensured and 12-hourly until the patient is ambulant or can be re-established on an oral regime. Small doses of heparin activate antithrombin III which inhibits factors X and thrombin. Particular care must be taken with haemostasis and drains inserted where necessary.

Surgicel is inserted in the sockets, or for larger bone cavities, surgicel soaked in Russel viper venom (Stypven) and the wound carefully sutured. Excess bleeding as a result of surgery and the coumarin anticoagulants can usually be controlled in an emergency by packing and suturing. If it is serious the patient should be fully investigated, i.e. haemoglobin, full blood count, prothrombin time or thrombotest, whole blood clotting time (WBCT), thrombin time (TT) or activated partial thromboplastin time (APTT). With controlled anticoagulant therapy, the WBCT and TT are 2–3 times normal and the APTT 1–2 times normal. Serious or severe, continued bleeding may require further reversal of the anticoagulation. This can be done by giving phytomenadione (vitamin K_1) 2·5–10 mg by slow i.v. injection. However, this will take up to 12 hours to be effective and will disturb further anticoagulant therapy for days or weeks. Therefore in such an emergency fresh frozen plasma will provide more immediate control. These measures are not without risk of precipitating venous thrombosis. It should be rare that oral surgical haemorrhage cannot be controlled by local measures.

Aspirin, and other protein binding drugs, alcohol, co-trimoxazole, metronidazole, etc., potentiate the effects of warfarin. Some drugs which increase liver microsomal activity like barbiturates antagonize the effect of warfarin. A formulary should be consulted before prescriptions are given to these patients.

Deep vein thrombosis with embolism is rarely a complication of head and neck surgery although it can be encountered with multiple injuries involving the pelvis and femora. If the risk is anticipated, especially in patients over

50 years and heavy smokers, again a prophylactic subcutaneous heparin regime should be used (5000 units s.c. 12-hourly).

If deep vein thrombosis is detected then a full anticoagulant regime is required as follows: a loading dose of 5000 units of heparin intravenously followed by a continuous infusion of 40000 units over 24 hours or 10000 units intravenously every 6 hours. Simultaneously the patient is started on warfarin 10mg daily for 3 days then adjusted to the maintenance dose of 3–10mg a day maintaining a prothrombin time of 2–3 times the control. It should be measured daily from the fourth day of treatment.

Warfarin is teratogenic and should not be used in the first trimester of pregnancy.

ORAL CONTRACEPTIVES

Oral contraceptive tablets contain either a mixture of oestrogen and progestogen or progestogen alone. The oestrogen/progestogen tablets vary in the amount of oestrogen which they contain from $20 \mu g$ oestrogen to $50 \mu g$ oestrogen. One of the side-effects of both types of contraceptive pill is venous thrombosis and thrombo-embolism. The risk is less the lower the oestrogen content but is also a potential problem with the progestogen only preparation. In the case of the lower dose oestrogen combined preparation and the progestogen only tablets precise adherence to regularity and timing of doses is important if they are to be effective. Many women using this form of contraception now take tablets containing $30-35 \mu g$ oestrogen.

Deep vein thrombosis starting in the calves and propagating upwards is a possible complication of surgery or even confinement to bed and the risk of this is increased by the contraceptive pill. Pulmonary embolism from such thrombi is serious and is a potential cause of sudden death in the postoperative period. Permanent damage to the venous return of the leg can result also. Smoking increases the risk of venous thrombosis for women using the pill.

Patients who are to have elective in-patient surgery preferably should not take oral contraceptives for 4 to 6 weeks preoperatively and of course should be advised to use alternative methods of contraception during the next (postoperative) menstrual cycle. Some women do not admit to taking contraceptive pills for a variety of reasons. Often they are part of their normal way of life and not considered medication. Sometimes they feel that the environment at consultation prior to admission is not private enough. To avoid having to delay a major elective procedure these factors should be considered at preoperative visits.

Quite a proportion of women due for more minor in-patient surgery will only disclose their use of the contraceptive pill at the time of admission. Where the procedure will not last longer than, say, 1–2 hours and where the patient will be fit enough to get up and move around the next day experience shows that the risk of venous thrombosis is very small. In all such cases the pill should be stopped on admission and until the appropriate starting day in the next cycle and an alternative method of contraception used until after the fourteenth tablet in the next cycle. Preferably the patient should consult the doctor or clinic prescribing the tablets for expert advice.

Some patients will attempt to maintain the course of tablets despite the anaesthetic and surgery from their own supplies. This is to be discouraged as a failure to take the tablets regularly or at the correct time or if one is vomited up it can lead to a lack of effectiveness and an unwanted pregnancy.

Certain drugs interfere with the effectiveness of oral contraceptives. Of particular importance to dentists is the interaction of antibiotics, particularly ampicillin, barbiturates and carbamazepine. A formulary should be consulted before drugs are prescribed for patients on the pill.

Oestrogens may be prescribed for other reasons, for example, during the menopause, for men with metastatic carcinoma of the prostate and occasionally for women with carcinoma of the breast. Discussions with the doctor prescribing the oestrogens is indicated to evolve an appropriate regime.

Support at the ankles by plastic foam wedges during the surgery to prevent pressure on the calves, leg exercises and early mobilization are general measures to reduce deep vein thrombosis. Low-dose heparin can be used as a prophylaxis against venous thrombosis and pulmonary embolism and can be used where the patient has not stopped taking the contraceptive pill at the proper time and where delay to the operation is not appropriate, or where a risk seems possible even with a short procedure. Heparin 5000 units is given subcutaneously and repeated every 12 hours until the patient is ambulant. However, heparin even in this dose will increase the amount of oozing at operation and can produce unsightly haematomas at the site of the injection. Haemostasis can usually be effected with care in soft tissue wounds, but postoperative oozing from cut bone and consequent haematoma formation is a risk.

SMOKING

Patients should be encouraged to reduce the amount they smoke before operation and if possible to stop completely for some days beforehand, a week or ten days if possible. Smoking increases the incidence of postoperative chest infection, venous thrombosis and embolism, and can increase vascular spasm or reduce the blood supply to pedicle and free flaps.

HYPOTENSIVE AGENTS

A variety of drugs are used to control hypertension either singly or in combination. They control the blood pressure by a number of different mechanisms. At one time it was considered best to withdraw hypotensive treatment before a general anaesthetic because the peripheral vasodilatation induced by the anaesthetic drugs could increase the fall in blood pressure. With currently used drugs it is mostly safer for patients to continue with their medication, rather than to present the anaesthetist with an uncontrolled hypertensive. Indeed, withdrawal of some drugs results in rebound hypertension. In general such patients are best referred to hospital, even for a short general anaesthetic, so that they can receive the care of an experienced anaesthetist.

The use of local anaesthetics in normal quantities is not contraindicated but prilocaine with felypressin may be preferred and local anaesthetic solutions containing noradrenaline should be avoided. Hypertensive patients of course tend to ooze more than normotensive individuals during surgery and hypertension can be one cause of postoperative haemorrhage.

TRICYCLIC ANTIDEPRESSANTS

Noradrenaline is released as a neural transmitter at postganglionic sympathetic nerve terminals. Part of the released noradrenaline is inactivated by catechol-ortho-methyltransferase and some escapes into the circulation, but 85 per cent is taken up again into the nerve terminal to be used again. This active pump mechanism is inhibited by competitive binding by tricyclic antidepressants, leading to an increase in circulating noradrenaline.

A large number of tri- and tetracyclic antidepressants are available. There is a risk of ventricular dysrhythmias and of a rise in blood pressure if injections containing adrenaline or noradrenaline are given to these patients. Hypertension is a particular hazard with noradrenaline and this vasoconstrictor particularly should be avoided. Local anaesthetic solutions containing felypressin may be used with safety for these patients.

Withdrawal of tricyclic antidepressives before a general anaesthetic is usually not in order because the effects of the drug persist for 2-3 weeks. If it is withdrawn for such a period of time, relapse of the depression is likely and there will be a further period of 10-14 days before control is re-established after recommencing treatment.

MONOAMINE OXIDASE INHIBITORS (MAOI)

Monoamine oxidase modulates the release of noradrenaline at sympathetic nerve terminals by inactivating noradrenaline within the terminal. It is also present in the liver and gastrointestinal tract where it detoxicates dietary amines such as tyramine. It is for this reason that certain items of food precipitate headache and hypertension in patients taking monoamine oxidase inhibitors. Because of the dietary restrictions required MAOI have declined in popularity and have been partly replaced by tricyclic antidepressives.

Adrenaline in local anaesthetic solutions does not present a hazard for patients taking MAOI. However, noradrenaline is released and in large amounts by sympathomimetic amines like amphetamine, ephedrine, phenylephrine and isoprenaline and these substances must not be prescribed. Tricyclic antidepressants also must not be given with MAOI.

Morphine and other opioids can also precipitate a hypertensive crisis and pethidine results in severe hypotension. The inactivation of monoamine oxidase by MAOI is irreversible and persists for up to 14 days after withdrawal of the drug so that prescription precautions apply during this time. These patients often carry a treatment card which indicates which drug they are taking and a series of precautions which the patients must follow.

LITHIUM

Certain lithium salts are prescribed for patients with manic-depressive illnesses. The therapeutic range is quite narrow and special care is required to avoid toxicity. Sodium depletion and vomiting can potentiate the effect of lithium and result in toxicity. Short out-patient procedures are unlikely to require changes in medication but the anaesthetist may require the drug to be discontinued a week before major in-patient surgery. The patient's psychiatrist or physician prescribing the lithium should be consulted.

ANTICONVULSANT DRUGS

There is a great temptation to stop anticonvulsant therapy for epileptics when undergoing surgical procedures, particularly if they have no recent history of fits. Unfortunately both the procedure and the abrupt withdrawal of the medication may precipitate a seizure postoperatively. Epileptics are normally continued on their anticonvulsant regime for an operation under general anaesthesia. The preoperative dose is given orally as usual with minimum water and then parenterally until the patient can swallow without being sick postoperatively. Despite the administration of sedation or anaesthetic drugs fits are more likely to occur in the postoperative period.

Epileptic patients who have taken their tablets should be treated normally for oral surgery under local anaesthesia. Even so, occasionally a patient will have a fit as a result of the stress of attending. Recovery is usually spontaneous with general care and a rubber ring between the teeth during clonic contractions prevents tongue biting. Should status epilepticus supervene, intravenous diazepam may be given slowly (not methohexitone or thiopentone which excite the motor cortex). However, respiratory arrest

PORPHYRIA

This is an inborn error of porphyrin synthesis which occurs in several forms. Sufferers normally carry a warning card. It is particularly important not to give either thiopentone or methohexitone to them.

HEREDITARY RED CELL ABNORMALITIES

Certain abnormalities of red cells are important to the oral surgeon because either drug therapy or anaesthetics can present particular problems.

ENZYME DEFICIENCY

Glucose-6-phosphate dehydrogenase (G6PD) is the first enzyme in the hexose monophosphate shunt of the Embden–Myerhoff glycolytic pathway from which erythrocytes gain most of their metabolic energy. This shunt services the enzymes glutathione reductase and glutathione peroxidase which protect erythrocytes against oxidation damage. If G6PD is absent this protective mechanism is reduced and certain drugs in substantial concentration can injure the red cells. High doses of sulphonamides, antimalarials and aspirin, phenacetin and chloramphenicol taken during infective illnesses can result in haemolysis. It is an X-linked recessive disorder affecting mainly negroes and particularly those in East and West Africa where the incidence may reach 20 per cent in males and 4 per cent in females.

HAEMOGLOBINOPATHIES

Haemoglobin is composed of two pairs of polypeptide chains and four haem molecules. Each polypeptide chain is folded to enclose one of the haem molecules. During fetal life and the first few weeks after birth, human erythrocytes contain haemoglobin F.

The globin in haemoglobin F is composed of 2α polypeptide chains and 2γ chains ($\alpha 2 \gamma 2$). Normal adult haemoglobin comprises mostly haemoglobin A, formed by 2α and 2β chains ($\alpha 2 \beta 2$) with some A2 ($\alpha 2 \delta 2$).

In one group of conditions certain amino acids in the polypeptide chains of some abnormal haemoglobins are substituted by others. There are several hundred such variants, only a few of which are of clinical significance. They are either designated by a capital letter of the alphabet or the name of the locality where they were discovered. Sickle-cell anaemia is the most important of this group in respect of therapeutic hazards.

In another group the gene for one type of polypeptide chain is either missing, or defective, or its translation is defective. Consequently one pair of polypeptide chains is either absent or incomplete. The β and α thalassaemias are the most frequently encountered examples of this group.

Sickle-cell Disease

A normal adult has the haemoglobin genotype A,A. Sickle-cell trait, the heterozygous state, has the genotype A,S and homozygous sickle-cell disease, S,S. Some patients, heterozygous for the sickle-cell conditions, have haemoglobins other than A present, such as C, D and E. Haemoglobin synthesis is inherited from both parents and expressed as a mosaic. Thus if both parents are heterozygous a quarter of the offspring are likely to be normal, a further quarter will have sickle-cell anaemia and the remainder sickle-cell trait.

When haemoglobin S is deoxygenated, the molecules of haemoglobin S becomes cross-linked to form elongated pseudo-crystalline 'tactoids' which distort the red cell into the 'sickle' shape. Although the change is reversible with reoxygenation, permanent deformation of the red cell envelope occurs after repeated sickling. The presence of haemoglobin F strongly inhibits tactoid formation but the presence of C as haemoglobin SC facilitates their formation. The change is likely to occur in sinusoidal vessels or capillaries where blood flow is sluggish. Sickle cells render the blood more viscous and they obstruct capillaries resulting in infarction.

Trait patients may appear healthy. As the presence of HbS confers a degree of resistance to malaria (which is not enhanced by the homozygous state) this accounts for its prevalence in the areas in which this disease is endemic and its persistence in negroes. However, even trait patients may experience sickling with relative anoxia occurring, for example, during the induction of general anaesthesia, in inadequately pressurized aircraft or in a limb prepared for bloodless field surgery by the use of a tourniquet.

Two major complications face homozygous sickle-cell disease patients: a severe haemolytic anaemia and infarction crises. Normally the patients have only 8–10 g/dl haemoglobin. Episodes of sequestration of red cells lead to rapid further falls in haemoglobin level. Viral infections can even precipitate an aplastic anaemia. The spleen and liver are enlarged and red marrow hyperplasia enlarges medullary spaces and produces bossing of the skull. Infarction crises in bone or spleen result in severe pain, fever, malaise and jaundice. Secondary infection in bone infarcts results in osteomyelitis. Infarction of renal papillae leads to haematuria, and mesenteric infarction to an abdominal emergency.

Investigation

A simple blood film from an homozygous patient is likely to contain a few sickle cells, but a film from a 'trait' patient will be normal. However, blood from a heterozygous patient mixed with a sodium metabisulphate solution and allowed to stand, covered with a coverslip, for twenty minutes will show sickling. The Sickledex test is done using blood from a finger prick in small tubes, one containing the test specimen and the other acting as control. After 5 minutes, with a positive result cayenne-pepper-like clumps of red cells can be seen when the tube is viewed against a white background. This is convenient as a surgery screening test.

Neither the Sickledex test nor the slide test differentiate between haemoglobins AS, SS, SC, SD, SE or S thalassaemia. Positive patients or patients about whom the clinician is suspicious on clinical grounds should be referred to a haematologist and a haemoglobin electrophoresis performed which will distinguish these various conditions. The patient should be issued with a card stating the exact abnormality to avoid repeated investigation and near relatives should be investigated where this has not already been done. A simple haemoglobin estimation to determine the degree of anaemia should not be forgotten.

Treatment

Both sickle-cell trait and sickle-cell disease patients can be treated under local anaesthesia, but large volumes of solution containing the higher concentrations of adrenaline which might cause appreciable tissue cyanosis should not be used.

Where a general anaesthetic or inhalation sedation is required referral to hospital is advisable, so that an experienced anaesthetist can give the anaesthetic. Inhalation sedation or a short general anaesthetic with adequate oxygenation is usually safe for trait patients on an out-patient basis. Homozygous patients are usually admitted and the haemoglobin level checked. In some still ambulatory patients it can fall as low as 5 g/dl as these patients become habituated to a relative anaemia. Preoperative transfusion will then be necessary.

Special precautions to ensure pre-induction oxygen saturation and to avoid any episodes of restricted oxygen intake are important. Anaemic patients may not exhibit clinical cyanosis as the amount of reduceable haemoglobin may be insufficient to produce a colour change. Dehydration and electrolyte depletion must also be avoided.

β-Thalassaemia

The condition is found commonly in the Mediterranean area and particularly among certain island populations. In β-thalassaemia part or all of the β polypeptide chains are not synthesized. The heterozygote thalassaemia minor produces a mild anaemia but little disability. The homozygous condition is serious as the patient is unable to synthesize haemoglobin A ($\alpha 2 \beta 2$) because β chains cannot be formed. There is a profound anaemia from soon after birth with increased destruction of abnormally shaped red cells. Production of haemoglobin F ($\alpha 2 \gamma 2$) which contains no β chains, continues beyond the neonatal period and increases to form 30–40 per cent of circulating haemoglobin. Despite red marrow hyperplasia the child cannot survive for long unless transfused, but repeated transfusion soon leads to haemosiderosis. There is bossing of the skull due to subperiosteal haemopoiesis and massive hepatosplenomegaly.

Diagnosis
There is almost always thalassaemia among the other members of the family. Thalassaemia minor patients have a mild iron refractory hypochromic anaemia. A blood film will demonstrate microcytes and red cells are resistant to osmotic lysis. On electrophoresis there is a raised haemoglobin A2 ($\alpha 2 \delta 2$) fraction. The thalassaemia major patients are small for their age, are obvious chronic invalids and almost always already under the care of a haematologist or paediatrician. They are anaemic, indeed profoundly so. A blood film will demonstrate severe red cell dysplasia and erythroblastosis. Haemoglobin electrophoresis will reveal an absence of haemoglobin A and raised haemoglobin F. Both parents will have thalassaemia minor.

Heterozygous patients can be treated normally in practice but multiple extractions and oral surgery other than the removal of the roots of a single tooth or straightforward impaction are best undertaken in hospital. General anaesthetics are best given at a hospital.

Routine restorative work can be managed in practice for the homozygous patient. They are particularly susceptible to infection and present obvious difficult management problems so that admission for any oral surgery is essential.

α-Thalassaemia

This condition is encountered mainly in South-East Asia. Two variants occur, one with severe and the other with mild inhibition of α chain production. Heterozygotes rarely present a clinical problem. Homozygotes of the mild form require management in hospital. Homozygotes of the severe disease die *in utero*.

DRUG ALLERGY

Hypersensitivity to drugs is likely to occur in patients with a history of general allergy, i.e. atopy which usually takes the form of hay fever, asthma or eczema. The most common sources of drug reaction are penicillin, sulphonamides, aspirin and antitetanus serum, but few drugs are free of allergenic potential.

In all cases the medication must be stopped and the patient treated as follows:

1. For skin rashes which are urticarial, maculopapular, morbilliform, vesicular, bullous or eczematous an oral antihistamine should be given such

as chlorpheniramine maleate 4 mg, 3–4 times a day. Very irritant lesions may also be treated with 1 per cent hydrocortisone cream.

2. For erythema multiforme, consisting of conjunctival, orolabial and urethral inflammation together with the cutaneous target lesion rash should be treated immediately with high doses of corticosteroids, e.g. dexamethasone 4 mg or prednisone 20 mg, 8-hourly, reducing the dose gradually after seven days.

3. Angioedema can be treated with an oral antihistamine or 10–20 mg chlorpheniramine maleate by intramuscular or slow intravenous injection. If severe and involving the respiratory tract adrenaline 0·5–1 ml of 1 : 1000 (equivalent to 0·5–1 mg) should be given intramuscularly. Simultaneous intravenous hydrocortisone sodium succinate 100 mg should be given. Where the airway remains obstructed tracheal intubation or even a tracheostomy will be required.

4. Asthma can be treated with salbutamol which is a beta 2-adrenoreceptor stimulator producing bronchodilatation and can be given by aerosol inhalation 100–200 μg (1–2 puffs) 4-hourly, by tablet 2–4 mg, again 4-hourly, or by slow intravenous injection of 250 μg. If not available aminophylline 250–500 mg may be given by slow intravenous injection over 15 minutes or a 360 mg suppository may be tried. For severe asthma, 100 mg hydrocortisone sodium succinate must be given intravenously together with oxygen.

5. Serum sickness consisting of fever, arthralgia, rashes and lymphadenopathy should be treated like erythema multiforme.

6. Anaphylactic shock in which many features of the above occur together with hypotension should be treated with 0·5–1 mg adrenaline i.m. (the dose can be doubled if the patient is unconscious), hydrocortisone 100 mg i.v., oxygen and intravenous Hartmann's solution to maintain the blood pressure.

PREVENTION OF ORAL AND DENTAL DISEASE

A positive approach to the prevention of the two major dental diseases is an integral part of normal patient management in dental practice. Of course patient education in preventive measures by the dentist should also embrace other oral diseases where there are known controllable aetiological factors.

Patients, and in the case of a child, the patient's family, faced by the problems created by debilitating or disabling conditions tend to conserve their emotional and physical energies by neglecting some of the less important aspects of daily life. They have got to be convinced of the need for a conscientious attitude to dental and oral preventive measures or they may consider these of low priority.

The prevention of dental disease in the normal person will avoid unnecessary and sometimes hazardous complications. For many patients with chronic disease not only are the consequences of progressive dental disease more serious, but both the oral disease and its treatment can be potentially life-threatening.

SUGGESTED READING

Bailey B.M.W. and Fordyce A. M. (1983) Complications of dental extractions in patients receiving warfarin anticoagulant therapy. *Br. Dent. J.* **155,** 308–310.

British Medical Association and the Pharmaceutical Society of Great Britain (published annually) *The British National Formulary.*

Goodman A. and Gilman L.S. (1985) *The Pharmaceutical Basis of Therapeutics,* 7th ed. New York: Macmillan.

Laurence D. R. and Bennett P. N. (1980) *Clinical Pharmacology,* 5th ed. Edinburgh, London and New York: Churchill Livingstone.

Seymour R. A. and Walton J. G. (1982) Analgesic efficacy in dental pain. *Br. Dent. J.* **153,** 291–298.

INDEX

Abscess(es)
  buccinator muscle and 143
  bursting 170
  causes 123
  with collateral oedema 172–3
  drainage of 167–70
  encapsulated chronic 163
  management of patients with 172–3
  opening 149–50, 154, 169
  osteomyelitis following 180, 200–1
  sinus formation 170, (Fig. 6.22) 171–2
  see also under specific sites
Abseal 274
Acetylsalicylic acid 344
Acoustic neurinoma 338
Actinomycosis 71, 187, 197, (Fig. 7.8) 198–9, 219
  chronic 172
Actinomycotic infections 216
Acyclovir 217, 337
Adenoid cystic carcinoma 331
Adrenal
  cortex atrophy 354
  steroid production inhibited 352
Adrenalectomy 352
Adrenaline injection 113
Adrenals, destruction of 352
Agranulocytosis 334
AIDS 228–31
  antibodies 230
  carriers 229
  infections from, prevention 230–1
  transmission 230
Air motors, surgical 20–1
Airway, protection of patient's 23
Alarm clock headache 340
Albers–Schönberg's disease 201
Alcohol as disinfectant 232
Alcohol injection 334
Alcoholism 178
Allergy
  aspirin 344
  dressings 342
  drugs 209, 342, 364–5
  penicillin 223
  sulphonamides 216
  upper respiratory tract 235
Allografts 116
Alpha-thalassaemia 364
Alveolar abscess 218
  acute 121–5, 174
  chronic 123

Alveolar abscess (cont.)
  differential diagnosis 180, 182
Alveolar bone
  atrophy 114
  file 93
  fractures 93
  loss 110
Alveolar
  cysts, median 272
  osteitis 318
    acute 174–8
  process mucosa, soft-tissue swellings of 297
Alveolar ridge
  fibrous enlargement, surgical treatment 97–8
  orthognathic surgery for 119
  remodelling 110–11
Alveolar wounds 30
Alveolectomy 94
Alveolitis sicca dolorosa 174
Alveolotomy, inter-septal 94
Ameloblastoma 59, 286, 305
  aspiration 281
  cystic 276
  marsupialized 287
Aminoglutethimide 352
Aminoglycosides 213
Ammonium compounds, quaternary 233
Amoxycillin 210, 222–3, 224, 244
Amphetamine 360
Amphotericin B 217
Ampicillin 210, 358
Amyloid infiltration 312
Anaemia
  in infancy 363
  sickle cell 362
Anaerobes 123, 218
Anaesthesia
  dolorosa 337
  general 19–20
    diabetic under 350–1
    in Ludwig's angina 141
    preparation for 20
  local 6–7, 12–13, 190
    in apicectomy 257–8
  of nerves 70
  for wisdom teeth removal 60
Analgesia, prolonged opioid 346
Analgesics 343
  narcotic 345
  non-steroidal anti-inflammatory 343–4

INDEX

Anaphylactic shock 365
Aneurysm, internal carotid artery 339
Aneurysmal bone cyst 272–3
Angina pectoris 333
Angio-oedema 313, 365
Angioneurotic oedema (*Fig.* 6.16) 157–8
Ankylosis
  extra articular 325
  of impacted canine 82
Antibiotic therapy 208–9
  abscesses 124, 163
  actinomycosis 172, 199
  canine fossa infection 161
  cavernous sinus thrombophlebitis 166
  inadequate 209
  infratemporal fossa infections 166
  intermaxillary fixation 224–5
  Ludwig's angina 141
  osteomyelitis 180, 218–19
  osteoradionecrosis 218–19
  parapharyngeal space infection 153
  pericoronitis 127
  post-apicectomy 260
  pre-radiation prophylaxis 189–90, 192
  prophylactic 220–2
  quinsy 154, 332
  sinusitis 220
  soft tissue infections 166–8
  submasseteric infection 149
  tetanus 231–2
  upper lip abscesses 157
Antibiotic-resistant microbes 210
Antibiotics 208, 210–16
  allergy to 364
  antagonistic 209
  contraindications 209
  interacting with contraceptives 358
  placebo response to 326
Anticoagulants, oral 355–7
Anticoagulation, aspirin contraindicated 344
Anticonvulsant drugs 306–7, 360
Antidepressants 343
  anxiolytic 319
  tricyclic 9, 319, 324, 340
Antifibrinolytic agents 177
Antifungal drugs 217
Antimalarials 361
Antiseptic bath 20
Antiseptics 24
Antitetanus serum allergy 364
Antiviral drugs 217
Antral lining, exposure 248
Antroliths mistaken for roots 251
Antrostomy 73
  intranasal 244

Antrum
  carcinoma 331
  large, cyst and 279
  maxillary 331–2
  unerupted teeth displaced into 247
Anxiety 321, 323
Aortic valves, biscupid 222
Aortic valvular disease, degenerative 222
Apical
  abscess 123
    chronic (*Fig.* 6.1*a*) 122
  cyst 260
  elevators 45
  granuloma 255, 257
  periodontal cyst 270–1, 277
    marsupialization (*Fig.* 11.3) 286
  root canal obstruction 257
  seal, faulty 260
  thrombosis, 254
Apicectomy 257–61, 262
  in cyst closure 290
  flap incision for 30–1
  infection after 158
  with retrograde seal 260
Arsenic trioxide 194
Arterial graft patients 223
Arterial malformation 281
Arteriovenous malformation 281
Arteritis
  giant-cell 340–1
  temporal 340–1
Arthritis
  acute 318
  infective 318
  juvenile rheumatoid 318
  rheumatoid 319
    acute 318
  traumatic temporomandibular 318–19
Arthrography, temporomandibular joint 325
Arthromyalgia, facial 319, 322–6, 326, 331, 340
Aseptic necrosis of bone 193–4
Aspirin 343–4, 361
Assistants, training of 8
Asthma 365
Atropine 348
Auriculotemporal
  nerve avulsion 336
  syndrome, Frey's 336
Autoclaves 9

Bacterial resistance 209
Bacteroides melaninogenicus 218

INDEX

Barbiturate 358
Basal cell naevus syndrome 268
Bath
  antiseptic 20
  preoperative 20, 24
Benzylpenicillin 208–10
Beta-thalassaemia 363–4
Betamethazone 354–5
Bicuspid aortic valves 222
Black silk, suturing 18
Bleeding, postoperative 73
Bleeding disorders, aspirin contraindicated 344
Blood
  infected 225
  pressure, postoperative fall 354
  supply to mandible 178
  transfusions, multiple 226
Bone
  aseptic necrosis 193–4
  cancellous 255
  cysts (*Fig.* 11.1) 264–5, 272–4
    solitary 295
  density 58
  destruction 256
    cancellous 279
    cortical 279
    radiographs of 254–5
  file, alveolar 93
  formation
    and destruction 174
    new, subperiosteal 148
  fractures, alveolar 93
  graft donor sites, preparation 24
  grafting in cyst enucleation and closure 293–4
  grafts 21, 115
  hypovascularity 187
  infection, childhood 179–80
  inflammation 174
  necrosis 194
  pain 318
  plates, miniature 115
  sclerosed 176
Bone removal
  around impacted canine 79
  from fractured root 46–50
  impacted 3rd maxillary molar 72
  impacted lower premolar 85
  inferior dental canal and 58–9
  supernumeraries 89
Bone-cutting instruments 14–16
Bony ridge augmentation 114–16, (*Fig.* 5.9) 117
Borrelia vincentii 180

Bridge, odontalgia with fitting 326
Bruxism 319, 323–4
Buccal
  advancement flap, oroantral fistula closure by 241, (*Fig.* 9.1) 242–4
  mucosa, swellings of 298, 308–10
  rotation flap, oroantral fistula closure by (*Fig.* 9.3) 246–7
  space 143, (*Fig.* 6.10) 144
    haematoma in 144
    infection 144, (*Fig.* 6.11) 145, 148, (*Fig.* 16.21) 165
Buccinator muscle 142–3
Buccolingually orientated teeth, impacted 56
Bucket handle deformity 115
Buprenorphine 346
Burning tongue 330
Burs
  bone-cutting 14, 47–8
  in impacted canine exposure 82
  irrigation of 16
  rose-head 85–6
  tungsten carbide tapering fissure 65
    in separation of whole crowns 67
  use for mandibular 3rd molar extraction 63

Cachageusia 329
Caffey's disease of bone 204
Calcifying odontic cyst 268–9
Calculus 300, 302–3, 331
  deposits 111
Canal, inferior dental, damage during bone removal 58–9
Cancerophobia 310, 328
Candida albicans 214, 217, 300
Candidiasis 229
  chronic hyperplastic 310
Canine
  bone removal around 79
  displaced, surgical repositioning 83
  fossa 158, (*Fig.* 6.17) 159
    infection 159, (*Fig.* 6.18) 160
  impacted lower, removal of 83–4
  impacted maxillary 73–4
    buccal approach 77–8
    elevation 79–80
    examination 74
    leaving in place 81
    palatal approach 78–81
    radiology 74–5
    reasons for removing 75–6

369

INDEX

Canine (cont.)
    removal (Fig. 4.8–9) 76–81
    surgical exposure 81–2
    suturing after extraction 78, 80–1
    lower, over-eruption 83
    maxillary, monitoring development of 74
    see also Unerupted canine
Carbamazepine 333–4, 358
Carbenicillin 211
Carbuncle 160
Carcinoma 236, 311
    adenoid cystic 331
    antrum 240, 332
    in cyst linings 287
    metastatic 205, 318
    nasopharyngeal 337–8
    squamous cell 193
    tongue 330
Cardiac
    arrest 5
    transplant patients 224
Caries 59–60
    cervical 190
    comforter (Fig. 6.1a) 122
    radiation 188–9
Carotid artery, aneurysms of internal 339
Carotid sheath 131
Catgut 18, 36, 89
Causalgia 335
Cavernous sinus
    infection 166
    thrombophlebitis 155–6, 160, 166
Cavity, irrigation 170
Cellulitis 124, 128, 169, 173
    acute facial 179
    due to upper lip infection 156
    orbital 160, 179
    poultice increasing spread of 167
    right sublingual space (Fig. 6.7) 139
Cephalgia, histamine 340
Cephalosporins 212, 218, 220
Cervical
    caries 190
    fascia, deep 130
    sympathectomy 336
Cetrimide 233
Cheek chewing 323
Cheilitis
    grandularis apostomatosa 312
    granulomatosa 312
Chemical necrosis 194
Chemotherapeutic agents 208
Chemotherapy 208, 343–9
    cytotoxic 194
    prophylactic regimes 222–32

Chemotherapy (cont.)
    oral 222
    parenteral 222–3
Childhood
    aspirin not under 12 years 344
    bone infection in 179–80
    emotional disturbances 323
    enucleation in 284–5
    mandibular osteomyelitis in 180,
        (Fig. 7.1, 4) 181–4
    ocular abnormalities in 268
    osteomyelitis in 199–200
    periostitis in 202
    psychosomatic pain 322
    rheumatoid arthritis 318
    tetracycline therapy in 214
Chisels 14–15
    in impacted canine exposure 82
    in impacted mandibular 3rd molar removal 62–3
    in removal of fractured root 48
Chloramphenicol 224, 361
Chlorhexidine 220–1, 232–3
Chlormethiazole 349
Cholesteatoma 338
Choramphenicol 214–15
Chromic gut 18–19
Clavulanic acid 211
Cleidocranial dysostosis, impaction caused by 52
Clindamycin 215
Clinical management of infection 218–20
Clobezam 334
Clostridium difficile 216
Clostridium tetani 231–2
Clotrimazole 217
Cluster headaches 340
Co-trimoxazole 216
Coagulation diathermy 20–1
Cocaine 347
Codeine 345
Condylar head
    adhesions or gross osteophytes 325
    surgery 320, 325
Condylar shave, high 320
Congenital epulis 305
Congenital heart disease 222
Connective tissue, loose, breaking down 34–5
Constipation, 346
Contraceptive, oral 357–8
Coronary by-pass history 223
Cortical
    bone destruction 279
    hyperostosis 179

INDEX

Cortical (*cont.*)
  infantile 204
  osteomyelitis 201
Corticosteroids 352–5
Coumarins 355–6
Coupland's chisel 48
Cranial
  base lesions 338
  fossa lesions, middle 339
  fossa tumours, posterior 338
Crestal incision 28–30
Crohn's disease 311–12
Crown, odontalgia with fitting 327
Crowns
  acid etched cementation of orthodontic bracket to 82
  tungsten carbide tapering fissure burs in separation of 67
Cryotherapy 334, 336
Cumine scaler 45
Curettes 17
Cyclosporin A 306
Cystic ameloblastoma 276
Cystic carcinoma, adenoid 331
Cysts 237, 263
  apical 260
  apical periodontal 270, 277, (*Fig.* 11.6) 291
    marsupialization (*Fig.* 11.3) 286
  aspiration 281
  biopsy 282
  bone 272–3
    aneurysmal 273–4
    solitary 295
  carcinoma in linings 287
  clinical presentation 277–8
  closure 287–9, 292
    with bone grafting 293–4
  dental 162
  dentigerous 87, 263, (*Fig.* 11.1) 264–8, 277–8, 280–1
  dermoid 275
  in edentulous jaws 96
  enlargement 275–6, 278, 280, 284
    osmotic theory 276
  enucleation 287, (*Figs.* 11.4–5) 288–9, (*Fig.* 11.6) 291–5
    with bone grafting 293–4
    in childhood 284–5
    and decompression 292
    instruments for 289–90
  eruption 265–6
  fissural (*Fig.* 11.1) 264–5, 271–2, 272, 295
  fluid electrophoresis 281

Cysts (*cont.*)
  follicular 263, 265
  gingival 274
  globulomaxillary 271
  impaction against 52
  incisive canal 269–70
  incisive papilla 270
  inclusion 271–2
  infected 123, 318
  investigation 278
  jaws 263, (*Fig.* 11.1) 264–5
  large
    antrum differentiation 279
    enucleation 293
    mandibular fractures after removal 294
  malignant change 279
  mandibular 290
  marsupialization 276, 283–4, (*Figs.* 11.2–3) 285–7
  maxillary 278–9
    incisor 286
  median
    alveolar 272
    dermoid 272
    palatine 271
  multilocular 280
  nasolabial 270–1, 280
  nasopalatine 269–70, 280, 294–5
  ododontic 263, 265
    calcifying and keratinizing 268–9
  periapical 255–7, 277, 279–80
  periodontal 263, (*Fig.* 11.1) 264–7, 278, 281
  periosteal 293
  postoperative follow-up 295
  radicular 266–7
  radiology 278–80
  ramus 293
  small 294
  treatment 282–3
  upper lip 158
Cytomegalovirus infections 149
Cytotoxic chemotherapy 194

Dacryocystitis neonatorum 179
Deciduous molar, buried 87
Deciduous teeth
  apical periodontal cysts from 277
  upper incisors, trauma to 89
Dental disease, prevention of 365–6
Dentigerous cysts 87, 263, (*Fig.* 11.1) 264–6, 267–8, 277–8, 280–1

371

INDEX

Denture
  hyperplasia 3
  intolerance 328, 329
Denture-bearing area 93
  decrease in 111
  irregularities in 96–7
    alveolar ridge remodelling 110–11
    bony ridge, augmentation 114–16
    floor of mouth, lowering 113, (*Fig.* 5.8) 114
    frenal and fibrous bands 98–9
    maxillary tuberosities 100–1, (*Figs.* 5.2–3) 102–3
    muscle attachments 106, (*Fig.* 5.6) 107–8
    ridges 96–8
    tori 103, (*Figs.* 5.4–5) 104–6
  sulcus deepening 111–13
Denture-induced
  granuloma 299, (*Fig.* 12.2) 300
  hyperplasia 108–9
    removal (*Fig.* 6.7) 109–10
Dentures
  discrepancies in jaws' relative position and 119
  elderly patients' 118
  established wearers' problems 95–6
  granuloma due to 203
  horseshoe shaped 104
  immediate 93
    fully-flanged 95
    one-stage replacement 94–5
    two-stage replacement 93–4
  loss of retention 95
  modifying to fit new sulcus 112
  pathological lesions under 96
  persistent intolerance of 95–6
  pressure ulcers from 95
  prosthodontic considerations before extractions for 92–3
  removal of unerupted canines before fitting 75
  retained roots under 96
  short lingual frenum displacing 100
  surgical preparation of mouth for 92
  temporary, smoothing inside of 93
  unerupted teeth under 96
Depression 321–4
Depressor origins damage in sulcus deepening 112
Depth of tooth, assessment of 56–7
Dermoid cysts 275
  median 272
Dexamethasone 70, 354–5
Dextranomer 178

Diabetes 178
  mellitus 341, 349–52
Diabetic
  coma 351
  neuropathy 336
  vasculopathy, ischaemic necrosis in 338
Diabetics
  pre-, intra- and post-operative management 351–2
  under general anaesthesia 350–1
Diagnosis 1, 3–4
  differential 3
Diamorphine 346
Diathermy forceps 21
Diazepam, 347
Dichloralphenazone 348
Diguanides 232–3
Dindevan 355
Diphenylhydantoin 305
Disinfectants 228, 232–3
Disinfection
  chemical 9
  hand 10
Disto-angularly impacted teeth 56–7
Doxycycline 244
Drainage
  abscesses 167–70
  acute infratemporal fossa infections 165
  Ludwig's angina surgery 142
  parapharyngeal abscess 153
  periapical abscess 257
Dress 10
  theatre 21–2
Dressings 19
Drills 16
Droperiodol 347
Drug addicts 178, 226
  intravenous 229
Drug-induced gingival hyperplasia 305–6
Drugs 343
  allergy 342, 364–5
  failure to respond 343
  interaction 343–4, 356, 358
Dysaesthesia, oral 328–9
Dysphagia, painful 332

E. coli 211, 213
Eagle's syndrome 332
Ear infection, middle 332
Electric laboratory type motors 20
Elevation
  bone removal prior to 58
  forceful 70

INDEX

Elevation (*cont.*)
  impacted canine 77, 79–80
    lower 83
  impacted lower 3rd molar 61, 65
  impacted teeth 57
  impacted upper 3rd molar 72
Elevators 16–17
  apical 45
  application 50–1
  inferior dental nerve at risk from 71
  lingual nerve at risk from 70
  periosteal 14, 29, 31, 35, 61, 70
Embolism, pulmonary 357
Emergencies 5, 19
Emotional disturbances, childhood 323
Emotional illness 321
Emphysematous pulmonary disease 192
Endarteritis, obliterative 176, 187
Endocarditis 216
  bacterial 221
  infective 222
Endodontic
  osseous implants 261–2
  paste, removal of periapical 262
  therapy, orthograde 256
Endorphin 343
Endosseus implants 118
Endosteal implants 123
Enkephalins 343
Envelope flaps 28–9
  suture 69
Enzyme deficiency 361
Epanutin hyperplasia 307
Ephedrine 360
Epileptics, surgery for 360–1
Epstein's pearls 271
Epulides 298–9
  congenital 305
  fibrous (*Fig.* 12.1) 298–9, 302
  giant cell 303, (*Fig.* 12.5) 304–5
  pregnancy (*Fig.* 12.4) 302–3, 306
Ergotamine tartrate 340
Erupt, failure of tooth to 52
Eruption cysts 265
Erythema
  multiforme 365
  post-irradiation 188
Erythromycin 212, 218, 220, 222, 224
Ethyl alcohol 232
Eugenol 177
Eusol 233
Ewing's sarcoma 205
Examination 2
Excavators
  bi-angled spoon 45

Excavators (*cont.*)
  large 17, 35
Exodontia 16
Exostoses, developmental 103, 105
Extraction
  excess trauma during 176
  impacted lower canine 83–4
  with local anaesthetic and vasoconstrictor 175
  mandibular 3rd molar 61–70
    burs for 63
    examination prior to 54
  maxillary molars, oroantral fistula in 236–7
  odontalgia with 327
  osteomyelitis complicating 176, 200–1
  of partly erupted wisdom teeth 59–60
  pre-radiation 189–91
  in preparation for dentures 92–3
  resorption after 110
  socket toilet after 68
  split-bone technique 63, (*Figs.* 4.2–7) 64–9
Eyes
  pain in region of 332
  protection of patient's 10, 23

Facial
  arthromyalgia 319, 322–6
  deformity 21
  pain, atypical 326–8
Family history 2
Felypressin 13, 241
Fentanyl 347
Fibrinolytic alveolitis 174
Fibro-epithelial polyps 300, (*Fig.* 12.6) 306–9
Fibroblastoma 305
Fibromas 307, 309
Fibromatosis
  gingivae 306–7
  von Recklinghausen's 309
Fibromatous enlargement of maxillary tuberosities 307
Fissural cysts (*Fig.* 11.1) 264–5, 271–2, 295
  median mandibular 272
  non-odontontic 269–72
Flaps
  raising 28–9
  reflection 29, 30–1, 46, (*Fig.* 3.1) 47
  rhomboidal 258
Flucloxacillin 210–11

INDEX

Foliate papillae, inflamed 310
Follicular
 cysts 76, 263, 265
 formation 72
Food impaction 121, 300
Food withheld before general anaesthetic 20
Forceps
 angled 17
 artery 17, 21, 108
 contouring 16
 diathermy 21
 dissecting 18
  toothed 17
 extraction 16–17
 upper roots pattern 84
Foreign bodies 71, 123, 239
Formaldehyde 232
Fractured root
 elevation of 48, (*Fig.* 3.2) 49–50
 elevation application (*Fig.* 3.2) 49, 50–1
 infected 43
 leaving 43
 localization 45–6
 removal
  by forceps 43–4
  non-surgical 44–5
  in preparation for dentures 92
  surgical 45, 46–50
Fractures 21, 123, 318
 after large cyst removal 294
 apex 257
 cranial base 338
 jaw 21
 styloid process 332
 tuberosity 73
  maxillary 252–3
 with unerupted teeth removal 71
Frenectomy 98–9, 100
Frey's auriculotemporal syndrome 336
Fucidin 215

Gangrene 128
Garre's osteomyelitis 148
General practitioner, notification of operation to 26
Genial
 muscle mass, displacement downwards 108
 tubercles, removal of 107–8
Giant cell
 arteritis 340–1
 epulis 303, (*Fig.* 12.5) 304–5

Giant cell (*cont.*)
 granuloma 158, 274, 303–4, 310
Gingival
 cysts 274
 diffuse enlargements 305–7
 fibromatosis, hereditary 306–7
 granulomas, pyogenic 305
 hyperplasia 311
  drug-induced 305–6
Gingival margin
 avoided in outlining flap 29
 examination before removal of 3rd molar 53–4
 incision 28
 protection in impacted canine exposure 82
 suturing 93
Gingival mucoperiosteum, thick, retaining for denture support 93
Gingival swellings 297–307
Gingivectomy 306–7
Gingivitis
 pregnancy 303
 ulcerative 176
  Vincent's 125
Gingivostomatitis, herpetic 127
Glands, swollen salivary 330
Glaucoma, acute 332
Globulomaxillary cyst 271
Glossitis, median rhomboid 309–10
Glossodynia 328, 330
Glossopharyngeal neuralgia 332, 334
Glossopyrosis 329, 331
Gloves 10
 against infection 230–1
Gloving (*Figs.* 1.3–4) 22–3
Glucocorticoids 353–4
Glucose-6-phosphate dehydrogenase 361
Glutaraldehyde 232
Gorlin and Goltz syndrome 268
Gouges 15, 48
Gout 318–19
Gradenigo's syndrome 338
Grafting
 bone 115
 sandwich 115
 skin 21, 24, 114
Grafts, bone, in cyst enucleation and closure 293–4
Gram-negative bacteria 232–3
Granular-cell myoblastoma 305, 311
Granulation tissue, infected 111
Granuloma 109–10
 apical 255, 257
 denture-induced 299, (*Fig.* 12.2) 300–1

374

INDEX

Granuloma (cont.)
  giant cell 158, 274, 303–4, 311
  localized destructive 312
  malignant 312
  periapical 237, 244
  pregnancy (Fig. 12.4) 302–3, 306
  pulse 203
  pyogenic (Fig. 12.3) 301–3, 309
    of tongue 309
Gray's syndrome 214
Gum polyp 299
Gut 18–19

Haemangioma 148, 310
  capillary 305
  intramedullary cavernous 281
Haematoma 35–6, 148
  after suturing 77–8, 80
  postoperative 73
  prevention 110, 244
Haemoglobinopathies 361–2
Haemolysis 361
Haemophilus influenzae 212, 214
Haemorrhage 5
  postoperative 359
Haemostasis in lingual frenum excision 100
Halitosis, obsessional fear of 328–9
Halogens 233
Hamartoma, dental 305
Hands
  preparation 10
  scratched or cut 231
Head support for operation 23
Headache
  alarm clock 340
  Cluster 340
  see also Migraine
Heart disease
  congenital 222
  ischaemic 332
Heart valve
  disease 221
  prosthetic 222
Heparin injections 355–8
Hepatitis, viral 225
  accidents 227
  carriers 224–5
  immunity to 228
  infection from 224, 226–7
  instruments' sterilization or disinfection 228
  operative procedures 226–7

Heroin 346
Herpes simplex, ulcerating 229
Herpes zoster 194, 337
Herpetic gingivostomatitis 127
Hexachlorophane 233
Hibitane 221
Histamine cephalgia 340
Homosexuals 226, 229
Hooks, skin 18
Hopkins ridge augmentation 116, (Fig. 5.9) 117
Horizontally impacted teeth 56
Horten's syndrome 340
Hospital, discharge from 26–7
Hospitalization in soft tissue infection cases 169
Human skeletal growth factor (HSFG) 174
Hydrocortisone sodium succinate 353–4
Hydrogen peroxide injections 194
Hydroxylapatite
  blocks in bony ridge 116
  cones in sockets 111
  granules in subperiosteal pockets 116
  subperiosteal injection of particulate 97
Hygiene, oral 10
Hygienist, dental 26
Hyoid bone (Fig. 6.2e) 133
Hyoscine 348
Hyperaemia, reactionary 260
Hypercementosed molar roots 252
Hypercementosis 176
Hyperostosis, infantile cortical 204
Hyperparathyroidism, giant cell epulides in 304
Hyperplasia 307
  denture-induced 108–9, (Fig. 5.7) 109–10
  drug-induced gingival 305–6
  epanutin 306
  fibro-epithelial, of tongue 309
  gingival 311
  pseudoepitheliomatous 311
Hyperplastic
  candidiasis, chronic 310
  papilla 298
Hypertension 358–9
Hypertrichosis 306
Hypochlorites 233
Hypochondria 321
Hypochondriacal neurosis, monosymptomatique 329
Hypogammaglobulinaemia 129
Hypoglycaemia 349–52
Hypophysectomy 352

INDEX

Hypotensive agents 358–9
Hypothyroidism, impaction caused by 52
Hypovascularity 187
Hysteria 321

Ibuprofen 345
Idoxuridine 217
Impacted teeth 52
  canines, *see* Canines, impacted
  dentigerous cysts on 266
  molars
    1st and 2nd 87
    see also Molars, impacted mandibular *and* maxillary; Premolars
Impacted wisdom teeth, pain and 315
Impaction of teeth
  degree of 57
  disto-angular 56–7
  horizontal 56
  palatal 74
  vertical 56–7
Implant
  endodontic osseous 261–2
  procedures 118–19
Impressions 94–5
  with oroantral fistula 240
Incisions 28–31
  closing 35, 40
Incisive canal cysts 269–70
Incisive papilla cysts 270
Incisors
  dilacerated 89–90
  imbrication, 3rd molar eruption and 59
  lateral, abscesses arising from 161, (*Fig.* 6.19) 162
  malpositioned 88
    maxillary 88
  retained pulpless deciduous 52
  upper deciduous, trauma to 89
Inclusion cysts 271–2
Indomethacin 178
Infantile cortical hyperostosis 204
Infants
  non-accidental injury 205
  osteomyelitis 179
Inferior dental
  canal, damage during bone removal 58–9
  nerve, risk to during extraction 71
Inflammation, persistent 172
Inflammatory agents 174
Infraorbital lining, safeguarding in exposing antral lining 248

Infratemporal fossa 163, (*Fig.* 6.20) 164
Inhalations 244
Instruments (*Fig.* 1.1) 11–12, 11, 34–5
  bone-cutting 14–16
  for major surgery 20–1
  preparation 8
  sterilization 9
  suturing 17–18
Insulin injection 349
Interdental papillae, division of 28
  septa
    removal 94
    smoothing for dentures 93
Intermaxillary fixation 224–5
Interosseous wires at fracture site 115
Intracranial
  infection 166
  lesions 338
  neoplasms 333
Intratemporal fossa infection 164, (*Fig.* 6.21) 165–6
Iodine 233
Iodophors 233
Irradiation
  morbidity after 187–91
  therapy 176
Irrigation 16
  cavity 170
Ischaemia 187
Ischaemic
  heart disease 333
  necrosis in diabetic vasculopathy 338
Isoprenaline 360
Isopropyl 232

Jacobsen's nerve, intracranial section of 336
Jaw fractures 21
Jawbone, resistance to infection 174
Jaws, painful movement of 319
Joint
  primary organic disease 318–20
  replacement, patients 224
  temporomandibular functional disorders 320, 322–6
Juvenile rheumatoid arthritis 318

Kaposi sarcoma 231–2
Keratin pearls 271, 274
Keratocyst formation 72

INDEX

Keratocysts 263, 267–8, 271, 275–6, 278, 280–1, 284, 287, 292–3, 295
Ketosis 350
Knots
  infections from 41
  tying surgical 38, (*Fig. 2.1*) 39, 41

Labial flap, pyramidal 89
Labial frenum, excision of 98–9
Langhan's giant cell granuloma 158
Lateral pharyngeal
  abscess, differential diagnosis 154, (*Table* 6.1) 155
  space (*Fig. 6.13c*) 150, 152–3
Leucoplakia of oral mucosa 230
Light, operating 8
Lignocaine 13, 334
Lincomycin 215
Lingual
  flap retrctors 70
  frenum, excision of 100, (*Fig. 5.1*) 101
  lymphoid tissue 310
  nerve
    risk to during extraction 70
    safeguarding in incision 33
    pain 330
    thyroids 210
Lip, upper, infection (*Figs. 6.14–16*) 155–8
Lip chewing 323
Lipoma 148, 309
Lips, lubrication in major surgery 25
Lithium 360
Loose teeth, anaesthesia and 53
Ludwig's angina 128, 139 (*Figs. 6.8–9*) 140–2
  drainage 168
Lymph node enlargement 311
Lymphadenopathy (PGL) syndrome 229
Lymphangiomas 310
Lymphokine osteoclast activating factor (OAF) 174
Lymphoma 29, 203, 205

Malignant
  granuloma 312
  otitis externa 338
  tumours 318
  ulcers 330
Mallet 15
Malocclusion 323–4

Mandible
  arthritis following blow to 318
  blood supply 178
  cysts of 278, 290, 293
  median fissural 272
  potentially infected spaces related to 132, (*Figs. 6.2–7*) 133–9
  severe pain in left 332–3
  surgical access to 32
  see also Molar, impacted mandibular, removal
Mandibular
  abscess 144
  edentulous ridge, incision along 28
  molar, *see* Molar, impacted mandibular 3rd
  nerve fibres, division of 334
  retrognathism 320
  space infections 132–48, 149–55
  differential diagnosis 148–9
Marsupialization of cysts 276, 283, (*Figs. 11.2–3*) 283–4, 285–7
Masseter muscle 146–7
Mastication stresses, pain due to 319
Masticatory mucosa
  breach in 99
  stable 112
Maxilla
  gumma 195, (*Fig. 7.7*) 196
  potentially infected spaces (*Figs. 7.14–21*) 155–66
  surgical access to 33
Maxillary
  alveolar process, exposure of 28
  antrum 331–2
  cysts 278–9
    large 286, 290
    median alveolar 272
  impacted 3rd molar, *see* Molar, impacted maxillary
  incisors, malpositioned 88
  nerve fibres, division of 334
  pain 331
Maxillary sinus 236, 240
  irrigation 240
  periapical abscesses in relation to 163
  spontaneous expulsion of root from 250
  tooth or root displacement into 247–8
  removal of 248, (*Fig. 9.4*) 249–51
Maxillary sinusitis, acute 160
Maxillary supernumeraries 88–9
Maxillary tuberosities
  enlarged 100
  bony 100–2
  fibromatous 307

377

INDEX

Maxillary tuberosities (*cont.*)
  fibrous 102, (*Figs.* 5.2–3) 102–3
  fractured 252–3
Mefanamic acid 345
Melkersson–Rosenthal syndrome 312
Meningitis, post-traumatic 224
Meniscectomy 3220
Meniscus, anterior dislocation 325
Mental analgesia 318
Mental nerve
  damage in sulcus deepening 112
  injury by incision 32
  preservation during buccinator detachment 113
  syndromes, neuralgia from 334–5
Mental retardation, fibromatosis gingivae associated with 306
Mentally handicapped children 226
Mepivacaine 13
Merkerson–Rosenthal syndrome 158
Mesial caries A.A. (*Fig.* 6.1*b*) 122
Mesio-angular teeth, impacted 56–7
Mesiodens 87, 89
Metastatic carcinoma 318
Methyl morphine 345
Metoclopramide 349
Metronidazole 168, 175, 177, 180, 211–13, 215, 218, 220, 224–5
Miconazole 217
Microbiology 169–70
Microcysts 271
Midazolam 347–8
Migraine 315, 339–40
  dental 328
Migrainous neuralgia, facial 340
Mitchell's trimmer 17
Mitral valve prolapse 222
Molars
  2nd deciduous, premature extraction 52
  ankylosed 87
  buried deciduous 87
  impacted 1st and 2nd 87
Molars, impacted mandibular 3rd
  bone removal 62–3, 65
  diseased 59
  disto-angular, removal 65, (*Fig.* 4.3) 66
  elevation of 57–8, 61, 70
  examination 53–5
  horizontal, removal 67, (*Figs.* 4.6–7) 68–9
  mesio-angular, removal 65, (*Figs.* 4.4–5) 66–7
  orientation 55–6
  patient assessment 52–3

Molars (*cont.*)
  removal 52, 59–60
    anaesthesia 60
    bone density and 58
    complications 70
    envelope flap incision 61, (*Fig.* 4.1) 62
    flap suture after 69
    investigation prior to 60
    lubrication of retractors and elevators 61
    prophylactic 60
    radiological assessment 55–8
    socket toilet after 68
    split-bone technique 63, (*Figs.* 4.2–7) 64–9
    surgical technique 61–70
  root relationship to inferior dental canal 58–9
  root shape 57–8
Molars
  impacted maxillary 3rd, removal 71–3
  mandibular 3rd
    bleeding from 144
    displacement causing parapharyngeal infection 152
    pericoronitis associated with 125–6
  mandibular 4th 88
  maxillary 3rd, infections of 165
    abscesses involving 160–1
    extractions 236–7
    tuberosities, fibromatous enlargement of 308
  periapical infection 143
  removing palatal root of upper 44
  root
    amputation and sealing 260–1
    blind elevation of lower 3rd 45
    hypercementosed 252
  second, distal periodontal pocketing 71
  supernumerary teeth in region of 88–9
  unerupted maxillary 3rd removal, tuberosity fractured in 252
Monoamine oxidase inhibitors 324, 359–60
Monocyte cell factors (MCF) 174
Mononucleosis 125
Morphine 346, 349, 360
  methyl 345
Mouth
  lowering floor of 113, (*Fig.* 5.8) 114
  props 20
  substantial swelling of floor of 169
Mucoperiosteal flaps 30, 78–9
Mucoperiosteum, raising 33

INDEX

Mucosa radiopacity 235–6
Multiple sclerosis 339
Mumps 149, 330
Myelomatosis 311
Mylohyoid
  muscle (*Fig. 6.2d*) 133, (*Fig. 6.3*) 134,
  ridge resection 106, (*Fig. 5.6*) 107, 113,
  (*Fig. 5.8*) 114
Myoblastoma, granular cell 305, 311
Myofascial pain dysfunction syndrome
  322–6

Narcotic analgesics 345
Nasal furuncle 156
Nasolabial cysts 270–1, 280
Nasopalatine cyst 269–70, 280, 294–5
Nasopharyngeal
  carcinoma 337–8
  tumour 332
Needle holders 17, 36–7
Needles
  contaminated 151
  curved 36–7
  disposable 13
  half-circle cutting 80–1
  radium 191
  suturing 18, 36
Neomycin 213
Neoplasm
  intracranial 333
  malignant, 172
  upper lip 158
Neoplastic disease 205
Nerve avulsion 336
Neural morbidity in bony ridge augmentation
  116
Neuralgia
  atypical facial 326–8, 333, 336, 340
  glossopharyngeal 334
  mental nerve 335
  migrainous facial 340
  paroxysmal 319, 333, 343
    trigeminal 333
    in youth 339
  post-herpetic 337
  primary 333–4
  psychogenic atypical facial 332
  secondary 334–5
  splenopalatine 340
  trigeminal 315
  vidian nerve 340
Neurilemmomas 309
Neurinoma 309

Neurinoma (*cont.*)
  acoustic 338
Neuroblastoma 205
Neurofibroma 309
Neurofibromatosis, plexiform 309
Neurofibrosarcoma 309
Neuroleptanalgesia 347
Neuropathy, diabetic 336
Neuropraxia 70
Neurosis 321
Neurosis, mono-symptomatique
  hypochondriacal 329
Neurovascular bundle
  avulsion of inferior dental 336
  damage during bone removal 59
  division of 78
  preservation 33–4
  retarding cyst enlargement 278
Nibblers, bone 15
Nitrazepam 348
Noradrenaline 359
Nurses, postoperative care by 26
Nutrient vessels, thrombosis of 178
Nystatin 217

Occlusal trauma, repeated 121
Occlusion, examination prior to 3rd molar
  removal 54
Ocular abnormalities 268
Odontalgia, atypical 317, 326–8
Ododontogenic cyst 263, 265
  calcifying and keratinizing 268–9
Odontomes 123
  impaction against 52
Oedema 124, 126
  angioneurotic (*Fig. 6.16*) 157–8
  in cavernous sinus thrombophlebitis 166
  forehead 160
  gangrene due to 128
  glottis 141
  Ludwig's angina 142
  periodontal membrane 254
  periorbital 73
  postoperative 40
  quinsy 154
  radiopacity 235
  upper lip 158–9
Oestrogens 357–8
Omnopon 346
Operation site preparation 10–11
Operative procedures
  diabetics 351–2
  where corticosteroids given 353

INDEX

Ophthalmia neonatorum 179
Ophthalmoplegia 166
Opioids 360
  endogenous 343
Oral disease, prevention of 365–6
Oral mucosa, soft-tissue swellings of 297
Orientation of teeth 55–6
Oroantral fistula 73, 163, 236–9
  chronic 239–40
  closure of 241, (*Figs.* 9.1–3) 242–7
Orthognathic surgery 119
Osmotic theory of cyst enlargement 276
Osseous
  implants, endodontic 261–2
  integrated implants 118
  tumour 202
Osteitis
  acute alveolar 174–8
  alveolar 318
  localized 174
  petrous temporal 338
Osteoarthritis, temporomandibular joint 319–20, 333
Osteomycosis, chronic hypertrophic 199
Osteomyelitis, 71, 176, 178–80, 318
  actinomycotic 197, (*Fig.* 7.8) 198–9, 219
  acute 218
    pyogenic, of mandible 180, (*Figs.* 7.1–5) 181–4
  childhood 180
  chronic 185–7, 218
  cortical 201
  following submasseteric abscess 147–8
  Garre's 200
  infants' 179
  intramedullary 201
  involucrum of 174
  localized (*Fig.* 7.5) 184, 188, 197
  neoplastic simulations 205
  non-pyogenic 194–9
  non-suppurating sclerosing 200
  in osteopetrosis 201
  in Paget's disease 200
  sclerosing 196
  squestrectomy in 185
  subperiosteal 201
  syphilitic 194–5, 195
  tuberculous 196–7
  typhoid 197
Osteopetrosis 201
Osteoporosis 195
Osteoradionecrosis 187–9, (*Fig.* 7.6) 191–3, 216, 219
Osteotome 15

Osteotome (*cont.*)
  tooth splitting with 71
Osteotomy
  Hopkins sandwich 116, (*Fig.* 5.9) 117
  horizontal sandwich 116
  Le Fort I level, incision in 31
  Obwegeser–Dalpont sagittal split 193
  visor 115
Otitis externa 332
  malignant 338
Over-eruption of lower canine 83
Overdentures 110
Oxygen concentration 192

Pacemakers 223
Packing material 19
Paget's disease 176, 199, 338
  osteomyelitis in 200
Pain
  atypical facial 326–8
  bone 318
  control 343
    placebo response 343
    postoperative 26
  episodic 317
  eye region 332
  investigation 315
  maxillary 331
  orofacial 315
  patient's history of 315–17, 321
  psychogenic 315–16, 321–2, 326–7, 343
  relief 319–20
  sharp 316–17
  starting point 315
  treatment, empirical 315–16
  trigeminal 338
  vascular 339–41
Palatal
  access 33–4
  impaction 74
  mucoperiosteal flap 89
  mucoperiosteum 161
  mucosa
    graft 112
    plate protection 113
    swellings of 298, 307–9
  rotation flap, oroantral fistula closure by (*Fig.* 9.3) 246–7
  subperiosteal abscess 161, (*Fig.* 6.19) 162
  transposition flap, oroantral fistula closure by 244, (*Fig.* 9.2) 245–6
Palatine artery, division of 33

INDEX

Palatine cyst, median 271
Palsy, facial 312, 337
Papaveretum 346
Papilla, hyperplastic 299
Papilloma (*Fig.* 12.7) 308
Paracetamol 339, 344–5
Parapharyngeal
  abscess, differential diagnosis 154, (*Table* 6.1) 155
  space infection 152–3
Paratyphoid fever 197
Parotid
  fascia 130
  painful 331
  swellings 149
Paroxysmal neuralgia 319, 343
  in youth 339
Patient
  age of, teeth extraction and 52–3
  with arterial grafts 223
  assessment for surgery 52–3
  with cardiac transplants 224
  with chronic liver disease 226
  with coronary by-pass 223
  discharge from hospital 26–7
  discussion of difficult surgery with 261
  dying 347
  elderly 116–18
  extra-European 226
  family history 321
  follow-up arrangements 27
  general health 1
  high-risk, prophylactic regime 223
  history 1–2, 342
  of pain 314–16
  with joint replacement 224
  management of, in abscess cases 172–3
  multiple blood transfusions history 226
  oral hygiene instruction 10
  past medication 342
  postoperative care 25–6
  preparation 7
    for major surgery 20, 23–5
  preventive education 365–6
  smoker 357–8
  social history 322
  tattooed 226
Penicillin 210–11, 218
  allergy 212, 223, 364
Pentazocine 345–6
Peptic ulceration, aspirin contraindicated 344
Periapical
  abscess 257
  acute 121–5, 255

Periapical (*cont.*)
  osteomyelitis following 180, 200–1
  pus spreading from 146
  related to maxillary sinus 163
  cyst 255–7, 277, 279–80
  endodontic paste removal 262
  granuloma 237, 244
  infection
    molar 143
    soft-tisue infections due to 128
  lamina dura, loss of 254–5
  radiolucency 255
Pericoronal abscess 123
Pericoronitis 59–60, 72, 125–8, 151, 218, 265
  of 3rd molar 144
  acute, quinsy complicating 153
  submasseteric abscess due to 146
  ulcerative 127–8
Periodontal
  abscess
    acute 121, 123
    primary acute 317
  cyst 263, (*Fig.* 11.1) 264–7, 275–6, 278, 281
    apical 270–1, 277
      marsupialization (*Fig.* 11.3) 286
    developmental lateral 274–5
  disease, maxillary sinusitis due to 163
  membrane, oedema of 254
  pocketing 60, 71
Periodontalgia, idiopathic 327–8
Periodontitis 317–18, 327
Perioral tissues, incision in 34
Periosteal
  cyst 293
  damage during sulcus deepening 112
  elevators 13–14, 21, 29, 31, 35
  incision 32, 33–4
Periostitis 196, 201–3
  actinomycotic 219
  chronic 203
  ossificans 200
Peritonsillar
  abscess 153–4, 332
    differential diagnosis 154 (*Table* 6.1) 155
  space (*Fig.* 6.1*b*) 150
Perpenazine 349
Pethidine 345, 349
Petrous temporal osteitis 338
Phantom bite syndrome 328–9
Pharyngeal
  space
    abscess in lateral 131

381

INDEX

Pharyngeal (cont.)
  lateral (Fig. 6.13c) 150
  sucker 19
Pharynx, substantial swelling of side of 169
Phenacetin 361
Phenindione 355
Phenol injections 194
Phenolics 233
Phenoperidine 347
Phenothiazine 324, 329
Phenoxymethylpenicillin 210
Phenylephrine 360
Piperacillin 211
Pituitary tumours 339
Pizotifen 340
Plaque 300
Platybasia 338
Pneumatosis cystoides intestinales 263
Pneumocystis carinii Pneumonia (PCP) 229
Polymers, synthetic 36
Polymyalgia rheumatica 341
Polyp
  fibro-epithelial 300, (Fig. 12.6) 306–9
  gum 299
  pedunculated fibro-epithelial 300
  prolapsed 240
  pulp 299
  tongue 309
  vascular antral 302
Porphyria 361
Post-herpetic neuralgia 337
Posterior cranial fossa tumours 338
Postoperative
  bleeding 5
  care 25–6
  feeding 221
  infection 158, 218
  medication 348
  oedema 40
Poultices 167
Pregnancy
  ergotamine tartrate contraindicated in 340
  gingivitis 303
  granuloma 306
  tumour (epulis or granuloma) (Fig. 12.4) 302–3
  warfarin contraindicated 357
Premedication 347
Premolar region, supernumerary teeth in 88–9
Premolars
  impacted lower

Premolars (cont.)
  examination 84
  leaving in situ 86
  radiography 84
  removal 84–6
  impacted maxillary 86–7
  with inclined apices 86
Preoperative procedure 7–12
Pretracheal fascia 131
Prevertebral fascia 130
Prilocaine 13
Promethazine hydrochloride 348
Propionic acid derivatives 345
Proplast sponge in subperiosteal pockets 116
Prostaglandins 174
Prosthetic heart valve 222
  prophylactic regime 223
Proteus vulgaris 211
Pseudomonas aeruginosa 211, 213
Psoriasis 318
Psychogenic
  atypical facial neuralgia 332
  oral dysaesthesia 95
  pain 315–16, 321–2, 326–7, 343
  dysfunctional 322
Psychosis, hypochondriacal 329
Psychosomatic pain 322
Pterygomandibular space (Fig. 6.13) 150–1, (Fig. 6.20) 164
  abscess 151–2
    differential diagnosis 154, (Table 6.1) 155
  infection 151, (Fig. 6.21) 165
Pulmonary disease, emphysematous 192
Pulmonary embolism 357
Pulp
  infection, treatment 256–7
  infective necrosis of 121
  inflammation 254, 327
  necrosis 354–7
  pain 316–17
  polyp 299
Pulpitis, acute 163
Pus, sites of accumulation 131–2
Pyriform aperture wires 115

Quinsy 153–4, 332

Radiation caries 188–9
Radicular cysts 266–7

INDEX

Radiofrequency thermocoagulation 334
Radiographs
  cysts 278–80
  calcifying ododontic 269
  dry socket 177
  enlarged tuberosities 101–2
  impacted mandibular 3rd molar removal 55–6
  occlusal 54, 74–5, 202
  oroantral fistula 238–9
  osteomyelitis (*Figs.* 7.1–5) 181–4, 186–7
  osteoradionecrosis (*Fig.* 7.6) 191
  periapical 54–5, 74–5
  periostitis 202
  prior to extractions 92
  pulp infection 254
  sinusitis, 235–6
  of supernumeraries 88–9
  toothache 318
  unerupted premolar 84
  see also Tomography
Radiotherapy
  impaction caused by 52
  malignant granuloma 311
  morbidity after 187–91
  prophylaxis 189–91
Radium needles 191
Ramsay Hunt syndrome 337
Ramus
  cysts 293
  enlargement 149
  frame implant 119
  infection following submasseteric abscess 147–8
Record of major operation 25
Red cell abnormalities, hereditary 361
Resorption
  burrowing 96
  irregular 96–7
Respiratory
  failure 5
  tract infection 126
Restorations, loose or lost 316
Retractors 13
  double-ended 21
  lingual flap 70
  tongue 20–1
Retrognathism, mandibular 320
Reye's syndrome, aspirin in causation 344
Rheumatic valvular disease 222
Rhinitis, allergic 235
Rhinitis, non-allergic vasomotor 326
Ribbon gauze 19
Rongeurs, bone-cutting 15

Root
  antrolith mistaken for 251
  displacement into antrum 248, 250–1
  filling
    faulty 256–6
    preoperative 282, (*Fig.* 11.6) 291
  fractured, removal in preparation for dentures 92
  hypercementosed 73
  residual, *see* Fractured root
  resorption 75–6
  retained, dentures and 96
  retention
    accidental 111
    deliberate 110–11
    giant cell epulis related to (*Fig.* 12.5) 304
  pain and 315
  sections, intracranial 336
  shape 57
  spontaneous expulsion from maxillary sinus 250
Root-canal therapy 173
Roots, separation of 48, (*Fig.* 3.2*d*) 49
Rotation of teeth, supernumeraries causing 88
Rubella immunization, arthritis reaction to 318
Rugines 35

Salivary
  fistula 172
  glands
    swollen 330
    tumours 331
  sand 329
Salmonella 197, 214
Sandwich grafting 115
Sarcoid 311–12
Sarcoma 148
  Ewing's 205
  Kaposi 231
Scalpel 13–14, 21
Schwannoma 309, 338
Scissors 18
  dissecting 21
  suturing 17–18
Sclerosants 194
Sclerosis, disseminated 333, 339
Scrub technique 21–2
Sedation 347–8
  night 348–9

INDEX

Self-inflicted lesions 329
Serum sickness 365
Sialoadenitis 218, 331
Sickle cell
　anaemia 361
　crisis 318
　disease 194, 362–3
　trait, 362–3
Sinus
　excision 172
　formation 170 (*Fig.* 6.22) 171–2
　see also Maxillary sinus
Sinusitis 163, 220, 235–6
　acute 331
　chronic 326, 331
　maxillary 235
　　acute 160
Sjögren's disease 149, 329
Skin graft 21
　periosteal 114
　sites
Skin hooks 18
Skin incisions 21
Skin rashes 365
Skull fractures 224
Sluder's syndrome 340
Smoking 357, 358
Social history 2
Socket
　dressing 177–8
　dry 174–6, 318
　infection 71, 176
　rocking to expand 92
　suppurative infection of 71
　suturing gingival margins 93
　toilet 68
Soft tissue
　abscesses, use of heat in 167
　infection
　　hospitalization with 168
　　management 218
　　spreading 128–31
　swellings of 311–12
　see also Swellings
Splenopalatine neuralgia 340
Splinting, fractured tuberosity 253
Splints 21, 115, 190
Split bone technique 57
　for impacted mandibular 3rd molar
　　removal 63, (*Figs.* 4.2–7) 64–9
Split skin graft in sulcus deepening
　　112–13
Split tooth 316
　latent 327
Staphylococci 128

Staphylococcus aureus 178–9, 180,
　　211–12, 215, 232–3
　penicillin resistant 209
Staple implants 118–19
Sterilization 8–9
　dry heat 9
　following viral hepatitis surgery 228
Steroids 353–5
　intra-articular 320
Still's disease 318
Streptococcus viridans 123, 216, 221–2
Streptomycin sulphate 213
Stress 321, 324, 329
Students 5
　errors 22–3
Styloid process, elongated 332
Sublingual space (*Fig.* 6.6) 137
　infections 138, (*Figs.* 6.7–8) 139–40
Submandibular space (*Fig.* 6.3) 134
　infections 134–5, (*Figs.* 6.4–5) 136–7
Submasseteric
　abscess 146, (*Fig.* 6.12) 147
　infections
　　differential diagnosis 148–9
　　treatment 149–50
　space 145
　swellings 148
Submental
　sinus (*Fig.* 6.22) 171
　space infections 132, (*Fig.* 6.2)
　　133
Submucosal dissections 112
Subperiosteal
　implants 118, 123
　new bone formation 148
　osteomyelitis 201
Suction 8
　tips 19
　tubes 19
Sulcoplasty 115–16
Sulcus
　deepening 111–13, 115
　mucosa folds 99
Sulcus tissue
　incisions in 30
　unerupted canine in 82
Sulphadiazine 216, 224
Sulphonamides 177, 208, 216, 361
　allergy 364
Supernumerary teeth 87–9
　anterior maxillary 89
　extraction 88–9
　inverted palatally placed 88
Suppurative infection 128
Surgeon, preparation of 8

384

INDEX

Surgery 4–7
  contraindications 53
  difficult 261
  elderly patients and 117–18
  major 19–27
  record 25
  oral contraceptive before 357–8
  orthognathic 119
  preparation 20, 23, 220
  under local anaesthetic 7
Surgical repositioning of displaced tooth 83
Surgicel 356
Suture scars 40
Suture-cutting scissors 18
Sutures
  absorbable 37, 41
  atraumatic 36
  braided 37
  buccal advancement flap 243
  continuous 40–1
    horizontal mattress 31
  envelope flap 69
  interrupted 40
  materials for 18–19, 36–7
  mattress 41
  polyglactin 36, 113
  removal 41–2, 69
  resorbable 113
  under tension 30–1
Suturing 35, 37–8, (*Fig.* 2.1) 39–42
  instruments 17–18
  sulcus tissue adhesion due to 71
  while bleeding continues 77, 80
Swabs 19, 25
Swellings
  buccal mucosa 298, 307–9
  floor of mouth or side of pharynx 169
  gingival 297–307
  oral mucosa 297–8
  palatal mucosa 298, 307–9
  tongue 298, 309–11
Sydenham's chorea 222
Sympathectomy, cervical 336
Syphilis 187
  acquired 195, (*Fig.* 7.7) 196
  neonatal 195
Syphilitic osteomyelitis 194–5
Syringes 16
  local anaesthetic 12–13

Taste abnormallities 328
Temgesic 346

Temporal arthritis 340–1
Temporomandibular joint
  arthritis, traumatic 318–19
  arthrography 325
  dysfunction syndrome 322–6
  functional disorders 320
  osteoarthritic 319–20, 333
  surgery 336
Tetanus 231–2
Tetracycline 177, 209, 213–14, 218
Thalassaemia 363–4
Thermocoagulation, radiofrequency 334
Thrombo-embolism 357
Thrombophlebitis 129, 148
  cavernous sinus 166
  due to upper lip infection 156
  injection site 347–8
  in soft tissue infection 153, 160
Thrombosis
  apical 254
  deep vein 355, 356–7
  nutrient vessels 178
  vasa nervorum 318
Thyroid, lingual 210
Tic douloureux 333, 335, 339
Ticarcillin 211
Tinnitus 322, 344
Tissue
  dividing 35
  space abscess 173
Tissue-dissection scissors 18
Titanium screw-type implants 118
Tomography
  rotational 55, 75, 84, 92
  unerupted upper 3rd molars 72
Tongue
  burning 328
  carcinoma of 330
  pain 330
  retractors 20
  swellings of 298, 309–11
Tongue-tie 100
  in edentulous patient 100, (*Fig.* 5.1) 101
Tonsils, painful 332
Tooth, lack of vitality 256
Toothache 317
Torus 103–5
  lingual 105
  mandibularis 105, (*Fig.* 5.5) 106
  palatinus, removal 103, (*Fig.* 5.4) 104–5
Towels, in major surgery preparation 25
Tracheostomy 221
  in Ludwig's angina 142

INDEX

Traumatic temporomandibular arthritis 318–19
Treatment, selection of 6
Treponema pallidum 194–5
Tricyclic antidepressants 359–60
Trigeminal
  nerve compression 334
  neuralgia 315
  pain 338
  paroxysmal neuralgia 333
Trolley, surgical 12
Trotter's syndrome 337
Tubercles, genial, removal of 107–8
Tuberculosis 187
Tuberculous osteomyelitis 196–7
Tuberosity
  fibromatous enlargement of 307
  fractured maxillary 252–3
  fragments 73
Tumour
  in edentulous jaws 96
  osseus 202
Typhoid fever 197

Ulcer
  malignant 330
  pressure 95
Ulceration
  factitious 329
  peptic, aspirin contraindicated 344
Ulcerative gingivitis, acute 176
Ultrasound, reducing postoperative morbidity 70
Unerupted 3rd molar, extraction, tuberosity fractured in 252
Unerupted canine
  extraction 76–81
  leaving in situ 81
  radiological examination 74–5
  reasons for removing 75–6
  surgical exposure 81–2
  transplantation 82–3
Unerupted mandibular premolars 84, 86
Unerupted teeth 52
  cyst enucleation and 295
  dentigerous cysts on 266
  dentures and 96
  displacement into antrum 247
  removal of permanent 90

Unerupted teeth (*cont.*)
  supernumeraries causing 88
  transplantation 82
Uveitis 310

Vancomycin 215–16, 223
Vascular disease, ergotamine tartrate contraindicated in 340
Vascular pain 339–41
Vasoconstriction
  in apicectomy 258, 260
  excessive 175
Vasoconstrictors, felypressin 241
Vasomotor rhinitis, non-allergic 326
Vertically orientated teeth, impacted 56–7
Vicryl 18–19
Vidian nerve neuralgia 340
Vincent's organisms, ulcerative pericoronitis due to 127–8
Vincent's ulcerative gingivitis 125
Von Recklinghausen's neuro-fibromatosis 309

Warfarin 355–7
  contraindicated drugs 356
Washing 10
  of patients 24
Wegener's granulomatosis 312
Wire cutters, theatre 21
Wiring kit 21
Wisdom teeth
  impacted
    covered by denture 60
    mandibular 3rd molar and 53
  removal of partly erupted 60
Wisdom tooth, displacement into antrum 73
Wounds
  alveolar 30
  infection of moist unhealed 221

Yaws 187, 196

Z-plasty 99–100
Zovirax cream 217

Part Two

PREFACE

THIS *Outline of Oral Surgery* is written as a guide for postgraduate and senior undergraduate students and for practitioners with a special interest in oral surgery. It is not intended as a textbook for the established consultant in the speciality, for in a book of this size it is impossible to consider the subject in the necessary detail.

The field of oral surgery covers a wide range of topics and in a work of this nature it is impossible to discuss the entire speciality. Space has therefore been devoted to the more important aspects of oral surgery, but even so it has been necessary to divide the work into two volumes. Although these two books are complementary, each volume is more or less complete in itself. Part I is mainly devoted to the practical aspects of minor oral surgery and should be of value to all dental practitioners who perform surgery, while Part II deals with the needs of the dental surgeon working in a hospital.

At the request of the publisher, fractures of the mandible and middle third of the facial skeleton have not been discussed as these subjects have been dealt with elsewhere in the Dental Practitioner Handbook series, and illustrations have been cut to a minimum in order to reduce costs.

It is the authors' sincere hope that this *Outline of Oral Surgery* will be of help to students preparing for undergraduate final examinations and for higher examinations in dentistry.

H.C.K.
February, 1975　　　　　　　　　　　　　　　　　　　　　　　　G.R.S.
L.W.K.

CONTENTS

Chapter		Page
I.	The Case History	1
II.	Clinical Examination of a Patient with a Pain, a Lump, or an Ulcer	5
III.	Some Additional Examinations carried out when Investigating a Lesion	12
IV.	The Differential Diagnosis of Swellings of the Neck	24
V.	Skin Incisions in Oral Surgery	36
VI.	The Management of Haemorrhage in Oral Surgery	40
VII.	Some Non-malignant Lesions in and around the Jaws	60
VIII.	Benign Soft-tissue Cysts	81
IX.	Giant-cell Lesions of the Jaws	89
X.	The Odontogenic Tumours and Odontomes	99
XI.	Histiocytosis 'X' and Malignant Granuloma	116
XII.	Some Premalignant Conditions of the Oral Cavity	121
XIII.	The Clinical Diagnosis of Oral Malignancy	129
XIV.	The Treatment of Malignant Neoplasms	135
XV.	Some Methods used in the Surgical Correction of the Jaws in Cases of Facial Deformity	148
XVI.	The Replacement of Bone	184
XVII.	Some Skeletal Diseases of Interest to the Oral Surgeon	195
XVIII.	The Major Salivary Glands	216
XIX.	Diseases of the Temporomandibular Joint	232
XX.	Nerve Injuries of Interest to the Oral Surgeon	245
XXI.	Some Non-pyogenic Infections of the Soft Tissues	250
XXII.	The Fungal Diseases	254
XXIII.	The Management of some of the Foreign Bodies seen in and around the Jaws	261
	Index	269

ACKNOWLEDGEMENTS

THE authors' sincere thanks are due to Miss B. Richardson, of the Eastman Dental Hospital for much painstaking work in arranging and typing the manuscript of the first edition. We are also grateful to Mrs. B. Rayiru and Mrs. A. McMahon for typing and arranging the revised reprint. We should like to thank Miss P. Burgess, of the Photographic Department of the London Hospital, and Mr. J. Morgan, of the Photographic Department of the Eastman Dental Hospital, for their skilled photography. The illustrations *Figs.* 27, 28, and 29 are by Professor G. Seward and his co-authors are sincerely grateful. *Figs.* 14, 15, and 16 were originally published in *The Dental Practitioner and Dental Record* (**18,** 83–98, 1967), and the authors would like to thank John Wright and Sons Ltd., Bristol, for permission to reproduce them. *Figs.* 38, 39, 40, and 41 were published in *Oral Surgery, Oral Medicine and Oral Pathology* (**25,** 670–678, 1968, and **25,** 810–816, 1968), and we should like to thank the C. V. Mosby Co., St. Louis, for permission to include them. *Figs.* 9 and 10 were published in the *British Journal of Oral Surgery* (**3,** 36–47, 1965) and *Fig.* 32 was published in the same journal (**5,** 99–105, 1967), and the authors are indebted to E. & S. Livingstone Ltd., Edinburgh, for permission to use them.

Finally, we should like to express our sincere thanks to Mr. L. G. Owens, B.Sc., Publishing Director of John Wright of Bristol, for inviting us to write this work and for his great help and guidance in its preparation.

AN OUTLINE OF ORAL SURGERY, PART II

Chapter I
THE CASE HISTORY

THE art of taking an accurate case history is probably the most important single step in the diagnosis of a medical or surgical condition. Sometimes the disorder may be diagnosed from the history alone as many diseases have a characteristic story, but in every instance valuable diagnostic clues can be obtained and these leads may be followed up during the actual physical examination of the patient.

A case history may be divided into the following sections:—
1. The patient's name, age, occupation, address, and the address of his doctor and dental surgeon.
2. The nature of the complaint in the patient's own words.
3. The family history.
4. Personal or social history.
5. History of past diseases.
6. History of the present illness.

The order in which the information is obtained and recorded can vary due to personal preference, for example the history of the present illness may be placed after the complaint and before the family history, etc.

If the case to be examined falls within the province of the dental surgeon, it is unnecessary to consider each of the sections in the detail that a consultant physician would employ, but the same general scheme of history-taking should be followed and the detail may be adapted to the dental surgeon's requirements.

1. The importance of taking the patient's name, age, address, and doctor's address is too obvious to be commented upon. The patient's occupation is always of great interest and if it involves work with such substances as lead, mercury, arsenic, bismuth, etc., it may furnish a valuable clue to what might otherwise be an obscure oral condition. In this respect it is always worth while finding out exactly what people do at their place of employment. For instance, a worker in a lead paint factory may be engaged on clerical duties well away from any possible contamination.

2. The Complaint.—The nature and duration of the presenting symptoms should be considered briefly under this heading. Sometimes the patient will complain of several separate symptoms, in which case they should be listed, but with the major complaint first. Ask the patient: (*a*) 'What seems to be the main trouble?', (*b*) 'How long have you had this complaint?'

The nature of the complaint and its duration should be recorded in the patient's own words, but be careful to avoid using the patient's own diagnosis, i.e., neuralgia, sinus trouble, etc. Such diagnoses are usually incorrect and may lead the clinician astray. Re-frame the question and discover exactly what the patient does complain about, i.e., 'pain on the left side of the face which has been present for two months'. The complaint, therefore, represents the headings for the more detailed history of the present illness.

3. Family History.—The physician is interested in the health and medical history of all near relatives of the patient: the grandparents, parents, brothers, sisters, and any children. The wife or husband is, of course, not a blood relation, but their health may be relevant because of its impact on the spouse or perhaps because the illness may be infectious. If any member of the family is dead, the age at the time of death and the cause of the death are of importance. It is wise to inquire after all members of the family in turn. Often patients will assure you that there is no one ill in the family, and on further questioning it will be found that several members of the family have died from tuberculosis or some other disease.

Long or short lives, mental instability, epilepsy, migraine, high blood-pressure, diabetes, and some malignancies are sometimes found to occur in certain families, while in well-known hereditary diseases such as haemophilia, and some congenital abnormalities, a study of the relatives is essential for the establishment of a diagnosis.

The state of the health of the patient's children or a history of miscarriage or sterility may furnish valuable clues to such diseases as congenital syphilis. Much information in the family history is irrelevant, but some of the facts obtained may furnish conclusive evidence for a diagnosis.

The oral surgeon is interested in the family history in such conditions as haemophilia and congenital anomalies such as clefts of the lip or palate, congenital syphilis, emotional instability, etc.

Too much time should not be spent upon this part of the history, but only experience of case history taking will enable the clinician to decide whether it will prove a fruitful source of relevant information. Inquiry into the family history should never be omitted.

4. Personal History.—This part of the history enables the physician to build up a picture of the patient's background and much valuable information can be obtained by systematically covering the patient's entire life. The impact of the patient's disease and its treatment on his own life, his work, and the well-being of his family should be discovered.

a. School life: Did he play organized games? (Conditions such as congenital heart disease preclude normal activity at this age.) What was his age on leaving? What standard of education was reached?

b. Occupation: Here the physician wants to know the exact type of work in which the patient engages. Is he exposed to physical or mental strain? Is he exposed to weather or to noxious elements such as chemicals, dust, or fumes? Does he work with X-rays? Does he work long hours? Does he stick to one job or has he tried many? Does he like his work? These last two questions may give some clue as to the patient's mental state and give some idea whether the condition which is troubling him is of psychosomatic origin.

Every dental surgeon knows the difficult patient with the obscure pains or temporomandibular joint trouble. These symptoms may sometimes represent an escape mechanism.

c. Recreation: Does he take regular exercise? i.e., a man who plays football every weekend is probably a good risk for an out-patient general anaesthetic, etc.

d. Habituation to drugs: Few patients seen are drug addicts in the generally accepted sense of the expression, but many people habitually take sleeping tablets, tonics, or laxatives, or consume large quantities of alcohol. Many mysterious allergic rashes can be traced to such a source and excessive alcohol may lead to a vitamin-B deficiency, for alcoholics obtain their calorie requirements from the alcohol and do not feel the need for additional food.

e. Environment: The effect of a patient's home conditions on his general health cannot be over-emphasized and it is also of interest to know whether he lives in the town or the country.

f. Meals: Is he eating an adequate quantity of suitable food? Has he any food fads which might lead to a deficiency in the diet? Most patients will say that they have a normal diet. If there is a possibility of some deficiency disease being present, it is as well to ask the patient to describe the meals eaten during a typical day, and judge for yourself.

g. Holidays: Does he take regular holidays? Many symptoms can be ascribed to overwork and to too little time off.

h. Has he lived abroad? Could the condition be due to some tropical disease? Air travel increases the possibility of tropical disease being seen in countries where such conditions were previously unknown.

i. Worries: Has the patient either financial or domestic problems and what is his attitude to these worries? Does he think he is suffering from a serious disease such as cancer? It is always a good plan to ask the patient what he thinks is wrong with himself.

It may take both time and tact to elicit the relevant information. A proper rapport needs to be established before the patient will confide in the clinician. The key to an otherwise inexplicable problem may not be revealed until the patient has been seen several times.

5. Previous Diseases.—Inquire of the patient what *diseases*, *operations*, or *accidents* he has sustained and list them in chronological order. Always give the dates and do not write 'three years ago', etc.

Never accept the patient's diagnosis such as neuralgia, rheumatism, etc. Get him to describe the symptoms and judge for yourself.

Pay attention to time spent in hospital, what treatment was given, and whether the patient made a full recovery. Some diseases, such as rheumatic fever or chorea, are more likely to have left severe sequelae when the case has not been dealt with seriously, rather than when a history of strict bed-rest in hospital is obtained.

Patients often dismiss past illness in a light-hearted fashion. Put your questions as to illness in several ways. Have you ever been ill? Have you ever been under the doctor? Have you ever been in hospital? If you draw a blank on all these questions, ask incredulously, 'Have you *never* had anything the matter with you at all?' Occasionally the patient will then grudgingly admit that he had a bit of a touch of the rheumatic fever for a month or so, but never had anything *he* really calls an illness!

Direct questioning is often necessary to obtain a history of disease which the patient feels carries with it a social stigma, such as venereal disease or mental illness.

6. History of the Present Complaint.—This part of the story must be gone into in complete detail. It is best to start by asking, 'When were you last completely fit?', and then get the patient to tell the story in his own fashion. Never ask leading questions, for some patients are very suggestible and can readily be talked into a whole series of new symptoms. Ask what was the first thing that he noticed wrong. What other symptoms have occurred? What seems to be the main trouble now? What makes it better or worse? What treatment has he had and does it help? How much does this trouble incapacitate him (her)? What does the patient think he is suffering from?

Finally, ask about—Appetite, Weight, Bowel habits, Micturition, Sleep. And whether the patient has: Shortness of breath, Cough, Chest pain, Swollen ankles.

And whether any of these have been altered in any way since the onset of the illness.

If the patient is female, ask about menstruation. Menstrual history is recorded as 13 5/28 etc., that is,

$$\text{Age of onset in years} \; \frac{\text{Length of period in days}}{\text{Length of time between periods in days}}$$

The clinician must always consider whether the patient is a good witness and whether his statements can be relied upon. He will soon learn to assess such characters as the hysteric who sits back with a happy smile and describes his excruciating pains and unbearable sufferings.

Time spent in taking a case history is always well spent and the more skilled the physician or surgeon, the more time will he devote to this part of the examination. When the case history has been competently taken, the clinician is well on the way to a correct diagnosis before he even begins the actual physical examination of the patient.

When writing the patient's case notes or preparing a case history for publication, the facts should be recorded under the headings and in the order already listed. However, when interrogating a patient it is prudent to discuss the history of the present illness immediately after ascertaining the nature of the patient's complaint. The conversation then naturally leads on to the history of past diseases, personal history, and finally the family history. This is a matter of common sense, for a patient who is anxious to explain all about his illness is unlikely to see the relevance of explaining why his grandparents died. Taking the case history in this manner has the added advantage that when the family history is eventually discussed, the clinician will know whether it has any special relevance to the case under discussion.

CHAPTER II

CLINICAL EXAMINATION OF A PATIENT WITH A PAIN, A LUMP, OR AN ULCER

AFTER an accurate case history has been taken, the clinical examination is carried out. This consists of:—
 1. A general physical examination of the patient.
 2. A local examination of the lesion which carefully elicits all its clinical characteristics.

The majority of the patients who consult an oral surgeon complain of either a pain, a lump, or an ulcer. Each of these conditions have their own special characteristics which must be carefully elucidated by the clinician.

PAIN

Pain is a subjective symptom and unlike a lump or an ulcer which can be examined and assessed, in the case of a pain the clinician must rely on the description given by the patient. In the case of a pain, therefore, the history is of paramount importance. Careful consideration of the description of the pain frequently suggests the likely cause and the likely site of the cause. The clinician will direct his examination accordingly. With the account of a pain may go a story of associated phenomena—facial swelling, discharge, anaesthesia or muscular weakness, for example. The physical signs relevant to these complaints should also be sought at the examination.

There are ten questions which must be asked about any pain:—

1. Its Character.—Pains may be described as dull, sharp, throbbing, burning, etc. Patients with pain of psychosomatic origin often give bizarre descriptions of the pain, likening it to icy cold, red hot, or feathers running up and down their face, etc.

2. The Severity.—Owing to the varying degrees of pain threshold in different individuals, the intensity of a pain is difficult to ascertain accurately, for agony to one patient may be described as moderately severe by another. Relief afforded by a mild analgesic drug such as aspirin 300–900 mg. is a helpful indication of the degree of severity, for a pain which can be adequately controlled by a low potency analgesic preparation is not particularly severe. If more powerful analgesics such as pethidine 50–100 mg. are required to assuage the pain its severity must be correspondingly worse.

Interference with sleep is also a reliable guide to a pain's severity, for if the patient's sleep is not disturbed the pain cannot be too severe. Patients with pain of psychosomatic origin always exaggerate the pain and describe it as unendurable agony, but smile happily as they describe their symptoms. They usually complain of inability to eat or sleep, but invariably appear well rested and nourished. The patient's G.P. may well be helpful in providing background information about the patient. Great caution must be exercised before labelling a pain as psychosomatic in origin and even after such a diagnosis has been made, the patient should still be treated with great sympathy and understanding. The pain might be imaginary to the clinician but it is real enough to the patient.

3. Date of Onset.—The date of onset of a pain is of great importance and while most pains are of recent onset some may have been present for years. The likelihood of finding a previously unsuspected cause where the pain has been present for many years tends to be poor. Conversely the disease is clearly not of serious prognosis or progressive if the symptoms have remained unchanged over a long period of time.

4. Is the Pain Continuous or have there been Remissions?—Pain is seldom absolutely continuous, for even the most excruciating pains are relieved by occasional short remissions. Most patients with pain of psychosomatic origin describe it as continuous without any remissions.

5. Is it Increasing or Decreasing in Severity?—A pain which is increasing in severity will obviously require urgent investigation while a pain which is rapidly improving may allow a certain degree of procrastination on the part of the clinician. Of course, sometimes the pain persists at a uniform level.

6. Where is the Point of Maximum Intensity?—The most satisfactory method of ascertaining the point of maximum intensity of a pain is to get the patient to point to where it hurts most!

7. Area to which Pain spreads.—The pain usually spreads from the point of maximum intensity to involve the surrounding area to a greater or lesser extent. For instance, pain from an abscess on an upper canine may be most intense over the apex of the canine, but the entire side of the face may ache at the same time.

8. Area to which the Pain radiates.—The area to which a pain radiates is of considerable diagnostic significance. For example, the pain of coronary thrombosis is substernal, but the pain characteristically radiates down the left arm. In the mouth, pain from a carcinoma of the side of the tongue spreads to the ear on the same side and pains from infected lower 3rd molars often radiate in the same way. It must not be forgotten that pain in the mouth may be referred from one jaw to the other on the same side. In some cases the whole pain is ascribed by the patient to the site of radiation, so that the question of a referred pain should also be considered.

Hysterical subjects and other patients with pain of psychosomatic origin often describe pains radiating to areas to which it would be anatomically impossible. For instance, they may state that the pain radiates across the midline to involve the opposite side of the jaw.

9. What makes the Pain Worse?—Much useful information can be obtained by ascertaining what makes the pain worse or what aetiological factors are involved. For example, the excruciating pain of trigeminal neuralgia may be triggered off by a light touch on the face, while other pains are described as occurring when the patient is tired or worried. Pains which are produced when hot or cold drinks or foods are taken usually point to a purely dental origin. The pain of acute maxillary sinusitis is frequently exacerbated by biting, bending, lifting, straining, and by jarring movements.

10. Are there other Symptoms?—Local ones such as intra- and extra-oral swelling, discharge, bad taste, halitosis, discomfort on swallowing, and interference with mastication.

When the clinician has accurate information concerning the ten points enumerated in this examination, the pain can usually be accurately described and its possible aetiology ascertained.

Another way to prepare to examine a patient for the cause of a pain is to decide:—

1. The Nerve Involved.—In oral surgery it is usually the trigeminal, with the exception of pain over the angle of the mandible which may involve the great auricular, pain at the back of the tongue or in the throat which may be glossopharyngeal, or pain in the lower jaw associated with a tightness in the chest which may be cardiac in origin.

2. Whether the Pain is Peripheral, Proximal, Intracranial, or Intracerebral in Origin or whether it conforms to None of these Patterns.—If the cause is peripheral only one branch of the nerve will be involved.

If the cause is proximal, more than one branch will be involved; possibly more than one division, though this is uncommon.

If the cause is intracranial, more than one division may be involved and in advanced lesions there may be signs of a rise in intracranial pressure.

If the cause is intracerebral then there may be neurological deficits to be demonstrated on the other side of the body, due to involvement of the long tracts.

If the pain is due to trigeminal or glossopharyngeal neuralgia, Horton's syndrome, or is hysterical, it will not conform properly to any of the patterns.

3. The Pathological Process to be looked for.—Pain due to pulp disease or its sequelae is at some stage in its evolution intermittent and altered by hot and cold stimuli and the causative tooth becomes tender to bite on late in the course of the attack.

Pain due to gingivitis and periodontal abscesses tends to be constant and soreness or a tender tooth appears early on. A periodontal type of pain with a swollen cheek and limitation of opening suggests pericoronitis of a 3rd molar. Bilateral maxillary pain, pain and tenderness involving several maxillary teeth, and supra-orbital headache suggest sinusitis. If there is epiphora or a blood-stained discharge, carcinoma of the maxilla should be considered. Temporomandibular joint pain can radiate across either mandible or maxilla, but is often associated with a click in the joint or limitation of opening without swelling. Trigeminal neuralgia and Horton's syndrome have a characteristic pain pattern and negative findings on examination.

The Examination of a Lump

Before carrying out a local physical examination of any lump or mass it is essential to ascertain:—

1. How long the swelling has been present.
2. Whether it is getting larger.
3. Whether there is any possible cause for the swelling, i.e., trauma, etc.

As far as the local examination of the lump is concerned, the most important facts to ascertain are as follows:—

1. The Exact Anatomical Situation of the Mass.—Lumps may arise from skin, subcutaneous tissues, muscle, tendon, nerve, bone, blood-vessels, or an organ, and if the examiner is unable to ascertain the exact structure from which the mass arises then any attempt at differential diagnosis is likely to prove grossly inaccurate. For example, a swelling at the angle of the mandible may appear to originate from the hard tissues and the clinician will consider the possibility of a cyst, ameloblastoma, etc., when, in fact, the lump is arising from the soft tissues and is, indeed, a sarcoma of the masseter muscle.

Deciding the exact anatomical location of any mass or swelling is probably the most important single step taken in the physical examination and diagnosis of a lump.

2. Are the Associated Lymph-nodes Enlarged?—Whenever a lump or mass is examined, careful palpation of the associated lymph-nodes must be carried out. This important step must never be omitted. In fact, in the clinical investigation of an oral lesion, it is prudent to examine the cervical nodes first before inspecting the mouth, lest this vital stage in the local physical examination be overlooked once the clinician becomes engrossed by the findings in the oral cavity. The tender enlarged lymph-nodes associated with an inflammatory process are readily differentiated from the rock-hard nodes of a metastasizing malignancy.

3. Is the Swelling Single or Multiple?
4. The Shape and
5. The Size of any mass which is readily discernible.
6. The Surface of the Mass.—The surface of a mass may be smooth, lobulated, or irregular.
7. The Edge.—The edge of a lump may be clearly defined or diffuse, fading into the surrounding tissues as do most lumps or masses of inflammatory origin.

8. The Consistency.—The consistency of lumps or masses is defined surgically as *soft*, as in the case of the lipoma; *firm*, which is the consistency of a fibroma; *cartilage hard*, as in the pleomorphic adenoma; *bony hard*, as exemplified by the osteoma; *rock hard*, as seen in malignant lymphatic nodes; *rubbery hard*, which is the classic description of the consistency of the affected nodes in Hodgkin's disease. These descriptions of the consistency of lumps are surprisingly helpful and have been used by countless generations of surgeons.

9. Is the Lump Tender or Warm on Palpation?—Tenderness on gentle palpation is a valuable physical sign, for while it can be elicited with inflammatory lumps, neoplasms are commonly painless unless they just happen to be secondarily infected. The site of an acute inflammation is usually warmer than the adjoining areas.

10. Is the Lump Attached to the Skin?—During the physical examination of a lump an attempt should be made to move the skin over the lump to ascertain if the skin is tethered to it. The skin overlying an abscess may be fixed firmly to the inflammatory mass and a similar condition may occur with superficial malignancies. Of the benign lesions, the sebaceous cyst is characteristically tethered to the skin by the punctum of the sebaceous gland from which it arises.

11. Care must be taken to ascertain whether the Lump arises from Deeper Structures.—Can the overlying tissues move separately from it in any way. It is frequently helpful to get the patient to tense adjacent muscles to see whether the lesion is attached to them. In the differential diagnosis of a swelling at the angle a soft mass partly within a muscle may be extruded during contraction and regress into the muscle again as it relaxes.

12. Is Fluctuation Present?—Fluctuation is a valuable physical sign indicating the presence of fluid within a lump. It is elicited by placing the tips of two fingers on the lump. When pressure is applied to the mass with one finger, a transmitted upward impulse is felt with the other finger-tip. A variation of this method, which can only be employed with large tumours, is to place two finger-tips of one hand on the mass and then press between these two fingers with the tip of a finger of the other hand. The transmitted impulse will be felt with the finger-tips of the opposite hand. It should be remembered that a false positive sensation may be felt if these tests are carried out on each side of the longitudinal axis of a muscle. A useful variation of this test can be carried out with fluid-containing cysts of the jaws even when they are covered with an appreciable thickness of bone. Firm intermittent pressure with the thumb over the suspected cystic area in the buccal sulcus will produce a transmitted pulsation which can be detected by the finger-tip of the other hand placed on the opposite side of the alveolar process in the palate or on the lingual side of the mandible.

13. Are there Signs of Inflammation Present?—The classic signs of heat, redness, swelling, and pain are indicative of either an inflammatory swelling or secondary infection in a non-inflammatory mass.

14. Transillumination.—The only readily transilluminable swelling of the head and neck is the cystic hygroma, but this test can sometimes be applied to nasolabial cysts.

15. Is there an Impulse on Coughing and Crying?

16. Does the Lump pulsate?—There are three types of pulsation which may occur in lumps:

a. The mass may be pulsatile, i.e., the entire mass pulsates. This is best exemplified by the aneurysm.

b. Transmitted pulsation occurs when the mass rests on a large artery. When such a mass is palpated, an impulse is felt which is transmitted from the artery. Salivary adenomas in the palate may sometimes transmit the pulsation of the greater palatine artery.

c. A mass lying deep in the tissues may displace an artery so that it lies superficially upon the mass. On palpation the mass will appear to pulsate though the clinician is, in fact, palpating an artery.

17. Any Mass may produce Pressure Effects on:—

a. Arteries: Pressure on arteries is evidenced by diminution of the pulse and in extreme cases by coldness of the dependent part and eventually by gangrene.

b. Veins: Pressure on veins may produce cyanosis and oedema on the distal side of the vessel.

c. Nerves: Pressure on nerves may produce paraesthesia, anaesthesia, or paralysis, etc.

d. Neighbouring organs: Pressure may be exerted by a mass on any neighbouring organ. In the head and neck two structures commonly affected in this way are the trachea and the oesophagus, with resultant respiratory embarrassment and dysphagia.

18. The Colour of the Lump.—This may be a helpful diagnostic sign.

Reddening may suggest an inflammatory aetiology, while a bluish swelling which blanches on pressure is most probably a haemangioma.

19. The General Condition of the Patient.—Massive swellings associated with cachexia of the patient are usually indicative of malignant neoplasms. Carcinoma of the head and neck does not commonly cause a severe deterioration in the patient's nutritional state until the terminal stages of the disease, unless the tumour involves the gastro-intestinal tract and mechanically interferes with ingestion and deglutition of food. Massive inflammatory swellings will produce a toxic effect on the patient. In these days, tuberculoma of the tongue or other oral tissues are rare in the extreme in this country, but are not in some others. Such lesions occur only in the advanced stages of the disease.

Examination of an Ulcer

Before carrying out any local examination of an ulcer, ascertain whether there is any known exciting factor such as trauma, etc., and also establish the duration of the ulcer.

So far as the local physical examination of the ulcer is concerned, start the examination by palpating the dependent lymph-nodes associated with the ulcer. This essential step is best carried out at the onset of the examination in case it is inadvertently omitted.

With regard to the actual ulcer, ascertain:—

1. The Situation of the Ulcer.—Many ulcers occur in characteristic situations, for example the rodent ulcer at the side of the nose and beneath the eye, and the carcinoma of the tongue at the side of the tongue, while the gummatous ulcer often occurs at the junction of the hard and soft palates. Some indication of the nature of an ulcer may be obtained from its situation alone.

2. Is the Ulcer Single or Multiple?

3. Note the Size of the Ulcer.

4. Examine the Shape of the Ulcer.—Ulcers may be round, oval, crescentic, serpiginous, irregular, punched-out, etc.

5. Note the Base of the Ulcer.—The base of an ulcer may be indurated, soft, or fixed to deeper structures. Marked induration or fixation to deeper structures may be indicative of malignancy.

6. The Floor of the Ulcer may be covered by:—
 a. Granulations. These may be red, pale, or flabby and may or may not bleed.
 b. The floor may be smooth.
 c. It may be covered with slough, membrane, scab, etc.
 d. The floor may be adherent to soft parts or bone.
 e. The floor may be fungating as seen in some clinical varieties of malignant disease.

7. The Edge of the Ulcer may be:—
 a. Undermined (as seen in tubercular ulcers).
 b. Punched-out (as found in gummatous ulcers).
 c. Rolled (as characteristically occurs in rodent ulcers).
 d. Rolled, raised, and everted (as characterized by malignant ulcers).

8. The condition of the parts surrounding the ulcers must be examined.

EXAMINATION OF PAIN, LUMP, OR ULCER

They may be inflamed, healthy, oedematous, pigmented and, in some instances, the adjoining area may have impaired sensation.

Most long-standing areas of ulceration are surrounded by zones of pigmentation and this condition is well exemplified by the varicose ulcer over the internal malleolus. When the region surrounding an ulcer is anaesthetic, as on the sole of the foot with a tabetic ulcer, the area of anaesthesia is, of course, largely responsible for the ulceration, for the normal response to pain is absent and existing irritation is therefore ignored by the patient. Similar ulcers may be seen in the palate after alcohol injection of the trigeminal ganglion.

9. If there is a discharge from the ulcer, its colour, and smell should be noted and a bacteriological smear taken for culture.

10. Is the Ulcer Painful?—Inflammatory and traumatic ulcers are usually painful while tuberculous ulcers in the mouth are often extremely painful, but in the early stages most malignant ulcers are painless. However, when the malignant ulcer becomes established and increases in size it may cause extreme discomfort.

11. The General Condition of the Patient must always be considered.—Patients become very cachetic when a malignant ulceration involves the gastro-intestinal tract. Tubercular ulceration of the mouth may be associated with pulmonary tuberculosis, while severe ulceration in the oral cavity may occur in diabetes, leukaemia, uraemia, agranulocytosis, scurvy, syphilis, etc.

One final point: Be cautious about handling ulcers you do not understand with ungloved fingers. Always wash your hands well after examining an ulcerated mouth.

Chapter III
SOME ADDITIONAL EXAMINATIONS CARRIED OUT WHEN INVESTIGATING A LESION

ALL patients admitted to a ward routinely have their temperature, pulse, and respiration rates recorded. They are weighed and their blood-pressure is measured, and routine blood investigations include their haemoglobin, differential white cell-count, sedimentation rate, and Wassermann reaction.

THE TEMPERATURE

A patient's normal temperature is 98·4° F. or 37° C. when taken in the mouth. Axillary temperatures are about ½° lower and rectal temperatures about 1° higher than the mouth reading. Rectal temperatures are usually taken in infants, for it is unsafe to place a thermometer in the mouth of most young children, as they usually chew the glass. There may be slight variations from the normal bodily temperature due to meals, hot baths, etc., and the evening temperature is usually 1° F. higher than the morning temperature. The temperature may fall as low as 95° F. in severe shock and pyrexia occurs in all fevers.

THE PULSE

The pulse should be felt in both wrists, for there may be variations between the sides. The normal adult pulse-rate is usually 72 per minute, but it is more rapid in children, being about 140 at birth and gradually becoming slower with age until it reaches the adult rate at about 15 years of age. In old age the pulse becomes slower and may be 55–65 per minute. Bradycardia is also seen in some athletes. Tachycardia occurs following exercise and also in fevers, thyrotoxicosis, and emotional upsets.

The rhythm of the pulse tends to increase with inspiration and decrease with expiration and when this alteration is marked the term 'sinus arrhythmia' is used. This condition is comparatively common in young adults. Common irregularities are extra systoles which are of no clinical significance and which disappear with exercise. A more sinister irregularity is atrial fibrillation which is described as an 'irregular irregularity'. This is an irregularity which generally occurs with serious heart disease and is commonly associated with mitral stenosis, thyrotoxicosis, and ischaemic heart disease.

BLOOD-PRESSURE

The blood-pressure is measured with a sphygmomanometer. The average blood-pressure in a group of healthy adults tends to increase with age and is 120/80 at about the age of 20 years, rising to about 160/90 at the age of 60 years. There are, however, wide variations in the blood-pressures within such a group of adults, but for life insurance examinations and similar medical examinations, 150/90 is usually taken as the upper limit of normal. Moderate elevations of the systolic pressure are of less clinical significance than rises in the diastolic pressure. Gross elevation of the blood-pressure is always a matter of concern and necessitates a full clinical examination. About 80 per cent of cases of hyperpiesis are due to essential (idiopathic) hypertension and 19 per cent to renal disorders. Rare diseases such as Cushing's syndrome, phaeochromocytoma, or coarctation of the aorta account for the remainder of the causes. Malignant hypertension carries an especially grim prognosis.

Fall in blood-pressure is found in collapse, shock, and following severe haemorrhage. Hypotension in the elderly is seen following cerebral or cardiac catastrophes, and in this age-group is an especially valuable sign in the diagnosis of the so-called 'silent coronary'.

RESPIRATORY RATE

The normal respiratory rate is 16–20 per minute and like the pulse-rate it is faster in children and slower in old age. An increase in the rate of respiration occurs following exercise and in fever, thyrotoxicosis, etc., while the rate decreases during sleep and under the influence of narcotic drugs. Cheyne-Stokes respiration consists of an apnoea followed by respirations which increase in magnitude to a maximum and then diminish until apnoea occurs again. This type of respiration is found in grave illness such as cerebral haemorrhage, meningitis, uraemia, etc.

WEIGHT

A patient may be above or below the normal weight, but more important are rapid alterations in the weight. Loss of weight is a presenting symptom in diabetes, pulmonary tuberculosis, thyrotoxicosis, etc., and is also seen in its extreme form in anorexia nervosa and malignant disease which affects the gastro-intestinal tract. An increase in weight is most commonly caused by over-eating which is often due to an emotional factor, but it is also seen in pregnancy and in all conditions where fluid retention occurs in the body.

Particularly sad is the sudden increase in weight which occurs in patients with extreme cachexia due to malignant disease which has become widely disseminated throughout the body. This increase is, of course, due to ascites and is frequently a terminal event.

HAEMATOLOGICAL INVESTIGATIONS

Haemoglobin.—The average haemoglobin content of normal blood is 14·8 g. per 100 ml. (Haldane 14·6 g. per 100 ml.), but variations in men from 13·56 to 18 g. per 100 ml. and in women from 11·56 to 16·4 g. per 100 ml. are seen. The figure of 14·8 g. per 100 ml. is usually taken as an arbitrary 100 per cent in most laboratories, but as there is some controversy on this point, the haemoglobin should always be expressed in grams per 100 ml.

The Red-cell Count.—The red-cell count tends to be inaccurate unless the counting is done by an experienced and careful worker, but the information is only required in some obscure anaemias. Iron deficiency can be more readily diagnosed by the Mean Corpuscular Haemoglobin Concentration (MCHC). The normal red-cell count is subject to wide variations. Normal for men is 5·4 million $\pm 0·8$ and in women 4·8 million $\pm 0·6$. As the red-cell count, except in very experienced hands, is an inaccurate measurement, the indices derived from it, i.e., colour index, mean corpuscular haemoglobin, and mean cell volume, are correspondingly inaccurate.

The opinion of a haematologist on the appearance of the red cells is much more valuable than a red-cell count. The mean cell diameter is 7·5 µ ± 0·3 µ and is the same for men, women, and children, though at birth it is 8·6 µ and falls to 7·4 µ at six months.

Haematocrit Value (Packed cell volume).—This is the volume occupied by red cells in 100 ml. of centrifuged blood and is normally about 45 ml. per cent.

Mean Corpuscular Haemoglobin Concentration (MCHC).—This value is obtained by dividing the haemoglobin in grams per 100 ml. by the packed cell volume in ml. per 100 ml. and then multiplying by 100. The normal is 32–38 g. per cent and values below this figure invariably indicate the need for iron therapy. The MCHC is the most reliable evidence for the recognition of iron-deficiency anaemia.

Mean Corpuscular Volume (MCV).—The mean corpuscular volume is the average volume of a single red cell in cubic microns and is obtained by dividing the packed cell volume in ml. per 1000 ml. of blood by the red cells in millions per c.mm. The normal is 78–94 c.µ. The MCV is therefore an indication of the size of the red cell in three dimensions.

Colour Index.—The colour index is obtained by dividing the haemoglobin percentage by the red-cell count expressed as a percentage of the normal figure of 5 million and therefore indicates the mean haemoglobin content of a single red cell. The normal figure is 1.

Red Cell Appearance and Abnormalities.—

Reticulocytes.—Reticulocytes normally form 1·5 per cent of the total red-cell count but up to 6 per cent is normal in children. They are found when increased marrow activity occurs, particularly in pernicious anaemia when treatment is started. They are also present after acute or chronic bleeding.

Nucleated Red Cells.—Nucleated red cells are not normally seen but occur in any very severe anaemia and in leukaemia, multiple myeloma, carcinomatosis, pernicious anaemia, and in newborn infants.

Punctate Basophilia.—Punctate basophilia is not normally present, but occurs in lead poisoning.

Sickle Cells.—Sickle cells occur in sickle-cell anaemia and are usually seen during suboxygenation.

Polychromasia.—Variable staining of the red blood-cells occurs during conditions of increased marrow activity.

Anisocytosis.—A condition where the red blood-corpuscles are unequal in size.

Poikilocytosis.—An alteration in the shape of the red cells.

Anisochromia.—Which denotes irregular staining.

These last three are all seen in severe anaemia.

White Cells.—The normal total white-cell count is 4000–11,000 c.mm. There is a leucopenia in haemopoietic disorders such as aplastic anaemia, aleukaemic leukaemias, pernicious and iron-deficiency anaemias. It also occurs in bacterial infections, such as typhoid, brucellosis and in any overwhelming pyogenic infection, as well as in many virus diseases such as influenza, measles, rubella, etc. The white-cell count can also be depressed as a result of drugs and toxic chemicals such as benzene, nitrogen mustard, thiouracil, chloramphenicol, amidopyrine, phenylbutazone, etc.

The *Polymorphonuclear Leucocyte Count* is normally 35–75 per cent of the total count and is raised in all acute infections and following trauma, blood-loss, and after cardiac infarction. It is also raised in rheumatic fever, rheumatoid arthritis, gout, and polyarteritis nodosa. The polymorph count is greatly raised in myelogenous leukaemia, but the cells are, of course, abnormal. The polymorphonuclear leucocyte count is lowered in acute leukaemia and as a result of drug therapy with thiouracil, amidopyrine, gold, and arsenic and occasionally with sulphonamides. The condition is known as 'neutropenia', and an extreme reduction is called 'agranulocytosis'.

The *Lymphocyte Count* is normally 15–60 per cent of the total and is raised in pertussis, lymphocytic leukaemias, and in glandular fever where there are abnormal forms. The lymphocyte count is lowered in whole body radiation exposure. The lymphocytes are increased and the polymorphs decreased in children as compared with adults as a normal state of affairs.

Monocytes usually account for 2–9 per cent of the total count and the count is raised in all protozoal infections and in monocytic leukaemia. It is also raised in infective mononucleosis or glandular fever.

Basophils normally constitute 0–2 per cent of the total white count and are rarely increased to any considerable extent.

Eosinophils account for 1–6 per cent of the total count and are raised in all parasitic diseases and intestinal worm infestations as well as in some allergic diseases such as asthma and urticaria.

Bleeding Time.—The normal bleeding time by Duke's method is 2–7 minutes. It is raised in idiopathic and symptomatic thrombocytopenia and in secondary non-thrombocytopenic purpuras and Von Willebrand's disease. The bleeding time is normal in haemophilia, Christmas disease, hereditary telangiectasia, anaphylactoid purpuras, and is usually normal in prothrombin deficiency.

Clotting Time.—The clotting or coagulation time is usually measured by the Dale and Laidlaw method and the normal is 1 minute 40 seconds. The clotting time is increased in haemophilia and Christmas disease, but it may be normal during their quiescent periods. It is also raised in conditions of fibrinogen deficiency and in patients being treated with anticoagulant therapy such as heparin, etc. The clotting time is normal in all purpuras.

Red Cell Sedimentation Rate.—The Westergren method is usually used and the normal for men is 3–5 mm. in 1 hour and women 4–7 mm. in 1 hour. It has recently been recommended that the upper limit of normal should be: men 15 mm./hour, women 25 mm./hour (below 50 years) and men 20 mm./hour, women 30 mm./hour (above 50 years).

The sedimentation rate is raised in any condition of raised plasma fibrinogen or of increased or abnormal globulins. This test is especially useful for assessing the progress in rheumatic fever, pulmonary tuberculosis, and rheumatoid arthritis. However, a normal E.S.R. cannot exclude serious disease and if the test is normal, it may engender a false sense of security in the clinician. On the other hand, a high sedimentation reading may occasionally prevent an erroneous diagnosis of psychosomatic illness being made. The sedimentation rate is especially high in multiple myelomatosis, carcinomatosis, and polyarteritis nodosa.

Examination of the Urine

The normal daily urinary output in a healthy adult is about 1500 ml. but it may vary between 400 and 3000 ml. depending upon fluid intake and loss by sweat, etc. It is important to maintain an adequate fluid intake and urinary output in all hospitalized patients and to ensure satisfactory levels a fluid balance chart is kept. This record is especially important in cases of facial fracture, when pain on deglutition may discourage the patient from drinking and in the unconscious or semi-conscious patient who is being fed via a transnasal gastric tube or by intravenous fluids. It should be remembered that following a severe accident or operation there is an impairment of water excretion which lasts for 24–36 hours and is characterized by a low output of urine which has a high specific gravity. A high fluid intake is required for patients on sulphonamide therapy to prevent crystalluria and again a fluid balance chart must be kept.

Specific Gravity.—The specific gravity of urine is measured with a hygrometer and varies between 1024 and 1032.

Proteinuria.—Protein in the urine may be due to an infection of the urinary tract (cystitis, pyelitis, etc.) or to excess protein leaking from the blood to the urine across the glomerular membrane. Albumin has the smallest molecule and leaks most easily, but all fractions of the plasma proteins appear in the urine if the glomerular leak is severe.

Proteinuria is found in every variety of renal disease, but the quantity present is not related to the severity of the disease. It should be remembered that a trace of protein may be seen as a contaminant in routine urine specimens especially in women, and whenever possible a catheter specimen should be sent for examination.

Bence-Jones Proteose.—Bence-Jones proteose is the name given to a protein precipitate which occurs at 55° C. and disappears at 85° C. when a urine specimen is heated in a water bath. The condition occurs in multiple myelomatosis.

Cells in Urine.—If 10 ml. of urine are centrifuged and the deposit examined under a $\frac{1}{6}$th objective occasional cells may be seen. This test should be carried out in cases of suspected subacute bacterial endocarditis when excess red cells may be seen as a result of minute emboli in the uriniferous tubules, and in patients under protracted sulphonamide therapy when crystalluria will also produce multiple red cells in the urine.

Blood in Urine.—The urine of all accident cases, especially the first specimen passed after the injury, should be examined for blood which may indicate damage to some part of the urinary tract. Patients with facial fractures caused by accidents while riding two-wheeled vehicles are especially liable to damage to the urethra from the saddle. If in a patient with a fractured pelvis a drop of blood appears at the urethral meatus and a ruptured urethra is suspected, the patient should not be encouraged to pass urine until a surgical opinion has been obtained. If the urethra is torn across, extravasation of urine could follow an attempt to pass it.

Glycosuria.—The presence of glucose in the urine in large amounts or on repeated tests gives rise to a suspicion of diabetes mellitus, especially if acetone is also present. It should be remembered that glucose may be present in the urine following subarachnoid haemorrhage and is also found in early specimens of urine from patients who have sustained a severe fracture of the middle third of the facial skeleton.

WASSERMANN REACTION, KAHN TEST, V.D.R.L., AND PRICE'S PRECIPITATION REACTION

Of the standard tests for syphilis, the Wassermann reaction is a complement-fixation method, the Kahn and V.D.R.L. (Venereal Disease Reference Laboratory) tests are flocculation reactions, and Price's precipitation reaction is a precipitation with antigen test.

These tests form a useful screening measure for syphilis. The V.D.R.L. slide test is claimed to be more specific for syphilis than the W.R. and Kahn methods. The tests are expressed as positive, negative, or doubtful and they become positive about four weeks after the primary infection or one week after the chancre appears. Tests for syphilis before this time are carried out by dark ground illumination examination of a smear of the chancre when the *Treponema pallidum* are seen. True positive reactions occur in bejel, pinta, leprosy, sleeping sickness, and yaws, as well as in syphilis. False positive reactions occur in about 1/3000 normal people as well as in 20 per cent of cases of *Leptospiro-ictera haemorrhagica* (rat bite fever) and relapsing fever. False positive reactions are seen in bacterial infections such as leprosy (50 per cent of cases), advanced tuberculosis, scarlet fever and pneumococcal pneumonia, protozoal infections such as acute malaria (100 per cent of cases), and virus infections such as virus pneumonia, glandular fever, infective hepatitis, vaccinia, mumps (20 per cent of cases), measles, lymphogranuloma venereum (2–5 per cent of cases), as well as in certain miscellaneous conditions such as the collagen diseases.

False negative reactions occur in about 10 per cent of patients with tertiary syphilis, particularly in tabes dorsalis. False negative results seldom occur in active cardiovascular disease.

RADIOLOGY

Radiology plays an important role in the differential diagnosis of lesions of the jaw. Most pathological conditions of the mandible or maxillae can be satisfactorily demonstrated by routine radiography, but occasionally special radiographical techniques are required to elucidate some particular facet of the case under investigation.

Routine Radiography.—

*The Lower Jaw.—*The routine radiographs required for a lesion of the mandible are:—
 1. Left and right oblique lateral jaw views of the appropriate regions.
 2. The postero-anterior jaws view.
 3. The true lateral.
 4. Intra-oral periapical views.
 5. An occlusal view.
 6. Modified reverse Towne's (to show condylar necks).
 7. Temporomandibular joint views with the mandible in the open and closed positions.

The Upper Jaw.—
 1. Occipito-mental views. The standard view is taken with the radiographic base line at 45°, but other tilts such as 15° are sometimes used. Also the tube may be tilted caudally 30° for the 30° O.M.

2. Postero-anterior jaws view, penetrated for the maxilla.
3. Intra-oral periapical views.
4. True, lateral, or oblique occlusals.

One or more of these radiographs will usually demonstrate any bony lesion of the upper and lower jaw in a satisfactory fashion, but occasionally they must be supplemented by radiographs which make use of additional radiographical techniques. Some of these special X-ray examinations are:—

1. Tomography.—Tomographs are used to demonstrate lesions at varying depths in the body. Using a technique whereby both the film and the X-ray source move at the time of exposure, only the layer of the body which is stationary relative to both is shown on the film and all other parts are blurred. Radiographs can be taken to depict layers at 0·5 cm. and 1 cm. intervals through the thickness of the part under investigation and the depth of a cavity in, for example, the lung can then be estimated. The routine postero-anterior radiograph of the chest would, of course, only show the area of the lesion. In the jaws the tomogram is principally used to demonstrate intra-capsular fractures of the condyle which cannot be seen with any clarity on the P.A., oblique lateral, and modified reverse Towne's views. Tomograms are sometimes used to demonstrate the exact size and shape of lesions such as an osteoma in the maxillary sinus or to search for destruction of the bony wall as evidence of the presence of a carcinoma.

2. Soft Tissue Radiographs.—These are very helpful in showing the exact relationship of the soft tissues to the underlying bone. They are employed for assessing the degree of deformity in skeletal anomalies such as prognathism and they are also used for orthodontic investigations.

3. Pantomography.—Pantomography is useful for demonstrating the upper and lower teeth on a single X-ray film. Rotational tomography uses similar principles to planar tomography except that curved layers are recorded. One centre (concentric) or two or three centres (eccentric) of rotation or a continuously varying centre of rotation which follows a semi-elliptical path may be used to demonstrate the whole of the upper and lower dental arches on one film. These machines can also be used to produce tomographic views of the nasal sinuses and temporomandibular joint.

4. Bite Wing Films.—In the bite wing film attention is directed principally to the crowns of the teeth. The technique is mainly used for demonstrating carious lesions, but is also valuable for assessing early periodontal bone loss.

5. Stereoscopic Radiographs.—To produce a stereoscopic effect, two radiographs are taken of the same area but at a slightly different angle to each other, the difference between the positions of the X-ray tube representing the distance between the eyes. These films are placed on two viewing boxes which are fixed facing each other at either end of a six-foot viewing table. In the centre of the table, exactly between the viewing screens, are two plane mirrors with their mirrored surfaces facing the viewing screen at each end of the table. These central mirrors are hinged together at their anterior edges and the clinician stands facing this anterior edge. By manipulating a simple screw device which pushes the distal edge of the mirrors apart, the mirrors can be angled so that the films in the viewing box come into focus stereoscopically. This form of investigation enables the exact relationship of the fragments in fractures of the middle third of the facial skeleton to be studied. For small films a prismatic stereoscope, which is like a pair of binoculars, can be used.

6. Cineradiography.—Cineradiography has been used to study the movements of the tongue and palate in speech and deglutition. It is especially useful for observing variations of the normal in such conditions as the cleft palate.

7. The Use of Radio-opaque Materials.—The principle of using radio-opaque materials in conjunction with routine or special radiographs can be applied in many ways:—

a. Radio-opaque Probes.—Soft silver probes can be inserted down sinuses in the jaw prior to taking radiographs in order to demonstrate the path, depth, and extent of the sinus. The same principle can be used by inserting one or more needles into the tissue in order to localize a foreign body such as a broken needle in the soft tissues.

b. Localization of Roots using a Removable Appliance.—In order to localize roots in the upper or lower jaw some authorities use a wax plate containing metal markers which can be placed over the alveolus prior to taking radiographs. The position of the roots can then be ascertained in relation to the metal markers and the plate is removed prior to surgery.

c. Sialography.—Neohydriol solution can be injected into the ducts of glands in order to demonstrate the glandular structure. By this method such conditions as duct stricture or dilatation, glandular dilatation (sialectasis), and intra-glandular space-occupying lesions can be demonstrated. (*See* The Major Salivary Glands, p. 216.)

d. Barium Swallow.—In this technique postero-anterior and lateral radiographs are taken as a patient swallows a solution containing barium. This technique demonstrates deviations, strictures, space-occupying lesions, and foreign bodies in the oesophagus. It is an invaluable technique for demonstrating a radiolucent foreign body such as a broken acrylic denture impacted in the oesophagus.

e. Following the marsupialization of a large cyst the cavity can be packed with cotton-wool soaked in lipiodol. Used in conjunction with routine radiographs of the jaw, this will demonstrate the exact area involved by the cyst and follow-up radiographs will show any regression of the lesion. The injection of radio-opaque material into maxillary cysts prior to operation is not particularly helpful in delineating the extent of the cyst, for it obscures the adjacent bony structures and the lipiodol could, of course, be injected in error into the maxillary sinus.

f. Angiography.—The injection of a radio-opaque material into blood-vessels is useful in the head and neck for demonstrating aneurysms. The material used is Hypaque which is completely inert. At one time radio-active materials such as diadrast and thoratrast were used, but they carried a risk of causing a sarcoma of spleen and should not be employed.

Arteriovenous shunts occasionally occur in the mandible, especially at the angle and they may resemble a residual cyst, for they appear as a radiolucent area in the jaws.

g. The Exploration of Sinuses and Fistulae.—Water-soluble radio-opaque media can be injected into external sinuses and fistulae on the face and neck and a postero-anterior and lateral radiograph will clearly demonstrate the path and extent of the track. This technique is invaluable for demonstrating thyroglossal and branchial fistulae.

Additional Blood and Serological Tests

Glucose.—The normal fasting glucose or blood-sugar is 70–120 mg. per 100 ml. and the blood glucose is raised in diabetes mellitus, Cushing's syndrome, haemochromatosis, and subarachnoid haemorrhage. It is also raised in various other conditions such as acute pancreatitis, Wernicke's encephalopathy, etc., which are of little dental interest. There is, however, often a raised glucose level following severe head injury and raised levels are often seen in fractures of the middle third of the facial skeleton immediately after injury. In such cases the blood-sugar level returns to normal within a few days.

In all cases where glycosuria is present, a full glucose tolerance test should be carried out for one random test is of little value.

Glucose Tolerance Test.—The glucose tolerance test is represented as a 2-hour curve showing the response to 50 g. of glucose by mouth. A fasting blood-sugar together with a urine examination for sugar is made and then the patient is given 50 g. of glucose by mouth. Further glucose and urine examinations are carried out at 1 hour and 2 hours and the results plotted as a curve.

The normal fasting level is 70–120 mg. per 100 ml. which rises by 30–60 mg., but not above 170 mg., the normal renal threshold. At 2 hours the normal reading will be about 120 mg. A level of less than 170 mg. at 1 hour excludes frank diabetes.

Paul-Bunnell Test.—The Paul-Bunnell test is a serum agglutinin test and when agglutination at serum dilutions of 1/128 occurs it is diagnostic of glandular fever (infective mononucleosis). Positive results can also be obtained with trypanosomiasis.

Blood-urea.—The normal blood-urea is 15–40 mg. urea per 100 ml. and it is raised (azotaemia) in primary renal disease and other conditions with impaired renal function. Hence, an increased blood-level is to be expected in acute and chronic glomerulonephritis, chronic bilateral pyelonephritis, and renal tubular necrosis. The blood concentration is also elevated in lower urinary tract obstruction due to prostatic obstruction, increased tissue protein metabolism associated with a negative nitrogen balance (e.g., in fevers, thyrotoxicosis, wasting diseases, diabetic coma, or after a major operation) and in extra-renal uraemia due to impaired renal circulation and dehydration.

Blood Uric Acid.—The normal blood uric acid is 1·5–3·9 mg. per 100 ml. and a high level is suggestive but not diagnostic of gout.

It is also raised in any condition where there is excessive breakdown of cell nuclei such as carcinomatosis, polycythaemia, chronic myeloid leukaemia, and often in pernicious anaemia.

Alkaline Phosphatase.—The normal alkaline phosphatase in adults is 4·5–12 units per 100 ml. by the King-Armstrong method and 1·5–4 units per 100 ml. by the Bodansky method. Higher values, up to 25 King-Armstrong units, are normal for children. The alkaline phosphatase is raised in Paget's disease, hyperparathyroidism (when there are bone changes), carcinomatosis metastasizing to bone, rickets, osteomalacia, renal rickets, fibrous dysplasia, and in patients with healing fractures. The highest readings are seen in Paget's disease, especially during the active phase of the disease.

Acid Phosphatase.—The normal acid phosphatase is 1–3 King-Armstrong units per 100 ml. or 0·5–1·5 Bodansky units. It is raised in metastasizing carcinoma of the prostate as well as in osteogenesis imperfecta and marble bone disease. It is also raised in any condition where there is a very high serum alkaline phosphatase.

Serum Calcium.—The normal blood or serum calcium is 9·6–10·9 mg. per 100 ml. and it is raised in hyperparathyroidism, vitamin D intoxication, sudden immobilization as after fractures, idiopathic hypercalcaemia of infants, and after excessive milk or alkali therapy. It is also raised in some malignant diseases involving bone such as multiple myeloma, skeletal metastases, etc. The serum calcium is lowered after total parathyroidectomy.

Inorganic Phosphates.—The normal value of the serum inorganic phosphates is 2–4 mg. per 100 ml., but these are slightly raised in infancy.

The inorganic phosphates are raised in renal failure from any cause and values over 8 mg. per 100 ml. indicate severe renal failure. They are also raised in vitamin D overdosage, in acromegaly, and in cases of diminished parathyroid function.

The inorganic phosphate level is lowered in hyperparathyroidism, Fanconi syndrome, and in conditions caused by a vitamin-D deficiency, i.e., rickets and osteomalacia.

Biopsy

The term 'biopsy' is most frequently used to indicate the removal of tissue and its histological examination. It is the least equivocal of all the diagnostic procedures performed in the laboratory and it should be carried out whenever a suspicious lesion is encountered.

Excision and Biopsy.—Where the clinician is reasonably certain on clinical grounds that a lesion is benign it should be excised and sent for histological examination.

Incisional Biopsy.—If the lesion under examination is extensive, if its nature is uncertain or if it is suspected that it might be malignant, then an incisional biopsy is the method of choice. This consists of removing one or more portions of representative tissue from the lesion. The material should be taken from the edge of the lesion so as to include some normal tissue. In taking a margin of normal tissue unnecessary risks of spreading the lesion should be avoided. However, care must be taken to ensure that an adequate amount of the abnormal tissue is included. Where the lesion is very small an adequate sample may include all the visible part. Obviously no attempt should be made to remove a curative margin on the assumption that it is malignant as this may cause unnecessary mutilation. Care must be taken, however, to record accurately the pre-biopsy appearance and a decision on treatment must be made while the site is still clearly visible in the patient. Three modifications of the incisional biopsy are the punch biopsy, the needle biopsy, and curettage.

Punch biopsy is performed with a surgical instrument which punches or bites out a portion of tissue. It has no advantage over the incisional biopsy and can result in the material being bruised or otherwise damaged.

Needle or drill biopsy has been employed for obtaining material from deep-seated lesions, but histological diagnosis of such material is difficult and it has a very limited place in oral surgery.

Curettage biopsy suffers from the same disadvantage for again the material obtained tends to be damaged and unsuitable for histological examination. For the same reason any manipulation and grasping of the specimen during excisional or incisional biopsy must be minimal so as to preserve the tissue structure intact.

Dangers of Biopsy.—The spreading of tumour cells along lymphatic and vascular channels by biopsy is a possibility and gross manipulation of a tumour may possibly increase the number of cells released. However, the risk of spreading cells from a malignant tumour during a biopsy is secondary to establishing a diagnosis so that correct treatment can be instituted. Other dangers of biopsy are haemorrhage, infection, and failure of the tissue to heal.

Haemorrhagic tumours should be biopsied with extreme caution and intra-oral biopsies of tumours such as an adamantinoma may result in an infected area in the mouth which is slow to heal. This might preclude the insertion of an immediate bone-graft following resection of the portion of mandible containing the tumour. Nevertheless the most direct approach to the mass is appropriate to avoid opening unnecessarily the tissue planes of the face or neck.

Aspiration Biopsy.—Aspiration biopsy is a most valuable investigation and should be carried out on all cystic and fluctuant lesions. It is a simple examination and causes the patient minimal inconvenience. Local analgesic is injected over the lesion after which a wide-bore needle attached to a 10-ml. syringe is inserted into the lesion. Inability to aspirate usually indicates that the lesion is solid. Aspiration of air in the molar region of the upper jaw indicates that the needle is in the maxillary sinus and is a valuable method of differentiating the sinus from a suspected cyst. Aspiration of air from a cystic lesion in the lower jaw usually indicates a solitary bone cyst (traumatic, haemorrhagic, etc.). Aspiration of pus indicates an abscess or an infected cyst and aspiration of chronic abscesses around the jaws often confirms the diagnosis of actinomycosis. Keratin, which has the clinical appearance of pus without its unpleasant smell, denotes the presence of a keratocyst (primordial) while periodontal and dentigerous cysts contain straw-coloured fluid containing cholesterol crystals. Aspiration of blood denotes a haemorrhagic tumour or a blood-vessel. The inspissated material contained in a dermoid cyst is aspirated with extreme difficulty. Aspiration of cyst contents may prove to be an important aid to the diagnosis of the odontogenic keratocyst. If the aspirate is subjected to electrophoresis a soluble protein level below 4 g. per 100 ml. is very suggestive of keratocyst, whereas a level above 5 g. per 100 ml. favours apical, dentigerous, or other non-keratinizing cysts. An even simpler aid to diagnosis is to examine a stained film of the cyst fluid to demonstrate keratinized squames.

Oral Cytology.—Cytological examination for tumour cells was first described by Papanicolaou (1946) as a diagnostic procedure in the detection of uterine malignancy. Scrapings are taken of the suspected lesion, after which the cells obtained are smeared on to a clean slide, stained and examined. The report is based on the morphological features and staining quality of the cells.

The technique can be applied to oral lesions, but should be employed as an adjunct to, and not a substitute for, biopsy as it is not so uniformly reliable as the excisional or incisional biopsy.

Postal Regulations.—If biopsy specimens are sent by post the postal regulations must be complied with.

REFERENCE

PAPANICOLAOU, G. N. (1946), 'Diagnostic Value of Exfoliated Cells from Cancer Tissue', *J. Am. med. Ass.*, **131,** 372.

Chapter IV
THE DIFFERENTIAL DIAGNOSIS OF SWELLINGS OF THE NECK

SWELLINGS of the neck may be conveniently divided into three main groups: (1) Lymphatic swellings, (2) Cystic swellings, (3) Other swellings.

LYMPHATIC SWELLINGS OF THE NECK

The cervical lymph-nodes are arranged in two main groups:—

1. A Circular Group around the base of the skull which includes the submental, submandibular, pre- and post-auricular, parotid, retropharyngeal, and occipital lymph-nodes. Above this level there is the isolated facial gland on the cheek.

2. The Vertical Chain of Nodes running down the neck. These consist of a relatively unimportant *superficial chain* which includes the anterior jugular, prelaryngeal, pretracheal, and paratracheal, and a deep chain which is arranged in four main groups according to the level at which they lie and their relation to the internal jugular vein. They are:—

a. The upper anterior deep cervical lymph-nodes in the upper part of the anterior triangle in front of the jugular vein.

b. The upper posterior deep cervical nodes in the upper part of the posterior triangle.

c. The lower anterior group in the lower part of the anterior triangle.

d. The lower posterior group which lie in the posterior triangle along the posterior belly of the omohyoid.

In examining enlarged lymph-nodes of the neck, attention must be given to:—

1. Pain.—Pain is usually only severe in acute pyogenic lymphadenitis.

2. The Age of the Patient.—For example, the predominant cause of enlarged cervical nodes in childhood is chronic upper respiratory tract infection and tuberculosis, while in old age secondary carcinoma is a more likely diagnosis.

3. The Duration.—The duration of the enlarged gland characterizes the swelling as acute, subacute, or chronic. For example, an acute swelling of short duration is almost certainly pyogenic in origin. A subacute swelling may, for example, be tubercular or syphilitic, while chronic swellings may possibly be tubercular or neoplastic.

4. The Number of Nodes Involved.—The number of nodes involved may give some indication of the aetiology. Numerous nodes are involved in infective mononucleosis, leukaemia, etc., while solitary nodes may be due to lymphosarcoma and secondary carcinoma. Whenever more than one cervical node is enlarged, an examination must be carried out for lymphadenopathy elsewhere in the body, for the condition may be generalized.

5. The Site of the Nodes.—The site of the enlarged nodes is especially helpful where lymph-node enlargement is of pyogenic aetiology, especially when the source of the infection is in the mouth.

DIAGNOSIS OF SWELLINGS OF THE NECK

6. The Consistency of the Enlarged Glands.—The consistency of the enlarged gland may be of diagnostic significance. The enlarged gland in Hodgkin's disease feels rubbery, the secondary carcinoma feels rocky-hard, enlargements due to pyogenic infection are tender and relatively soft while the glands of tuberculosis may be fluctuant or matted together.

The primary cause of a cervical lymphadenopathy must be sought in the area drained by the gland or glands in question. However, if there is a generalized lymphadenopathy involving axillary, inguinal glands, etc., there is more likely to be a generalized systemic cause for the lymphatic enlargements.

When the occipital or post-auricular glands are enlarged, the scalp is examined. The submental glands drain the lower lip, the lower incisor area, and the tip of the tongue and part of the floor of the mouth, the submandibular glands drain much of the face, the mouth, and anterior two-thirds of the tongue excluding the tip. The upper anterior cervical glands are usually involved from the fauces and pharynx. In the case of a pyogenic infection, the instigating focus of infection may have healed and search should be made for a scar or other evidence of recent infection. Difficulty may be experienced in secondary involvement of the cervical glands with carcinoma, for the primary lesion may be extremely small and may be merely a crack in the lip or a minute ulcer in the vallecula or the piriform fossa. The primary lesion may also be hidden in the nasopharynx, subglottic region, or the paranasal sinuses. Malignant lesions in the nasopharynx are notoriously difficult to find. The skin should be examined for rashes which are seen only fleetingly in such diseases as rubella and tularaemia, but are more obvious in secondary syphilis. Other investigations include the temperature, which may be raised in infective mononucleosis, tularaemia, etc., while a blood examination establishes a diagnosis of leukaemia and infective mononucleosis. However, many lymphadenopathies require special investigations in order to elucidate their aetiology, and the Wassermann reaction for syphilis, the Paul-Bunnell test for infective mononucleosis, and the examination for viral antibodies are obvious examples of this group.

7. The Histology and Bacteriology of the Nodes.—Should a diagnosis not be possible after the above measures, then a few drops of sterile saline may be injected into one of the nodes and aspirated. The aspirate can be used to produce a smear, or it can be cultured or used for guinea-pig inoculation. In this way various causative bacteria may be isolated including the tubercle bacillus.

Excision of a node for biopsy should be performed where histological examination is necessary. In such a case it may be helpful to send half of the specimen unfixed for bacteriological examination.

Examination of an Enlarged Lymph-node should include:—

Aspiration { Smear, Culture, Guinea-pig inoculation } Pyogenic organism, Tubercle

Excision of a node or biopsy: half for histological examination and half for bacteriological examination.

Classification

Lymphatic swellings of the neck may be pyogenic, viral, tubercular, syphilitic, or malignant in origin.

1. Pyogenic Origin.—Pyogenic lymphadenopathy may arise from the lips, incisor region, and chin when the submental glands are involved. Infection from the face, mouth, and front of tongue usually involves the submandibular glands while the upper anterior cervical group of glands are involved from a focus in the fauces and pharynx. A not uncommon cause of extensive cervical lymphatic enlargement is a septic focus in the scalp, and the hair of the head of a child should always be searched for head lice when painless glands of recent origin are found involving the occipital chain of glands or the superficial cervical glands on either side of the neck. The infective source may be a septic cut or scratch and it is prudent to remember that pediculosis capitis is by no means uncommon and gives rise to extensive septic involvement of the scalp through scratching. Grossly enlarged lymphatic glands may break down and suppurate.

2. Viral Origin.—

German Measles (rubella).—This mild disease practically always produces enlargement of the cervical nodes which persists long after the rash, which may be transient, has disappeared. Although a harmless disease which is never fatal, it may give rise to congenital deformities in the developing foetus if the mother is affected during the first four months of pregnancy. The history of a mild febrile illness with a macular type of eruption lasting 1-3 days may help to make the diagnosis in an otherwise inexplicable lymphadenopathy. Identification of the rubella virus during the first three days of the illness is now feasible by means of a haemagglutination-inhibition procedure.

Infective Mononucleosis (glandular fever).—This common disease usually affects young adults. There is low protracted pyrexia and general malaise often associated with a sore throat. Many cases present with severely affected gums which may be erroneously diagnosed as ulcero-membranous gingivitis. A generalized lymphadenopathy develops which can sometimes be prolonged and recurrent. The diagnosis is confirmed by the blood picture, for there is a raised lymphocyte count and atypical mononuclear cells are plentiful in the film. Additional confirmation of the diagnosis is made with the Paul-Bunnell test which is positive in about 90 per cent of cases.

Cat Scratch Fever.—This febrile disease is transmitted to man by a scratch or bite from an apparently healthy cat. It may also enter the body through scratches made by thorns, wood splinters, or fishbones. The causal agent is a virus of the lymphogranuloma-psittacosis group. An ulcer occurs at the site of inoculation and a low-grade fever develops together with a regional adenitis which may be extremely protracted. Occasionally the glands break down and suppurate—often with sinus formation. Recovery is gradual. The only diagnostic test is the positive skin reaction obtained by intradermal injection of heated pus obtained from another case or from the patient himself. Frei antigen gives a negative reaction.

Tularaemia.—This highly infectious disease is normally enzootic in rodents. The clinical disease in man is characterized by a focal ulcer at the site of infection with marked lymphadenopathy, and severe constitutional symptoms. The condition is caused by the *Pasteurella tularensis* and diagnosis is made by recovery of the organism from the primary lesion or lymph-nodes.

Glanders.—This disease is due to an infection with *Pfeifferella mallei* (*Malleomyces mallei*) and occurs in horses and similar animals, but rarely may be transmitted to man. There is severe ulceration at the site of infection and enlargement of the cervical lymph-glands which may suppurate. The constitutional symptoms are severe. Diagnosis is by isolation of the causative organism.

Toxoplasmosis.—Toxoplasmosis in adults due to *Toxoplasma gondii* (a protozoan) often presents as a lymphadenopathy of the cervical lymph-nodes. The glands are smooth and mobile and may be mistaken for those in Hodgkin's disease. There is malaise but no fever. Diagnosis can be difficult and culture has only been successful in living cells. A complement-fixation test and a dye test using the patient's serum can be carried out by certain public health laboratories. The intraperitoneal inoculation of white mice with infected biopsy or autopsy tissue will cause infection in which *T. gondii* can be recovered.

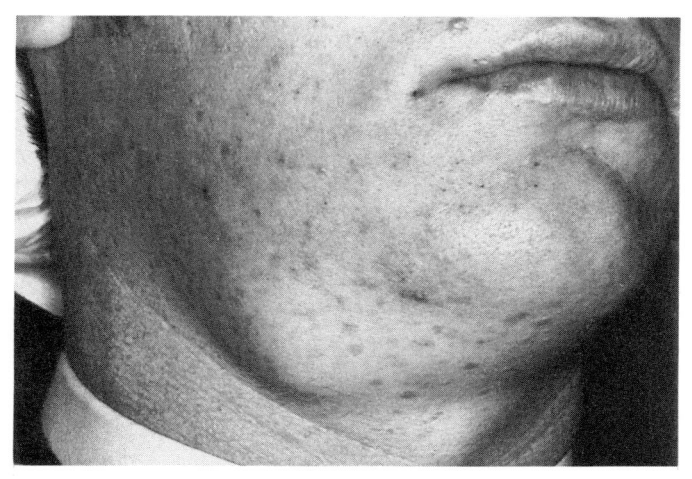

Fig. 1.—Tuberculous abscess.

3. Tubercular.—

Tuberculosis.—Tuberculous cervical lymphadenitis usually arises from an initial infection in the tonsillar crypt and spreads to the cervical lymph-nodes. These may become chronically enlarged and heal by fibrosis and calcification, but they may break down and caseate (*Fig.* 1). Initially the glands may be discrete, but when they become large they may become matted together and form an indurated mass.

Occasionally when they undergo caseous necrosis the pus tracks through the fascial planes to form a superficial cold abscess at some distance from the involved node. This is known as a 'collar-stud abscess'. Tuberculous cervical adenitis is seen in patients who have no immunity to tubercular infection and is often diagnosed in patients from Southern Ireland and from Norway. In such individuals the Mantoux test is often negative. Diagnosis is made either by biopsy of an affected lymph-node or by aspiration biopsy of a broken down lymph-gland when the characteristic acid-fast organisms of the tubercle bacillus are seen. The diagnosis may be confirmed in doubtful cases by animal inoculation. Occasionally the primary focus is on the gingivae and the submandibular nodes are affected. The primary oral lesion is granular, flat, and pale red and resembles a capillary haemangioma in appearance. Pressure with a glass slide may reveal 'apple jelly' nodules.

In some countries tuberculous lymphadenitis is becoming less frequent, and being replaced by unclassified or anonymous mycobacterial infections which also cause cervical lymphadenitis. The distinction is not merely academic. In addition to the eventual culture of the mycobacterium responsible, differentiation from classic tuberculosis can often be made by showing lack of contact with known cases of tuberculosis, lack of evidence of tuberculous foci elsewhere in the body, especially in chest radiographs, and the greater skin sensitivity to PPD (Purified Protein Derivative)-B (from unclassified mycobacteria) than to PPD-S (from *Mycobacterium tuberculosis*).

4. Syphilitic.—

Syphilitic Lymphadenopathy.—Enlargement of the cervical lymph-glands is seen in primary syphilis when the chancre is in the mouth or on the lips. There is a generalized enlargement of the submental, submandibular, pre-, and post-auricular, and the occipital glands, a condition known as a syphilitic collar. The glands are usually non-tender and discrete. Confirmation of the diagnosis of syphilis at this stage is made by dark-ground illumination of a smear taken from the suspected chancre in which the *Treponema pallidum* can be identified. It should be remembered that at this stage the Wassermann reaction will not be positive.

In the secondary stage of syphilis there is a generalized lymphadenopathy and again the individual glands are discrete, non-tender, and freely mobile. At this stage there may be an accompanying skin rash with mucous patches in the mouth or condylomata and the Wassermann and Kahn reactions are positive.

5. Malignant.—

Leukaemia.—Leukaemia is a disease characterized by proliferation of abnormal leucopoietic tissue throughout the body. It is divided according to the type of leucocyte affected into myeloid, lymphocytic, and monocytic varieties, but they all present a similar clinical picture in the acute phase. They occur at any age but are most common in young patients and at the start about a third of the patients are aleukaemic. The onset is sudden with fever, sore throat, bleeding mouth and the patient is gravely ill. In approximately one-third of patients, lymph-node enlargement is the first sign of acute leukaemia, generalized in the lymphocytic form but it may be inconspicuous in the myelocytic type. There may be ecchymosis, petechiae, and an enlarged spleen. The blood picture may show a raised white-cell count or it may be aleukaemic, but the most important feature is that the white cells are abnormal forms. This may lead to difficulty in distinguishing which of the white cells are predominantly affected during the acute stage.

There is a severe reduction in the red-cell and platelet count and the patient is markedly anaemic. The disease is fatal within a matter of days, weeks, or months.

Chronic Myeloid Leukaemia.—Chronic myeloid leukaemia occurs in early adult life and middle age. It usually presents as a progressive tiredness due to the anaemia together with a dragging feeling in the abdomen due to the enlarged spleen.

The total white count with abnormal forms is in the region of 500,000–1 million associated with a reduced red-cell count and haemoglobin.

Chronic Lymphatic Leukaemia.—Chronic lymphatic leukaemia occurs in late middle age and has a reasonable prognosis. The lymph-nodes in the neck are markedly enlarged. The blood picture is similar to that seen in myelogenous leukaemia, but the cells affected are small lymphocytes.

Hodgkin's Disease (lymphadenoma).—Hodgkin's disease is a progressive and fatal disease of lymphoid tissue characterized by lymph-node swellings which are first localized and later generalized, accompanied by splenomegaly and progressive cachexia.

The disease starts in a superficial group of lymph-glands, but eventually all the lymph-nodes in the body may become affected. In a majority of cases the first symptom is an enlargement of a cervical lymph-node. The glands are painless, rubbery, and firm. Diagnosis is made by biopsy of an affected gland when Virchow and Dorothy Reed cells are seen. Eosinophilia is seen in about 10 per cent of cases, but is of little diagnostic significance.

Lymphosarcoma.—Lymphosarcoma may affect any lymphatic tissue, but is more common in the neck. The glands affected may be single or multiple and histologically the tumour is seen to be composed of lymphoblasts. Diagnosis is by biopsy.

Secondary Carcinoma.—An enlarged cervical lymph-node in an adult patient over 40 years old is likely to have a sinister significance, and is frequently a sign of malignant neoplasia. Indeed, it has been widely taught for many years that all painless swellings of the neck are malignant unless proved otherwise. It is also important to realize that in middle-aged individuals, non-specific lymphadenitis is not uncommonly related to a nearby malignant tumour which has not actually invaded the node.

Secondary carcinoma in the neck, as elsewhere in the body, takes the form of a rocky hard swelling of one or more lymph-nodes. The swelling is painless and in time becomes fixed to the surrounding tissues. Eventually it penetrates the overlying skin and may fungate. Enlargement of a cervical lymph-node in relation to a known primary lesion is not necessarily due to a secondary neoplasm, for it may be a pyogenic lymphadenitis.

Malignant enlargement of cervical lymph-nodes may precede the diagnosis of the primary lesion which may be in the nasopharynx or some similar location where it cannot be readily detected. According to Aird (1957), in one-third of all nasopharynx tumours neck swelling is the first symptom.

Malignant Melanoma.—Malignant melanoma is a rare tumour of the head and neck, but if the patient lives long enough, metastases will occur in the lymph-glands of the neck. These secondary deposits may be blackish in colour.

In childhood various neoplastic conditions produce enlargement of the lymph-nodes. Leukaemia is probably the commonest and after that lymphosarcoma, especially in the first decade of life. Hodgkin's disease and other lymphomas account for a small proportion of cervical masses.

Drugs.—Lymphadenopathy may be a rare complication of anticonvulsant therapy with the hydantoins and primidone, and the condition clinically and morphologically resembles a reticulosis. The exact mechanism by which the disease occurs is unknown, but the nature of the condition has been considered to be a hypersensitivity reaction.

Immunological Factor.—A symptom-complex can occur in young children characterized by generalized lymphadenopathy (involving the cervical nodes) and hepatosplenomegaly. This simulates a malignant lymphoma, and, although of unknown aetiology, it is suggested that this condition may be a primary immunological disorder.

Cystic Swellings of the Neck

1. The Sublingual Dermoid Cyst.—Sublingual dermoid cysts may be central or lateral, a classification originally described by Barker (1883). These cysts always originate above the mylohyoid but occasionally they may penetrate it (Seward, 1965). Usually such cysts give the appearance of a 'double chin', but occasionally there is considerable sublingual swelling. This intra-oral swelling is exacerbated if the cyst becomes infected. Under these circumstances the swelling of the floor of the mouth gives the appearance of a Ludwig's angina with the tongue pressed up against the roof of the mouth.

2. The Thyroglossal Cyst.—The thyroglossal cyst may present in any part of the thyroglossal tract in its course from the foramen caecum to the isthmus of the thyroid. The most common situations in order of frequency are: (*a*) Beneath the hyoid; (*b*) In the region of the thyroid cartilage; (*c*) Above the hyoid bone.

It is a midline swelling except in the region of the thyroid gland where the thyroglossal tract is pushed to one side, usually the left. According to Aird, 25 per cent are either to the left or right of the midline. As with all thyroid swellings, the thyroglossal cyst moves on swallowing but in addition the cyst also moves upwards when the patient protrudes the tongue. Very rarely the thyroglossal cyst can present in the mouth and interfere with speech. Thyroglossal cysts have a tendency to recurrent attacks of inflammation and may be mistaken for abscesses and incised. In this way a thyroglossal fistula may be formed. The thyroglossal cyst is often not noticed by the patient until middle or old age, but about 10 per cent are present in infancy (Aird, 1957).

3. Branchial Cyst.—The branchial cyst is said to arise from the second branchial cleft. The cyst is often seen for the first time between the ages of 20 and 25 years, but the swelling may present much later in life. Its position is characteristic in the upper part of the neck beneath the upper third of the sternomastoid muscle, protruding beneath its anterior border (*Fig.* 2). It is a smooth, globular, tense swelling and if the cyst becomes very large the patient may complain of discomfort, dysphagia, and even huskiness of the voice.

Many of these cysts are diagnosed as tubercular glands and clinically the differential diagnosis may be difficult. On aspiration of the branchial cyst, however, fluid containing cholesterol crystals is obtained. Occasionally a branchial cyst becomes infected and this increases its similarity to an abscess.

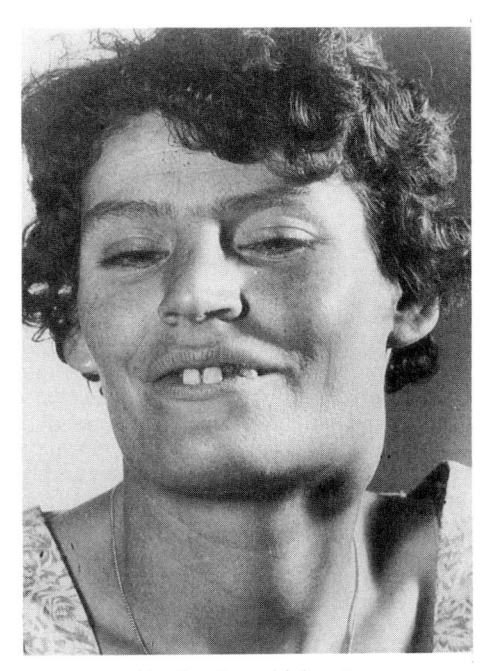

Fig. 2.—Branchial cyst.

4. Cystic Hygroma.—Cystic hygromas are formed by sequestration of the lymphatic endothelium of the jugular sac, the sequestrated endothelium retaining independently its power of irregular growth. The cystic hygroma may be present at birth or become manifest during infancy or childhood. It forms a soft translucent tumour usually situated in the lower third of the neck, but they can also occur in the axilla. When extremely large they may even interfere with labour.

It is the only tumour of the head and neck which is brilliantly translucent. The tumour may continue to grow during infancy, in which case it may interfere with respiration by compressing the trachea, and require urgent decompression by aspiration. At other times it may become infected and spontaneous regression may follow the successful treatment of this complication. Uncontrolled secondary infection, on the other hand, may be fatal. Pathological examination of the tumour shows an aggregation of cysts like masses of soap bubbles. These cysts are lined by endothelium and contain lymph and tend to infiltrate the underlying muscle layers.

Other Swellings of the Neck
(i.e., Non-Lymphatic and Non-Cystic)

1. Sternomastoid Tumour.—The sternomastoid tumour is a hard spindle-shaped tumour which occurs in the lower third of the sternocleidomastoid muscle and makes its appearance ten days to two weeks after birth. It is usually unilateral, but rarely bilateral tumours are present. The mass can be moved laterally but cannot be moved vertically up and down the muscle. After remaining quiescent for some weeks it decreases in size and tends to disappear before the sixth month. However, the patient may be left with a permanent torticollis (wry-neck). The sternomastoid tumour may be due to haematoma formation following birth trauma, or the lesion may be vascular in origin. Ischaemia of the muscle may be responsible and by some it is considered to be a pure fibroma. The permanent wry-neck becomes manifest at the age of about 4 years. If this is untreated, secondary cranial and facial asymmetry develops. Histologically the sternomastoid tumour is found to be a mass of fibrous tissue.

2. Cervical Rib.—Cervical ribs usually arise from the seventh cervical vertebra and in about half the cases they are bilateral. They may vary in size and extend from a complete rib to a fibrous band in the scalenus medius muscle. In some cases the rib ends in a large bony mass and in others the rib is connected to the scalene tubercle of the first rib by a fibrous band. A complete or incomplete cervical rib may be felt as a bony swelling in the neck and it may, of course, be unilateral or bilateral. Symptoms from cervical rib may be nervous or vascular. The sensory phenomena include pain, paraesthesia, and anaesthesia of the little and ring fingers, the ulnar border of the hand, and the forearm. There may be motor weakness which affects the small muscles of the hand and sometimes the flexors of the wrist and fingers. Some 5–6 per cent of patients suffering from neurological manifestations of cervical rib have vascular anomalies of the upper extremity. In the shoulder these may take the form of excessive pulsation and thrill of the subclavian artery above the clavicle, while distally there may be a weakness or obliteration of the radial pulse. The hand may exhibit pallor, cyanosis, paraesthesia, Raynaud's phenomena, acrocyanosis, or even gangrene of the finger-tips.

3. Lipoma.—Lipomas can occur anywhere in the neck and form soft lobulated tumours of varying size. They are most commonly seen bilaterally at the back of the neck beneath the occiput.

4. Carotid Body Tumour (Non-chromaffin Paraganglioma).—The carotid body tumour is a rare swelling which generally first becomes apparent in middle life. It is usually unilateral but may occur bilaterally. When this occurs the second swelling arises some time after the first. The tumour arises from the bifurcation of the carotid artery and is therefore localized to this area. After remaining localized for many years the tumour may metastasize. From its shape, lobulation, and colour, it has become known as a 'potato' tumour. The swelling is usually painless and symptomless, but compression effects are sometimes observed while some patients complain of attacks of faintness—the carotid sinus syndrome.

5. Branchial (Branchiogenic) Carcinoma.—'Branchial carcinoma' is the term used for a tumour lying deep to the upper part of the sternomastoid in a patient who apparently has no primary lesion. It is probable that all the so-called 'branchial carcinomas' are, in fact, metastases from a minute primary concealed in the nasopharynx, paranasal sinuses, pyriform fossa, etc., which can easily be overlooked. The more careful and exhaustive the examination made for inconspicuous primaries, the less frequently the diagnosis of branchial carcinoma is made.

6. **Aneurysm.**—Aneurysms of the neck are usually related to the common carotid artery and they produce a pulsatile swelling of the neck which may compress the trachea, oesophagus, larynx, or recurrent laryngeal nerve. A prominent carotid in an elderly subject should not be mistaken for an aneurysm.

7. **Neurofibromas.**—Multiple neurofibromas may be seen on the neck in Von Recklinghausen's neurofibromatosis and similar lesions will, of course, be seen elsewhere on the body.

8. **Carcinomatous Deposits in Left Supraclavicular Lymph-nodes.**—A rock-hard swelling of the left supraclavicular lymph-node indicates a carcinomatous metastasis from a gastric carcinoma. This physical sign is named after Troisier.

9. **Enlargements of the Thyroid Gland.**—Any enlargement of the thyroid gland is known as 'goitre'.

Classification of Enlargements of the Thyroid

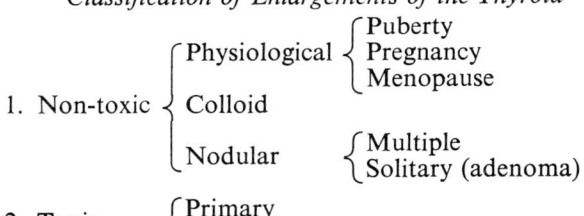

1. Non-toxic
   - Physiological
     - Puberty
     - Pregnancy
     - Menopause
   - Colloid
   - Nodular
     - Multiple
     - Solitary (adenoma)

2. Toxic
   - Primary
   - Secondary to an existing non-toxic goitre

3. Inflammatory
   - Acute pyogenic
   - Chronic
     - Tubercular
     - Syphilitic
     - Actinomycotic

4. Riedel's thyroiditis (Riedel's struma)

5. Hashimoto's disease (struma lymphomatosa)

6. Carcinomatous
   - Follicular
   - Papilliferous
   - Anaplastic

1. Non-toxic Goitres.—

a. Physiological Goitre.—The physiological goitre is almost exclusively confined to females and presents as a swelling in the neck in the thyroid region which requires no specific treatment as it usually subsides in the course of time. However, some of these parenchymatous goitres fail to subside completely and constitute a potential colloid goitre.

b. Colloid Goitre.—Colloid goitres are seen between the ages of 15 and 30 years and are usually physiological goitres which have failed to subside.

c. Nodular Goitre.—Nodular goitre is seen after the age of 30 years and the entire gland is studded with rounded swellings of varying size. Patients with colloid goitre tend to develop nodular goitres with age. Pressure on the trachea may occur especially if haemorrhage into one of the cysts occurs.

2. Toxic Goitre.—Toxic goitre may be primary or secondary and while symptoms often occur between 20 and 40 years, they may develop either earlier or later. The condition is more common in females and is usually characterized by exophthalmos and enlargement of the thyroid gland. Symptoms and physical signs occur in several bodily systems.

   a. Cardiovascular Signs and Symptoms.—
     i. Tachycardia.
     ii. Extrasystoles.
     iii. Raised pulse pressure.
     iv. Atrial fibrillation.
     v. Enlargement of the heart.
     vi. Systolic murmur.
     vii. Heart failure.

   b. Central Nervous System.—
     i. Irritability.
     ii. Fatigue.
     iii. Nervousness.
     iv. Manic depressive insanity.

   c. Gastro-intestinal Tract.—
     i. Voracious appetite.
     ii. Diarrhoea.
     iii. Vomiting.

   d. Metabolic.—
     i. Loss of weight.
     ii. Alimentary glycosuria.
     iii. Raised E.S.R.
     iv. Accelerated tendon reflexes.

   e. Genital.—
Amenorrhoea.

   f. Integumentary.—
     i. Lips are red due to vasodilatation.
     ii. Skin delicate, glossy, and moist.

   g. Eye Signs.—
     i. Exophthalmos.
     ii. Lid lag sign (von Graefe's sign).
     iii. Absence of wrinkling of forehead when head is bent down and patient looks up (Joffroy's sign).
     iv. Difficulty in convergence (Moebius's sign).

Examination of a Patient with an Enlarged Thyroid.—
1. Feel the gland which may be diffuse or localized, smooth or nodular.
2. Watch and feel the gland on swallowing.
3. Is the trachea displaced? Palpate and radiograph.
4. Is there a retrosternal extension? Percuss and radiograph.
5. Listen to breathing for stridor.

6. Examine the eyes. Remember that in secondary thyrotoxicosis positive eye signs are usually absent.
7. Feel pulse and measure blood-pressure. Look for tachycardia, atrial fibrillation, and raised pulse pressure.
8. Watch the outstretched hand for tremor.
9. Examine the condition of skin, nails, hair, and demeanour of the patient.
10. Ascertain whether there is paralysis of recurrent laryngeal nerve. Listen to voice and perform laryngoscopy.

3. Inflammatory.—The thyroid gland may be the seat of acute pyogenic infection or chronic infections of tubercular, syphilitic, or actinomycotic origin.

4. Riedel's Thyroiditis.—Riedel's struma or thyroiditis presents as a small stony, hard thyroid which often causes pressure symptoms. It cannot be differentiated from a scirrhous carcinoma on physical examination alone, and must be confirmed by operation and biopsy.

5. Hashimoto's Disease.—Hashimoto's disease or struma lymphomatosa usually affects middle-aged women and is becoming more common. The entire gland is enlarged and feels like india-rubber and is seldom tender on palpation. Confirmatory diagnosis from carcinoma of the thyroid gland is made by operation and histological examination.

6. Carcinoma of the Thyroid Gland.—Carcinoma of the thyroid gland shows wide histological variations, but three main types are seen:—

1. *Papilliferous:* This often occurs in young persons, frequently in a solitary node and may remain quiescent for long periods eventually metastasizing to the cervical lymph-nodes.

2. *Follicular:* This variety of carcinoma occurs in the middle-aged and is more malignant than the papilliferous variety and rapidly metastasizes to the bone and lungs via the blood-stream.

3. *Anaplastic:* This variety occurs in the elderly and often in a previously normal gland.

In some instances the primary carcinoma of the thyroid may remain small and be overlooked clinically. Eventually metastasis to a bone takes place. Metastases of a carcinoma may also exhibit sufficient secretory activity for the patient to present as a case of mild thyrotoxicosis.

REFERENCES

AIRD, I. (1957), *A Companion in Surgical Studies*, 2nd ed. Edinburgh: Livingstone.
BARKER, A. E. (1883), 'Sebaceous or Dermoid Cyst of the Tongue; Removal by Submental Incision; Cure', *Trans. clin. Soc. Lond.*, **16**, 215.
SEWARD, G. R. (1965), 'Dermoid Cysts of the Floor of the Mouth', *Br. J. oral Surg.*, **3**, 36.

Chapter V

SKIN INCISIONS IN ORAL SURGERY

SOME oral surgery operative wounds are opened through intra-oral incisions and these have been dealt with in Part I. To perform other procedures, the surgical field is approached through a skin incision. One of the major disadvantages of incisions in the skin of the face and neck as opposed to incisions in the mucous membrane of the mouth is that the healed scars are exposed to view. They are not even normally covered by clothing. Therefore, every care must be taken to see that the resulting scars are inconspicuous.

This objective can be achieved in a number of ways: firstly the incision can be placed in a relatively hidden area, such as within the hairline, or in the shadow of the lower border of the mandible. Secondly, the incision can follow Langer's lines. Incisions placed parallel to these lines of tension in the collagen fibres of the dermis do not gape and when they are sutured a thin scar is formed. Should incisions be placed at right angles to Langer's lines the wound edges are pulled apart and a broad, stretched scar is the result after the sutures have been removed. Thirdly, incisions should not be placed in a direction such that muscles which are inserted into, or attached to, the skin can pull on the edges of the wound and widen the scar. The best place for an incision is therefore in a skin crease, that is where there is a local excess of skin and where muscular activity tends to approximate the skin edges. Incisions so placed will, of course, be hidden in the skin crease, or one placed parallel to a skin crease will be mistaken for a further skin crease once the scar has completely matured. Lastly, the wound should be closed with care and sutured skilfully.

The skin creases, as a result of the manner of their formation, represent areas where muscular pull is absent. The direction of skin creases and lines at right angles to the direction of muscle pull do not necessarily follow Langer's lines, but the general direction is similar and conformity to one, or the other, will not seriously affect the quality of the final scar.

Certain factors out of the control of the surgeon mitigate against the formation of a cosmetically acceptable scar. It must, of course, be recognized that all soft tissue wounds heal by scar formation. The question is one of degree. Some persons have a propensity for the formation of hypertrophic or keloid scars. Such persons are more common in certain racial groups. As most older children and adults have suffered accidental cuts, or surgical incisions, such a likelihood can be ascertained by questioning the patient and by a physical examination. The distinction between a hypertrophic and a keloid scar is, to some extent, a matter of degree. Hypertrophic scars are unusually thick, prominent scars confined to the line of the incision. They remain a dusky red colour for longer than normal scars. Keloid scars are even more thickened and lumpy and the process spreads into the tissue adjacent to the margin of the wound.

Occasionally they reach enormous proportions. Mildly hypertrophic scars will flatten in time. The condition may be improved by the intradermal injection of triamcinolone and a jet injection device is ideal for this purpose. Keloid scars can be treated by excision, followed by a small dose of X-irradiations to the new wound as it heals.

Incisions in growing children tend to heal with a broad scar. A possible explanation is the increase in volume of the tissues beneath as a result of somatic growth so that the newly formed scar is stretched. Broad or hypertrophic scars also result when all the first three principles outlined above are transgressed because of the need to make the most direct approach to the operation site. Emergency tracheostomy when a vertical incision is made in the front of the neck is an example of such an occasion.

Before the surgeon puts knife to tissue he should plan the incision. In some situations it may be sufficient to visualize the site and extent of the cut. On the face it is advisable to map the incision out with pen and Bonney's blue. For incisions in the neck it is satisfactory to scratch the line of the cut with the back of the point, provided that the scratch is not carried too deep. Lengthy incisions should be cross-hatched at about three places with Bonney's blue on the face, or with scratches on the neck. Such marks help in the correct approximation of the wound edges at the end of the procedure.

The skin is incised at right angles to the surface except within the eyebrow where the cut should be angled along the line of the eyebrow hairs. Skin and subcutaneous tissue should be penetrated in one sweep if possible, down to the subjacent layer. The tissues should be separated on both sides of the wound over the surface of each succeeding layer and each is opened in turn. In this way, proper layer-by-layer closure is facilitated. Where the subcutaneous fat is thick a subcutaneous suture will be required and the wound edges should be undercut to a depth of about 2 mm., about 4 mm. deep from the surface. This will permit proper eversion of the wound edges without unnecessarily deep stitches and minor corrections can be made in the lie of the wound margins with the skin sutures. Such undercutting should be done as the wound is established, so that proper haemostasis has been ensured by the time that closure is undertaken. It is particularly important to undercut the opposite edge of a wound where one edge is raised as a skin flap. Unless both margins are equally mobile a nice closure is difficult. Undercutting is also necessary where there is oedema of the skin, as, for example, when osteomyelitis or certain fractures are operated upon. Otherwise the stiff skin is difficult to suture.

The skin edges of neck and facial wounds should not be grasped with dissecting forceps, tissue forceps, or towel clips or they will be crushed and damaged. Where a wound is to be open for some while it must be protected from organisms brought to the surface of the adjacent skin as the patient sweats. Plastic sprays, adhesive drapes, and skin towels should be applied to overcome this problem, particularly where bone surgery is involved. Where skin towels are applied, they should be sewn on with loosely tied horizontal mattress sutures and not clamped on with towel clips. Should a skin flap be everted as the tissues are retracted, a moist pack should be applied to the underside of the subcutaneous fat to prevent drying in the heat of the operating room.

The deep layers should be closed neatly with 3·0 or 4·0 plain catgut. Often a continuous suture is satisfactory, but the stitch should not be drawn up tight like a purse string and the knots should be buried on the deep surface of the layer. Skin hooks and 5·0 or 6·0 nylon on atraumatic curved cutting needles should be used to close the skin. Some surgeons prefer braided silk as it is softer and knots more easily. The stitches should enter not more than 2 mm. from the wound edge and pass to a depth of about 4 mm., embracing a greater width of subcutaneous tissue. Each edge should be dealt with separately so that accurate passage of the needle through the tissues is ensured. The suture should pass to the same depth through each wound margin to avoid overlapping or stepping of the skin and it must lie at right angles to the wound. When it is closed the wound surfaces should be approximated so that no dead spaces are left and the cut edges at the surface should be slightly raised in order to produce a final scar that is flat and level with the rest of the surface. A spray-on plastic dressing is sufficient since a dry wound stands the best chance of remaining uninfected, unless, of course, a pressure dressing is applied.

Neck Incisions.—Incisions in the neck are made to follow the skin creases. In general, therefore, they are horizontal or sloping somewhat downwards from behind forward. The major exception is the incision for a block dissection of neck which has a vertical component.

Incisions in the submandibular region are placed in, or parallel to, the skin creases. When the mandible is to be exposed they should be about 1 cm. below the lower border so that the final scar is in the shadow of the jaw. Regard should not be paid to the position of the mandibular branch of the facial nerve. The latter lies deep to the platysma. More posteriorly, it is deep to the deep fascia as well, so that if it is necessary to include the nerve in the upper flap the incision in the platysma can be adjusted to the appropriate level. It is in any case best to identify the nerve, regardless of he way the incision is made, so that it may be preserved.

In the submental region the skin creases run transversely, so it is difficult to join an incision posteriorly to one below the chin. Neither does a submental scar always heal to give a good aesthetic result. The midline of the mandible is best reached by a degloving incision made in the lower buccal sulcus, or by retraction forwards of a submandibular incision.

Peri-orbital Incisions.—Incisions are made in this region to expose the zygomatico-frontal region, the floor of the orbit and infra-orbital margin and the medial wall of the orbit. The zygomatico-frontal region can be exposed by an incision in the lateral end of the eyebrow carried backwards in the line of a crow's foot crease. An alternative is a V-shaped cut made just internal to the lateral margin of the orbit, in the lax tissue lateral to the upper and lower eyelids.

Medially an incision can be made medial to the supra-orbital notch and within the eyebrow. If necessary, such an incision can be extended across the root of the nose so as to expose the nasal bones.

Inferiorly the incision is usually made in a curve following the line of the infra-orbital margin. It should not encroach on the lateral third of the orbit or the lymphatic drainage from the lower lid is affected. For resections of the maxilla the incision runs through the upper lip, lateral to the philtrum, around the ala of the nose, and then up to the margin of the lower lid lateral to the lacrimal canaliculus. It is carried laterally through the lower conjunctival fornix and may be extended further laterally in a crow's foot crease (Crockett, 1963). Incisions involving the free margin of the lip should be broken by lateral cuts and sutured in a Z. Special care should be given to approximating the muscle layer. Both measures are necessary to prevent notching of the lip as the scar contracts. Stepping of eyelid incisions is also necessary to prevent a coloboma of the lid as the wound heals (Kazanjian and Converse, 1959). ... That is, the conjunctival incision is made a short distance to one side of the skin incision so that a step is created through the muscle layer.

Opposite the lower lateral rim of the orbit a radial incision is made. Such cuts not only follow the skin creases, but also do not interfere with the lymphatic drainage of the lower lid.

Pre-auricular Incisions.—Pre-auricular incisions are required to approach the zygomatic arch, temporomandibular joint, and parotid salivary gland. Such incisions should start within the hairline, slope backwards to the pinna, and follow the anterior attachment of the auricle on to the free margin of the tragus. From there they may be extended down and then back beneath the cover of the lobe of the ear. If further extension is required, it may be made backwards into the hairline again or downwards and forwards into a submandibular crease.

REFERENCES

CROCKETT, D. J. (1963), 'Surgical Approach to the Back of the Maxilla', *Br. J. Surg.*, **50**, 819.

KAZANJIAN, V. H., and CONVERSE, J. M. (1959), *The Surgical Treatment of Facial Injuries*, 2nd ed. pp. 72. Baltimore: Williams & Wilkins.

Chapter VI
THE MANAGEMENT OF HAEMORRHAGE IN ORAL SURGERY

Haemorrhage is encountered to a greater or lesser degree in all surgical operations and its management depends upon whether the patient is haematologically normal or suffers from some upset in the clotting mechanism. Anomalies of bleeding occur as a result of a diathesis or from some form of disease or drug therapy which adversely affects haemostasis.

The Management of Haemorrhage in the Normal Patient

Haemorrhage during the Operation.—The overwhelming majority of patients seen by the oral surgeon have a normal haemostatic mechanism and are not suffering from diseases or taking drugs whose effects might produce the problem of prolonged haemorrhage. Even so, excessive loss of blood during the operative procedure can only be avoided by meticulous attention to haemostasis. The management of haemorrhage during the operation can be considered under the following headings:—

1. Planning of the incision to avoid large blood-vessels.
2. The securing of bleeding vessels with haemostats.
3. Haemostasis through the application of pressure with swabs.
4. The use of haemostatic agents.
5. Hypotensive anaesthesia and vasoconstriction.

1. *Incision Planning.*—In the performance of any operation it is mandatory to plan the various incisions so that unduly large blood-vessels are not severed. Intra-oral and extra-oral incisions have already been discussed (*see* p. 17, Part I; p. 36, Part II), but it should be remembered that even in the normal patient haemorrhage may be profuse if the area to be incised is inflamed as a result of local infection. Once the wound has been opened further dissection should be conducted in such a manner that sizeable blood-vessels are identified and dealt with in a systematic fashion. This presupposes that the surgeon is adequately acquainted with the normal anatomy of the part.

2. *The Securing of Bleeding Vessels with Haemostats.*—The most effective haemostats for use in oral surgery are the curved or straight Halsted's mosquito artery forceps and no incision should ever be made through the skin unless an adequate number of haemostats is available for immediate use. Intra-orally the use of haemostats is somewhat limited, but occasionally a moderate-sized aberrant vessel is encountered in the cheek and has to be ligated, or one of the greater palatine arteries requires clamping. It is, of course, impractical to clamp the inferior dental artery within the bone and the use of haemostats on the lingual aspect of the mandible in the lower 3rd molar area is also unwise, since the lingual nerve may be included in the seized tissue which could lead to a protracted anaesthesia of the anterior two-thirds of the tongue. When operating on the face and neck, arteries and veins should, of course, be carefully

identified and, if they have to be divided, haemostats should be applied above and below the point at which they are to be incised before dividing the vessel. The tips of the curved haemostats should be applied so that the curve of the instrument causes the tips of the blades to face upwards and out of the wound so that each severed end of the vessel can be properly exposed by the assistant in order to facilitate the tying off of the vessel with catgut. Size 3·0 (metric size 2·5) catgut is satisfactory for most purposes in oral surgery. Many small vessels do not require tying and if the end of the haemostat is twisted a couple of times before removing it the haemorrhage will usually cease. Small vessels can also be sealed by briefly touching the haemostat with a diathermy set for coagulation before removing it from the vessel.

3. *Haemostasis through the Application of Pressure with Swabs.*—If bleeding points cannot be secured with haemostats, haemorrhage should be controlled by pressure from swabs and this is undoubtedly the most effective method for almost all intra-oral wounds. A dry gauze swab is packed into the wound over the bleeding area and digital pressure is maintained over the swab for a minimum of two and a half minutes. The normal coagulation time is just over two minutes and it is useless to expect to control haemorrhage from a wound by pressure with a swab for a shorter period than this. Pressure is a simple but most effective method of controlling haemorrhage, and the authors have witnessed bleeding from the maxillary artery successfully arrested in this manner. If there is a large raw area which is oozing blood, some operators prefer to use a hot, wet swab to control the haemorrhage. The swab is soaked in hot normal saline solution (temperature 48·8° C., 120° F.), and then it is well wrung out before applying it to the wound. This method is no more effective than the use of ordinary dry swabs and is dangerous when used in the mouth as the delicate tissues of the floor of the mouth may be scalded, especially if there is any excess fluid in the swab. Occasionally the haemorrhage shows a tendency to persist even after pressure with a dry swab for an adequate period of time. This can occur when an artery such as the inferior dental within its canal is incompletely severed and, therefore, the ends are unable to contract. In such circumstances a pack can be left in the wound. To reduce any risk of infection, half-inch (1·25 cm.) ribbon gauze soaked in Whitehead's varnish (benzoin 10 parts, storax 7·5 parts, balsam of Tolu 5 parts, iodoform 10 parts, and solvent ether to 100 parts) should be packed into the wound. The pack should be sewn into position to prevent its subsequent displacement and this precaution is especially important if the patient is being operated upon under general anaesthesia. Such packs will always control a persistent haemorrhage, but they should be removed within 48 hours if they have been packed into a bleeding tooth socket or they may give rise to a dry socket (alveolar osteitis).

4. *The Use of Haemostatic Agents.*—Every dental surgeon is familiar with the multiplicity of topical haemostatic agents which have at some time or other been advocated for the control of dental haemorrhage. Some of these materials, such as turpentine or tannic acid applied on gauze packs or cotton-wool, can be frankly dangerous and the authors have seen second-degree burns at the angle of the mouth and on the lips where the material has leaked over the face. The various commercial

preparations are often of dubious efficacy and obviously more costly than the dry gauze swabs which are infinitely more efficient. Thrombin and Russell viper venom will certainly precipitate clot formation when applied on a pledget of cotton-wool, but again both are expensive. One of the best of the commercially absorbable haemostatic agents is oxidized regenerated cellulose (Surgicel). Unlike most of the other preparations, it works very efficiently and as it is absorbable it can be safely buried in the tissues. Several absorbable gauzes and sponges act merely as a mechanical trap for fibrin and are otherwise inert. Surgicel partially dissolves to form acid products which coagulate plasma proteins together with haemoglobin so as to form a black, sticky clot. The pH of the mass remains acid and may theoretically interfere with normal clotting locally. However, this is not a practical disadvantage since the Surgicel clot is not formed by the normal physiological mechanism. Nevertheless, because of the low pH thrombin solutions should not be used with the gauze because the activity of the thrombin will be rapidly destroyed.

A purely mechanically acting haemostatic agent is Bone Wax (Horsley's) which consists of beeswax (yellow) 7 parts by weight, olive oil 2 parts, phenol 1 part. This substance is packed into bleeding bone ends to control the haemorrhage. Some operators still use this substance, but it should not be used with any frequency as appreciable quantities can result in the formation of wax granulomas.

5. *Hypotensive Anaesthesia and Vasoconstriction.*—Hypotensive anaesthesia can be employed when working under general anaesthesia in order to reduce operative haemorrhage to a minimum. In this technique the patient's blood-pressure is lowered by the anaesthetist through the use of hypotensive agents such as Arfonad and bleeding is greatly reduced. There are disadvantages to this procedure, for during the operation sizeable vessels may be cut without any obvious bleeding and, if overlooked, they are not then tied off with catgut. However, when the operation is over and the patient's blood-pressure is allowed to return to normal, such damaged vessels bleed profusely and the patient may have to be returned to theatre for haemostasis to be effected. There is also a risk of encouraging thromboses, especially in elderly patients with hyperpiesis, when the blood-pressure is lowered to such an extent, and the method itself is not without risk. Hypotensive anaesthesia should therefore be reserved for operations where excessive haemorrhage due to oozing can be anticipated or where visibility is of the utmost importance and a dry field cannot be obtained by other methods. In such cases it is of considerable value.

The use of vasoconstrictors: Vasoconstrictors are incorporated in local analgesic solutions in order to prolong their analgesic effects and they are employed when working under general anaesthesia in order to reduce capillary haemorrhage. The usual vasoconstrictor employed in local analgesic solutions such as Xylocaine (lignocaine) is 1/80,000 adrenaline, but in Citanest (prilocaine) the strength is 1/300,000 and this has been found sufficient in combination with this drug. Adrenaline is alleged, however, to produce undesirable cardiac arrhythmias, especially when a halogenated anaesthetic agent is employed. Further, when used as a vasoconstrictor to facilitate visibility during an operation, it has the disadvantage of producing local tissue cyanosis and acidity. Therefore, as the effect of the adrenaline passes off, a reactive hyperaemia occurs which potentially can result in postoperative haemorrhage and haematoma formation. However, according to Shanks (1963) Octapressin (felypressin) does not produce such undesirable sequelae during halothane anaesthesia and, used in a concentration of 0·03 I.U. per ml. with prilocaine 3 per cent, a satisfactory degree of vasoconstriction is obtained without the same risk of postoperative haemorrhage. Felypressin solutions without prilocaine are not generally available and have not, so far, been widely used as a surgical vasoconstrictor. Not more than 8–10 ml. of the 0·03 I.U. per ml. solution should be injected into an adult at one time.

Postoperative Haemorrhage.—Postoperative haemorrhage may be due to: (1) Failure to control haemorrhage at the conclusion of the operation; (2) A factor restarting haemorrhage in the early postoperative period; (3) Infection at the wound site leading to secondary haemorrhage.

1. *Failure to effect Haemostasis.*—Failure to effect adequate haemostasis at the conclusion of an operation comes under the heading of negligence and it causes great inconvenience to the patient, the nursing staff, and the operator. It is obviously more simple to deal with haemorrhage at the time of operation than have to contend with haemorrhage in the ward or in the out-patient department. No wound should ever be sutured until adequate haemostasis has been effected, for even though the haemorrhage may not be sufficiently severe to necessitate re-opening the wound in order to control it, the patient will inevitably bleed into the tissue planes of the neck and this results in an unsightly ecchymosis, or there may be haematoma formation of considerable dimensions. In the extreme case this could even result in fatal pressure on the trachea.

2. *Factors restarting Haemorrhage.*—Haemorrhage may start again during the first few hours after the operation. During this time haemostasis in the smaller vessels is largely due to contraction of the vessel and platelet thrombus and the mechanism monitoring the former is altering. Blood-clots, too, have not yet matured and contracted. Mechanical injury of the wound, application of heat to the wound inducing local hyperaemia, reactive hyperaemia resulting as the effect of adrenaline wears off, violent exercise with general peripheral vasodilatation and a rise in blood-pressure, or the consumption of a number of alcoholic drinks, perhaps for their analgesic or euphoric effect, again with general peripheral vasodilation, all may trigger off such a haemorrhage. A fit of coughing, as for example in response to a small trickle of blood or saliva, may produce venous congestion and restart substantial haemorrhage from the wound. The classic reactionary haemorrhage, of course, is that which supervenes with the rise in blood-pressure during the initial recovery from a severe operation.

3. *Infection at the Wound Site.*—Secondary haemorrhage is usually due to a partial division of a blood-vessel in combination with sepsis and according to Aird (1957) sepsis alone rarely causes secondary haemorrhage. Provided the operation is carried out with careful attention to asepsis and haemostasis and postoperative infection is prevented, secondary haemorrhage on the classic tenth day should largely be of purely historical interest.

One operation of interest to oral surgeons carries a particular risk of such a haemorrhage. This is the radical neck dissection. The carotid vessels are stripped clean of tissue on their superficial aspect. If the tri-radiate part of the suture line lies over these vessels and wound dehiscence occurs, there is a considerable risk of ulceration and rupture of a carotid.

Bleeding from a Tooth Socket.—Bleeding from an extraction socket is the most common postoperative haemorrhage encountered by the dental surgeon. As with other wounds bleeding may be a continuation of the primary haemorrhage, reactionary haemorrhage occurring after the passage of a few hours, or secondary haemorrhage occurring 7–10 days after the extraction.

The most common cause of persistent primary haemorrhage is *preexisting local inflammation* at the site of the wound. The sockets of teeth extracted for advanced periodontal disease are notorious for the way they bleed and the routine suturing of such sockets has much to commend it. *Hypertension* either as the patient's normal state, or as a result of the emotional stress associated with the extraction, is another cause. *Small puncture wounds* in the sulcus opposite an upper canine, or a lower second molar, due to a slip with an instrument, can damage the upper labial artery or the facial artery, respectively, and can be a cause of profuse, persistent haemorrhage which may be thought mistakenly to be coming from the socket.

All of the factors mentioned under Section 2 above may result in reactionary haemorrhage from a tooth socket. Secondary haemorrhage is fortunately a rare complication of tooth extraction. It is most likely to be seen where a patient develops a Vincent's acute ulcerative gingivitis during the days following the extraction. Because the haemorrhage under such circumstances is not severe, but may recur persistently, a defect in the haemostatic mechanism may be suspected rather than the true cause. The exhibition of antibiotics together with appropriate haemostatic manoeuvres will control the bleeding.

Treatment depends upon identifying the source of the bleeding. First, the patient's mouth should be washed out with cold water and adherent clot removed with a gauze swab, so that the bleeding socket can be accurately visualized and identified. The operator then places the thumb and forefinger on either side of the socket and applies pressure to the gingivae covering the buccal, lingual, or palatal alveolar process. If this pressure controls the haemorrhage, it implies that the source of the bleeding is in the gum and a suture across the socket will effect haemostasis by compressing the mucoperiosteum against the underlying bone. If such pressure fails to control the blood-flow it is obvious that the source of the haemorrhage originates within the bony cavity and some form of socket pack is required, i.e., Whitehead's varnish on ribbon gauze or one of the absorbable haemostatic agents such as gelatin sponge or Surgicel. Suturing across the socket will not control this type of haemorrhage, for the bleeding will continue in the depths of the socket, and as it is unable to escape from the socket owing to the suture it will extravasate into the tissue planes of the neck.

Haematoma Formation.—Postoperative haematoma formation is due to a combination of inadequate postoperative haemostasis or lack of drainage where this is appropriate. All potential dead spaces should be drained and pressure dressings applied to their flaps to discourage capillary ooze and the consequent accumulation of blood. In intra-oral surgery lack of drainage may be due to over-tight suturing of the wound. It may result in a considerable facial swelling which is tender on palpation. The condition is usually present on the first postoperative day and should be treated by removal of one or more sutures and evacuation of the haematoma possibly by aspiration with a sterile wide bore needle. In the mouth it is usually sufficient to institute an intensive régime of hot saline mouthbaths. These effusions of blood often become infected and if the patient has a pyrexia, suitable antibiotic therapy should be instituted. An infected haematoma inevitably leads to breakdown of the suture line and protracted healing of the wound.

The Haemorrhagic Diseases

The haemorrhagic diseases can be divided into three main groups: (1) Diseases where there is a defect in coagulation; (2) Diseases where there is a thrombocytopenia; (3) Diseases where there is an abnormality in the capillaries.

1. *Diseases where there is a Defect in Coagulation*

A defect in coagulation occurs in (*a*) haemophilia and its related diseases and (*b*) in conditions where there is hypoprothrombinaemia.

Coagulation.—The mechanism of the coagulation of blood is still imperfectly understood and the views expressed in this text are those of MacFarlane (1965). According to Professor MacFarlane the natural haemostatic mechanism is an interlocking mechanism of three processes: fibrin formation, platelet aggregation, and vascular contraction. Immediately after vascular injury the platelets adhere to the damaged tissue and to each other to build up a haemostatic plug which in the case of very small vessels is sufficient to stop bleeding, but in larger vessels must be reinforced by fibrin in order to withstand the blood-pressure. Vascular contraction is important as it reduces the diameter of the vessel and so helps to consolidate the haemostatic plug. The mechanism of vascular contraction is imperfectly understood but it may occur as a result of the direct effect of trauma on the muscle of the vessel wall or to nervous impulses, but it is also due to vaso-active substances, e.g. 5 hydroxytryptamine, 5HT, released by the platelets and to substances formed in the blood as a result of clotting. Platelet aggregation is probably due to adenosine diphosphate; a powerful platelet agglutinin which is known to be released in areas of damage and also by the platelets themselves when they are exposed to foreign surfaces or the action of thrombin.

Fibrinogen is a glycoprotein composed of three pairs of polypeptide chains, α, β and χ. Thrombin is a proteolytic enzyme which removes first of all 19 amino-acids from one end of both α chains and then more slowly 14 amino-acids from one end of both β chains. The remainder of the molecule forms the fibrin monomer which polymerizes end to end to form a soluble polymer, fibrin Ia. Insoluble fibrin Ib is precipitated by Factor XIIIa which results from the action of thrombin on Factor XIII. Thrombin is generated from prothrombin by the action of thromboplastin now called prothrombinase. Prothrombin is therefore a pro-enzyme. Prothrombinase is generated by the combination of Factor Xa (which results from the activation of Factor X) with the phospholipid platelet Factor 3 (PF3) and Factor V in the presence of calcium ions.

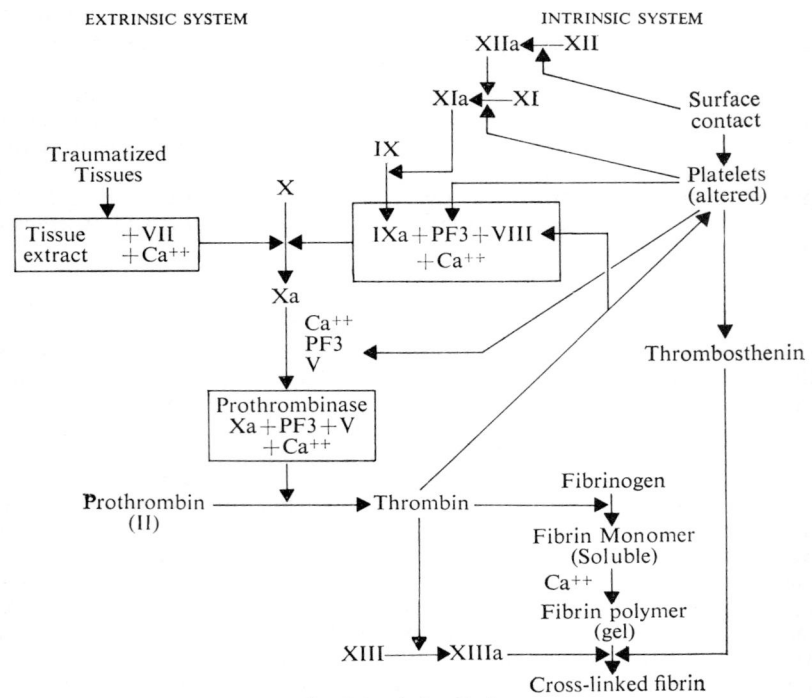

```
EXTRINSIC SYSTEM                    INTRINSIC SYSTEM
                              XIIa ◄— XII
                         XIa ◄— XI
                                              Surface
                                              contact
                      IX                    Platelets
   Traumatized        X                     (altered)
    Tissues
                           IXa + PF3 + VIII
   Tissue    + VII              + Ca++
   extract   + Ca++
                     Xa
                    Ca++
                    PF3
                     V
                  Prothrombinase
                   Xa + PF3 + V
                     + Ca++
                                              Thrombosthenin
                              Fibrinogen
   Prothrombin ——————► Thrombin ——————►
      (II)                    Fibrin Monomer
                              (Soluble)
                              Ca++
                              Fibrin polymer
                              (gel)
              XIII ———► XIIIa
                              Cross-linked fibrin
```

The Coagulation Pathway
(after Boulton, 1973)

Two systems may activate Factor X to Xa: the so called extrinsic system, and the intrinsic system which is formed in normal blood which has been left to stand. In the body both systems probably function together.

In the extrinsic system a phospho-lipo-protein is released from traumatized tissue and combines with Factor VII in the presence of calcium ions. This molecular complex then activates Factor X as described above. In the intrinsic system Factor IXa produces another macro-molecule with PF3 and Factor VIII in the presence of calcium ions. Factor IX is activated to Factor IXa by Factor XI which itself is activated, either by platelets which have been altered by contact with exposed collagen, or by Factor XIIa which arises as a result of the contact of Factor XII with a foreign surface, all this in the form of a 'cascade' reaction (MacFarlane, 1965):

$$\begin{aligned}
XII &— XIIa \\
XI &— XIa \\
IX &— IXa \\
VIII &— VIIIa \\
X &— Xa \\
II &— thrombin \\
I &— fibrin
\end{aligned}$$

Once thrombin is formed it too induces the release of PF3 so that the two processes of clotting and platelet aggregation are interlocked (*see diagram on* p. 52).

Each of these clotting factors may be deficient as a result of hereditary defects or disease or the action of drugs. The most important are haemophilia due to a deficiency of Factor VIII, Christmas disease which is due to deficiency of Factor IX, and deficiencies of Factors V and VII. A review of the blood clotting mechanism and haemostasis in general is to be found in a paper by Boulton (1973).

a. Haemophilia

Haemophilia has an incidence of 1 or 2 per 100,000 of the population and it is caused by a deficiency of antihaemophilic globulin (AHG or Factor VIII) in the plasma. It is inherited as a sex-linked recessive character appearing only in males and is transmitted to them by clinically normal female carriers. All sons of haemophiliacs are free from the haemophiliac gene and all daughters are carriers. When a female marries a normal man half the sons are haemophiliacs and half the daughters are carriers. If a haemophiliac carrier marries a haemophiliac it is possible for their daughter to be a haemophiliac. A case of female haemophilia has been reported by Gilchrist (1961).

The defective gene on the X chromosome causes a deficiency of Factor VIII which can be complete or partial. If the level is 25–50 per cent of normal the patient has no trouble unless he suffers from major trauma. Minor injuries do not bleed abnormally owing to the fact that haemostatic function is quantitative and what is enough for minor injuries is insufficient for major trauma. At levels of 10–25 per cent more serious bleeding occurs after minor injuries and below 10 per cent bleeding into muscles and joints occurs. The blood coagulation time is normal with Factor VIII levels above 1–2 per cent, but the severe haemophiliac usually has 0 per cent Factor VIII. Of the severe haemophiliacs most cases appear to have a plasma factor which cross-reacts with human Factor VIII, but a few do not. This implies that there are two populations of haemophiliacs: the larger one having a non-functioning Factor VIII analogue and a smaller one which does not even produce the abnormal Factor VIII. These latter patients are particularly liable to develop Factor VIII antibodies as a result of transfusions.

Symptoms of Haemophilia.—The principal symptoms are persistent bleeding after cuts and abrasions and especially after tooth extraction. There is also bleeding into the large joints especially the knee-joint.

The Investigation and Management of a Haemophiliac requiring Oral Surgery.—

The History.—The medical history of an adult haemophiliac will leave no doubt in the mind of the clinician concerning the diagnosis, for it will consist of numerous accounts of severe bleeding episodes following trivial trauma, most of which will have resulted in the patient being hospitalized.

Clinical Examination.—Clinical examination of the patient usually reveals evidence of haemarthrosis in the form of limitation of movement of large joints such as the knee, and in more recent episodes there may be evidence of swollen painful joints and possibly swollen areas elsewhere in the body. The bleeding is deep in the tissues and ecchymosis is not a prominent feature. The patient may also give a history of episodes of haematuria and haematemesis.

Selection of Time for Operation.—A study of the medical history will show that the bleeding episodes tend to be grouped together and are separated by periods when the patient appears to have been relatively free of the disease. An intelligent adult haemophiliac can usually be relied upon to inform the clinician when he is in a 'good phase' and if surgery is contemplated, it is prudent to select such a time.

Diagnosis.—The investigation of a suspected case of haemophilia requires the services of a skilled haematologist, and once the missing factor in the coagulating mechanism has been identified the patient can be rendered fit for surgery by injecting the missing factor intravenously. The clotting time in haemophilia is not prolonged until the level of AHG falls below 1 per cent and a relatively normal reading could prove most deceptive to the surgeon. The only safe test for haemophilia is to estimate the AHG level in the patient and this requires the services of a specially equipped laboratory.

Treatment.—The treatment of haemophilia is essentially a problem for the haematologist, first, by diagnosing the exact nature of the disorder, and then, by replacing the missing factor in the blood, it may be possible to render the patient relatively normal so far as the surgery is concerned. The blood level of Factor VIII can be raised by the injection of various substances, but the effect is short-lived. The preparations which contain Factor VIII are:—
1. Fresh whole blood.
2. Fresh or frozen plasma.
3. Cryoprecipitate prepared from human plasma.
4. Freeze-dried animal AHG (antihaemophilic globulin).
5. Freeze-dried human AHG (antihaemophilic globulin).

Fresh whole blood and plasma have low concentrations of Factor VIII and as one can only give a certain volume without overloading the circulation, only a limited blood level can be attained. Even when fresh blood containing its full complement of Factor VIII is used, it cannot be transfused into the patient quickly enough to achieve a level of Factor VIII which will bring about haemostasis. The policy, therefore, should be to give blood transfusions only to replace blood-loss and not to use as a source of Factor VIII. The best Factor VIII level which can be attained with whole blood is 5–7 per cent and with frozen or fresh plasma 15–20 per cent. By using human AHG a level of 50–60 per cent can be obtained and a level of 60–100 per cent can be attained by using animal AHG. There is a shortage of human AHG and the supplies are inadequate for the demand, but animal AHG which is derived from ox or pig blood is readily available. Unfortunately, this material is a foreign protein and is antigenic, and if treatment with this agent is unduly protracted the patient will develop resistance and there will also be a loss of therapeutic effect and probably an allergy will develop. Animal AHG should, therefore, be reserved for emergencies, for a second course of the drug would probably result in anaphylaxis.

Cryoprecipitate and fresh frozen plasma are the preparations usually used to cover exodontia. Of the two preparations, cryoprecipitate is the more concentrated (anything from 5 to 15 times more concentrated) so that higher blood levels of AHG are more easily obtained and there is less risk of overloading the circulation, particularly in a child. Further, cryoprecipitate can be given intravenously with a syringe, while fresh frozen plasma requires an intravenous infusion. Cryoprecipitate is prepared by freezing fresh plasma and re-thawing in a controlled manner at $+4°C$. so that AHG and fibrinogen are precipitated. Plastic bags containing 5–20 ml. of plasma are in use and concentrations are between 15 and 45 New Oxford units per ml. Each pack will, on average, increase the level of Factor VIII in the blood of a 70-kg. man by $3\frac{1}{2}$ per cent so that about 8–10 packs may be needed preoperatively. While much AHG is lost in the preparation the technique is comparatively simple compared with the preparation of dried human AHG. The excess of fibrinogen does not normally matter.

The half-life of injected Factor VIII in the body is about 12 hours and 24 hours after an injection it will be down to a quarter of its immediate postinjection level. According to MacFarlane (1965) a level of 20 per cent Factor VIII falling to 5 per cent is adequate for minor injuries and single tooth extractions (i.e., use of plasma). More serious traumas such as multiple extractions require 40 per cent falling to 10 per cent which can be achieved with human AHG. Major trauma or surgery will probably require a 100 per cent Factor VIII level, and therefore animal AHG will have to be used. It should be stressed, however, that most patients become resistant to treatment with the particular animal AHG within 7–10 days of starting treatment and their Factor VIII response after transfusion of the dose gradually diminishes.

Management of the Haemophiliac undergoing Oral Surgery.—The management of the haemophiliac is essentially a haematological problem which consists of an exact diagnosis of the condition followed by the replacement of the missing factor. There are, however, certain additional steps which should be taken by the oral surgeon. The most likely operation to be performed is, of course, the extraction of a tooth or teeth, for no one would advocate more major surgery unless it was absolutely vital. Every effort should be made to conserve teeth and no more extractions should be carried out than are absolutely essential.

Anaesthesia.—In some ways local analgesia is preferable to general anaesthesia, for bleeding could occur at the back of the throat and the region of the glottis as a result of passing an endotracheal tube. In some cases a nasal inhalation anaesthetic after full premedication is satisfactory, in others a nasopharyngeal tube is used, or an orotracheal tube is passed in the relaxed patient under direct vision. Mandibular block injections are absolutely contra-indicated in view of the danger of persistent haemorrhage into the parapharyngeal tissues. Death following a mandibular block injection for conservative treatment has been reported (Parnell, 1964). Local infiltration causes bleeding at each point where the needle is inserted and the only absolutely safe site for injection is down the periodontal membrane. This is painful and infection could be introduced by the needle, but it gives good analgesia and the area is to be disrupted by the forceps beaks anyway.

A haemorrhage plate should be constructed prior to operation, not to control the haemorrhage, which it is incapable of doing, but to protect the blood-clot from the trauma of food and the patient's tongue during the postoperative period. The tooth to be removed should be extracted as atraumatically as possible, after which the sides of the socket are gently squeezed together. The socket should not be sutured, for not only would the needle wounds bleed but blood which could not escape into the mouth would merely be directed down the fascial planes of the neck. If the patient does bleed postoperatively it is preferable for the blood to flow into the mouth where it can be seen and be treated. A small pledget of cotton-wool soaked in Russell viper venom should be placed over the socket or Surgicel can be used for the purpose, after which gentle pressure is maintained until coagulation occurs.

It should be remembered that unless the patient has a 0 per cent concentration of AHG, coagulation will eventually occur and if, for example, the coagulation time is half an hour, gentle pressure for just over half an hour will eventually succeed in staunching the flow. Normally the missing factor will, of course, have been replaced by the intravenous route shortly before operation and so coagulation can be confidently expected in a comparatively short time. The patient is returned to the ward and subjected to the following régime:—

1. The patient should be nursed in the sitting position.
2. The patient should be on absolute bed-rest.
3. To prevent breakdown of the clot by muscular movement, the mandible should be immobilized by applying a barrel bandage.
4. A lukewarm liquid diet should be ordered.
5. The patient should not have hot drinks or any form of alcohol.
6. The patient is best in a room on his own so that the bleeding is not started by excessive talking.
7. Visitors should be kept away for the same reason.
8. In order to endure this régime, the patient should be sedated with phenobarbitone 30 mg. b.d.

Additional booster doses of Factor VIII (e.g., cryoprecipitate) should be administered daily and the patient must be hospitalized until five days have elapsed without bleeding. It need hardly be added that such analgesics as aspirin are absolutely contra-indicated in view of the danger of severe haematemesis and even in small doses aspirin is known to impair platelet function, and this added haemostatic defect in the haemophiliac can make him prone to bleed. As an alternative to aspirin as an analgesic, paracetamol or dihydrocodeine may prove effective.

EACA.—In recent years epsilon aminocaproic acid (EACA), an antifibrinolytic substance, has been used to increase the stability of the clots formed after extractions in haemophiliacs. EACA has been used in combination with various local measures but without AHG replacement, and also in combination with AHG replacement. The drug is not free from possible unpleasant side-effects, but no treatment in haemophiliacs is without risk (Cooksey and others, 1966; Reid and others, 1964). Tranexamic acid reduces plasminogen activity by competitive inhibition and it also reduces the activity of preformed plasmin. Pell (1973) suggests that as it is a safer drug than EACA it should be used in preference to the latter in the treatment of haemophiliac bleeding.

If the patient has Christmas disease or an absence of Factor V or VII, the necessary modifications are made to this treatment.

Christmas Disease.—Christmas disease has the same inheritance and clinical features as haemophilia, but the Christmas factor (Factor IX) is much more stable than antihaemophilic globulin and stored blood can be used in its treatment. As in the case of haemophilia some patients appear to have an inactive material which cross-reacts antigenically with the normal factor, that is Factor IX. A few cases do not have this abnormal material. Some cases have a factor which appears to inhibit both normal Factor IX and normal Factor VII *in vitro*. These cases have been designated Haemophilia B.M. Cryoprecipitate does *not* contain Factor IX and is not appropriate in the treatment of Christmas disease. Fresh frozen plasma or, if they are available, Factor IX concentrates are used. As the half-life of Factor IX is 2½ days, smaller amounts of infusion material are required.

Factor V Deficiency is inherited in some families as a dominant trait, but is extremely rare. It can be treated with fresh blood.

Factor VII Deficiency is seen in patients under anticoagulant therapy and occasionally in advanced liver disease. Treatment is with stored blood.

Other Deficiencies.—From time to time patients with a deficiency of other factors—for example, Factor X (Quast and others, 1971) and Factor XI (Williams, 1972)—are reported. Such cases are rare and specialist advice by a haematologist is necessary to unravel their diagnostic problems.

b. Conditions in which there is a Hypoprothrombinaemia

Prothrombin is produced in the liver and vitamin K (napthaquinone) is required for its synthesis. Factors VII, X, and IX also require the presence of vitamin K for their production in the liver. There are two sources of vitamin K—an exogenous source in the diet and an endogenous source from the intestines where it is synthesized by certain bacteria. Vitamin K is not properly absorbed in the absence of bile-salts. Clinical prothrombin deficiency is therefore seen in:—

1. Newborn babies in whose intestines the vitamin-K-forming organisms have not yet become established, i.e., haemorrhagic disease of the newborn. This condition can be largely prevented by giving intramuscular vitamin K either to the mother before birth or to the baby as soon as it is born.

2. Patients with obstructive jaundice who should also be given vitamin K analogues if any surgical operation is contemplated, otherwise serious haemorrhage can occur.

3. Patients in whom the vitamin-K-forming organisms have been greatly reduced as a result of protracted therapy with broad-spectrum antibiotics, or who are 'washed-out' through severe dysenteries. In these patients vitamin K production may be inadequate and so again haemorrhage may occur. The conditions also can be corrected by administering water-soluble vitamin K analogues.

4. Patients with severe liver damage as a result of hepatitis, multiple metastases, etc., in whom again there is a failure to produce prothrombin,

but this condition is not wholly dependent on the lack of vitamin K and may be improved, but cannot be corrected by its administration.
  5. Conditions of extreme malnutrition.
  6. Patients receiving an oral anticoagulant.
  7. Patients suffering from fatty diarrhoea, e.g., coeliac disease and sprue.
  8. Patients who have a rare form of congenital hypoprothrombinaemia. Such patients are on maintenance doses of vitamin K for life.

The main importance to the oral surgeon of all these conditions is that he should be aware of the possibility of severe haemorrhage following even minor surgery when working upon any of these categories of patients. Water-soluble vitamin K analogues given i.m. for three days preoperatively may be helpful in such cases—except, of course, for patients on phenindione, etc., where vitamin K_1 (phytomenadione) given intravenously is usually advocated for the emergency reversal of the anticoagulant effect. Frequently all that is needed is to stop treatment with the anticoagulant, but if urgent reversal of the anticoagulant is required fresh frozen plasma should be given. This measure is safer and rather more constant in its effect than the administration of vitamin K. Whatever treatment is used the effect should be monitored by prothrombin time tests.

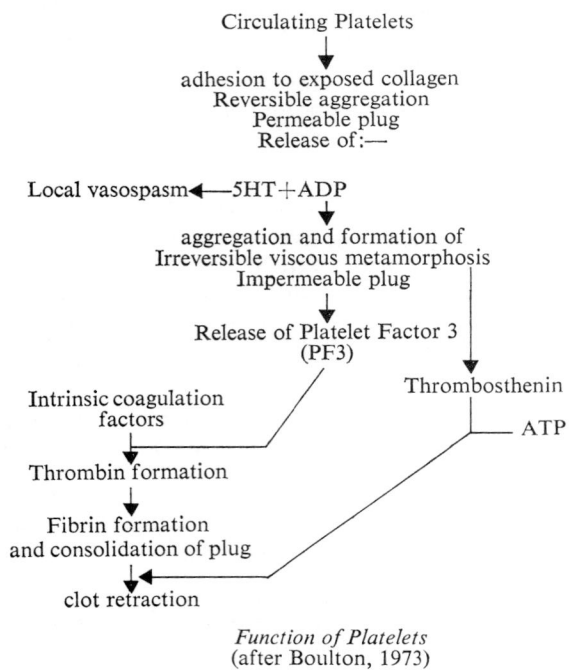

Function of Platelets
(after Boulton, 1973)

2. Diseases where there is a Thrombocytopenia

Essential Thrombocytopenia (Idiopathic Thrombocytopenic Purpura).—This is a rare disease of young adults characterized by episodes of skin qurpura, epistaxis, and alimentary and uterine haemorrhage. The platelet count is low (below 40,000 per c.mm.) and the bleeding time is prolonged but the coagulation time is normal. The Hess test is strongly positive. As a result of recurrent haemorrhages the patient may have an iron-deficiency type of anaemia. In some patients the spleen is palpable.

Treatment is by splenectomy, but this carries a high mortality if carried out during the acute phases of the disease. Adrenocortical steroids may also be used in treatment and these must be considered if surgery is contemplated.

Bleeding in thrombocytopenia is excessive after even minor trauma so that tiny wounds such as needle punctures can bleed for prolonged periods, or give rise to a spreading haematoma (Seward, 1962). Widespread bruising and petechial haemorrhages are also characteristic of a platelet deficiency or abnormality rather than a clotting defect. Boulton (1973) lists the following drugs which may cause thrombocytopenia:—

1. Those associated with pancytopaenia:

Cytotoxic drugs	Tolbutamide
Gold	Chlorpropamide
Chlorthiazides	Organic arsenicals.

2. Those causing selective thrombocytopenia:

Quinidine	Phenobarbitone
Quinine	Butobarbitone
Digitoxin	Cephalothin sodium
	Salicylates.

There are also a number of diseases in which the platelets are normal in number but abnormal in function. For example, part of the cause of bleeding in Von Willebrand's disease is due to defective platelet adhesion, and in Glanzmann's disease, or thrombasthenia, there is a defective platelet aggregation in the presence of ADP and defective clot retractions (Wood, 1973). Skilled haematological testing is required to sort out these abnormalities.

In thrombocythaemia the number of platelets is increased. If their function is normal a hyperthrombotic state exists. If they are abnormal the patient bleeds abnormally. In macroglobulinaemia the platelets tend to become coated with protein and their function is impaired.

3. *Diseases in which there is an Abnormality of the Capillaries*

Purpura may be seen in any of the acute fevers, especially meningococcal infections, and can also occur as a result of drug sensitivity with agents such as heavy metals, sodium salicylate, isoniazid, thiouracil, chlorpromazine, etc. Senile purpura occurs in elderly people and purpura also occurs as a result of avitaminosis (scurvy).

Anaphylactoid Purpura

The Schönlein-Henoch syndrome is characterized by purpura and allergic manifestations such as urticaria, joint pains, joint swelling, and angioneurotic oedema which also affects the gut causing intestinal colic. Henoch's purpura is associated with abdominal colic and Schönlein's purpura with joint pains, but both conditions may occur in the same patient. Severe haemorrhage may occur when operating on patients suffering from these conditions.

The Ehlers-Danlos Syndrome

The Ehlers-Danlos syndrome (E.D.S.) was originally described by Van Meekeren in 1682. Ehlers (1901) described the hyperelastic skin, skin haemorrhages, and loose jointedness, while Danlos (1908) reported the cutaneous pseudotumours and peculiar scarring. The syndrome is inherited as an autosomal dominant trait and the condition is said to be more common in males. The basic defect in E.D.S. is unknown. Wechsler and Fisher (1964) carried out histochemical and electron microscopy investigations without elucidating the basic defect, but most authors consider it to be a collagen defect. Jansen (1955) considered that the cross linkages between the collagen fibres were defective.

Clinical Features.—

Fragility of the skin: The skin has a velvety feel and is hyperelastic and brittle. Minor trauma results in gaping wounds of the skin which are difficult to suture because the sutures tear out.

Scarring: When the lacerations heal they form thin papyraceous scars which, instead of contracting, tend to spread.

Hyperextensibility of the skin: In pronounced cases the skin can be pulled into large folds, but when it is released it snaps back into its normal position.

Hypermobility of the joints: Joints may be extremely mobile (double-jointed). Thexton (1965) reported a case who had to have bilateral condylectomy following repeated dislocations of the mandible. This characteristic of joint hypermobility is shared with Marfan's syndrome, osteogenesis imperfecta, and some cases of cleidocranial dysostosis.

Pseudotumours: Resolving haematomas and excessive scarring form 'pseudotumours' over prominences such as the elbows and knees.

Subcutaneous spherules: These small, hard, mobile nodules occur in the subcutaneous tissues. They are said to be fat lobules which have a fibrous tissue capsule and later they become calcified and are rendered radio-opaque.

Excessive bruising: After minimal trauma there is extensive ecchymosis and haematoma formation.

Protracted bleeding after extractions: Protracted post-extraction haemorrhage has been reported by Tobias (1934), Johnson and Falls (1949), and Jacobs (1957), but in the 9 cases described by Barabas and Barabas (1967) only one suffered from post-extraction bleeding. Five of their 9 cases were subjected to a haematological examination which included bleeding time, whole-blood clotting time, one-stage prothrombin time (Quick's method), serum prothrombin consumption index, thromboplastin generation test, antihaemophiliac globulin assay, clot retraction, and the Hess test for capillary fragility. The Hess test was positive but all other tests were negative, including the case in which post-extraction haemorrhage had occurred.

Von Willebrand's Disease

Von Willebrand's disease has also been known as 'pseudohaemophilia' and was first described in 1926. It is transmitted as an autosomal dominant and occurs as frequently in men as in women. It is a haemorrhagic disorder characterized by a protracted bleeding time thought to be due to capillaries which do not contract normally and there is an associated deficiency of antihaemophilic Factor VIII. The abnormal capillaries may be seen with a dissecting microscope in the nail bed. Platelet adhesion is also reduced. Infusions of plasma or cryoprecipitate not only correct the Factor VIII deficiency but also correct the platelet abnormality. Following such an infusion the patient's own Factor VIII synthesis temporarily increases. Curiously the infusion of haemophiliac plasma will also stimulate Factor VIII synthesis. Patients suffering from Von Willebrand's disease are subject to exacerbations and remissions of their condition. Viral infections particularly may incite an exacerbation and surgery should be avoided during these illnesses. Haemorrhages follow trivial trauma and menorrhagia, haematoma formation, epistaxis, and gingival bleeding may occur. The bleeding tendency may improve in middle or old age. Treatment is effected by the administration of fresh blood or plasma.

Hereditary Haemorrhagic Telangiectasia
(Osler-Weber-Rendu Disease)

Hereditary haemorrhagic telangiectasia (H.H.T.) is not a true intrinsic bleeding state and in patients suffering from the disorder all the currently recognized haematological investigations are within normal limits. The disease involves the cutaneous, visceral, and mucosal surfaces and the disease is characterized by its familial occurrence and is transmitted as an autosomal dominant, both sexes being affected equally. The disease was first described by Sutton in 1864, who reported epistaxis as a disease or a prime symptom of a diseased state. In 1865 Babington described a disorder characterized by epistaxis which he had traced through five generations and in 1896 Rendu referred to the disease as 'pseudohaemophilia', a familial condition with epistaxis. However, Osler (1901) first provided a full clinical description of the disease, while Weber in 1907 made a clear-cut distinction between H.H.T. and the haemophilias. Hence, the eponym 'Osler-Weber-Rendu Disease'.

Clinical Features.—The diagnosis is made on the basis of the clinical triad of the characteristic telangiectatic lesions, a hereditary incidence, and a haemorrhagic diathesis. The angiomatous skin or mucous membrane lesions may be punctiform, spider-like, and nodular, and may all bleed when traumatized. There is a wide distribution of the telangiectases including the lips, tongue, nose, and more rarely the brain, spinal cord, gastro-intestinal tract, lungs, eye, bladder, and uterus. The defect has usually been attributed to a purely mechanical defect in the vessels. These fragile vessels are liable to rupture when subjected to minimal trauma. Ullman (1890), however, regarded the telangiectases as a new capillary formation of vessels. The haemorrhagic episodes are usually of short duration, but may occur so frequently that the patient becomes anaemic. However, some patients have a protracted bout of bleeding. The disease usually presents as recurrent epistaxes in youth with the cutaneous manifestations appearing in the second and third decades. The disease tends to become progressively more severe with age and many of the symptoms of the elderly sufferer are attributable to chronic anaemia. The disease is of particular interest to oral surgeons for the lips, tongue, cheeks, and floor of the mouth are the areas most commonly affected. The lesions present as tiny bright red or violaceous raised haemangiomas about 2 mm. in diameter which blanch on pressure. Even the minor trauma sustained during conservative dental treatment can lead to haemorrhage from one or more lesions through their surfaces being abraded. Protracted haemorrhage is unusual, but Killey and Kay (1970) reported a case in which a palatal lesion bled profusely on two separate occasions, and in 1908 Phillips reported a fatality following the use of a toothbrush on the gingival tissues.

Treatment of a telangiectatic area which tends to bleed persistently is effected by cautery excision, but this method is, of course, impractical when it comes to dealing with all the lesions present in the mouth. Nasal intubation for endotracheal anaesthesia is, of course, contra-indicated owing to the risk of a severe epistaxis.

Acute Fibrinolytic States in Surgery

One cause of acute failure of haemostasis during surgical operations is pathological fibrinolytic activity.

The fibrinolytic enzyme system or plasminogen–plasmin system is believed to have a physiological role complementary to that of the coagulation system in maintaining an intact, patent, vascular system. It is believed that the two systems are in a state of dynamic equilibrium, the coagulation system sealing with a fibrin plug any solution in continuity of the system and the fibrinolytic enzyme then removes such fibrin deposits after endothelial repair has been effected. The main components of the fibrinolytic enzyme system are plasminogen, plasmin, activators, and inhibitors. Plasminogen is normally an inert plasma globulin which is converted by activators to plasmin, a proteolytic enzyme which can digest many proteins including fibrinogen, fibrin, antihaemophilic globulin (AHG), and Factor V. The activators of plasminogen include a plasma activator, tissue activators present in high concentrations in lungs, prostate, thyroid, and uterus, and certain bacteria which can also produce plasminogen activators. Urinary activators may play a part in producing the ooze of blood which may take place from the gland bed after a prostatectomy. Surgeons have been aware for many years that fear increases haemorrhage and that sedation can be an aid to haemostasis. While the elevation of blood-pressure which accompanies fear may be one mechanism by which this occurs, fibrinolysis may also play a part because fear can cause the liberation of plasminogen activators.

Normal plasma probably contains inhibiting mechanisms to control the small amounts of plasminogen in the tissues. If large amounts of plasminogen activator are suddenly released into the circulation, plasminogen is suddenly converted into plasmin. This overwhelms the antiplasmin mechanism and the presence of free plasmin in the circulation results in digestion of fibrinogen, Factor VIII, and Factor V and a grave coagulation defect occurs. The products of fibrinolysis are also capable of interfering with the polymerization of fibrin and the formation of a clot. This condition may occur in thoracic surgery, especially when the heart-lung machine is employed, but it can also occur as a result of transfusing a patient with blood which is contaminated with bacteria. Certain bacteria (cryophilic) can actually breed in the chilled state in which blood used in transfusions is stored. A transfusion with such blood would result in a surgical disaster. EACA has been used in the treatment of this condition, combined, of course, with massive replacement transfusion.

Plasmin therefore removes fibrin after endothelial repair of a break in a vessel and probably in the tissues as well as a normal event. Fibrinolysins produced by bacteria also act in a similar fashion, but to facilitate the spread of the organisms through the tissues. Plasmin activators may be used to promote the removal of unwanted clot, as in venous thrombosis and pulmonary embolism, and fibrinolysins have been tried as a means of cleaning wounds and as a way of reducing postoperative swelling.

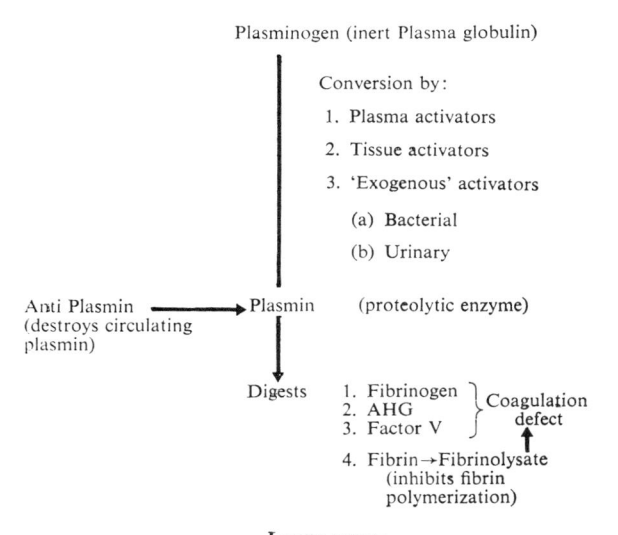

Plasminogen (inert Plasma globulin)

Conversion by:
1. Plasma activators
2. Tissue activators
3. 'Exogenous' activators
   (a) Bacterial
   (b) Urinary

Anti Plasmin ⟶ Plasmin (proteolytic enzyme)
(destroys circulating plasmin)

Digests
1. Fibrinogen ⎱ Coagulation
2. AHG   ⎰ defect
3. Factor V
4. Fibrin → Fibrinolysate
   (inhibits fibrin polymerization)

LEUKAEMIA

Leukaemia is generally regarded as a neoplastic process, but its exact aetiology is unknown. The part which viruses play in human disease is uncertain. It is a disease characterized by abnormal proliferation of leukopoietic tissue throughout the body and it is classified according to the type of leucocyte which is affected into lymphatic, myeloid, and macrocytic varieties.

Acute Leukaemia.—The clinical picture in acute leukaemia is similar in all varieties. It can occur at any age, but it is more common in children. During the early stages of acute leukaemia there is usually a leucopenia and this is associated with low red-cell and platelet counts. Recurrent infective lesions and purpuric manifestations occur at this stage. The onset is usually sudden with fever, sore throat, and bleeding from the mouth and nose. The patient is pale and has a generalized lymphadenopathy and is obviously severely ill. There is usually tenderness on palpation over the sternum and the diagnosis is confirmed by examination of the bone-marrow, when abnormal varieties of white cells are seen. Protracted post-extraction haemorrhage can be a presenting symptom and the authors have seen several cases which have been diagnosed in this fashion. Postoperative bleeding can be anticipated in all types of chronic leukaemia and especially in the terminal stages of leukaemia when the patient becomes aleukaemic and there are severe haemorrhages and infections.

Anticoagulants and Surgery.—Anticoagulants are used in the treatment of a variety of thrombo-embolic conditions such as myocardial infarction and pulmonary and venous thrombosis, and the oral surgeon is increasingly confronted with the problem of having to carry out surgery on such patients. Minor surgery can be safely effected provided the patient is having a correct normal or slightly reduced maintenance dose of an anticoagulant drug, but many patients presenting for surgery have not been adequately supervised and have a higher than necessary or desirable level of the anticoagulant. In such patients severe postoperative bleeding can be anticipated.

Prior to oral surgery, the patient's anticoagulant level must be correctly regulated and this is confirmed by measuring the prothrombin level. This is done by:—

1. Owren's thrombotest method, when the value should be 7–15 per cent of normal.

2. Quick's test, where the level should be 15–30 per cent of normal.

3. Prothrombin and proconvertin method, when it should be 10–25 per cent of normal.

Provided that the patient's therapeutic level is within range of normal, forceps extractions can be undertaken without undue risk of postoperative haemorrhage. The reflection of flaps and multiple extractions necessitate a reduction in anticoagulant dosage. It is dangerous in some patients to stop the anticoagulant therapy prior to operation, for sudden withdrawal of the drug may lead to a tendency to an overswing towards thrombosis which may have serious and even fatal consequences. This phenomenon, which is especially liable to occur when anticoagulants of the dicoumarol group are suddenly discontinued, has been termed 'anticoagulant rebound' or 'rebound thrombosis' and may possibly be due to excessive concentration of Factor VIII.

REFERENCES

AIRD, I. (1957), *A Companion to Surgical Studies*, 2nd ed. Edinburgh: Livingstone.
BABINGTON, B. G. (1865), 'Hereditary Epistaxis', *Lancet*, **2**, 362.
BARABAS, G. M., and BARABAS, A. P. (1967), 'The Ehlers-Danlos Syndrome', *Br. dent. J.*, **123**, 473.
BOULTON, F. E. (1973), 'A Review of Haemostasis', Suppl. to *Lond. Hosp. Gaz.*, **76**, No. 1.
COOKSEY, M. W., PERRY, C. B., and RAPER, A. B. (1966), 'Epsilon-aminocaproic Acid Therapy for Dental Extractions in Haemophiliacs', *Br. med. J.*, **2**, 1633.
DANLOS, H. (1908), 'Un cas de cutis laxa avec tumerus par contusion chronique des condes et des genoux', *Bull. Soc. fr. Derm. Syph.*, **19**, 70.
EHLERS, E. (1901), 'Cutis laxa, neigung zu hemorrhagien in der haut, lockerung mehrerer artikulationen', *Derm. Z.*, **8**, 173.
GILCHRIST, L. (1961), 'A Case of Female Haemophilia', *Proc. R. Soc. Med.*, **54**, 813.
JACOBS, P. L. (1957), 'Ehlers-Danlos Syndrome', *Archs Derm.*, **76**, 460.
JANSEN, L. H. (1955), 'Le mode de transmission de la maladie d'Ehlers-Danlos', *J. Génét. hum.*, **4**, 204.
JOHNSON, S. A. M., and FALLS, H. F. (1949), 'Ehlers-Danlos Syndrome: A Clinical and Genetic Study', *Archs Derm.*, **60**, 82.

KILLEY, H. C., and KAY, L. W. (1970), 'Hereditary Haemorrhagic Telangiectasia', *Br. J. oral Surg.*, **7**, 161.
MACFARLANE, R. G. (1965), 'The Haemostatic Defect in Haemophilia and its Temporary Correction', *Proc. R. Soc. Med.*, **58**, 251.
OSLER, W. (1901), 'Family Form of Recurring Epistaxis', *Bull. Johns Hopkins Hosp.*, **20**, 63.
PARNELL, A. G. (1964), 'Danger to Haemophiliacs of Local Anaesthesia', *Br. dent. J.*, **116**, 183.
PELL, G. (1973), 'Tranexamic Acid—its Use in controlling Dental Postoperative Bleeding in Patients with Defective Clotting Mechanisms', *Br. J. oral Surg.*, **11**, 155–164.
PHILLIPS, S. (1908), 'Case of Multiple Telangiectasia (shown for Dr. Sidney Phillips by Sir F. Semon)', *Proc. R. Soc. Med.*, **1**, 44.
QUAST, U. R., SIBINGA, T. A., and WIJNJA, L. (1971), 'Stuart-Prower Factor Deficiency in Oral Surgery', *Br. J. oral Surg.*, **9**, 146.
REID, W. O., LUCAS, O. N., FRANCISCO, J., and others (1964), 'The Use of EACA in the Management of Dental Extractions in the Haemophiliac', *Am. J. med. Sci.*, **248**, 184.
RENDU, M. (1896), 'Epistaxis répétées chez un sujet porteur de petits angiomes cutanes et muqueux', *Bull. Mém. Soc. méd. Hôp. Paris*, **13**, 731.
SEWARD, M. H. (1962), 'An Unusual Presentation of Acute Leukaemia', *Dent. Practit.*, **13**, 143.
SHANKS, C. A. (1963), 'Intravenous Octapressin during Halothane Anaesthesia', *Br. J. Anaesth.*, **35**, 640.
SUTTON, H. G. (1864), 'Epistaxis as an Indication of Impaired Nutrition and of Degeneration of the Vascular System', *Med. Mirror*, **1**, 769.
THEXTON, A. (1965), 'A Case of Ehlers-Danlos Syndrome presenting with Recurrent Dislocation of the Temporomandibular Joint', *Br. J. oral Surg.*, **2**, 190.
TOBIAS, N. (1934), 'Ehlers-Danlos Syndrome', *Archs Derm.*, **30**, 540.
ULLMAN, K. (1890), *Arch. Derm., Syph.*, **35**, 195.
WEBER, F. P. (1907), 'Multiple Hereditary Developmental Angiomata of the Skin and Mucous Membranes', *Lancet*, **2**, 160.
WECHSLER, H. L., and FISHER, E. R. (1964), 'Ehlers-Danlos Syndrome', *Archs Path.*, **77**, 613.
WILLIAMS, J. L. (1972), 'Plasma Thromboplastin Antecedent Deficiency', *Br. J. oral Surg.*, **10**, 126.
WOOD, N. (1973), 'Management of Extractions in a Case of Glanzmann's Disease', *Ibid.*, **11**, 152.

Chapter VII
SOME NON-MALIGNANT LESIONS IN AND AROUND THE JAWS
Papilloma

The papilloma is one of the more common benign neoplasms of the oral cavity and occurs with equal frequency on the cheek, soft palate, fauces, posterior wall of the pharynx, and tongue. They may be pedunculated or sessile and consist of keratinized epithelium on a connective tissue base. They are particularly common in children and young adults and in this age-group may be caused by the same virus that produces the multiple warts on the hands. They are usually single, occasionally multiple, pale pink to white in colour, irregular and often exhibit finger-like processes or have a knobbly or cauliflower-like surface. They are usually only a few millimetres in diameter, but may occasionally reach about 1 cm. in size. The surface over them is usually unbroken.

Treatment.—Treatment is by surgical extirpation and excision is effected through an incision round the base of the tumour. The incision need only be sufficiently deep to allow complete removal of the base of the attachment. Any haemorrhage from the base of the tumour can be controlled by a mattress suture or by electrocautery, after which the wound is allowed to granulate. However, if an elliptical incision is used the edges of the wound can be undermined to allow primary closure.

Fibroma and Fibrous Overgrowths

Fibrous overgrowths of the oral mucosa are comparatively common, but the majority of these are hyperplastic in origin and the true fibroma is a relatively rare tumour in the mouth. Barker and Lucas (1967) reviewed 171 fibrous lesions of the oral mucosa and in this series they excluded lesions due to denture irritation. There were 62 lesions from the cheek, 39 from the lip, 45 from the palate, and 25 from the tongue. Histological examination showed that 169 of the lesions were hyperplasias and only two of the lesions possessed a distinct capsule confining a mass of collagen fibres which differed both in character and size from those of the surrounding tissue. According to Barker and Lucas only these two lesions conformed to the generally accepted textbook definition of a fibroma.

The true fibroma is a firm, pink, sessile or pedunculated slow-growing tumour which cannot be differentiated on other than histological grounds from the more common fibrous overgrowths seen in the mouth. Fibrous hyperplasias in the mouth may be single or multiple and occasionally attain a considerable size. These benign tumours can be sessile or pedunculated and the pedunculated variety often occur in the palate where they may cover its entire surface, constituting a severe impediment to denture construction. The sessile variety are often found on the gingiva and may contribute to loss of teeth from caries as they tend to act as a food trap. Large fibrous overgrowths may become traumatized and ulcerated when they come into contact with teeth of the opposing jaw (*Figs.* 3, 4) and occasionally they become partially ossified, a fact which may be demonstrated by radiographs. The 'fibro-epithelial polyp' is a popular term for hyperplastic lesions of the palate, cheek, lips or tongue. The condition resembles a fibroma, but it is simply non-neoplastic reparative scar tissue (*Fig.* 5).

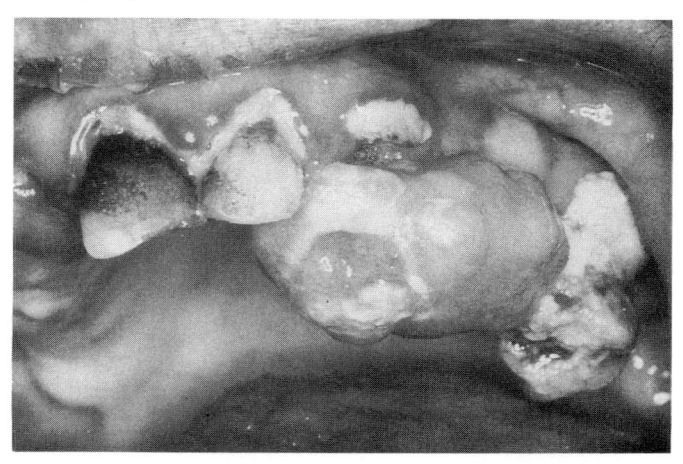

Fig. 3.—Fibrous epulis which has been traumatized by the opposing teeth in the lower jaw. The oral hygiene is poor.

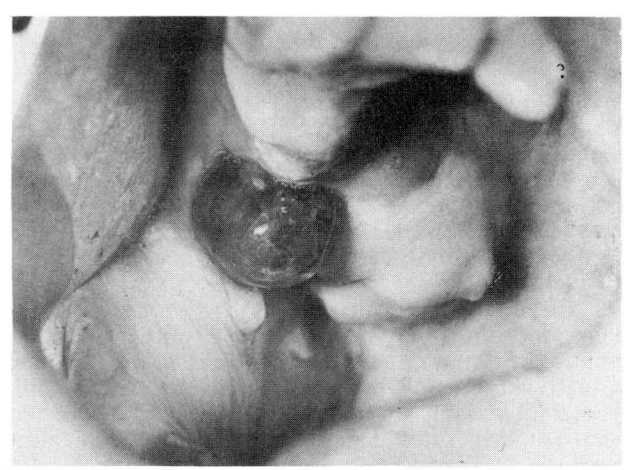

Fig. 4.—A prolapsed antral polyp; not to be confused with a fibrous or giant-cell epulis. The lesion is soft and a blunt probe can be introduced into an antro-oral fistula by the side of the peduncle.

Treatment.—Excision of a fibroma or a local fibromatous overgrowth is a simple matter, especially if the lesion is pedunculated. An incision is made round the base of the mass at mucosal depth and the lesion is dissected off the underlying tissues. A stitch passed through the mass to act as a handle facilitates the dissection. If a small raw area results it can be left to granulate, but the wound edges of a larger area should be undermined to allow primary closure. In the palate haemorrhage may be brisk, but can be controlled with a mattress suture.

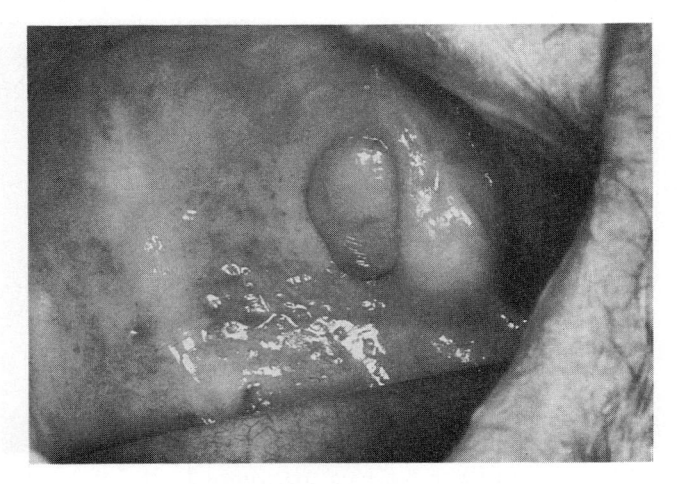

Fig. 5.—Fibro-epithelial polyp in the palate.

FIBROMATOSIS GINGIVAE

Fibromatosis gingivae (hereditary gingival fibromatosis) is a rare condition in which a diffuse mass of fibrous tissue is present within the gingivae of the upper and lower jaw. The mode of transmission of the disorder is usually a dominant trait, but occasionally it is the result of a new mutation. Although the hyperplasia is usually the only abnormal finding, there may be other associated defects particularly hypertrichosis, the onset of which may be at birth or puberty and is unrelated to the time of appearance of the gingival lesion. The second most frequent association is mental retardation. Clinically the condition is characterized by a firm painless nodular overgrowth of the palatal or gingival tissues of one or both arches. The tissue is pink in colour and very firm. The condition usually begins with the eruption of the permanent dentition, occasionally with the eruption of the deciduous dentition, and rarely is present at birth. According to Rushton (1957) a few cases have arisen in adult life. The lesional hypertrophic tissue may cover the whole or part of the dentition and even prevent the eruption of teeth into the mouth, although they erupt through the alveolar crest in the normal way. Histologically there is an increase in submucosal fibrous tissue. This syndrome is not only a diagnostic possibility when patients with gingival hyperplasia present with concomitant idiopathic hirsutes or mental retardation, but also when individuals show even more infrequent features of the disorder such as epilepsy, large ears, nasal abnormalities, and defective limb appendages.

Treatment.—Treatment is by a gingivectomy-type surgical removal of the excess tissue in order to expose the teeth and correct what is often a marked cosmetic deformity. The tissue seldom recurs if the excision has been radical.

GINGIVAL HYPERPLASIA FOLLOWING DRUG THERAPY

Fibrous hyperplasia of the gingiva may occur as a result of therapy with Epanutin or Dilantin Sodium (diphenylhydantoin), which is used as an anticonvulsant in the treatment of epilepsy. This side-effect only occurs in a minority of patients under treatment and it only affects areas where teeth are present. The gingival enlargement is lumpy with a smooth surface which is pink, firm, and shows no tendency to bleed. The enlargement may become so gross that the occlusal surface of the teeth is enveloped. At this stage ulceration from opposing teeth may occur and there is usually secondary infection.

Treatment.—Treatment is by surgical removal of the excess tissue in a gingivectomy type operation. If the patient continues the drug therapy recurrence is almost inevitable unless meticulous attention is paid to oral hygiene, but following removal of the teeth the condition will not recur.

DENTURE HYPERPLASIA

Denture hyperplasia or denture granuloma occurs as a response of the underlying tissues to a mobile, ill-fitting denture (*Fig.* 6). It may be

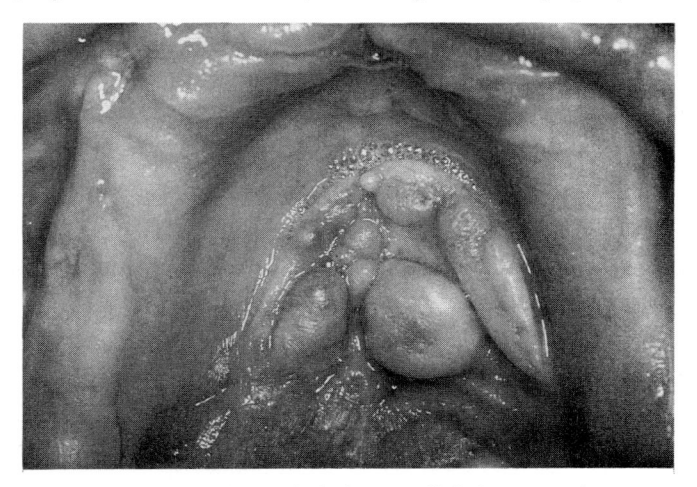

Fig. 6.—Denture hyperplasia from an ill-fitting upper denture.

localized or generalized and in some instances both the upper and lower ridges merely consist of several successive masses of fibrous tissue. Often the denture granuloma presents two flaps of tissue with a deep groove between, in which the flange of the denture fits. One flap of tissue lies against the fitting surface of the denture and may fill the gap left as the original ridge shrinks. The other flap overlaps the flange on the outer aspect. The course of events leading to the formation of a denture granuloma is probably as follows. There is repeated ulceration of the tissues where the flange presses into the sulcus. As a result of the irritation, there is a proliferation of granulation tissue particularly from each edge of the ulcer, so starting the two flap arrangement. Sometimes the underlying bone is affected by the denture trauma and becomes resorbed so that the ridge is soft and spongy. This happens especially in the upper incisor area when the full upper denture is opposed by the six standing lower incisor teeth. Occasionally a localized denture granuloma may be due to the denture cutting into the underlying tissues as a result of a cyst or other neoplasm growing within the bone. The possibility of a carcinoma of the maxillary antrum must always be considered when a denture granuloma occurs in the buccal sulcus in the upper molar area in a patient who has hitherto worn the upper denture without irritation of the underlying tissue.

Treatment.—Treatment of denture hyperplasia in the first instance should consist of leaving the denture out and this often results in quite a remarkable regression of the gingival hyperplasia. If the dentures are old or ill-fitting new dentures must be constructed. Residual masses of denture granuloma should be excised. The incision should be made at mucosal depth after which the mass is held up with toothed forceps or a series of transfixing sutures and dissected off the underlying tissues with McIndoe's scissors. If possible, primary closure of the wound should be carried out after undermining the edges of the wound with blunt-ended scissors. If the raw area is too extensive for primary closure it should be covered with a split skin-graft.

BILATERAL FIBROUS ENLARGEMENT OF THE TUBEROSITY

This condition has been described as symmetric gingival keloids (Rahb, 1936); diffuse fibroma of gums (Buchner, 1937); symmetrical hyperplasia of gingiva (Axhausen, 1940); (Linderman, 1941); fibroma of palate tuberosity (Straith, 1942); fibroma of tuberosity of maxilla (Cook, 1950), and fibroma symmetrica gingivalis (Fogh-Andersen, 1943).

The condition consists of bilateral hard fibromatous masses in the tuberosity region of the palate. While mild cases are not rare, sizeable examples are relatively uncommon. In a review of the literature, Fogh-Andersen (1943) found 40 cases, 27 occurring in men and 13 in women. The tumours are often present early in life, many being diagnosed in childhood. They may enlarge slowly, giving rise to impairment of tongue movements. With large lesions this can lead to speech difficulties and the impaction of food on the upper surfaces of the masses where it cannot be reached by the tongue. These are two reasons why the patients themselves seek medical advice. The only other symptoms described are gagging or retching (Beers Morrison, 1953) and pain on mastication due to the lesions impinging on the lower teeth and becoming ulcerated (Hiebert and Brooks, 1950). More often, it is the dental surgeon who advises their removal as a preliminary to the construction of dentures.

Fogh-Andersen describes a case where mother and daughter were affected, but a hereditary predisposition is not proved. He also describes a case where there was an associated mandibular protrusion. Most recorded cases mention associated dental sepsis in the region either from roots or abnormally placed teeth. It has been suggested that dental sepsis may play a part in causing enlargement of the tumour, but it can also be argued that the growing lesion may produce food traps around the teeth and result in extensive caries. The masses may also be responsible for abnormal positioning of the teeth if they happen to be present when the teeth are erupting.

The fibromatous masses are smooth, firm, pale pink in colour, and are usually sessile. They may become ulcerated on their undersurface by impinging on the lower teeth. In some cases the masses are so large they almost meet in the midline. Not infrequently the retromolar pad and the lingual gingivae in the lower molar region are also enlarged in the more marked cases. Such a finding suggests a possible relationship to fibromatosis gingivae, but if this is so it is curious that it is the palatal and lingual tissues which are involved.

Hiebert and Brooks (1950) suggest that they may become necrotic due to poor blood-supply and state that sarcoma may supervene. They also mention that the mass may become so enlarged that deglutition and even respiration are impaired.

Treatment.—Treatment is by surgical excision. As the fibromatous tissue is firmly adherent to the mucosa covering the area there is no plane of cleavage between the two and it is difficult to strip the mucosa from its surface.

Some authorities advocate excision of the masses subperiosteally, followed by fulguration of the cortex of the bone. They make no attempt to salvage the mucous covering. It would seem logical to raise a flap on the surface of the mass and use it to cover the raw defect, but this is difficult to achieve except in the edentulous patient as the underlying fibrous tissue is bound down to the surface epithelium and there is no tissue plane for dissection. If this operation is attempted, care must be taken to avoid damaging the greater palatine vessels or the flap will undergo necrosis. Excellent results can, however, be achieved by merely slicing the mass with a scalpel to restore the normal contours of the palate. This leaves an extensive raw area which can be left to granulate and epithelialize or can be grafted. The epithelium can be shaved off the surface of the part to be trimmed before the operation proper is started. This is stored in a swab moistened with saline until paring of the tuberosity has been completed and haemostasis obtained by firm pressure. A previously-constructed acrylic plate is lined with gutta-percha in the operation area and the pieces of graft assembled in a strip of tulle gras of appropriate size and shape. The graft is then applied to the raw area as a patch graft and held in place by the plate for 10–14 days.

NEUROFIBROMATOSIS

'Neurofibromatosis' is a term applied to a number of pathological conditions in which tumours of neurofibromatous material may occur singly or in various combinations. An inheritance factor may be detected in some instances and Freeman and Standish (1965) state that 41 per cent of cases show an inherited transmission. These tumours are slow-growing, cause pressure resorption of bone, do not have a capsule, and are radio-resistant. In either the solitary or generalized forms of the disease sarcomatous degeneration may occur and the incidence is about 8–15 per cent. Malignant change tends to follow chronic trauma or incomplete surgical excision.

Nerve-sheath tumours are not particularly common, but Heard (1962) collected 264 cases. There are numerous classifications of the condition and Aird's (1957) is both simple and comprehensive: (1) Generalized neurofibromatosis of Von Recklinghausen; (2) Plexiform neurofibromatosis; (3) Cutaneous neurofibromatosis; (4) Elephantiasis neuromatosa; (5) Solitary neurofibroma; (6) Neurofibrosarcoma.

1. Von Recklinghausen's Neurofibromatosis.—Generalized neurofibromatosis is a widespread thickening of nerves and tumour formation within them which may or may not be accompanied by plexiform and cutaneous forms of the disease or by elephantiasis. The essential feature of the disease is a proliferation of the cells of the nucleated sheath of Schwann and the tumours have been called 'Schwannoma', 'neurilemmoma', and 'neurinoma'. The nerves are thickened and present elliptical bulges. The tumour may displace the nerve-fibres to one side so that it can be shelled out easily, or it may grow among the fibres so that extirpation of such a mass leads to a neurotmesis. The tumours are greyish yellow or grey and they may undergo cystic degeneration. Although neurilemmomas are usually a part of Von Recklinghausen's disease, they can be solitary. The generalized tumours are most commonly distributed on the arms, legs, chest, back, and neck. Changes in the skeleton occur in 7 per cent of cases of generalized disease, there being osteoporosis, hyperostosis, or subperiosteal cysts.

Clinical Features.—Tumours appear in childhood and are seldom present at birth, and the skin manifestations vary from coffee-coloured freckles (*tâche-au-lait*) to extensive pigmentation of a limb. The tumours tend to grow at puberty and increase in size only slowly in adult life. The swellings are elliptical or fusiform and their long diameter lies along the axis of the nerve. The tumour is usually freely movable laterally, but not mobile in the line of the nerve. The swellings are firm in consistency and painless, and anaesthesias and paralyses are absent, though if the tumours occur in a confined bony space they may give rise to facial pain, deafness, and anaesthesia of the face or paralysis of the muscles of mastication.

Treatment.—If the disease is generalized, excision of all the tumours is impractical and surgery should be confined to selected tumours which are causing symptoms or are particularly unsightly.

2. Plexiform Neurofibromatosis.—Half of the cases of plexiform neurofibromatosis are associated with the generalized form of the disease. In this condition anastomosing branches of one or more contiguous nerves or plexus of nerves are thickened, fusiform, and beaded to form a dense mass which may be confined to the soft tissue or invade muscle. The neck, head, and extremities are commonly affected and the swelling may be large and pendulous (pachydermatocele). When it affects the scalp it may hang down over the face like an apron. The tumour may involve the face producing a hemifacial hypertrophy, and this may close the eye, block the external auditory meatus, and produce an enormous soft-tissue swelling

of the face. When the condition occurs in the mouth the teeth may be covered.
Treatment.—Treatment is by surgical excision, though the mass will probably recur.

3. **Cutaneous Neurofibromatosis.**—Multiple soft fibrous swellings occur on the face and in the mouth. They never occur on the palms of the hands or soles of the feet.
Treatment.—Treatment is by surgical excision of unsightly or inconvenient tumours.

4. **Elephantiasis Neuromatosa.**—This variety of neurofibromatosis becomes apparent at puberty or, if already present, undergoes a growth spurt at this time. The cutaneous tissues of the scalp undergo a massive increase in size, become pendulous, and may require surgical excision. Bones in the affected part may be either enlarged or thinner and more delicate than normal. The enlarged bones are involved by the neurofibromatous process and are greatly thickened. Knobbly outgrowths may be formed. The bony trabeculae are irregularly arranged and the condition may be mistaken for fibrous dysplasia of bone, although the bone is more radio-opaque than that found in the latter condition.

5. **Solitary Neurofibroma.**—These tumours are histologically similar to those found in the generalized form of the disease. They are rare in childhood and usually arise after 20 years of age. They arise anywhere in the body. It is an uncommon oral lesion, and Bhaskar (1966) found only 26 cases recorded in the files of the United States Army Institute of Dental Research. He described 2 further cases occurring in the palate.
Treatment.—Treatment is by surgical excision if the lesion in the mouth is interfering with mastication or the fitting of a denture.

6. **Neurofibrosarcoma.**—Neurofibrosarcoma may develop as malignant degeneration in a pre-existent neurofibroma of either the local or generalized form and the incidence is in the region of 8–15 per cent.

Appearances in the Mouth.—Neurofibromas may present as soft, pedunculated swellings of cheek, tongue, or palate with sessile masses on the gum. Deeper lesions produce a fusiform swelling, often soft and lobulated, in the substance of the cheek, tongue, or palate. In the first two sites they may be mistaken for lipomas because of their softness. Plexiform masses which involve the gingivae can prevent the eruption of teeth and when neuromas affect the inferior dental or infra-orbital nerves, the canals are enlarged. If the bone of the jaws is involved, there may be a uniform or lobulated enlargement. The overlying skin may be pigmented.

LIPOMA

The lipoma is a benign tumour composed of mature fat cells. The fat cells are histologically similar to normal fat cells but metabolically dissimilar, for on a starvation diet fat is not lost from a lipoma.

They are commonly found in the subcutaneous tissues, but are extremely rare in the mouth. Bernier (1947), in a review of 1822 benign swellings of the mouth, recorded only 3 lipomas and 1 fibrolipoma. Geshickter (1934) found only 3 oral tumours in a series of 490 lipomata. The oral lipoma is a sessile or pedunculated, painless, slowly-growing mass arising from the submucous connective tissues of the cheek, buccal sulcus, floor of the mouth, and lips. They are very soft and may exhibit pseudo-fluctuation. The lipoma is yellowish in colour and feels freely mobile within the tissues when palpated. Lipomas may be single or multiple and the patient may also have multiple lipomas distributed over the subcutaneous tissues of the limbs and trunk. Gray (1961) reported a case of a man with multiple lipomas in various parts of the body including one in the cheek. Myxomatous degeneration and calcification sometimes occur in lipomata of long duration, but although this is seldom seen in the mouth, occasional cases are reported. Lipomas of the cheek must be distinguished from herniation of the buccal pad of fat through the buccinator.

Treatment.—Treatment is by excision and, owing to its definite capsule and comparative avascularity, this is usually easy. If the excised tumour is sectioned it has a characteristic bright yellow colour.

Granular-cell Myoblastoma

In 1926 Abrikossoff described a series of 5 cases presenting with lesions on the tongue which he called 'myoblastic myoma' in the belief that the granular cells in the tumour were adult striated muscle-fibres which were degenerating as a result of trauma or inflammation. In 1931 he discarded this concept and suggested that the tumour cells were derived from myoblasts, a view previously suggested by Klinge (1928). Similar single lesions had previously been reported as rhabdomyoma and xanthoma, but it was Abrikossoff's series of 5 cases which established the connexion with striated muscle. The exact histogenesis of these tumours is not established and this has resulted in a multiplicity of synonyms such as 'Abrikossoff's tumour', 'congenital epulis', 'granular-cell myoblastoma', 'myoblastic myoma', 'uniform myoblastoma', and 'embryonal rhabdomyoma'.

Incidence.—It is a comparatively rare tumour. Crane and Trenblay (1945) collected 157 cases from the literature and Kerr (1949) added a further 35. Simon (1947) reported 6 cases, Powell (1946) published a further 3, and Bernier (1947) reported 17 cases. Kerr (1949) reported 9 cases and Bret-Day (1964) described 5 cases. Most of the reports in the literature, however, refer to single examples of the tumour.

Clinical Features.—Two clinical types are observed: the so-called congenital epulis in the neonate and infant. These produce pedunculated or sessile lumps on the alveolar process which are usually large in proportion to the size of the mouth. In the adult the lesion lies usually within the substance of the part. The tumours are most frequent in the third, fourth, and fifth decades but may occur at any age. The highest incidence is on the tongue, alveolar process, and skin, although they can arise on any part of the body. They are often small, elevated tumours with a greyish-white smooth surface and are usually symptomless. On palpation they are found to be firm and non-tender and may show an increase in size. They may be identified clinically by their pallor when they occur subepithelially. The tumours are usually benign, but malignant varieties have been reported. The overlying epithelium may show marked downgrowths of the rete pegs which must not be mistaken for carcinoma in a biopsy.

Treatment.—Treatment is by local excision and recurrences have been reported when removal was incomplete.

MELANOTIC NEUROECTODERMAL TUMOUR OF INFANCY

Histogenesis.—Krompecher (1918) is reported to have been the first to draw attention to this tumour which he regarded as a 'congenital melanocarcinoma'. Other writers have preferred to call the condition 'melanotic epithelial odontome' (Mummery and Pitts, 1925), 'retinal anlage tumour' (Halpert and Patzer, 1947), 'pigmented congenital epulis' (MacDonald and White, 1954), and 'melanotic neuroectodermal progonoma' (Stowens, 1957), since these names accord more closely with the respective authors' concept of their aetiology.

Stowens (1957) and Willis (1958) present evidence against the tumour cells being either neural cells or neuroglia, and argue convincingly against an origin from the retinal anlage. Willis goes on to show in the material that he examined parts of the dental lamina and proliferating strands of odontogenic epithelium. The latter was identified as such by the formation in parts of columnar cells and by the production of a stellate reticulum arrangement. From this odontogenic epithelium sprouts of pigmented epithelium arose which were continuous with that seen in the neoplasm. He thus confirms similar observations made previously by both Krompecher (1918) and Mummery and Pitts (1925). Willis was also successful in demonstrating dendritic pigmented cells between the tumour epithelium.

Kerr and Pullon (1964) reviewed previous cases in detail, added new cases and supported their odontogenic origin. Pontius (1965) also contended that in his case neoplastic cells originated directly from an enamel organ.

Borello and Gorlin (1966) again reviewed the literature and presented a case in which some 6–8 times the normal amount of vanilmandelic acid was being excreted in the urine. When the tumour was removed the urinary level of this substance fell to normal. Since other tumours with which vanilmandelic acid in excessive amounts is excreted in the urine include neuroblastomas, ganglioneuroblastoma and phaeochromocytoma these authors suggest an origin from neural crest cells. They also accepted that certain tumours found in sites outside the jaws were histologically the same. Such tumours have been found in the anterior fontanelle (Clarke and Parsons, 1951), the shoulder (Blanc, Rosenblatt, and Wolff, 1958), the epididymis (Eaton and Ferguson, 1956), and the mediastinum (Misugi and others, 1965).

Both Neustein (1967) and Hayward, Fickling, and Lucas (1969) examined histological material in detail including the electron microscopical appearances of the cells. They could not support the contention that some of the tumour cells were epithelial. Further, Koudstaal and co-workers (1968) compared the enzyme pattern of the cells with that of malignant melanoblastoma, paragangliomas and phaeochromocytomas and that of the small tumour cells with neuroblastoma cells. They concluded that both types of tumour cell in the melanotic jaw tumour were of neural crest origin.

The current view is therefore that these tumours are of neural crest origin and the preferred name is melanotic neurectodermal tumour of infancy. The odontogenic epithelium found in the jaw tumours, but not in those from other sites, is considered to be from the normal dental lamina and included secondarily in the tumour mass as it grows.

What remains to be considered are the accounts of multicentric tumours like those of Jones and Williams (1960) where each appeared to be related to a separate tooth germ and that of Pontius (1965) where it seems two separate lesions were seen. Should these be discounted as recurrences of incompletely removed tumours, or should the relationship to the tooth germs be considered fortuitous? It should perhaps be remembered that by far the majority of these lesions occur in the jaws—more in the maxilla than the mandible—and that neural crest cells appear to contribute to the development of the teeth. They probably induce the overlying epithelium to form enamel organs and may themselves form odontoblasts and pulp cells. Indeed Langdon (1970) has noted a relationship between conical teeth, absent teeth and delayed eruption with Rieger's syndrome and incontinentia pigmentosa—two developmental defects affecting neural crest. The relationship with the jaws and with the tooth germs may not therefore be entirely fortuitous.

Clinical Findings.—Infants within the first year to 18 months of life are affected often within the first six months and maxillary lesions are more common than mandibular ones. There is an expansion of the alveolar ridge which can increase in size quite rapidly. After a while the pigmented nature of the lesion can be appreciated through the overlying mucosa. Radiography reveals a rounded cavity expanding the jaw and containing or displacing a developing tooth or teeth.

At operation a grey to black soft or firm tumour mass is found. Mostly it lies in a smooth bony cavity, but may be more firmly attached in places. In some circumstances the overlying bone, often subperiosteal new bone, is pigmented, indicating invasion by the growth. In other cases finger-like processes of tumour penetrate the adjacent medullary bone. Because it is pigmented the tumour tissue can be identified and curetted out.

Histology.—Large cuboidal cells with a vesicular nucleus form groups and strands through the mass. The abundant cytoplasm is heavily pigmented. Smaller cells with deeply staining nuclei form similar groups, and sheets of elongated and stellate cells form arrangements which were mistaken for neuronal and neuroglial elements.

Some of the cuboidal cells outline irregular cystic spaces several of which contain small darkly staining cells. The whole is in a poorly vascularized fibrous stroma. In serial sections of jaw lesions the elements of dental lamina described by Willis and others may be discovered. Invasion of adjacent medullary bone spaces is to be seen.

Treatment.—Careful enucleation is the treatment required. While care should be taken to remove heavily involved bone and any pockets of tumour, a conservative approach should be followed. Any marked damage to the jaw at this age will, of course, produce a disfiguring deformity as the child grows up. Any tooth germs present within the lesion will be included in the specimen, often along with the successional germ. Adjacent teeth, however, should be spared.

Prognosis.—In spite of the poor prognosis normally associated with invasive and pigmented neoplasms, with this particular variety the prognosis is good. In some instances, there may be a single local recurrence which results from a failure to remove a pocket of tumour, but further enucleation and curettage is all that is required to effect control. Even where invaded bone must have been left behind, a good result has been obtained. In a case described by Battle, Hovell, and Spencer (1952) a melanotic tumour was seen involving the right body of the mandible in a child of 6 weeks of age. It was enucleated but recurred 6 months later. The mass then was so large the situation was considered hopeless and no further treatment was given. The patient was seen at the age of 6 when only a localized mass in the 3̄| region was present. This was removed and the continued presence of the tumour confirmed. It seems, therefore, that this condition may regress spontaneously, but it would be taking unnecessary risks to treat all cases expectantly as by its enlargement the tumour damages adjacent structures.

HAEMANGIOMAS

Haemangiomas are developed as proliferations of the embryonic vascular network and are congenital in origin. They are red or bluish in colour and all exhibit the characteristic physical sign of emptying on pressure. This physical sign is best demonstrated by pressure with a glass slide when they are seen to blanch. They may occur anywhere in the body and the most common sites in the mouth are the lips, tongue, buccal mucosa, and palate. They can be divided into capillary and cavernous types.

Capillary Haemangioma

These include the capillary haemangioma, the telangiectasis, the port wine stain, and the spider naevus.

1. Capillary Haemangioma.—The capillary haemangioma of skin is also known as the 'cutaneous naevus', 'haemangioma simplex', or 'salmon patch', and consists of a red network of small capillaries radiating from a central punctum which is the artery supplying the tumour. It lies flat with the surrounding skin and may occur on any skin surface. The lesion may be multiple and varies in size, but it is usually strictly unilateral. The strawberry patch is a capillary haemangioma which is raised above the surface. It is bright red, lobulated, and often grows rapidly. This variety often ulcerates.

Telangiectasis.—Telangiectasis is a dilatation of normal capillaries rather than a developmental anomaly and it includes the spider naevus. These are single or multiple bright red lesions about the size of a pinhead with several tiny thread-like arteries radiating away from them. They are often seen in patients with liver insufficiency. They are found in the immediate periphery of scarring of the skin which has followed irradiation. Spider naevi disappear on death (Aird, 1957).

Hereditary haemorrhagic telangiectasia (H.H.T.) (*Fig.* 7) is not a true intrinsic bleeding state and in affected persons it is usual to find that the currently recognized haemostatic factors are present at normal levels. The disease, which is known to involve cutaneous, mucosal, and visceral structures, is characterized by its familial occurrence and is transmitted as an autosomal dominant affecting both sexes equally. The diagnosis of the disorder is made on the basis of the clinical triad of characteristic telangiectatic lesions, hereditary incidence, and haemorrhagic diathesis. Nevertheless, a positive family history is not always forthcoming. The

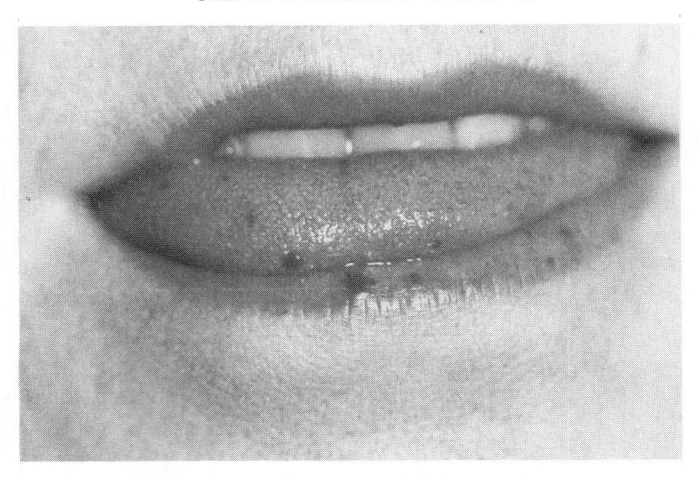

Fig. 7.—Hereditary haemorrhagic telangiectasia.

angiomatous skin or mucous membrane lesions pathognomonic of this malady fall into three types—punctiform, spider-like, and nodular—all of which tend to bleed when traumatized. The nodular type is tumour-like and may reach 2–3 cm. in diameter. There is, of course, a wide visceral distribution of the telangiectases.

Occasionally bleeding from the mouth may be severe, and alarming incidents including a fatality have been reported following the use of a toothbrush on the gingival tissues. If the gingivae are involved, the patient should be warned of the extra need for care during oral hygiene, but it is patently obvious that in the absence of a correct diagnosis bleeding may be wrongly attributed to periodontal disease. Regular conservation treatment will prevent injury to adjoining oral lesions from sharp, abraded carious teeth, but dental surgeons must be circumspect during the preparation and restoration of teeth and when using other instruments in the mouth to avoid damage to the oral mucosa. Conservative management for dental bleeding includes the topical application of haemostatic agents (e.g., gelatin sponge), diathermy, and the use of pressure packs. Blood transfusion is essential in cases of severe blood-loss and iron replacement therapy is indicated to correct anaemia produced by chronic bleeding.

Port Wine Stain.—Port wine stain is a pink, blue, or purple haemangioma of the skin produced by a generalized telangiectasis of the capillaries. These lesions are often seen on the face and in the mouth. Clinically there are two varieties—the smooth and the lumpy—depending whether the surface is heaped up. They often involve the entire side of the face and extend posteriorly to involve the palate and other areas of the mouth. Sometimes these ipsilateral tumours extend backwards to involve the leptomeninges over the posterior parietal and occipital lobes, which later in life may become calcified, producing at first a focal (Jacksonian) epilepsy and later a hemiparesis. This is known as the 'Sturge-Weber syndrome' or 'encephalofacial angiomatosis'.

Campbell de Morgan Spot.—The Campbell de Morgan spot is a bright red capillary naevus about 2 mm. in diameter. It develops on the trunk in middle age and was at one time wrongly associated with cancer.

Treatment.—Small haemangiomas can be treated by touching them with a stick dipped in trichloracetic acid or by electrocautery or cryotherapy. It is impractical to treat multiple spider naevi due to liver insufficiency, but they disappear if the liver condition can be corrected. Many of the extensive capillary haemangiomas present at birth tend to improve with age and some disappear entirely. Such lesions should therefore be kept under observation and treatment carried out only when further improvement appears unlikely, or in the rare event of the tumour enlarging. Capillary haemangiomas of the skin of the face are best disguised with a cosmetic cream such as Covermark and with such treatment the facial lesions are almost undetectable. For this reason treatments such as radiotherapy should be avoided as they spoil the texture of the surface and render subsequent treatment with disguising creams less effective. The 'lumpy' capillary haemangioma cannot be treated by camouflage with creams, and the area must be excised and grafted with skin.

The small lesions in the mouth in hereditary haemorrhagic telangiectasia are often inadvertently traumatized during routine dental treatment and occasionally they are responsible for a severe spontaneous haemorrhage from the mouth. It is impractical to excise all such lesions, but troublesome areas can be satisfactorily extirpated by cautery. The 'strawberry patch' lesions are best treated by injecting them with a bland sclerosing solution such as boiling saline solution. Capillary haemangiomas in the mouth may involve the alveolus and severe haemorrhage may occur as a result of tooth extraction. Cautery to the bleeding surface is the best way of dealing with this problem.

Haemangiomas may be treated also by cryosurgery. Large lesions should be treated by multiple sessions. Small lesions within the oral cavity can be dealt with by one or two freeze/thaw cycles on one occasion. Capillary haemangiomas of the skin are best dealt with by multiple short (10-second) freezes at fortnightly intervals so as to avoid scarring (Leopard and Poswillo, 1974). Pressure on feeding vessels to reduce the blood-flow and injections of vasoconstrictor can be used to potentiate the effect of the freeze.

Cavernous Haemangioma

The cavernous haemangioma is a raised red or bluish lesion which can be of any size, and it can occur anywhere on the body. It empties on pressure. On the face and in the mouth they are often very extensive and involve, for example, the entire tongue (*Fig.* 8). These hamartomas may undergo thrombosis and become swollen and painful during an actual episode of thrombosis. In these circumstances a lesion in the cheek may be mistaken for an inflammatory swelling but it must be recognized for what it is and not incised. Subsequently calcification in the thrombi produces phleboliths which can be mistaken for salivary calculi. Tumours present at birth have a tendency to regress in size and, therefore, no immediate treatment is indicated. The child should be kept under observation, and fortunately in some instances the haemangioma will disappear more or less

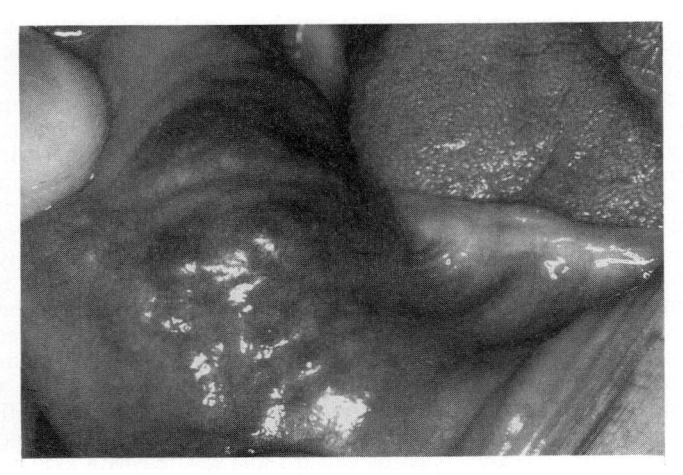

Fig. 8.—Cavernous haemangioma of lip.

completely. In other cases the lesion may remain stationary in size or in rare instances they may become larger.

Treatment.—When the lesion remains unchanged and no further improvement can be anticipated, or if it tends to enlarge, treatment should be advocated. Very small cavernous haemangiomas may be excised or treated by cautery, but the larger lesions should be injected with a sclerosing solution; the safest solution to use is near-boiling normal saline. It may be necessary to inject the haemangioma on more than one occasion, but the final result is usually quite satisfactory. Treatment with radiotherapy has been used in the past, but there is danger of adjacent growth centres in the bone being affected, leading to a growth failure. If the teeth are irradiated during the formative period they will be deformed and stunted, while there is the further possibility of the treated soft-tissue area breaking down at a later date through infection.

Traumatic Haemangioma.—As a result of a bite and damage to a vessel in the cheek or lip a haematoma forms. The haematoma cavity becomes lined with vascular endothelium to form a small localized cavernous haemangioma. It should be noted that there is no increased vascularity in the surrounding tissues. If unsightly, or if it is bitten again and bleeds, it may be excised quite simply and safely.

Central Haemangiomas.—Cavernous haemangiomas may be central in the mandible and maxilla and may present as destructive bone lesions with a radiographical appearance resembling that of a benign cyst. Surgical interference may lead to severe blood-loss and even death from exsanguination. Broderick and Round (1933) reported a case of fatal haemorrhage after tooth extractions in a patient with a cavernous haemangioma of the maxilla. Kroh (1926) described a patient who bled to death minutes after extraction of a loose tooth and at autopsy a cavernous haemangioma of the mandible was found. Smith (1959) summarized the literature up to 1959 and in a series of 20 cases of central haemangioma of the mandible described 3 in which the haemorrhage was fatal. Central cavernous haemangiomas are rare. Shira and Guernsey (1965) found only 41 cases recorded in the literature.

Diagnosis.—Diagnosis of a central haemangioma of the jaw prior to surgery is obviously of paramount importance and aspiration biopsy should be carried out when there is the slightest doubt concerning the exact nature of a radiolucent area in the mandible or maxilla. In some such lesions there is an arteriovenous shunt and a bruit may be heard on auscultation over the area. This physical sign was present in the case recorded by Shira and Guernsey (1965). A transmitted pulsation in a loose tooth is suggestive of an arteriovenous communication. Many cavernous haemangiomas of the mandible are particularly extensive and the entire jaw may be occupied by a multicystic radiolucent lesion having a soap-bubble or trabeculated appearance. Carotid angiography with hypaque is useful to demonstrate arteriovenous shunts into central haemangiomas of the jaws. Often, though not always, the blood-vessels in the overlying tissues are dilated and increased in number.

Mode of Presentation.—Most cases of central cavernous haemangioma are diagnosed as a result of investigation of an atypical radiolucent area in the jaws found during routine radiography. There is usually little expansion of the bone, but occasionally a pulsatile swelling may be present in the overlying soft tissues. The case described by Davies (1964) had a small pulsating mass behind the lower right 2nd molar. The clinical features may include a pulsating type of pain in the jaw. Spontaneous haemorrhage may occur in some instances and occasionally patients have experienced several haemorrhagic episodes. Davies (1964) described the bleeding as 'spurting' rather than a general ooze. Profuse haemorrhage following dental extraction is another obvious mode of presentation. The haemorrhage is of the character of that from a large vein. It is like water running from a tap and quite unlike the normal bleeding socket.

Radiology.—There are usually multilocular areas of bone resorption which produce either a soap-bubble or trabeculated appearance. Adjacent medullary spaces and vascular canals are widened so that the irregular outline has an indefinite border which blends into the normal architecture of the bone.

Treatment.—Treatment is required if spontaneous haemorrhage occurs or if teeth in relation to the haemangioma require extraction. The presence of a pulsatile soft-tissue tumour due to penetration of the bone also constitutes a potential hazard to the patient, and is a further indication for treatment. The lesions vary in their degree of vascularity: some appear to be capillary in nature, others solid in that the vascular channels are closed, and yet others are partially occluded with clot. It is lesions such as these which have been biopsied or treated by local surgery without danger. The dangerous ones are composed of venous sinusoidal vessels or arteriovenous malformations.

Some central cavernous haemangiomas respond favourably to radiotherapy and this may be carried out prior to surgical extirpation of the lesion. The latter is always a hazardous procedure. Unilateral clamping of the external carotid artery with arterial nooses or bulldog clamps may be indicated prior to operation, but this measure does not necessarily control the jaw haemorrhage (Moose, 1957; Packard and Baxter, 1960; Davies, 1964; and Shira and Guernsey, 1965). Bilateral ligation should not be practised since this leads to atrophy of the tongue. Resection of the affected portion of the jaw may be indicated and Shira and Guernsey (1965) successfully resected an extensive cavernous haemangioma of the mandible. Haemorrhage from the bone-ends was eventually controlled with bone wax.

Most of the cases in the literature have been treated either by radical surgery, which usually involves hemimandibulectomy, or by radiation.

Should a tooth be extracted, unknowingly, from a jaw affected by a central haemangioma, the operator will be in no doubt as to what has happened. The haemorrhage is torrential and requires rapid action if the patient is not to die. Appropriate pressure will control all haemorrhage. Clean gauze is packed into the socket until sufficient pressure can be applied so that the haemorrhage is controlled. An acquaintance of the author tells of packing 15 feet of 1-inch ribbon gauze (4·5 metres of 2·5 cm.) through a molar socket to arrest haemorrhage in a case he encountered.

OSTEOMA

This benign neoplasm may consist of compact or cancellous bone and is either endosteal or periosteal in location. True osteomas should show persistent growth and enlargement. The periosteal compact or ivory osteoma is a smooth, hard, painless lump which is usually sessile but may occasionally be pedunculated. The cancellous osteoma is composed of trabeculae of lamellar bone and covered with a thin layer of subperiosteal bone. They can occur anywhere on the jaws and may be single or multiple. Favoured sites are the angle of the mandible, the mental tubercle region, and the canine fossa. Radiologically they appear as a well-circumscribed dense radio-opaque mass.

Treatment.—If the osteoma is cosmetically unacceptable or if it interferes with the satisfactory construction of a denture it should be removed. Such a case was reported by Seward (1965). Pedunculated osteomas are easily removed by severing the base of the pedicle but the sessile osteoma can either be separated from the underlying bone or, if this would leave an unacceptable defect in the bone, the osteoma can be pared down and the normal jaw contours re-established. The latter treatment should be reserved for tumours which show little tendency to enlarge.

In the event of recurrence and with osteomas which have shown a tendency to enlarge, the tumour together with a small area of adjacent bone should be removed with a chisel or bur.

Torus Palatinus.—The torus palatinus, a developmental anomaly, is a slow-growing sessile compact exostosis which occurs in the midline of the hard palate and when it becomes large it tends to become lobulated. It is comparatively common and, when large, interferes with the satisfactory construction of a full upper denture and should be removed. This is carried out following a surgical approach through a midline incision from behind forwards which in the incisor area diverges on each side to form a Y. The mass can also be exposed through an incision made round the crest of the upper ridge which allows a large palatal flap to be reflected. The torus palatinus is of dense compact bone and is best sectioned with a bur and then removed with a vulcanite bur. Following excision the area is smoothed with a large round bur. Attempts to remove the torus with a chisel may result in fracture of the hard palate.

Incidentally, *exostosis* is a reactive hyperplasia or local enlargement, or an abnormal enlargement of a normal anatomical excresence. Growth is not usually progressive particularly if the stimulus is removed. The term 'exostosis' should not be confused with *endostosis*. The latter is a reactive sclerosis within the bone which is not encapsulated and which ceases to enlarge after a time.

Periosteal Cancellous Osteoma.—The periosteal cancellous osteoma may also occur anywhere around the jaws and it is often pedunculated. Radiographs show a cancellous mass surrounded by a thin layer of compact bone. Its removal is facilitated by the fact that it is easily sectioned with a chisel.

Torus Mandibularis.—The torus mandibularis is a cancellous exostosis found on the lingual side of the mandible in the region of the premolars. Like the torus palatinus, it varies in size and shape but is usually bilateral. It constitutes a formidable impediment to the construction of a lower denture and is easily removed by chisel or bur through an incision of suitable length made along the crest of the lower ridge.

Endosteal Osteoma.—The endosteal osteoma is usually located in the mandible and may attain a considerable size. The so-called 'endosteal osteoma' of the nasal sinuses (Rawlins, 1938) is of course subperiosteal in origin, although occurring within the sinus cavity. Small osteomas are usually symptomless and are discovered as an incidental finding on routine radiography. However, when they increase in size they extrude from the mandible and large osteomas of this type have been reported by Fickling (1951), Gilbert (1954), Uhler (1957), and Cooke (1957). Treatment is by surgical removal and, following adequate surgery, recurrence is rare. Endosteal osteoma must be differentiated from reactive bone sclerosis and the gigantic type of cementoma.

Multiple Osteomas.—In 1943 Fitzgerald reported the case of a woman with bony exostoses, desmoids, and multiple polyposis of the colon, and in 1936 Thoma reported the case of a patient with bony tumours of the jaws and fibroids of the skin. Unaware of these earlier reports, Gardner and co-workers (1953; 1962) described a family with multiple osteomas especially of the facial bones, together with epidermoid and sebaceous cysts of the skin, multiple polyposis of the large bowel, and desmoids or fibromas of the skin, and they established the condition as a syndrome. Gorlin and Chaudhry (1960) suggested that the syndrome might be a heritable disorder of connective tissue and it is now considered to have an autosomal dominant pattern.

The multiple intestinal polyposis of the colon and rectum, which has a marked tendency to undergo rapid malignant degeneration, is characteristic of the syndrome, but the condition differs from the Peutz-Jegher's syndrome in that there is no circumoral or intra-oral pigmentation and the polyps which are mainly restricted to the large bowel often become malignant. Multiple osteomas may be scattered through the calvarium and facial skeleton. They first appear at about the time of puberty and similar lesions may be seen in the long bones. In the case reported by

Rayne (1968) a ten-year follow-up radiological examination showed no increase in the size of the oral osteomas. Lucas (1964) states that it is unknown whether the peripheral osteoma is a neoplasm or a developmental anomaly. He also states that the osteoma does not recur after removal and it would therefore appear logical to suggest surgery to remove particularly unsightly or prosthetically inconvenient osteomas in patients with this condition. Dental anomalies including odontomas and multiple unerupted supernumerary and permanent teeth have been reported and bear comparison with those found in cleidocranial dyostosis, while the presence of many epithelial anomalies such as polyps, adenocarcinomas, sebaceous cysts, and odontomas may imply that there is an ancillary growth disorder of epithelium.

REFERENCES

ABRIKOSSOFF, A. (1926), 'Ueber Myome ausgehend von quergestreifter willkürlicher Muskulatur', *Virchows Arch. path. Anat. Physiol.*, **260**, 215.
— — (1931), 'Weitere Untersuchungen über Myoblastermyome', *Ibid.*, **280**, 731.
AIRD, I. (1957), *A Companion to Surgical Studies*, 2nd ed. Edinburgh: Livingstone.
AXHAUSEN, G. (1940), *Die allgemeine chirurgie in der zahn, mund-u-kieferheil-kunde*, p. 355. Munich: Lehmann.
BARKER, D. S., and LUCAS, R. B. (1967), 'Localised Fibrous Overgrowths of the Oral Mucosa', *Br. J. oral Surg.*, **5**, 86.
BATTLE, R. J. V., HOVELL, J. H., and SPENCER, H. (1952), 'Pigmented Adamantinoma', *Br. J. Surg.*, **39**, 368–370.
BERNIER, J. L. (1946), 'Myoblastoma', *J. dent. Res.*, **25**, 253.
— — (1947), 'Myoblastoma', *Am. J. Orthod.*, **33**, 548.
BHASKAR, S. N. (1966), 'Periapical Lesions: Types, Incidence and Clinical Features', *Oral Surg.*, **21**, 657.
BLANC, W. A., ROSENBLATT, P., and WOLFF, J. A. (1958), 'Melanotic Proponoma (Retinal Anlage Tumour) of the Shoulder in an Infant', *Cancer*, **11**, 959–962.
BORELLO, E. D., and GORLIN, R. J. (1966), 'Melanotic Neurectodermal Tumour of Infancy', *Ibid.*, **19**, 196–206.
BRET-DAY, R. C. (1964), 'Granular Cell Myoblastoma', *Br. J. oral Surg.*, **2**, 65.
BRODERICK, R. A., and ROUND, H. (1933), 'Cavernous Haemangioma', *Lancet*, **2**, 13.
BUCHNER, H. J. (1937), 'Diffuse Fibroma of the Gums', *J. Am. dent. Ass.*, **24**, 2003.
CLARKE, B. E., and PARSONS, H. (1951), 'An Embryological Tumour of Retinal Anlage involving the Skull', *Cancer*, **4**, 78–85.
COOK, T. J. (1950), 'Fibroma of the Tuberosity of the Palate', *Oral Surg.*, **3**, 33.
COOKE, B. E. D. (1957), 'Benign Fibro-osseous Enlargements of the Jaw', *Br. dent. J.* **102**, 55.
CRANE, A. R., and TRENBLAY, R. G. (1945), 'Myoblastoma', *Am. J. Path.*, **21**, 357.
DAVIES, D. (1964), 'Cavernous Haemangioma of Mandible', *Dent. Abstr., Chicago*, **9**, 501.
EATON, W. L., and FERGUSON, J. P. (1956), 'A Retinoblastic Teratoma of the Epididymis', *Cancer*, **9**, 718–720.
FICKLING, B. W. (1951), 'Osteoma of the Mandible', *Proc. R. Soc. Med.*, **44**, 56.
FITZGERALD, G. M. (1943), 'Multiple Composite Odontomes Coincidental with other Tumerous Conditions', *J. Am. dent. Ass.*, **30**, 1408.
FOGH-ANDERSEN, P. (1943), 'Fibroma symmetrica gingivalis', *Tandlaegebladet*, **47**, 145–149.
FREEMAN, M. J., and STANDISH, S. M. (1965), 'Facial and Oral Manifestations of Familial Disseminated Neurofibromatosis', *Oral Surg.*, **19**, 52.
GARDNER, E. J. (1962), 'Follow-up Study of a Family Group exhibiting Dominant Inheritance for a Syndrome including Intestinal Polyposis, Osteomas, Fibromas and Epidermal Cysts', *Am. J. hum. Genet.*, **14**, 376.
— — and RICHARDS, R. C. (1953), 'Multiple Cutaneous and Subcutaneous Lesions occurring Simultaneously with Hereditary Polyposis and Osteomatosis', *Ibid*, **5**, 139.

GESHICKTER, C. F. (1934), 'Diagnosis and Treatment of the More Common Diseases of the Oral Mucous Membrane', *Jl Dent.*, **8**, 96.
GILBERT, R. K. (1954), 'A Case of a Peripheral Ivory Osteoma of the Mandible', *Br. dent. J.*, **96**, 15.
GORLIN, R. J., and CHAUDHRY, A. P. (1960), 'Oral Manifestations of the Fitzgerald-Gardiner Syndromes', *Oral Surg.*, **13**, 1233.
GRAY, W. (1961), 'Oral Lipoma', *Br. dent. J.*, **110**, 55.
HALPERT, B. and PATZER, R. (1947), 'Maxillary Tumour of Retinal Anlage', *Surgery*, **22**, 837.
HAYWARD, A. F., FICKLING, B. W., and LUCAS, R. B. (1969), 'An Electron Microscopic Study of a Pigmented Tumour of the Jaw of Infants', *Br. J. Cancer*, **23**, 702–705.
HEARD, G. (1962), 'Nerve Sheath Tumours and Von Recklinghausen's Disease of the Nervous System', *Ann. R. Coll. Surg.*, **31**, 229.
HIEBERT, A. E., and BROOKS, H. W. (1950), 'Fibroma of the Palate', *Plastic reconstr. Surg.*, **5**, 532.
JONES, P., and WILLIAMS, A. (1960), 'A Case of Multicentric Melanotic Adamantinoma', *Br. J. Surg.*, **48**, 282.
KERR, D. A. (1949), 'Myoblastic Myoma', *Oral Surg.*, **2**, 41.
— — and PULLON, P. S. (1964), 'A Study of the Pigmented Tumours of the Jaws of Infants', *Ibid.*, **18**, 759–772.
KLINGE, F. (1928), 'Ueber die sogenannten unreifen nicht guergestenmyome myoblastenmyome', *Verh. dt. path. Ges.*, **23**, 376.
KOUDSTAAL, J., OLDHOFF, J., PONDERS, A. K., and HARDORK, M. J. (1968), 'Melanotic Neurectodermal Tumor of Infancy', *Cancer*, **22**, 151–161.
KROH, F. (1926), 'A Cavernous Angioma in Mandible', *Br. Dent. J.*, **47**, 566.
KROMPECHER, E. (1918), 'Zur Histogenese und Morphologie der Adamantinome und sonstiger Kiefergeschwulste', *Beitr. Pathol. Anat.*, **64**, 165.
LANGDON, J. D. (1970), 'Rieger's Syndrome', *Oral Surg.*, **30**, 758–795.
LEOPARD, P. L., and POSWILLO, D. E. (1974), 'Practical Cryosurgery for Oral Lesions', *Br. dent. J.*, **136**, 185–196.
LINDERMAN, A. G. (1941), *Die chirurgie des gesichtes der mundhohle under der luftwege.* Berlin-Wien, 71–72.
LUCAS, R. B. (1964), *Pathology of Tumours of the Oral Tissues.* London: Churchill.
MACDONALD, A. M., and WHITE, M. (1954), 'Pigmented Congenital Epulides of Neuro-epithelial Origin', *Br. J. Surg.*, **41**, 610.
MISUGI, K., OKAJIMA, H., NEWTON, W. A., KENETZ, D. P., and LORIMER, A. A. (1965), 'Mediastinal Origin of a Melanotic Progonoma in Retinal Anlage Tumour—Ultrastructural Evidence for Neural Crest Origin', *Cancer*, **18**, 477–484.
MOOSE, S. M. (1957), 'Sinusoidal Aneurism of the Mandible', *J. oral Surg.*, **15**, 245.
MORRISON, D. BEERS (1953), 'Bilateral Fibroma of the Palate', *Ibid.*, **11**, 330.
MUMMERY, J. A., and PITTS, A. T. (1925), 'Melanotic Epithelial Odontome in Child'. *Proc. R. Soc. Med.*, **19**, 11 (Reprinted *Br. dent. J.*, **47**, 121).
NEUSTEIN, H. B. (1967), 'Fine Structure of a Melanotic Progonoma or Retinal Anlage Tumor of the Anterior Fontanel', *Exp. Mol. Pathol.*, **6**, 131–142.
PACKARD, H. R., and BAXTER, W. F. (1960), 'Aneurism of the Right Maxilla', *J. oral Surg.*, **18**, 71.
PONTIUS, E. E. (1965), 'Multicentric Melanoameloblastoma of the Maxilla', *Cancer*, **18**, 381–387.
POWELL, A. (1946), 'Granular Cell Myoblastoma', *Archs Path.*, **42**, 517.
RAHB, H. (1936), *Dt. Zahn- Mund- u. Kieferheilk.*, **3**, 555.
RAWLINS, A. G. (1938), 'Osteoma', *Ann. Otol. Rhinol. Lar.*, **47**, 735.
RAYNE, J. (1968), 'Gardiner's Syndrome', *Br. J. oral Surg.*, **6**, 11.
RUSHTON, M. A. (1957), 'Hereditary or Idiopathic Hyperplasia of the Gums', *Dent. Practnr dent. Rec.*, **7**, 136.
SEWARD, M. H. (1965), 'An Osteoma of the Maxilla', *Br. dent. J.*, **118**, 27.
SHIRA, R. B., and GUERNSEY, L. H. (1965), 'Central Cavernous Haemangioma of the Mandible', *J. oral Surg.*, **23**, 636.
SIMON, A. (1947), 'Granular Cell Myoblastoma', *Am. J. clin. Path,.* **17**, 302.
SMITH, W. H. (1959), 'Haemangioma of the Jaws', *Arch Otolar.*, **70**, 579.
STOWENS, D. (1957), 'A Pigmented Tumour of Infancy: The Melanotic Progonoma', *J. Pathol. Bact.*, **73**, 43.
STRAITH, F. E. (1942), 'Fibroma of the Palatal Tuberosity', *Am. J. Orthod.*, **28**, 434.

THOMA, K. H. (1936), 'Osteodysplasia with Multiple Mesenchymal Tumours: Fibroma, Exotoses and Osteomas', *Orthodontia*, **22**, 1177.
UHLER, I. V. (1957), 'Massive Osteoma of the Mandible', *Oral Surg.*, **10**, 243.
WILLIS, R. A. (1958), 'Histogenesis of Pigmented Epulis in Infancy', *J. Pathol. Bact.*, **73**, 89.

Chapter VIII
BENIGN SOFT-TISSUE CYSTS

Dermoid Cysts of the Floor of the Mouth and Tongue

Dermoid cysts may be found in the midline of the floor of the mouth, in the midline of the tongue, and laterally in the gutter between the hyoglossus and mylohyoid muscles.

Midline Dermoid Cysts of the Floor of the Mouth.—In childhood midline dermoid cysts of the floor of the mouth may be found as small, yellowish spheres lying in the connective tissue beneath the lingual fraenum and just posterior to the mandible. As they increase in size they push apart the genioglossus muscles, moving deeper into the floor of the mouth and backwards into the tongue. They may be forced into this position by the tongue itself since the tongue occupies most of the space within the dental arches when the mouth is closed. (*Figs.* 9, 10.) Such cysts bulge

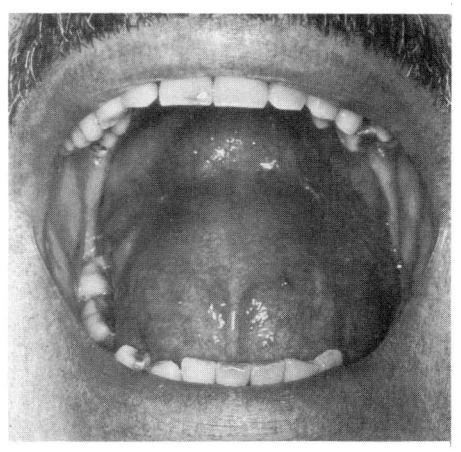

Fig. 9.—A median dermoid cyst of the floor of the mouth. The cyst is deeper in than the ranula, more firm to touch, and symmetrically disposed about the midline.

upwards and forwards towards the oral cavity as the mouth is opened and the mylohyoid and digastrics contract. When the mouth is closed they are displaced in the opposite direction producing a swelling in the submental region which the patient may mistake for a 'double chin'. A few cysts may develop rather more deeply in the tissues, that is between the genioglossi since they do not form the characteristic oral swelling.

Irrespective of their clinical presentation all median dermoid cysts of the floor of the mouth lie relatively close below the mucous membrane. As they increase still further in size, they pass downwards and backwards to the hyoid and epiglottis and separate the geniohyoid muscles to reach the mylohyoid. Some pass lateral to one of the geniohyoid muscles. A few squeeze part of their mass through the perforations in the mylohyoid muscles traversed by anastomotic branches between the submandibular and sublingual arteries. If they are left in situ beyond this stage they will cause an increase in size of the lower dental arch and then proclination of the lower incisors. Eventually it will prove impossible for the patient to close the mouth.

The lining epithelium may be plain, stratified, squamous epithelium (epidermoid type), or it may contain sebaceous glands and hair follicles (dermoid type). Some may have a small or substantial part of the lining composed of mucus-secreting and ciliated epithelium suggesting an endodermal origin. The dermal and epidermal varieties are filled with a

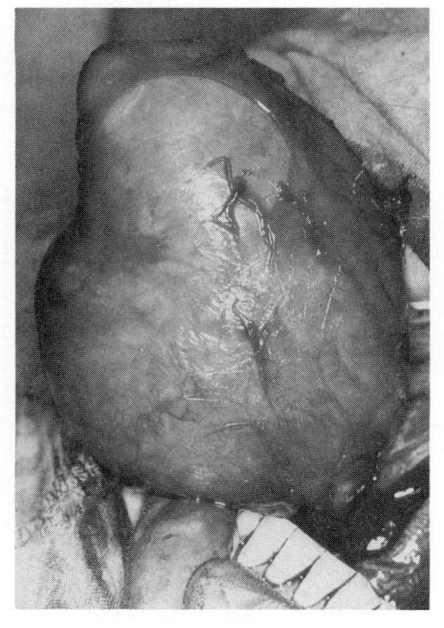

Fig. 10.—The same cyst at operation demonstrating the size of cyst which can be accommodated in the tissues at this site.

pultaceous mass of desquamated epithelial cells. The endodermal types are fluctuant and contain mucus. Because of the character of their lining epithelium, these lesions must arise close to the junction between ectoderm and endoderm and possibly between the paired contribution from the mandibular arch to the anterior two-thirds of the tongue.

Their removal is accomplished through an incision in the free edge of the lingual fraenum, from just behind the tip of the tongue down to its attachment to the mandible. A plane of cleavage is established between the cyst and the surrounding tissues. Any sizeable vessels crossing to the cyst are diathermized. Very large cysts must be opened once the dissection has progressed as far as possible around the periphery. The contents are aspirated and a finger inserted into the cavity so that the remainder can be separated in the same way as the sac of an inguinal hernia. That is, one finger is inserted into the cavity and indicates the site of the wall of the cyst while traction is applied to the lesion with the other fingers. It is then possible to separate the outside of the sac from the adjacent tissue with scissors without risk of tearing the sac or damage to adjacent structures. The wound is closed with vacuum drainage.

Dermoid Cysts of the Tongue.—Dermoid cysts occur as a rare entity in the midline of the tongue. They are, for the most part, of the epidermal type (Goldberg, 1965), but may have mucus-secreting, ciliated, or even gastric epithelium forming part of their lining indicating a mixed ectodermal and endodermal origin for the epithelium. Cysts in other locations about the tongue and floor of mouth with gastric and intestinal mucosa in the lining are described by Gorlin and Jirasek (1970). Treatment is by enucleation.

Lateral Dermoid Cysts of the Floor of the Mouth.—Lateral dermoid cysts arise in the gutter between the hyoglossus, geniohyoid, and genioglossus which lie medially, and the mylohyoid which lies laterally. They are positioned deep to the submandibular duct and lingual nerve and anterior to the stylohyoid ligament. Thus, they may arise from the ventral end of either the first pharyngeal pouch, or the first branchial cleft (Seward, 1965). Most lateral dermoids are lined by stratified squamous epithelium which may come either from ectoderm or endoderm, while some may be lined by ciliated, columnar epithelium which implies an endodermal origin. A few contain hairs (Cook, 1950; Duvergey, 1907) suggesting an origin from the first branchial cleft. Gold (1962) has described an example with a subepidermal lymphatic infiltration as is found in second-cleft branchial cysts, but this is exceptional.

When they are small, these cysts produce a fullness laterally in the sublingual sulcus and anteriorly in the submandibular region. At this stage they are deep in the tissues and not particularly close to either surface. Later they emerge behind the posterior end of the mylohyoid and displace the submandibular salivary gland to present as a prominent swelling in the neck. If left, they can push backwards medial to the mandible, up to the tonsil, and downwards to the sternomastoid muscle and the internal jugular vein.

Small cysts may be removed through an incision in the floor of the mouth lateral to the tongue after careful identification of the lingual nerve and submandibular duct. Larger cysts should be removed through a submandibular incision so that adjacent blood-vessels can be formally exposed.

Branchial Cyst

Branchial cysts may be found at the site of the second branchial cleft and pharyngeal pouch. Some more rare cysts found about the pharynx and neck may be related to the first and second pouches, the third and the fourth pouch (Wilson, 1955). The majority are lined by stratified squamous epithelium, but some of the deeper ones are lined by columnar epithelium. All have a subepithelial infiltration with lymphocytes.

Those developing from the second pharyngeal pouch present towards the back of the upper pole of the tonsil. Those developing from the second branchial cleft produce oval, fluctuant swellings emerging from beneath the anterior border of the sternomastoid, just below the angle of the mandible. In this situation they must be distinguished from a tuberculous abscess. Cautious aspiration through an oblique needle track may help to establish the diagnosis. Branchial cyst fluid often contains cholesterol crystals and tuberculous pus can be cultured or inoculated into guinea-pigs.

The treatment is excision.

Mucous Extravasation and Retention Cysts

These occur in two clinical forms about the mouth: small mucoceles or mucous cysts of the lips, cheeks, undersurface of tongue, and floor of mouth and the larger ranula.

Mucocele.—

Aetiology.—Formerly it was thought that these were all retention cysts resulting from the obstruction of the duct of one of the minor mucous salivary glands. Attempts to produce retention cysts by ligation of the duct of a salivary gland did not, however, result in the production of a cyst since acinar atrophy followed (Bhaskar, Bolden, and Weinmann, 1956; Standish and Shafer, 1957). In 1957, Standish and Shafer showed that the majority of mucous cysts did not have an epithelial lining, but that a mucus-filled cavity in the connective tissue communicated with a breach in the wall of the duct of an adjacent mucous gland. Other observers have confirmed these observations. Further experiments, in which the duct of a salivary gland was divided so that the secretions escaped into the tissues, resulted in the formation of similar cysts (Bhaskar and others 1956; Chaudhry and others, 1960). The majority of these lesions, therefore, result from damage to, or rupture of, the duct of a minor salivary gland such that mucus can escape into the tissues.

More recently Sela and Ulmansky (1969) have described small epithelium-lined cysts of minor salivary glands. These appear to constitute a dilatation, or saccular out-pouching, of the duct, and serial sections have revealed calculi within the duct. It seems, therefore, that with complete obstruction, pressure within the duct rises to a point where further secretion is prevented and acinar atrophy occurs. With incomplete obstruction, as by a calculus, secretion continues and dilatation of the duct eventually results.

Clinical Appearances.—Mucous cysts are usually superficial and only occasionally do they occur deep in the tissues. Superficial cysts appear as a circumscribed swelling which seldom exceeds 1–2 cm. in diameter. They form a tense or slightly flaccid swelling which has a bluish, greenish, or orange-yellow colour. The tense swelling is often inadvertently punctured by the patient's teeth, whereupon it bursts and discharges a gelatinous material. The lesion then subsides completely, only to fill up again over a period of time. Some patients deliberately bite, or puncture the cyst with a needle in order to get rid of it for a while. Deeply-placed mucous cysts are covered by normal mucosa, are more difficult to diagnose, and may be mistaken for a pleomorphic adenoma. Occasionally after rupture of the cyst, a sinus forms with a polyp of granulation tissue at the entrance. This is usually mistaken for a small fibro-epithelial polyp. Excision of the pedunculated swelling is invariably followed by its rapid recurrence. If, however, the cause of such a lesion is known, or the sinus closed by surgery and the reformed cyst observed before it can rupture again, then the correct diagnosis may be made. Provided that the causative mucous gland is then excised, a cure will result.

Histology.—The mucus extravasation cyst, in the early stages, is composed of pools of mucus lying in the connective tissue adjacent to a breach in the duct of a minor salivary gland. Granulation tissue is provoked and forms the first lining of the cyst. Some phagocytosis occurs both of the mucus and of some debris composed of desquamated epithelial cells from the duct. In time the granulations mature to form a fibrous capsule. The majority of such cysts remain without an epithelial lining, but in some cases epithelium from the duct migrates to line the wall partially. In others, flattened fibroblasts on the inner surface of the capsule may be mistaken for epithelial cells. The mucus retention cyst of Sela and Ulmansky is lined by a complete layer of duct epithelium.

Treatment.—The treatment is drainage of the mucus and excision of the salivary gland which is secreting the mucus. It is usual to remove the mucus by attempting to excise the entire cyst sac, but this is by no means easy. As has been seen in many cases, there is no definite sac, only pools of mucus, some of which may lie just beneath the mucous membrane of the mouth. Only the mature fibrous and epithelium-lined sacs can be removed, and these only provided that technical care is exercised. An incision is made in the mucosa to one side of the maximum eminence of the cyst and the cyst separated by gentle dissection with blunt-ended, fine scissors. A mixture of sharp and blunt dissection is necessary. The offending gland comes into view as the operation proceeds and is removed with the cyst. The resulting cavity is obliterated by the sutures as the wound is closed.

Ingenious operations in which alginate impression material is injected into the cyst cavity, or the cavity packed with ribbon gauze to facilitate marsupialization, are clearly unnecessary. Indeed, marsupialization is illogical since the majority of cysts are not epithelium-lined. Only if a fistula forms between the breach in the duct and the surface will the technique succeed, and this is usually prevented from happening by contraction and granulation of the connective tissue-lined cavity.

The Ranula.—The ranula is a thin-walled, bluish, transparent cyst which specifically occurs in the floor of the mouth beneath the tongue, blood-vessels in the mucous membrane course over the surface. The name arose because of the resemblance of the fully blown lesion to a frog's belly. (*Fig.* 11.)

It grows slowly and forms a painless, soft, fluctuant swelling, which usually occurs to one side of the midline, but may cross the midline as it enlarges. It is then constricted by the fraenum and may assume an hourglass shape. At first it is covered by mucosa of normal colour, but as it enlarges it takes on the classic appearance. Sometimes these cysts become sufficiently large to raise the tongue and if inadvertently punctured by the teeth or hard food they collapse with a discharge of mucoid material into the mouth. The ranula reforms when the puncture wound heals and it gradually refills with mucoid material. The stretched mucosa is always freely movable over the cyst. In some patients the submandibular duct passes over the surface of the ranula like a white cord.

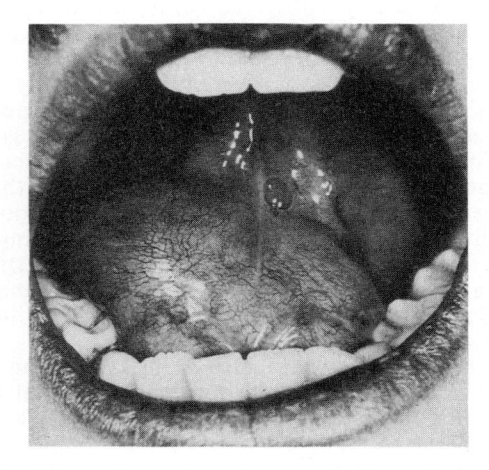

Fig. 11.—A typical ranula passing submucosally from right to left across the floor of the mouth. Note the dilated vessels which give the appearance resembling a frog's belly.

Two clinical forms of ranula are described: one is confined to the floor of the mouth and the other, the plunging ranula, passes back through the submandibular region and then down into the neck. In extreme cases it may almost reach the mediastinum.

Aetiology.—In the past there has been considerable controversy concerning the origin of these cysts. Obstruction of the duct of a salivary gland, inflammation or myxomatous degeneration of the sublingual salivary glands or the glands of Blandin and Nuhn were popular theories. A failure to understand their origin together with the incorrect notion that they were lined with epithelium led to many ineffective treatments and consequently recurrence was common.

Recently it has been realized that the ranula is an extravasation cyst, like the majority of the smaller mucoceles found on the lips and cheek. The only difference is that a larger gland, one of the sublingual glands, is involved and hence the volume of mucus saliva produced is greater. The anterior sublingual glands, either Bartholin's major sublingual or one of the minor sublingual glands, produce the ranula on the floor of the mouth. The posterior sublingual is the causative gland for the plunging ranula.

Histological Features.—These are similar to those of the mucocele. If a portion of the cyst sac is recovered it will be found to be composed of a thin layer of fibrous tissue. Not uncommonly a layer of cuboidal cells is seen, one cell thick on its inner surface. It is these which were mistaken for epithelial cells. Closer inspection shows them to be macrophages.

Treatment.—As long ago as 1897, Von Hipple advocated excision of the ranula complete with the sublingual gland and since then a number of authors have recognized this relationship to the sublingual gland. Crile (1957), for example, thought that excision of the cyst wall without removal of the gland resulted in recurrence and advocated simple drainage of plunging ranulas followed by excision of the appropriate sublingual gland. Whitlock and Summersgill (1962) eventually dealt successfully with a recurrent plunging ranula by excision of the sublingual gland and without a further attack on the cyst itself. Catone, Merrill, and Henny (1969) advocate formal exposure and removal of the sublingual gland.

A vasoconstrictor-containing solution is used to infiltrate the floor of the mouth and an incision made towards the lingual side of the plica sublingualis. As a first step the submandibular duct is identified and isolated. It is followed backwards and the lingual nerve found where it passes beneath the duct and a tape passed around it. Provided that the tissue lingual to the duct is not entered, the sublingual veins are not disturbed, and that the dissection is not carried deep to the submandibular duct and lingual nerve, neither the sublingual artery nor the hypoglossal nerve should be encountered.

The mucosal flap lateral to the incision is separated from the upper surface of the sublingual gland mass which can then be rolled medially off the surface of the mylohyoid muscle. Where the deep part of the submandibular gland is large, the lingual nerve tends to pass between the deep part and the duct as it travels forwards. Where the deep part is small, the posterior sublingual gland may be large and the nerve will pass obliquely under its posterior end from lateral to medial and will come into view again as the gland is rolled medially.

Final separation of the gland is from before backwards, lifting the anterior end out of the wound and completing the separation with a blunt dissector made by rolling cotton-wool pads tightly round the ends of closed artery forceps. Small vessels supplying the sublingual gland from the sublingual and submandibular arteries will be encountered and can be diathermized with care. The mucosa is then closed with few loose sutures.

The ranula itself is frequently ruptured and virtually vanishes at an early stage in the procedure, but this does not matter. If it does not do so, the sac can be separated and removed together with the gland.

Retention Cyst of Submandibular Duct

Complete obstruction of the submandibular duct, as for example by ligation, results in atrophy of the submandibular gland or, should the duct rupture at or behind the ligature, the production of a salivary fistula into the mouth or into the tissues. However, a case of congenital occlusion of the duct has been described which resulted in a cystic swelling in the floor of the baby's mouth (Beke, Tomaro, and Stein, 1963).

Ectopic Oral Tonsils

Knapp (1970) describes in some detail the appearances produced by oral tonsillar tissue. He describes round, oval, or bean-shaped elevations up to 1 cm. in length. Some are smooth and rounded, some flat plaques, and others nodular elevations. A few form yellowish globules which may discharge their contents on pressure.

The nodular lesions are hyperplastic lymphoid tissue around a tonsillar crypt. If the crypt becomes obstructed, keratin collects within to form a pseudocyst: the yellow globular lesion. Where the tonsils are traumatized they may be inflamed and hyperaemic, forming reddish elevations. Oral tonsils can be found on the soft palate, the tongue, and the floor of the mouth, either singly or in groups.

No treatment is required unless pseudocysts are formed which become infected. These may be either drained or excised.

OTHER ENTITIES

Lymphangiomas should not be mistaken for ranulas, since they often involve the dorsum of the tongue, are brownish and nodular, like the back of a warty toad rather than a frog's belly. Cystic hygroma may rarely involve the floor of the mouth, but involves the neck at the same time and is seen in the young infant. Curiously, although Fordyce's spots are common, sebaceous cysts are not seen. Even sebaceous adenomas of the buccal mucosa are rare, but Miller and McCrea (1968) have recorded such an occurrence.

REFERENCES

BEKE, A. L., TOMARO, A. J., and STEIN, M. (1963), 'Congenital Atresia of Sublingual Duct with Ranula', *J. oral Surg.*, **21**, 427.
BHASKAR, S. N., BOLDEN, T. E., and WEINMANN, J. P. (1956), 'Experimental Obstructive Adenitis in the Mouse', *J. dent. Res.*, **35**, 852.
CATONE, G. A., MERRILL, R. G., and HENNY, F. A. (1969), 'Sublingual Gland Mucus-escape Phenomenon: Treatment by Excision of Sub-lingual Gland', *J. oral Surg.*, **27**, 774.
CHAUDHRY, A. P., and others (1960), 'Clinical and Experimental Study of Mucocele (Retention Cyst)', *J. dent. Res.*, **39**, 1253.
COOK, J. T. (1950), 'Dermoid Cyst', *Oral Surg.*, **3**, 740.
CRILE, G. (1957), 'Ranulas with Extension into the Neck: So-called Plunging Ranulas', *Surgery, St Louis*, **42**, 819.
DUVERGEY, J. (1907), *Ann. Chir.*, **20**, 368.
GOLD, C. (1962), *Oral Surg.*, **15**, 1118.
GOLDBERG, A. F. (1965), 'Dermoid Cyst of the Tongue', *J. oral Surg.*, **23**, 649.
GORLIN, R. J., and JIRASEK, J. E. (1970), 'Oral Cysts containing Gastric or Intestinal Mucosa', *Ibid.*, **28**, 9.
KNAPP, M. J. (1970), 'Pathology of Oral Tonsil', *Oral Surg.*, **29**, 295.
MILLER, A. S., and MCCREA, M. W. (1968), 'Sebaceous Gland Adenoma of the Buccal Mucosa', *J. oral Surg.*, **26**, 593.
SELA, J., and ULMANSKY, M. (1969), 'Mucous Retention Cyst of Salivary Glands', *Ibid.*, **27**, 619.
SEWARD, G. R. (1965), 'Dermoid Cysts of the Floor of the Mouth', *Br. J. oral Surg.*, **3**, 36.
STANDISH, S. M., and SHAFER, W. C. (1957), 'Serial Histologic Effects of Rat Submaxillary and Sub-lingual Salivary Gland Duct and Blood Vessel Ligation', *J. dent. Res.*, **36**, 866.
VON HIPPLE, R. (1897), 'Ueber Bau und Wesen der Ranula', *Arch. klin. Chir.*, **55**, 164.
WHITLOCK, R. I., and SUMMERSGILL, G. B. (1962), 'Ranula with Cervical Extension', *Oral Surg.*, **15**, 1163.
WILSON, C. P. (1955), 'Lateral Cysts and Fistulae of the Neck of Developmental Origin', *Ann. R. Coll. Surg.*, **17**, 1.

Chapter IX

GIANT-CELL LESIONS OF THE JAWS

The Central Giant-cell Granuloma

The term 'giant-cell reparative granuloma' was coined by Jaffe in 1953, for the central, giant-cell lesion of the jaws, although the term has since been applied by others to the giant-cell epulis as well.

In order to understand Jaffe's concept of the giant-cell reparative granuloma, it is necessary to review the way in which it arose. Jaffe, Lichtenstein, and Portis and then Jaffe made a study of the giant-cell tumours of bone and noted that there was a marked difference in the behaviour of the lesions of long bones and those of the jaws. They noted that the long bone osteoclastoma was a treacherous lesion which often recurred and could metastasize. By comparison the jaw tumours were benign. When Jaffe investigated the two groups he found further differences. The long bone tumours tended to occur between 20 and 55 years of age, whereas the maximum incidence for the jaw lesion was between 10 and 25 years of age. Further, in histological sections from long bone lesions there were many giant cells evenly distributed throughout the tumour and varying degrees of atypicality of the stromal cells. In general there was no new bone formation. Sections from the jaw tumours showed a focal distribution of the giant cells and spicules of woven bone were frequent.

Because of its behaviour, Jaffe felt that the jaw condition was dysplastic rather than neoplastic and looked upon it as an abnormal granulation tissue, or tissue of repair. Hence, he coined the name 'giant-cell reparative granuloma'.

Since Jaffe's papers in 1953, our concept of this lesion has undergone further modifications. Most people agree that the term 'reparative' was unfortunate and could imply, to those who did not know the context in which Jaffe used it, that the natural history of the condition was biased towards repair. In fact, it seems to remain destructive and few would be courageous enough to observe one in the hope of spontaneous cure. Thus, mostly they are now called 'giant-cell granulomas', and the word 'reparative' has been dropped.

In support of the non-neoplastic nature of the condition is the realization that incomplete removal can result in a cure. The periphery is complex and even after careful enucleation small pockets of abnormal tissue can be left behind. These do not necessarily lead to recurrence. Further, it can be shown histologically that the marrow spaces adjacent to the major bone cavity are involved and these are not touched by simple surgery, yet a successful outcome is not affected. On occasions a generous biopsy has been known to stimulate healing. None of this is compatible with the natural history of even a benign neoplasm.

Jaffe's concept of the age of incidence has had also to be modified. Quite a number of cases of giant-cell granuloma have been observed in the age-group 25–40 years and some in patients as young as 2½–3 years and as old as 63 years.

Because a similar histological appearance is shared by a number of diseases of bone, the concept has grown up that they are all disturbances of the tissue which resorbs bone. Disturbances of a tissue which features multinucleated giant cells, thin-walled blood-vessels, a proliferation of a cellular, skeletal connective tissue, and histiocytes. Thus, the giant-cell granuloma can be looked upon as a dysplasia of the resorptive tissue of bone.

At various times it has been postulated that haemorrhage is the stimulus that incites the appearance of the giant cells. It is true that red cells are frequently seen in sections of surgical specimens and biopsies, but these are obviously spilt at the time of removal. It is also true that blood pigments can be found in the histiocytes, but even this is not surprising since the blood-vessels are so thin-walled. Indeed, in places the wall of a capillary may be replaced by a giant cell which 'collars' it, so that some leakage of red corpuscles in life could easily occur. There is, however, no evidence of appreciable phagocytosis of red blood corpuscles by the giant cell, nor are giant cells produced in other body tissues to deal with extravasated red cells.

There is, unfortunately, no histochemical difference between osteoclasts and foreign-body giant cells, but the constant association of the whole group of these lesions with bone makes it likely that these particular giant cells are osteoclasts.

It has been pointed out that the giant-cell granuloma favours the tooth-bearing part of the jaws and in particular regions which have supported primary teeth. This may be of diagnostic and possibly aetiological significance.

Females are said to be affected more often than males and the mandible more often than the maxilla. From their radiological appearances, central giant-cell granulomas can be subdivided into two types: those which appear to start in the medullary cavity and those which start subperiosteally.

The Central Medullary Type occurs almost exclusively in the tooth-bearing part of the jaws and produces an oval, or loculated, cavity in the bone. Marked resorption of the cortical plates takes place at an early stage in their development so that the transverse diameter of the lesion is often only a little less than its anteroposterior diameter. A thin layer of subperiosteal new bone covers the parts which have bulged beyond the original cortex. An important radiological characteristic of the sub-periosteal bone is that it is polyarcuate in outline as seen on occlusal radiographs.

Histologically the giant-cell granuloma consists of zones of the characteristic tissue, separated by septa rich in collagen fibres in which, in older lesions, woven bone is deposited. It is this lobulated structure, together with a marked ability to cause the resorption of adjacent bone and teeth, which accounts for its radiological features.

The lobulated surface results in a varying degree of ridging of the inner aspect of the bone cavity. In radiographs this produces a multilocular or cross-hatched appearance, particularly in the maxilla. New bone is laid down to form short, incomplete septa which run inwards from the indentations in the subperiosteal new bone. Where laterally directed X-rays pass tangential to these septa, linear shadows are produced in the periapical and oblique lateral jaw films which add to the multilocular appearance.

In the mandible early destruction of cortical bone results in dark, well-defined images in the lateral views which again can increase the appearance of loculation. Especially is this so if the subperiosteal new bone bulges laterally almost at right angles to the jaw surface so that a thin white linear image is cast, outlining the edge of the dark image.

In occlusal radiographs a Codman's triangle of new bone is seen at the junction of the subperiosteal sheet of bone with the old cortex. In some occlusal radiographs the raised periosteum appears to cover a greater area than the cortical perforation, though this could be a projection effect. Spicules of new bone other than those forming septa are often seen within that part of the lesion which bulges outside the original outline of the jaw.

Because little bone substance is removed by the intramedullary part of the cavity, the increased radiolucency which results in small and a well-marked periphery is seen only if the margin has a large radius of curvature.

Resorption of the roots of adjacent teeth is a frequent feature and where the surface of the lesion is lobulated several aspects of a root may be affected. Some giant-cell granulomas displace teeth as they increase in size while others loop up between the roots and come to surround them.

The Subperiosteal Type of giant-cell granuloma has the larger part of its bulk external to the normal contours of the jaw, but this does not preclude the involvement of the underlying bone to a considerable depth, especially

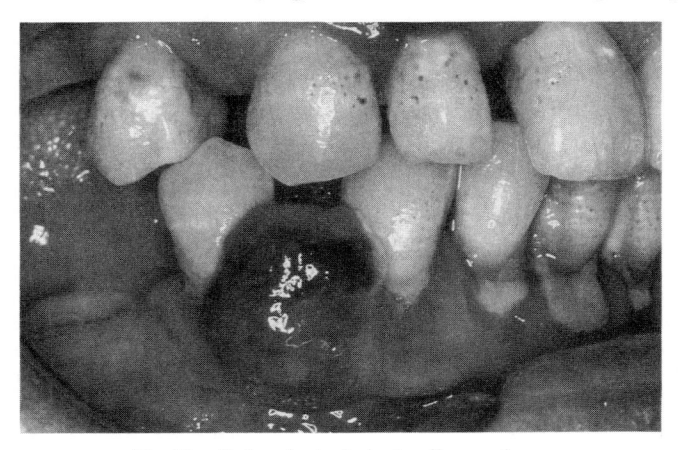

Fig. 12.—Subperiosteal giant-cell granuloma.

in the maxilla. Careful radiography will demonstrate a layer of subperiosteal new bone over at least part of the surface of the mass, though it may be less obvious than the subperiosteal bone formed over the extracortical expansions of the intramedullary type. (*See Fig.* 12.)

Because the cortex is attacked from the beginning, and often up to the greatest diameter of the tumour the lesion has a dark, punched-out appearance in radiographs. When seen in profile, fern-like or tufted arrangements of new bone trabeculae penetrate into the radiolucent centre of the mass.

A variant of the subperiosteal type occurs at the time at which the primary teeth are shed.

There is an excavation in the surface of the alveolar crest which may penetrate between and around the crowns of the permanent teeth. The alveolar process is bulged laterally on one or both aspects and a layer of subperiosteal new bone covers the lesion at these points.

The place where the primary teeth have been lost appears at first sight to be ulcerated. In fact, the tumour is covered by a thin epithelium, but the colour here contrasts with the pale mucoperiosteum on the lateral aspect. Apart from the expansion of the alveolar ridge only the presence of dilated, small vessels on the surface indicates the extent of the condition.

In some instances the permanent teeth erupt around the side of the mass and are further displaced and separated by it as it grows.

Radiographs are generally disappointing, give a poor indication of the size of the lesion, and may reveal few helpful diagnostic features. With care the successional teeth can be conserved, but a cautious prognosis is in order preoperatively, because of the difficulty in judging the extent of the process from the films. It is, of course, tempting to attribute the origin of these particular giant-cell granulomas to the tissue which is responsible for resorbing the deciduous teeth.

Treatment.—The treatment of the central giant-cell granuloma consists of enucleation of the lesion following adequate surgical exposure of the area and this can usually be effected through an intra-oral incision. Following removal of the mass the underlying bony walls and bed of the resulting cavity should be carefully curetted with a sharp Volkmann's scoop. Alternatively, a large rosehead bur can be used, skimming the surface to a depth of 0·5 mm. If this is done small pockets of lesional tissue will be uncovered and removed. These lie in irregular outpouchings of the bony cavity and are left behind as the main mass is removed. Neither important neurovascular bundles nor adjacent teeth should be unnecessarily hazarded by this procedure. Neither electrocoagulation as recommended by Kruger (1959) or thermal or chemical cauterization as suggested by Archer (1956) and Thoma (1962) is necessary, and are to be deprecated since they damage an unpredictable layer of bone which subsequently must be resorbed or sequestrated. If for a particular lesion it is felt that a margin of tissue should be removed, this should be outlined at the beginning, so that the mass is removed intact together with the appropriate margin.

Radiotherapy should not be used for giant-cell granulomas. In a small proportion of cases it is true that radiotherapy will destroy the lesional tissue, but curiously bony healing of the bony cavity does not occur. What is observed is that the margins and any septa become more distinct in the radiographs. Then after some years the lesion starts to grow again. One is then faced with the problem of treating a lesion lying in irradiated bone. Furthermore, radiotherapy should not, in general, be used for the treatment of benign conditions, particularly in the young and especially for tumours of bone where such treatment carries a risk of osteogenic **sarcoma** arising in 20–25 years.

The Osteoclastoma

The term osteoclastoma is now commonly reserved for the malignant neoplasm in this group of lesions. Presumably a benign neoplasm, the benign osteoclastoma, may also exist but there are, at the moment, no criteria by which it can be distinguished from the dysplastic giant-cell granuloma.

Only by their aggressive behaviour and, to some extent, by their histology, can neoplastic osteoclastomas be distinguished from giant-cell granulomas when they occur in the jaws. Indeed, the number of recorded cases which fulfil modern criteria for an osteoclastoma is small. Judging by these reports rapid growth, a poorly defined periphery in the radiographs, little evidence of new bone within the lesion, and little or no subperiosteal new bone over it are sinister features. The value of morphological differentiation between the neoplasm and granuloma is questionable, but certain histological features have been stressed. For instance, the giant cells in the osteoclastoma are stated to be more numerous and more evenly distributed in the spindle-cell stroma. These cells are also said to be of larger size than those of the granuloma, i.e., 50–100 μ, and contain 20–40 centrally placed nuclei. The nuclei may be vesicular or pyknotic and resemble those of the spindle cells. However, most of these characteristics are related to speed of growth and it is worth remembering that giant-cell granulomas can grow rapidly at times, particularly in the young and in pregnant women (McGowan, 1970).

Probably the most valuable criteria to look for are the usual histological characteristics of malignancy: increased nuclear-to-cytoplasm ratio, hyperchronic nuclei, variations in cell and nuclear size and abnormal mitoses.

Perhaps the most frequent malignant giant-cell lesion to involve the jaws is the giant-cell sarcoma seen in Paget's disease.

Treatment.—Once one becomes convinced that the lesion is a malignant osteoclastoma—that is, an aggressive neoplasm—then adequate radical surgery should be employed. The growth should be excised together with a wide margin. Radiotherapy may be necessary where palliative treatment is appropriate, or where tissue planes may have been contaminated by tumour cells during previous surgery.

The Periosteal Osteoclastoma

This lesion has also been described variously as peripheral giant-cell reparative granuloma, peripheral giant-cell tumour, giant-cell epulis, periosteal osteoclastoma, myeloid epulis, and osteoclastoma. The multiplicity of the designations applied to the condition indicate the prevailing confusion concerning its nature and aetiology. It was originally considered to be a true neoplasm but more recently the view has been advanced that it represents an unusual proliferative response of the tissues to injury. Histologically it resembles the giant-cell granuloma.

Clinical Appearance.—The periosteal osteoclastoma almost always occurs on the buccal or labial aspect of the gingiva or alveolar process and appears to arise from the mucoperiosteum (*Fig.* 13). Though unencapsulated, it is not infiltrative. The majority are located in the canine-premolar region, that part of the jaw which has borne deciduous teeth. In the past, the theory was advanced that a predilection for that site implied a proliferation of the osteoclasts which are normally involved in the shedding of the deciduous predecessors during the transition from a primary to a secondary dentition. However, this premise fails to explain the anomalous occurrence of some of these lesions in the posterior region of the jaws. The peripheral granuloma is sessile at an early stage, but later it becomes pedunculated. Its colour is usually purplish, dark red, or haemorrhagic, but its clinical appearance may vary and at times it may resemble a fibroma or even a pyogenic granuloma. The maximum diameter rarely exceeds 3 cm. and the consistency is soft or firm. Almost invariably the swelling is painless, but rarely it may become ulcerated due to trauma from opposing teeth or from the use of a toothbrush. When teeth are present, the granuloma protrudes from an interdental space and may

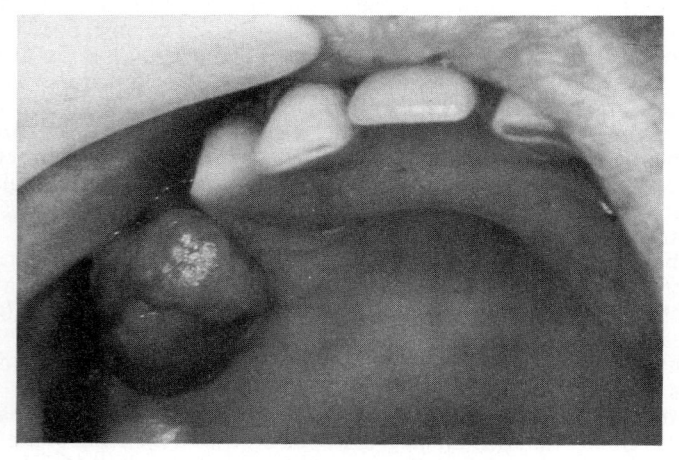

Fig. 13.—Periosteal osteoclastoma or giant-cell epulis; compare this lesion with the prolapsed antral polyp in *Fig.* 4.

cause divarication of adjacent teeth. In the edentulous patient it usually arises from the crest of the ridge. Increasing size of the lesion may cause interference with sleep or mastication. According to Bernick (1948) females are more commonly affected than males, but Cooke (1952) found that up to the age of 15 years the sexes were equally involved, although from 20 to 45 years there was a preponderance of affected females which represented 42 per cent of his series. A survey by Killey and Kay (1965) indicated that the mandible was more often involved than the maxilla.

Histology.—The lesion consists of a non-capsulated mass of tissue consisting of delicate reticular and fibrillar connective tissue stroma containing multinucleated giant cells. The latter are scarce and dispersed in concentric arrangements around foci of haemorrhage. Numerous capillaries are present and delicate trabeculae of osteoid or immature bone may be conspicuous.

Radiological Appearance.—A radiological examination will not have any specific value unless pressure resorption of the underlying bone has occurred. In such cases, intra-oral radiographs will reveal a sauceriform depression in the surface of the alveolar process which may be well-defined or have an irregular contour.

Treatment.—Treatment is by excision through an incision around the base of the lesion. Unlike the fibroma an excision a few millimetres wide of the obvious periphery is necessary to avoid the possibility of a recurrence but the adjoining teeth should be preserved unless pocketing has occurred interdentally. The surface of the alveolar bone underlying the lesion should be curetted. If a relapse does take place, extraction of the teeth in immediate proximity to the mass must be seriously considered and a vulcanite bur should be run over the surface of the bone to ensure that all the lesional tissue has been removed. The raw area of bone left after the excision should be covered over with a pack of ribbon gauze soaked in Whitehead's varnish. This is left in situ for about ten days, after which the area will be found to have granulated. The site of the periosteal osteoclastoma should be kept under observation at regular intervals, for many months, for some of these lesions show a marked tendency to recur. The periosteal osteoclastoma is sometimes found in patients suffering from hyperparathyroidism and in all such cases a serum calcium and phosphorus estimation should be performed.

Brown Tumours or Nodes

Peripheral or osteolytic central brown tumours or nodes occur in hyperparathyroidism and resemble the giant-cell granuloma both clinically and cytologically. Their incidence is difficult to assess from the literature, because most large published reviews of giant-cell lesions omit details of the proportion due to the endocrine disorder. In Killey and Kay's series of 23 cases, 3 were found to be central hyperparathyroid lesions. Dent (1962; 1966) recognizes three forms of hyperparathyroidism in addition to that due to carcinoma of the gland. These are primary, secondary and tertiary. Primary hyperparathyroidism is due to an adenoma or hyperplasia of the gland, secondary hyperparathyroidism is due to compensatory hyperplasia where there is phosphate retention or impaired calcium absorption, and tertiary hyperparathyroidism is due to an autonomous adenoma which arises in a case of secondary hyperparathyroidism. Secondary hyperparathyroidism is worthy of special note because usually the serum calcium is not raised in this form of the disease, At one time it was thought that there were two parathyroid hormones: one producing severe bone disease, a high alkaline phosphatase, and renal damage, and the other a high plasma calcium, low plasma phosphorus and their associated systemic disturbances, but a low alkaline phosphatase and less overt bone damage. This is no longer thought to be likely. The possibility of latent hyperparathyroidism must always be considered when giant-cell granulomas are diagnosed and particularly if there is a recurrence of the lesion after adequate excision, even though initial laboratory reports reveal that the relevant investigations of blood and urine produce results that are within normal limits. From the limited evidence available, it does seem likely that the jaw lesions can presage the onset of manifest hyperparathyroidism by a long period; in a case seen by the authors a time lag of one-and-a-half years occurred, and in another instance (Black and Ackerman, 1950) there was a lapse of thirteen years before the underlying parathyroid disease was detected.

Essential diagnostic blood determinations for hyperparathyroidism are the serum calcium, inorganic phosphorus, and alkaline phosphatase values. Excess calcium content in the urine can be determined by the Sulkowitch test which produces a cloudy reaction when positive, but some authorities are highly critical of this investigation, pointing out the high frequency of misleading results. Unfortunately, too, with localized skeletal manifestations of a parathyroid disorder, the alkaline phosphatase level is indecisive, often remaining at the upper limit of normal. McGeown (1961), however, has stressed that the serum calcium concentration is the most important single determination of parathyroid function, provided that the test is repeated three or four times, at intervals, in view of the observation that in hyperparathyroidism the serum calcium values fluctuate and often lie within normal limits. A small rise is significant, but as this can be concealed by increased inorganic phosphorus following exercise and a meal, the patient should be fasted overnight (Harris, 1966). Similarly, where there is a reduction in plasma protein, the loss of protein-bound calcium will also give a low figure. If the specific gravity of the plasma is less than 1·027, 0·25 mg. per cent is added to the calcium value for every unit by which the figure in third decimal place is less than seven, e.g., for a specific gravity of 1·023 add 1 mg. per cent. In contrast, venous stasis by raising the protein-bound calcium in the sample produces an artificially high value, so that a sphygmomanometer cuff must not be used in performing the venepuncture. Electrophoresis can also be employed to detect an abnormal protein picture.

Obviously early recognition of the disease is essential if irreversible renal damage is to be avoided in patients, and failure to identify a parathyroid abnormality in cases presenting with a peripheral granuloma is a well-known diagnostic pitfall. The clinical inquiry to assist in the exclusion or confirmation of hyperparathyroidism should be directed to the possibility of renal colic, lassitude, nausea, and vomiting.

Radiology.—The specific radiological signs of hyperparathyroidism may not even be present; only, in fact, an osteolytic area in the jaw identical in appearance to that of an endosteal giant-cell granuloma. Decreased definition of the bony trabeculae is supposed to be pathognomic and an inconstant dental sign of the disorder is partial loss or complete effacement of the lamina dura around the roots of the functioning teeth adjacent to the lesion. In X-ray films of the hands, subperiosteal resorption of the cortex of the phalanges is corroborative, and an abdominal projection is valuable in case of calcific changes in the kidneys. A lateral radiograph of the patella may also be helpful, for in hyperparathyroidism the softened patella appears to be wrapped round the femoral condyle. This phenomenon which is variously known as 'cloth cap patella' or 'Dixon's wrap-round sign', is due to a crush fracture in the bone produced by the pull of the quadriceps femoris.

Treatment.—Surgical removal of the over-active parathyroid tissue will allow the brown tumours to heal once the calcium metabolism is restored to normal.

CHERUBISM
(*Disseminated Juvenile Fibrous Dysplasia, Familial Multilocular Cystic Disease of the Jaws, or Familial Fibrous Swelling of the Jaws*)

Cherubism is the designation given to a familial giant-celled multicystic lesion of the jaws first described by Jones in 1933. The inheritance factor is an autosomal dominant gene and males appear to be affected twice as commonly as females. Thomas and Jones (1931) traced the condition back through five generations. At birth there is no evidence of this benign developmental abnormality and the facial deformity only becomes obvious at the age of about 2–4 years. This consists of a painless enlargement of both upper and lower jaws which develops rapidly up to the age of 7 years. The mandible is more frequently affected than the maxilla and the involvement is usually bilateral.

It is often dogmatically stated that the presence of bilateral changes is pathognomic of the condition, whereas, paradoxically, the youngest of Jones' original family was only affected on the left side. It is also pertinent to point out that the maxilla, too, may be only unilaterally enlarged. The extent of the lesions varies in size from changes restricted to the rami, tuberosities, and 3rd molar region to gross deformities of both jaws. A slower development of the deformity occurs between the age of 7 and puberty. The swellings in the jaws are firm and the mucosa overlying them becomes stretched and taut. Systemic manifestations are absent. After puberty the condition tends to regress with further maturation of the facial skeleton and eventually the cystic cavities are replaced with normal bone. Disappearance of the abnormality tends to occur at about the age of 22 years, but the authors have seen 2 patients aged 30 in whom there has been regression of the disease, but residual evidence of the original condition is still apparent on the radiographs. According to Jones (1965) enlargement of the local lymph-nodes is often present in early childhood. The lymphadenopathy regresses after the age of 5 years and has never been observed in adult patients either by Jones or by Caffey and Williams (1951). The enlargement is probably related to an upper respiratory tract infection.

The controversial matter of the 'heavenwards look' now appears to have been rationalized. Formerly, the extraordinary appearance of upturned eyes with exposed sclera between limbus and eyelid was attributed to the stretching of the skin overlying the expanded maxillary surface. It is now explained that this somewhat rare sign only occurs when the orbital floor is raised by a dome of dysplastic tissue which is continuous with the protuberant thickened anterior wall of the maxilla (Burland, 1962).

Intra-orally a diffuse swelling obscures the morphological distinction between the alveolus and body of the mandible. The palate may be almost obliterated by the gross enlargement of the tuberosities, and it is often narrowed in the anterior region. In places where the cortex is perforated, the swelling has a fleshy consistency. There is considerable interference with the normal development of both the deciduous and permanent teeth which may be absent due to premature exfoliation, displacement or failure to erupt. Agenesis of the 2nd and 3rd permanent molars is not uncommon, and McClendon, Anderson, and Cornelius (1962) reported supernumerary teeth in 1 of their patients and his paternal and maternal relatives. Ramon,

Berman, and Bubis (1967) reported a case complicated by gingival fibromatosis.

Radiographs demonstrate that the bones of the jaws are expanded and that there are multilocular radiolucencies especially in the ramus and body of the mandible and in the maxillary tuberosity. The antra may be completely obliterated and numerous unerupted teeth are seen. The radiolucent areas slowly fill in during the third decade, but some may persist until middle age. The lesions of this disorder are sometimes encountered in the long bones, metacarpals, and anterior ends of ribs. Some patients develop periosteal giant-cell lesions. There is no recognized abnormality of the serum calcium, phosphorus, or alkaline phosphatase levels.

Histology.—Histological examination of tissue from the lesions shows numerous giant cells arranged in groups around thin-walled blood-vessels in a fibrous tissue stroma. Epithelial remnants from developing teeth are sometimes seen scattered throughout the lesion and this may lead to an erroneous histological diagnosis of an odontogenic neoplasm.

Treatment and Prognosis.—It has been stressed that although the disease tends to progress rapidly in early childhood it tends to become static and even regress following puberty. Biopsy of the jaw lesions should be carried out to establish the diagnosis and if the condition is cosmetically unacceptable, surgical correction of the expanded jaw lesions can be carried out once the disease becomes quiescent.

REFERENCES

ARCHER, W. H. (1956), *Oral Surgery*. Philadelphia: Saunders.
BERNICK, S. (1948), 'Growths of the Gingiva and Palate. Connective Tissue Tumours', *Oral Surg.*, **1**, 1098.
BLACK, B. K., and ACKERMAN, L. V. (1950), 'Tumours of the Parathyroid', *Cancer, N.Y.*, **3**, 415.
BURLAND, J. G. (1962), 'Cherubism: Familial Bilateral Osseous Dysplasia of Jaws', *Oral Surg.*, **15**, 43.
CAFFEY, J., and WILLIAMS, J. L. (1951), 'Familial Fibrous Swelling of Jaws', *Radiology*, **56**, 1.
COOKE, B. E. D. (1952), 'The Giant Cell Epulis. Histogenesis and Natural History', *Br. dent. J.*, **93**, 13.
DENT, C. E. (1962), 'Parathyroid Disease', *Trans. med. Soc. Lond.*, **77**, 166.
— — (1966), 'Parathyroid Disease', *Ann. R. Coll. Surg.*, **39**, No. 3, 150.
HARRIS, M. (1966), 'Cherubism and the Osteoclastoma', *Oral Surg.*, **25**, 613.
JAFFE, H. L. (1953), 'Giant Cell Reparative Granuloma. Traumatic Bone Cyst and Fibrous (Fibro-osseous) Dysplasia of the Jaw Bones', *Ibid.*, **6**, 159.
JONES, W. A. (1933), 'Familial Multilocular Cystic Disease of Jaws', *Am. J. Cancer*, **17**, 946.
— — (1965), 'Cherubism', *Oral Surg.*, **20**, 648.
KILLEY, H. C., and KAY, L. W. (1965), 'Giant Cell Lesions of the Jaws', *J. int. Coll. Surg.*, **44**, 262.
KRUGER, G. O. (1959), *Textbook of Oral Surgery*. St. Louis: Mosby.
MCCLENDON, J. L., ANDERSON, D., and CORNELIUS, E. A. (1962), 'Cherubism— Hereditary Fibrous Dysplasia of the Jaws. Pathological Considerations', *Oral Surg.* **15**, 17.
MCGEOWN, M. G. (1961), 'Value of Special Tests of Parathyroid Function', *Proc. Ass. clin. Biochem.*, **1**, 46.
MCGOWAN, D. A. (1970), 'Central Giant Cell Tumour of the Mandible occurring in Pregnancy', *Br. J. oral Surg.*, **7**, 131.
RAMON, Y., BERMAN, W., and BUBIS, J. J. (1967), 'Gingival Fibromatosis combined with Cherubism', *Oral Surg.*, **24**, 435.
THOMA, K. H. (1962), 'Cherubism and Intraosseous Giant Cell Lesions', *Ibid.*, **15**, 1.
THOMAS, P. J., and JONES, W. A. (1931), 'Further Observations regarding Familial Multilocular Cystic Disease of the Jaws', *Br. J. Radiol.*, **11**, 227

Chapter X

THE ODONTOGENIC TUMOURS AND ODONTOMES

THE application of the term 'odontome' has varied considerably over the years. About 50 years ago it was used to cover all the abnormalities of the dental tissues whether developmental, inflammatory, or neoplastic. However, its present use is more restricted. Minor variations in size and number of the elements of a tooth are not now often described as odontomes, nor are the various odontogenic cysts, or those hamartomatous malformations and neoplasms which are largely composed of soft tissues. In general, the word is currently used for examples of the more extravagant variations in tooth morphology.

The term 'odontogenic tumour' is used for a group of lesions including the extreme morphological variants from the odontomes, together with the hamartomas and neoplasms of odontogenic tissues which have a large soft-tissue component to their structure. Some of these form cysts, but are separated from the other cystic odontogenic lesions for inclusion in this group because their epithelial component exhibits a growth and proliferation which is to a varying extent independent of the existence of a positive pressure within the cyst. Some other cystic lesions can be included because the lining is thick, the epithelium burrows extensively into the capsule of the cyst or induces odontoblasts to form.

Pindborg and Clausen (1958) proposed a classification of odontogenic tumours which recognized the inductive ability of odontogenic epithelium. This classification was used by Gorlin, Chaudhry, and Pindborg in their review article on the subject in 1961. The following classification is based on that of Gorlin, Chaudhry, and Pindborg.

ODONTOGENIC TUMOURS

Epithelial Odontogenic Tumours
With no inductive changes in the connective tissues
    Ameloblastoma
    Adeno-ameloblastoma
    Calcifying odontogenic epithelium tumour (Pindborg tumour)
With inductive changes in the connective tissues
    Ameloblastic fibroma
    Ameloblastic sarcoma
    Dentinoma (1) Fibro-ameloblastic type   (2) Mature type
    Calcifying odontogenic cyst
    Ameloblastic odontome
    Complex odontome
    Compound odontome
Mesodermal Odontogenic Tumours
    Odontogenic myxoma or fibromyxoma
    Cementifying fibroma.

The Epithelial Odontogenic Tumours
The Ameloblastoma.—

Origin.—The ameloblastoma seems almost certainly to be a neoplasm of odontogenic epithelium. Reasons for suggesting this are as follows:

1. No examples of this lesion have been reported from regions remote from the oral cavity. The so-called 'adamantinoma' of the tibia differs markedly from the condition found in the jaws, and only the craniopharyngioma resembles it histologically. Since the craniopharyngioma may arise from Rathke's pouch which derives from oral epithelium this latter similarity is consistent with the basic premise. A few have been reported in the soft tissue adjacent to the tooth-bearing parts of the jaws, but certain other odontogenic lesions are found in similar situations from time to time.

2. The epithelium bears a considerable histological similarity to that found in the bell stage of the enamel organ. The outer epithelium of the clumps is cylindrical and shows reversal of polarity like ameloblasts. The bulk of the rest of the cells resemble the stellate reticulum, but the innermost cells in the clumps of tumour cells have no counterpart in the normal structure. There are no cells resembling the stratum intermedium.

There are often sterile discussions as to whether this neoplasm should be regarded as benign or malignant. Some argue that it is not malignant since it virtually never metastasizes, unless subjected to repeated surgical trauma. It is suggested that as the ameloblastoma stems from odontogenic epithelium, which normally proliferates and penetrates into the jaws during odontogenesis, such behaviour is not necessarily that of a malignant neoplasm. However, it seems clear that a benign neoplasm should be encapsulated and readily enucleated and the ameloblastoma is not. Indeed, the degree to which it invades the tissues locally is such that recurrence is common, and eventual death of the patient from extension of the tumour into the skull a not uncommon occurrence.

The tumour normally arises centrally in the jaw, presumably from remnants of the tooth band. In some cases the lesion seems to stem from the alveolar epithelium, but since the tooth band developed originally from the oral epithelium this is quite reasonable. Fusion with the epithelium must, of course, be distinguished from origination.

As some examples have a dentigerous relationship to an unerupted tooth and may even form a unilocular cyst about the tooth, the suggestion is made that the ameloblastoma can arise from the epithelium lining a dentigerous cyst. In practice the validity of such claims can be difficult to assess. When the cells of an ameloblastoma are stretched over a large cyst they can closely resemble the epithelial cells which line simple odontogenic cysts. Only by careful comparison with the epithelium in the more solid part, the so-called 'mural ameloblastoma', will the observer realize that they also are ameloblastomatous. Another source of difficulty is the localized proliferations of odontogenic epithelium found from time to time within the capsule of dentigerous cysts. Should some of these take on a follicular form, it may require a pathologist of considerable experience to distinguish between innocent proliferation and an early ameloblastoma.

Incidence.—While there is no sex preference and no proved race incidence, there does seem to be a variation in the site most commonly involved in different races. In Europeans and North Americans over 70 per cent of lesions involve the molar and coronoid process region. In Nigerians, however, the anterior part of the lower jaw is the more commonly affected (Akinosi and Williams, 1968). The anterior part of the mandible is also rather more frequently affected in some Indians (Potdar, 1969). In all races maxillary lesions are the least frequent. It is not a particularly common neoplasm and the practising oral surgeon will see many more carcinomas than ameloblastomas.

When first seen, the patient is usually between 20 and 50 years, but children of 8 years and upwards and elderly people too may also be affected. It is difficult to gauge the age at onset, for although there is some variation in rate of growth, this is usually slow and sizeable tumours may have been present for many years.

Radiology.—The typical ameloblastoma is a truly multilocular lesion. That is, it is composed of several cystic compartments. The cysts vary in size and inspection of the periphery mesially, distally, buccally, and lingually reveals evidence of many small loculations in the periphery. Sonesson (1950) lays stress on the significance of a patchy sclerosis of the periphery and bony septa of an ameloblastoma. In some cases the lesion is composed of many comparatively small cysts, the microcystic or honeycomb variety of Worth (1938). These, particularly, exhibit considerable sclerosis of the adjacent bone.

Others have but one bony cavity and so may resemble simple cysts and encapsulated tumours. Differentiation on radiographical grounds is then most difficult. Such ameloblastomas may be composed of one large cyst with a more solid part somewhere in the periphery, or the entire bony cavity may be filled with tumour. Differentiation into solid and cystic forms is, however, not helpful, since most lesions have histologically detectable cysts and the number and size of the cysts seem to be related to age.

Differential radiographic diagnosis mainly involves the consideration of dentigerous and residual apical periodontal cysts, primordial cysts, fibromyxomas, and giant-cell granulomas. As has been said, unilocular lesions are difficult to differentiate. Some stress resorption of the roots of adjacent teeth, but while ameloblastomas tend to induce such resorption so do about one-third of sizeable simple cysts. Primordial cysts may be multilocular and the individual cysts are often of different size, but there are generally fewer locules than is the case with multilocular ameloblastomas. Sclerosis is not seen about the periphery of primordial cysts.

Both fibromyxomas and giant-cell granulomas create a single cavity with ridged walls and incomplete septa. The ridges and septa form straighter images than the walls of cysts and the periphery is lobulated but without the daughter cysts of the ameloblastoma. The fibromyxoma tends to produce a well-defined polyarcuate periphery and the giant-cell granuloma a less well-defined periphery. Resorption of tooth roots is common in relation to a giant-cell lesion.

Clinical Appearances.—The most frequent mode of presentation is an enlargement of the mandible. Multilocular examples may produce a knobbly enlargement and there is a tendency for the transverse diameter to be greater in proportion to the length than with simple cysts. Larger examples will produce a pale pink tumour mass with a granular surface, which bulges into the mouth. If it ulcerates the ulcer is dusky red and fleshy while the cut surface varies from pink to creamy white with sectioned cystic cavities.

Biopsy and Histology.—A biopsy must always be made to establish the diagnosis. Enough has been said about some of the difficulties which can arise in some cases and the opinion of a pathologist with experience of these lesions should be sought. In taking the specimen for histological examination the same rules as apply to the biopsy of malignant lesions should be followed. Representative samples from the more solid and non-ulcerated parts should be chosen if possible. Where an intra-bony lesion must be opened it should be approached by the shortest route, preferably through attached mucoperiosteum and through a wound which can be excised in toto should the subsequent diagnosis suggest that this is advisable. In particular, the wound must not widely open up tissue planes into which fragments of tissue or cyst fluid can escape. All surrounding tissues are copiously irrigated and aspirated dry with a clean sucker before the wound is closed.

Most ameloblastomas are composed of interlacing sheets and strands of epithelial cells surrounded by a fibrous stroma. Columnar cells showing reversal of polarity line the periphery of the strands and in the thicker parts the cells are joined only by the intercellular bridges so as to form a stellate reticulum-like arrangement. Where the network arrangement of tumour cell strands is predominant the appearance is described as 'plexiform' and where the cell masses are larger with a prominent stellate central mass of cells the pattern is described as 'follicular'. In the thicker masses squamous cell clumps may form, a few of which exhibit keratinization, parakeratinization, and ghostcell degeneration. In some otherwise typical neoplasms granular cells are to be found and a muco-epidermoid variant has been described by Hodson (1957). A few have a very vascular stroma and are described as haemangio-ameloblastomas. Both epithelium-lined and stromal cysts are formed.

Treatment.—In the past attempts have been made to approach the excision in a conservative manner. While in some cases this policy has been justified, it has resulted in far too high a recurrence rate for a neoplasm of this character. When recurrence does occur the neoplasm may remain undetected for many years, particularly if it is sited in the soft tissue planes. Incisions into the tumour and fragmentation of the mass during the operation predispose to seeding in the adjacent tissue planes. A proportion of recurrences are therefore inaccessible to further surgery and, after a protracted period of many years of increasing disability, result in death from intracranial extension, respiratory obstruction, or in cases where dissemination into the lungs has occurred, respiratory insufficiency.

Kramer (1963) provides the key to correct treatment. He has shown that the ameloblastoma can readily penetrate medullary spaces, but invades cortical bone with difficulty. It can also invade subperiosteal new bone. Thus, the tumour should be removed with a margin of approximately 1 cm. of cancellous bone where the periphery is in cancellous bone. Where original cortex survives, a subperiosteal excision is permissible;

but where the original cortex has been penetrated an extra-periosteal excision is necessary and where little or no bone remains over the tumour an adequate margin of soft tissues should be included.

In some patients a satisfactory removal will involve a partial thickness excision, in others a complete segment of jaw must be taken. If a high standard of repair is aimed at, few functional or cosmetic deficits should result. For the rare maxillary cases resection of the appropriate amount of maxilla is necessary. Since the periosteum contains large tumours within it for a considerable period of time, a successful *en bloc* removal may be possible, even where the lesion bulges into the pterygoid space, provided that the Crockett (1963) operation is employed. The lesion is radio-resistant and attempts to treat it by irradiation have produced some disastrous results. Follow-up should be for a minimum of 20 years, because the majority of recurrences do not manifest themselves until 10–15 years after surgery. Indeed, recurrences as late as 25 years after treatment are not unknown. If there is to be a hope of further successful treatment, recurrence must be detected early.

The Adeno-ameloblastoma.—The adeno-ameloblastoma is a benign encapsulated lesion which arises from odontogenic epithelium. Usually it has a central cavity and forms a thick-walled cyst, although occasional solid ones have been described. A dentigerous relationship to an anterior tooth is commonly observed. Most patients are less than 26 years of age, but examples in older age-groups are reported from time to time.

The lesion may be mistaken for a dentigerous cyst unless the calcified bodies in the lining are noted in the radiograph (*Fig.* 14). These form a layer of radio-dense spicules, at a distance internal to the margin of the

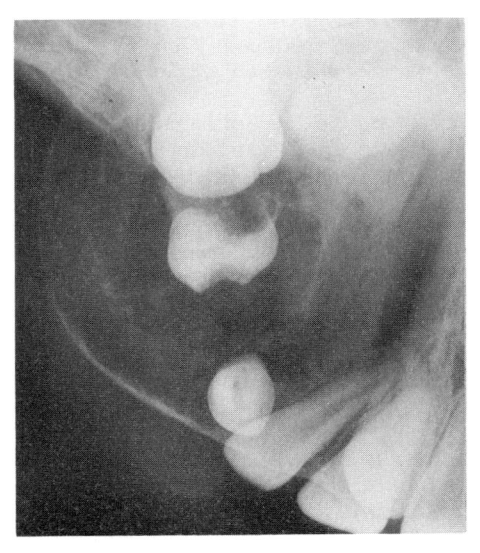

Fig. 14.—A lateral true occlusal radiograph of an adeno-ameloblastoma showing the calcified spicules distributed parallel to the periphery of the bony cavity.

bony cavity. This distance is uniform and represents the cyst capsule. In other cases the correct diagnosis may be suspected for the first time when an unusually thick cyst lining is found, perhaps with an eccentrically placed cavity. Approximately 2 cases have been described in females to every 1 in males.

Histology.—Great whorled masses of polyhedral epithelial cells accumulate and push into the capsule. A delicate vascular connective tissue penetrates between the masses. The epithelial cells separate to form a stellate reticulum. Within the masses columnar cells appear which surround small cystic spaces or form double rows of cells with an interval between. Some double rows are bent into an ox-bow shape. These cells show reversal of polarity characteristic of ameloblastomas and an eosinophilic material associated with reticulin fibres is formed within the lumen of the rings. Calcified globules, both single and in clumps, form in the epithelial masses and are the spicules seen in radiographs.

Treatment.—Simple enucleation is all that is required for this lesion which must not be confused with the ameloblastoma proper.

The Calcifying Odontogenic Epithelium Tumour (Pindborg Tumour).—Now that this neoplasm is more widely known, more frequent case reports are appearing, but it still remains a rare lesion. It arises usually from the reduced enamel epithelium of an unerupted tooth. The first indication of its presence, therefore, is a widening of the follicular space and a failure of the involved tooth to erupt. Where an unerupted tooth is not involved, it probably arises from remnants of the tooth band. While there is still a preponderance of examples from the mandible, the percentage of maxillary cases has increased.

Initially a circumscribed unilocular lesion is formed and at this stage enucleation is adequate treatment. Later a lobulated, or multilocular radiographic appearance is produced. Densely calcified spicules form clusters in the older parts of the lesion while the periphery is radiolucent. (*Fig.* 15.)

Histology.—Sheets of polyhedral epithelial cells are seen which invade the adjacent medullary bone and soft tissues. There is the usual fibrous stroma. In the older parts of the tumour eosinophilic globules appear and increase in size. They are concentrically laminated and soon become calcified. Adjacent globules fuse into a single mass and more material is added peripherally. The uncalcified material stains in a similar manner to ameloid (Ranløv and Pindborg, 1966), but is clearly related to the epithelial cells. It resembles globules found in relation to odontogenic epithelium in other locations and may be an aprismatic form of enamel (Seward and Duckworth, 1967a, b).

Treatment.—Enucleation is adequate for clearly circumscribed early lesions, but excision with a margin is required for advanced, multilocular lesions and those which exhibit invasive tendencies.

Ameloblastic Fibroma.—This comparatively uncommon odontogenic tumour is found during the first three decades of life. It is slowly growing and usually forms a unilocular cavity of simple outline, but may form a lobulated cavity with incomplete septa and so resemble the myxofibroma.

Histological examination reveals an encapsulated, dense, fibroma-like lesion in which strands and sheets of epithelial cells ramify. These are two

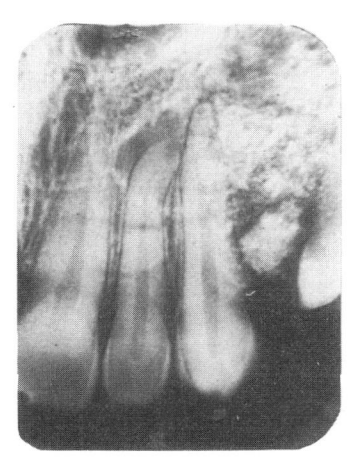

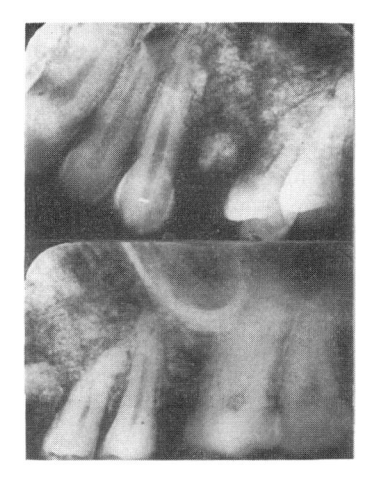

Fig. 15.—The clumped calcified spicules of high radiographic density and the irregular radiolucent margin of a calcifying odontogenic epithelium tumour.

cells thick for the most part and of a cuboidal or columnar shape. Terminal 'buds' may form on some of the strands where the cells increase in thickness and the central ones take on a stellate appearance. A cell-free zone occurs in the connective tissue adjacent to the epithelium.

Enucleation is adequate treatment, provided that care is taken to remove any outpouching of tumour if the periphery is irregular in shape.

Ameloblastic Fibrosarcoma.—The ameloblastic fibrosarcoma is a very rare odontogenic tumour composed of islands and strands of odontogenic epithelium in a cell-rich mesodermal stroma, the cells of which exhibit the histological features of a fibrosarcoma. The epithelium is indistinguishable from that in ameloblastic fibroma or ameloblastoma and it is probably a malignant variety of the ameloblastic fibroma. Most recorded cases have arisen in the mandible and the tumour is characterized by rapid growth and pain. An important diagnostic feature is that the pain has preceded the swelling in many instances and this has led to tooth extraction after which the tumour has extruded from the socket. Though the disease extends locally, despite surgical excision there are no recorded cases of the tumour metastasizing. This rare neoplasm is similar in histological appearance to the ameloblastic fibroma except that the fibrous tissue component is represented by a fibrosarcoma. The way in which this neoplasm should be fitted into the present classification is not clear If the basic neoplastic process is represented by the odontogenic epithelium and the fibromatous element the result of an inductive influence of the epithelium then it is not easy to see why it should undergo a malignant transformation. Alternative concepts are that the sarcoma is the definitive neoplasm, or that both elements are neoplastic. If the lesion is basically a fibrosarcoma arising within the alveolar process then it is conceivable that its presence could stimulate rests of odontogenic epithelium to proliferate. But should they proliferate to the degree seen in this particular neoplasm? If both elements are neoplastic then this is a 'mixed' tumour; a state of affairs which is contrary to the general philosophy of the classification. Another concept is that this is a collision neoplasm between two separate neoplasms. If this is so what happens to the stroma in which the odontogenic epithelium was proliferating? The treatment is radical surgery or radiotherapy depending on the particular case.

Dentinoma.—Two types of dentinoma are recognized by Gorlin, Chaudhry, and Pindborg (1961). The first resembles the ameloblastic fibroma save that odontoblasts are induced at the periphery of some of the sheets of epithelium. In some instances a stratum-intermedium-like layer is seen in the thicker bud-like parts of the epithelial cords. A tubule-free dentine or dentinoid is laid down by the odontoblast.

The second or mature type of dentinoma is composed of a laminated mass of dentinoid in parts of which some irregular dentinal tubules and enclosed odontoblasts may be found. The mass is usually opposed to the crown of an unerupted tooth in a similar fashion to certain complex odontomes. It is separated from the enamel of the tooth by the reduced enamel epithelium. Since odontoblasts cannot be formed without the inductive influence of epithelium, it is postulated that irregular, burrowing, cords of odontogenic epithelium initiated the dentinogenesis, perhaps originating from the external enamel epithelium of the enamel organ or from the adjacent tooth band. As the masses of dentine were deposited the epithelium was separated from any source of nutrition and died out. The mass of dentine therefore strangled the epithelium and stopped its proliferation in a manner resembling that seen in the complex odontome. Indeed, this type of dentinoma could be looked upon as a complex odontome in which the ameloblasts underwent sufficient histodifferentiation to induce the formation of odontoblasts, but not sufficient to lay down enamel or enameloid.

Both forms of dentinoma are very rare, are benign, and are treated by enucleation.

Calcifying Odontogenic Cyst.—Gorlin, Pindborg, Clausen, and Vickers (1962) and Gold (1963) independently drew attention to this entity. Certain odontogenic cysts have an epithelium forming the lining which has a basal layer of cuboidal or columnar cells. Some of the taller columnar cells exhibit reversal of nuclear polarity. In parts the epithelium increases markedly in thickness and undergoes the ghost cell type of degeneration. The ghost cells may subsequently calcify. Sometimes the ghost cell change can involve the full thickness of part of the epithelial lining. Where this happens the mass may be shed to leave an ulcerated surface. Should the degenerate mass remain in contact with the underlying connective tissue, it is invaded by granulation tissue and giant cells are formed which engulf the ghost cells. At other sites where the ghost cells come into contact with the connective tissue capsule, odontoblasts are induced and either an atubular dentinoid or tubular dentine is laid down.

Where no ghost cell change has occurred, the epithelium closely resembles that lining primordial cysts. The calcifying odontogenic cyst may therefore be related to the keratocysts since they can occur without a relationship to a formed tooth, or with a dentigerous or extra-follicular relationship to the crown of a tooth. Some may arise near the surface of the jaw so that only part of their circumference involves the bone or they may be found entirely in the soft tissues.

Again, like the primordial cyst some examples show some penetration of strands of epithelium into the capsule of the cyst, but this is comparatively uncommon. Occasional specimens, like that described by Duckworth and Seward (1965), are multilocular with some of the cysts having a very thick wall with deep penetration of large amounts of odontogenic epithelium into the fibrous capsule. The central cells in follicular expansions of these epithelial cords undergo both the ghost cell degeneration and calcification. Some of the cords of epithelium have a ring of early inductive changes in the adjacent connective tissue such as is seen in the ameloblastic fibroma. Both an atubular dentinoid and tubular dentine are induced. Enamel is not formed. It is such behaviour which can earn the calcifying odontogenic cyst a place in a classification of odontogenic tumours. A further matter of interest is the reports of two cases (Lurie, 1961; Duckworth and Seward, 1965) in which melanocytes were to be found in the tumours.

These lesions, like the adeno-ameloblastoma, should be suspected if dense calcified flecks or masses are detected forming an inner ring parallel with the inner surface of a bone cavity. A partially or completely extrabony lesion showing such calcifications is almost diagnostic. Simple enucleation cures.

Ameloblastic Odontome.—In 1952 Cahn and Blum postulated that soft odontomes which were left undisturbed might subsequently calcify to become complex odontomes. It is a fact that tumours can be found in young people which are largely composed of soft tissues and which pursue this course, but these would now be recognized as immature complex composite odontomes. The ameloblastic odontome can be clearly separated from these lesions (Seward and Duckworth, 1967a).

It is the diversity of histological and morphological differentiation of the dental tissues which characterizes the ameloblastic odontome. In places, normal tooth follicles and teeth of varying size and form are produced. Elsewhere tubular dentine and prismatic enamel are to be found in featureless masses characteristic of the complex odontome. Between these more highly differentiated tissues, masses of polyhedral epithelial cells are seen in a fibrous tissue stroma. Some parts of these develop the ring-like structures and swirled cell masses seen in the adeno-ameloblastoma. Elsewhere calcified globules appear in relation to the epithelial cells and are quickly fused into masses by further material which is formed in layers on their surfaces. Dentinoid or dentine with scanty tubules appears in large quantities near the original calcified material, which seems to be a form of enamel. The dentine increases in amount until it traps the epithelial cells which subsequently die.

In other sections, the proliferating epithelium has a resemblance to that seen in the plexiform and follicular types of ameloblastoma, and both epithelium-lined and stromal cysts may develop. All these are to be found within the mass irrespective of the patient's age and the size of the lesion and this again is of diagnostic importance.

Generally these tumours are encapsulated and can be enucleated, but in one or two cases a recurrence has been recorded. While the recurrences could be due to a failure to remove a pocket of tumour, it may be that in some examples the ameloblastic element is more aggressive and local invasion occurs.

On clinical grounds the ameloblastic odontome should be suspected where an otherwise radiolucent tumour contains large masses of calcified tooth substance. The appearance is particularly suggestive of this diagnosis if the patient is over 25 years of age—beyond the stage where an immature complex odontome might be found. (*Fig.* 16.)

Complex Odontome.—The complex odontome in its mature form is a conglomerate mass of dental tissues. The dentine is tubular dentine, however, and the enamel, prismatic enamel. Properly organized dental pulps and cementum are also formed. While by definition the mass does not in any way resemble a recognizable tooth morphologically, nevertheless the tissues may show some order. Regular plates of dentine and enamel are laid down and these may be arranged in a definite pattern. Common shapes are rectangular blocks of parallel plates, or a sphere of radially disposed plates.

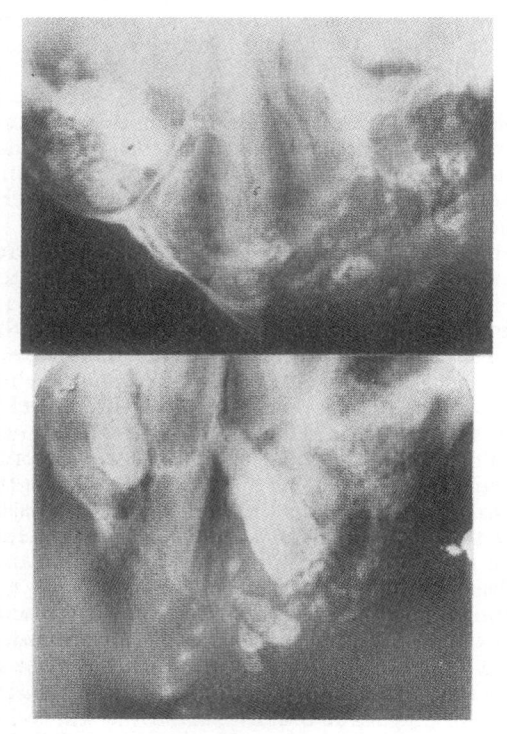

Fig. 16.—Radiographs of an ameloblastic odontome. Denticles, calcified masses, and calcified spicules lie in a mass of soft tissue. The bony cavity is well defined.

In its immature stage the lesion can be largely radiolucent and composed of a loose connective tissue penetrated by strands and sheets of odontogenic epithelium 2–3 cells thick and resembling those seen in the ameloblastic fibroma. However, when a follicular expansion is formed the epithelium rapidly differentiates into all the characteristic elements of an enamel organ and the normal stages of induction and odontogenesis occur. All that is lacking is a proper spatial arrangement such that a recognizable tooth is formed.

Some examples may continue to proliferate until past the normal time of tooth development, but all have ceased to grow by the early twenties. As the complex odontome ceases to grow, some consider it to be a hamartoma rather than a benign neoplasm. Others favour the neoplastic concept pointing out that the epithelium does not cease to proliferate of its own volition. It induces changes in the surrounding connective tissue so that calcified tissue is formed which traps the epithelium and prevents its further proliferation.

The dense laminated masses of the mature complex odontome are quite characteristic and easily recognized in radiographs. (*Fig.* 17.) Not infrequently they form over the crown of a developing tooth so that its eruption is prevented. Others appear to replace a tooth which is missing from the arch, and yet others occur in those parts of the jaw favoured by supernumeraries.

Their removal may present mechanical difficulties if they are large and if adjacent teeth are to be preserved, but there are no other problems with the mature tumour.

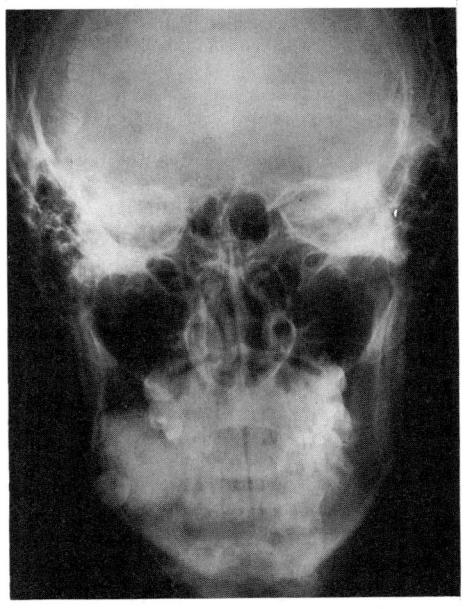

Fig. 17.—Postero-anterior radiograph showing a complex composite odontome.

If immature examples are removed, a limited recurrence can occur if part is overlooked, but as maturation and calcification take place its growth ceases and no great harm results.

Compound Odontome.—The compound odontome is somewhat similar to the complex odontome except that a higher degree of morphological differentiation is achieved and a number of denticles is formed. Surprisingly, large numbers may be found and it is not unusual to underestimate the number present from the radiograph. They vary greatly both in number and shape.

Careful removal of the denticles is in order, particularly if they are in a position to impede the eruption of a tooth of the normal series or to become infected. The usual precautions with regard to localization of the teeth and preservation of the adjacent normal teeth should be observed as in the removal of single supernumeraries.

THE MESODERMAL ODONTOGENIC TUMOURS

The Odontogenic Myxoma or Fibromyxoma.—

Aetiology.—If myxomatous change in other lesions such as chondromas, osteogenic fibromas, fibrous dysplasia, etc., is excluded there are virtually no records of fibromyxomas to be found at sites outside the jaws (Dahlin, 1957). Thus, while there is no positive evidence that these are odontogenic tumours some feel that this fact is sufficient to justify their place in the classification (Gorlin, Chaudhry, and Pindborg, 1961).

Histologically the tumour is composed of stellate cells with long processes which form a loose meshwork. A mucoid intercellular substance fills the spaces between the cells. Occasional strands of odontogenic epithelium may be found, but since these tumours occur in the jaws this may be a chance relationship. Similarly, too much cannot be made of the involvement of unerupted teeth, particularly wisdom teeth, since they often develop at a time when the 3rd molars are unerupted. Their growth is slow so that the most common age of presentation is the second and third decade.

It has been suggested that fibromyxoma of the jaws is an innocent tumour (Thoma and Goldman, 1947; Shear, 1959) and certainly it has a deceptively benign histological appearance, but its clinical behaviour is more suggestive of malignancy and its invasive nature has been recognized by Wawro and Reed (1950), Hayward (1955), Shafer and others (1963), and Killey and Kay (1964).

Clinical Features.—Fibromyxoma of the jaws is a rare tumour and it usually presents as a painless swelling of the bone or as an incidental radiological finding. It is alleged to arise more commonly in the second and third decades of life and to have a predilection for the posterior areas of the upper and lower jaws. It has a strong tendency to recur following operations such as local curettage and enucleation, but does not metastasize.

Radiological Features.—There are no diagnostic radiological features of the condition, but when it appears to be multilocular the straight septa divide the radiolucent image into square, rectangular, or triangular spaces, with a central portion traversed by fine, gracile trabeculations. This appearance has been likened by Sonesson (1950) to that of the strings of a tennis racket. As the tumour expands, the outer cortical plate first becomes a thin shell and finally it may be perforated.

Appearance at Operation.—The appearance of the fibromyxoma at operation is that of an ivory white tumour, which is firm in consistency with a smooth, lobulated, shiny surface. There is no evidence of encapsulation and prolongations of the tumour invade the surrounding bone and make dissection of the mass more or less impossible.

Differential Diagnosis.—Both clinical and radiological methods of examination sometimes fail to differentiate the fibromyxoma from such tumours as bone cysts, giant-cell granuloma, ameloblastoma, and fibrous dysplasia, and the only certain method of diagnosing the condition is by histological examination of the tissue.

Treatment.—In view of the fact that the behaviour of fibromyxoma is unpredictable and that it has a high recurrence rate even after local resection, it would seem prudent to avoid such treatment as local curettage or enucleation. Where the tumour is comparatively small and localized, a local resection of the tumour together with about 1 cm. of the normal surrounding bone may be carried out, after which a regular and careful follow-up should be instituted.

For the larger tumour a resection of the jaw is probably the only practical solution. There is no precise evidence concerning the response of fibromyxoma to radiotherapy. Shafer and others (1963) considered that the tumour was not radiosensitive, but Ackerman and Spjut (1963) suggested that fibromyxoma does, in fact, react to radiotherapy. However, Prossor (1963) feels that the prognosis can be improved by radiotherapy provided that it is carried out in conjunction with a wide surgical excision of the tumour, and this would appear to be the treatment of choice.

Cementifying Fibroma.—This condition is also known as multiple cementoma and periapical fibrous dysplasia. Although it was first recognized by Brophy in 1915 and described in detail by Stafne (1933, 1934, and 1943), by Ennis (1947), and by many others, knowledge of the condition still does not seem to be widespread. In its most common form periapical areas of bone destruction appear, presumably as a result of proliferation of the periodontal membrane. Any teeth may be involved, but anterior teeth are affected more than posterior and particularly the lower incisors.

After a while calcified spicules can be seen in radiographs in the centre of the radiolucencies. Histologically at this stage, the calcified tissues may have characteristics similar either to cementum or to woven bone. During these stages the lesions may be mistaken for inflammatory periapical lesions. In time the calcified masses increase and a radio-opaque mass is formed: either a knob of cementum attached to the root, a mass of cementum separated from the root by a reformed periodontal membrane, or even new trabeculae of bone so that only a slight alteration in bone pattern is to be seen. Obviously both difficulty in extraction of an involved tooth and infection of the socket are hazards associated with this condition.

Occasionally during the earlier stages one of these lesions will increase sufficiently in size to produce a deforming lump which requires surgical treatment.

The gigantic or gigantiform type of cementoma may be seen in two forms. In one form a large, relatively radiolucent lesion forms in which irregular masses of cementum are laid down. The condition is often mistaken for Paget's disease, but it should be noted that the cortex of the jaw remains normal: a state of affairs not found in Paget's disease. Following an extraction, infection sometimes supervenes, adding to the difficulties of reaching a correct diagnosis.

In the second form, large dense masses of cementum are to be found in the molar regions in each quadrant. There is a thin capsule about each mass separating it from the bone. When molar extractions are performed there is a considerable risk of the tumour becoming infected. If this happens, the whole lump must be removed. This can be a formidable undertaking since the knobbly surface indents the cortex of the jaw to such a degree that, in the mandible, undercut cavities are formed in the cortex. Releasing the mass by cutting away the bone may entail the removal of a considerable amount of mandibular bone at that site. Cutting up the mass itself is most difficult as it is immensely hard. In some cases resection of a length of jaw may be necessary. Typical cementoma lesions about the apices of the incisors may help in differentiating these masses from complex odontomes. Negroes seem particularly afflicted with the gigantiform cementoma.

Odontomes

As has been explained in the section on odontogenic tumours, the term 'odontome' has been variously applied. Minor variations in size and form are not now often referred to as odontomes and the hamartomas and neoplasms of dental tissues are usually grouped under the heading of odontogenic tumours. Only the more aberrant tooth forms, but ones in which prismatic enamel, tubular dentine, pulp, and cementum are formed and in which the structure reaches a finite size, are included under this heading. In this discussion the emphasis will be on points of surgical interest.

Gemination and Dichotomy.—In gemination two tooth elements which are separate at their coronal end subsequently become fused. Thus, there is at least a groove, or notch, marking the demarcation between the two occlusal surfaces or incisal edges. In some examples two separate crowns are supported on conjoined roots. Hitchin and Morris (1960) prefer the term 'connate' for these malformations and based their understanding of their formation on observations made on a strain of dogs in which connate incisors are common. They have shown that in these dogs stellate reticulum from adjacent enamel organs proliferates into the part of the tooth band which joins them so that one large enamel organ is formed.

Dichotomy is reduplication by division. A tooth germ splits into two parts during odontogenesis so that a single crown is supported on reduplicate roots. Crudely put: in gemination there are two crowns on one root and in dichotomy one crown on two roots. However, with dichotomy the crown of the tooth is often excessively large and there is no clear evidence that a different mechanism is involved from that producing the connate tooth.

The surgical importance of these forms is the mechanical difficulties which they may pose if their extraction is required. Also in some instances of gemination a conical tooth form is fused to a crown of normal shape.

When such a tooth is partially erupted it may appear that a supernumerary tooth is adjacent to a tooth of the normal series and displacing it. Should the conical element be palatal or labial to the part of normal shape the site of union may be difficult to demonstrate radiographically. Only when an attempt is made to extract the supernumerary may the true state of affairs be discovered.

Such an arrangement is also bad from a periodontal point of view as well as an aesthetic or orthodontic one. Of course, if the tooth can be root-filled an attempt can be made to remove the extra part surgically, sealing the opening into the pulp cavity of the parent part with amalgam and replacing the flap tight against the tooth.

Invaginated Odontomes.—Because the area of attachment of the invagination to the tooth bud is small, the invagination probably results from the proliferation of comparatively few ameloblasts in the case of coronal invagination or epithelial cells of Hertwig's sheath in the case of a radicular one. Again, proliferation is probably the mechanism by which the invagination is formed because the large size achieved by some invaginations would be impossible by a mechanism of local growth arrest with continued growth of the rest of the epithelial component of the tooth germ around it.

The invagination may be small as in the case of the *cingulum invagination*, so frequently seen in upper lateral incisors and less commonly in other upper anterior teeth. If it is rather larger the tooth is deformed, or conical, but has a normal apex and a *dens in dente* is formed. These again are not uncommon in the upper incisor region, especially among supernumerary teeth. Some have a slit-like opening at the surface and produce an invagination to one side of a tooth which has a comparatively normal crown.

Where the invagination is larger still, it passes through the 'apex' and the pulp cavity forms a circular slit around the invagination. The external form of the tooth is altered and enlarged so that the lesion is described as a *dilated odontome*. Probably all invaginations have imperfect enamel and dentine at the bottom. The deeper varieties have only grossly deficient dentine or even an aperture at the fundus.

Invaginations in posterior teeth are most uncommon. Some coronal ones have a sizeable surface opening. Certain examples originate from Hertwig's sheath and involve only the root of the tooth and these are largely to be found in molar teeth. Multiple invaginations can occur so that the specimen superficially resembles a complex odontome. Invaginated odontomes are of importance mainly because organisms can penetrate the bottom of the invagination and either destroy the pulp of a *dens in dente* or cause a periapical infection directly in a dilated odontome. Root-canal treatment is always difficult and in some cases impossible so their extraction is usually required once infection has supervened. Dilated odontomes and root invaginations then present a problem because of their shape and must be removed by open surgery.

Compound and Complex Odontomes.—These odontomes have been discussed in the section on odontogenic tumours.

The Evaginated Odontome.—Evaginated, 'Leong's' or 'Tratman's' odontomes are small tubercles or extra cusps to be found on the occlusal surface of posterior teeth, palatally in the cingulum region of canines, and rarely on the palatal aspects of upper incisors (Leigh, 1925; Tratman, 1950; Oehlers, 1956).

On posterior teeth they are to be found in or close to the fissures and therefore in the centre of the crown. Premolar teeth are most often affected and mongoloid peoples, such as Chinese, Malays, and Eskimos, are almost exclusively the subjects of these anomalies.

The tubercle is covered by enamel and under a thin layer of dentine has a prolongation of the pulp. They can be taller than the adjacent cusps and are frequently worn away or fractured off. Caries of the fissure rapidly involves the pulp and cavity preparation is hazardous. Thus in many cases the pulps become infected, hence the oral surgical significance of this condition.

REFERENCES

ACKERMAN, L. V., and SPJUT, H. J. (1963), *Tumours of Bone and Cartilage*. Section 2—Fascicle 4. Armed Forces Institute of Pathology.

AKINOSI, J. O., and WILLIAMS, A. O. (1968), 'Adamantinoma in Ibadan, Nigeria', *W. Afr. med. J.*, **17**, 45.

BROPHY, T. W. (1915), *Oral Surgery: A Treatise on the Diseases, Injuries, and Malformations of the Mouth and Associated Parts*. Philadelphia: Blakistons.

CAHN, L. R., and BLUM, T. (1952), 'Ameloblastic Odontoma: Case Report critically analysed', *J. oral Surg.*, **10**, 169.

CROCKETT, D. J. (1963), 'Surgical Approach to the Back of the Maxilla', *Br. J. Surg.*, **50**, 819.

DAHLIN, D. C. (1957), *Bone Tumors: General Aspects and an Analysis of 2,276 Cases*. Springfield, Ill.: Thomas.

DUCKWORTH, R., and SEWARD, G. R. (1965), 'A Melanotic Ameloblastic Odontome', *Oral Surg.*, **19**, 73.

ENNIS, LeR. M. (1947), *Dental Roentgenology*, p. 368. London: Kimpton.

GOLD, L. (1963), 'The Keratinizing and Calcifying Odontogenic Cyst', *Oral Surg.*, **16**, 1414.

GORLIN, J. R., CHAUDHRY, A. P., and PINDBORG, J. J. (1961), 'Odontogenic Tumours', *Cancer, N.Y.*, **14**, 73.

— — PINDBORG, J. J., CLAUSEN, F., and VICKERS, R. A. (1962), 'The Calcifying Odontogenic Cyst: A Possible Analogue of the Cutaneous Calcifying Epithelioma of Malherbe', *Oral Surg.*, **15**, 1235.

HAYWARD, J. R. (1955), 'Odontogenic Myxofibroma of the Mandible', *J. oral Surg. Anesth. Hosp. dent. Serv.*, **13**, 149.

HITCHIN, A. D., and MORRIS, I. (1960), 'The Inheritance of Connate Incisors in the Dog', *J. dent. Res.*, **39**, 1101.

HODSON, J. J. (1957), 'Observations on Origin and Nature of Adamantinoma with Special Preference to Certain Muco-epidermoid Variations', *Br. J. plast. Surg.*, **10**, 38,

KILLEY, H. C., and KAY, L. W. (1964), 'Fibromyxomata of the Jaws', *Br. J. oral Surg.*, **2**, 124.

KRAMER, I. R. H. (1963), 'Ameloblastoma: A Clinicopathological Appraisal', *Ibid.*, **1**, 13.

LEIGH, R. W. (1925), 'Dental Pathology of the Eskimoes', *Dent. Cosmos*, **67**, 884.

LURIE, H. I. (1961), 'Congenital Melanocarcinoma, Melanotic Adamantinoma, Retinal Anlage Tumour, Progonoma and Pigmented Epulis of Infancy: Summary and Review of the Literature and Report of the First Case in an Adult', *Cancer*, **14**, 1090–1108.

OEHLERS, F. A. (1956), ' Tuberculated Premolar ', *Dent. Practnr dent. Rec.*, **6**, 144.

PINDBORG, J. J., and CLAUSEN, F. (1958), 'Classification of Odontogenic Tumours', *Acta odont. scand.*, **16**, 291.

POTDAR, G. G. (1969), 'Ameloblastoma of the Jaws as seen in Bombay, India', *Oral Surg.*, **28**, 297.

PROSSOR, T. M. (1963), personal communication.

RANLØV, P., and PINDBORG, J. J. (1966), 'The Amyloid Nature of the Homogeneous Substance in the Calcifying Epithelial Odontogenic Tumour', *Acta path. microbiol. scand.*, **68,** 169.

SEWARD, G. R., and DUCKWORTH, R. (1967a), 'A Review of the Pathology of the Calcifying Odontogenic Cysts and Tumours', *Dent. Practnr dent. Rec.*, **18,** 83.

— — — — (1967b), 'A Study of the Pathological Calcified Materials in the Calcifying Odontogenic Cysts and Tumours', *Ibid.*, **18,** 125.

SHAFER, W. G., HINE, M. K., and LEVY, B. M. (1963), *A Textbook of Oral Pathology*, 2nd ed. Philadelphia: Saunders.

SHEAR, M. (1959), 'Central Myxofibroma of the Mandible', *J. dent. Ass. S. Afr.*, **14,** 424.

SONESSON, A. (1950), 'Odontogenic Cysts and Cystic Tumours of Jaws: Roentgendiagnostic and Patho-anatomic Study', *Acta radiol.*, Suppl. **81,** 36.

STAFNE, E. C. (1933), 'Cementoma: Study of 35 Cases', *Dental Survey*, **9,** 27.

— — (1934), 'Periapical Osteofibrosis with Formation of Cementoma', *J. Am. dent. Ass.*, **21,** 1822.

— — (1943), 'Periapical Fibroma; Roentgenologic Observations', *Ibid.*, **30,** 688.

THOMA, K. H., and GOLDMAN, H. M. (1947), 'Central Myxoma of the Jaw', *Am. J. Orthod.*, **33,** 532.

TRATMAN, E. K. (1950), 'Indo-European Racial Stock with the Mongoloid Racial Stock', *Dent. Rec.*, **70,** 63.

WAWRO, N. W., and REED, J. (1950), 'Fibromyxoma of the Mandible: Report of 2 Cases', *Ann. Surg.*, **132,** 1138.

WORTH, H. M. (1938), 'Radiological Findings in some Less Common Jaw Affections', *Proc. R. Soc. Med.*, **32,** 331.

Chapter XI
HISTIOCYTOSIS 'X' AND MALIGNANT GRANULOMA

Histiocytosis 'X'

'Histiocytosis "X" ' is a term suggested by Lichenstein (1953) to describe a disease of unknown aetiology which is characterized by enlarging solitary or multiple destructive aggregations of proliferating histiocytes. The disease is not hereditary and there is no racial predilection. Males tend to be affected more often than females and Blevins and others (1959), who reviewed a series of 27 cases which involved the oral tissues, found that 20 males were affected. There are three clinically distinct variations of the disease, but all three syndromes are believed to be manifestations of the same pathological process. All three types of histiocytosis 'X' are rare, and in the first instance are characterized by a proliferation of histiocytes with secondary storage of cholesterol in them and finally by fibrosis and scarring. The disease may be localized or generalized and the generalized form of the condition is chronic or acute.

Localized Histiocytosis 'X'.—In the localized variety of the disease there is a lesion, often single, known as an 'eosinophilic granuloma' which is confined to the skeleton, usually the skull, vertebrae, pelvis, or extremities. Bone lesions of this type develop rapidly and are also found in the jaws, especially in the mandible. Jaw lesions are, however, rare. Blevins and others (1959) studied 600 cases at the Mayo Clinic and found oral involvement in only 27 cases. Occasionally there may be more than one bone involved and Schwartz (1965) reported a bilateral mandibular lesion. During the histiocytosis proliferation phase there is an accumulation of leucocytes. The condition tends to appear in young children mostly in the 4–6 year age-group. It presents as a local tumour of bone and the overlying soft tissues are often red, painful, and swollen. When it occurs in the jaws the radiograph shows an expansion of the bone surrounding an irregular radiolucent lesion.

In children two clinical types of eosinophil granuloma are seen and in some cases both varieties may affect the same child, but at different times. One appears to start in the cancellous bone and produces a highly irregular bony cavity. Radiographically the jaw has a worm-eaten appearance with enlargement due to the destruction of the original cortex and deposition of subperiosteal new bone.

The other type affects the gingival margin to produce a red or pink granulation tissue. The teeth become loose and the radiograph reveals severe destruction of the alveolar bone. Eventually the teeth are denuded of bone and 'float' in the lesional tissue. Radiographically they appear to be suspended in space.

In the adult; deep, foul, chronic periodontal pockets are found with considerable alveolar bone destruction. These may increase to such a size that almost all the medullary bone is involved. Once secondary infection has supervened chronic osteomyelitis is simulated. In other instances spherical cavities not unlike those of residual or periodontal cysts are seen in the radiographs. When these are opened granulation tissue or a mixture of granulation tissue and infected necrotic material is found.

Both curettage and a low therapeutic dose of irradiation will effect a cure but as far as possible irradiation should be avoided in the child because of the effect on growth of the tissues. In the adult the choice depends in part on the extent of the lesion. Occasionally apparently traumatic lesions or a denture granuloma of the sulcus or tongue may resemble eosinophil granuloma. Simple excision cures them and Bhaskar and Lilly (1964) have shown that experimental damage to the tongue in dogs can reproduce these lesions.

Treatment.—Treatment is by excision and curettage. At operation a layer of new bone is found covering an irregular cyst-like cavity containing deep purplish-red soft tissue which tends to bleed vigorously. Following removal of the contents of the cavity, the lesion tends to fill in with new bone. The condition should be kept under review, for in some instances the disease progresses to the chronic or acute variety.

The Chronic Variety.—The chronic variety of the disease is known as 'Hand-Schüller-Christian disease'. This is a chronic disseminated histiocytosis 'X' in which there are multiple skeletal and visceral lesions usually with the classic triad of skull defects, exophthalmos, and diabetes insipidus. The granulomatous lesions, which contain histiocytes, eosinophils, and foam cells, occur in many sites including particularly the lymph-nodes, spleen, liver, brain, and bones. The disease usually begins in the first five years of life but may occasionally occur later in life, even in middle age. Its onset is insidious with skull defects, diabetes insipidus, and exophthalmos, though often only one of this triad of symptoms is present. The diabetes insipidus is due to involvement of the region of the hypophysis at the base of the brain. There is a hepatosplenomegaly and often a maculopapular rash over the face and trunk. The granulomata often affect the jaws and there may be swelling and ulceration of the gums leading possibly to extrusion of the teeth. Scattered tubercle-like lesions may occur in the lungs and there may be bronchopneumonia. Radiographs show punched-out lesions in the bones and spontaneous fractures may occur.

Treatment.—Local radiotherapy to the lesions which are causing symptoms is effective, and remissions have been reported with courses of prednisone 2–4 mg. per kg. body-weight for 6–8 weeks, which is then tapered off over an 8–10 week period (Scott, 1966). The diabetes insipidus requires treatment with pituitary hormone. The disease is relatively benign and protracted, but may carry a mortality-rate of about 13 per cent.

The Acute Form of Histiocytosis 'X'.—The acute form of the disease is known as 'Letterer-Siwe's disease' and it is a diffuse, and rapidly progressive disease. It occurs in early infancy, often before the age of two years, and leads to death within a few weeks. The spleen, liver, lymph-nodes, skin, lungs, and bone-marrow are heavily infiltrated. There is generalized lymphadenopathy, hepatosplenomegaly, anaemia, and a tendency to haemorrhage.

Treatment.—The disease is usually rapidly fatal, but attempts to treat the condition with corticosteroids and ACTH are under evaluation.

Malignant Granuloma and Wegener's Granulomatosis

Malignant granuloma or lethal midline granuloma and Wegener's granulomatosis, according to Mills (1967), are one and the same disease. Where this rare disease is primarily localized to the midline of the palate and nose it is called 'malignant granuloma' while the generalized disease involving changes in the respiratory system (necrotizing granuloma), kidneys (necrotizing glomerulitis), liver, spleen, and skin is termed 'Wegener's granulomatosis'. Only the malignant granuloma is of interest to the oral surgeon, though occasionally oral manifestations occur in the generalized type of the disease. Morgan and O'Neil (1956) reported a case of Wegener's granulomatosis in which oral and cutaneous manifestations were predominant features. Several cases have been recorded in which the presenting sign of the disease was an ulcerative stomatitis or the failure of a socket to heal. More recently Clarke (1964) has described a case of Wegener's granulomatosis in which the patient presented with a single oral ulcer, and Brooke (1969) has mentioned the possibility that granular purplish-red gingival enlargement may be an important and even pathognomic manifestation of the disease. The course of the condition is usually rapid, progressing to death in a few weeks or months.

Malignant Granuloma.—Mills (1958) reviewed 86 cases of malignant granuloma; 55 were male and 31 female. In 67 of these cases the disease began in the nose and in 19 patients it arose in the paranasal sinuses. Mills points out that many had a preceding nasal or paranasal infection; he regards this as a sensitizing phase preparatory to a hypersensitivity reaction. As the disease process extends, there is a progressive destruction of the nose, face, and pharynx.

Aetiology.—Williams (1949) considers that malignant granuloma is due to a dysfunction of the immune mechanisms responsible for granuloma formation. This leads to a vascular allergy and either the Arthus phenomenon occurs in the case of capillaries or periarteritis nodosa if the arterioles are affected. The hyperimmune tissues become necrotic because of obstruction to the blood-supply.

Symptoms.—The symptoms depend on the site involved and usually the nose becomes stuffy and blocked and this leads on to a watery or serosanguineous discharge. This prodromal stage lasts for one or two months, but may persist for several years. Later a swelling develops on the side of the nose or the inner canthus. If secondary infection occurs the face and periorbital tissues are grossly swollen and painful. There may be diplopia and anaesthesia of the cheek. In spite of these symptoms the patient remains healthy, a fact which has been commented upon by several observers. The nasal mucosa is swollen and covered with crusts and on removing them masses of what appears to be simple granulation tissue is revealed. There may be exposure of bone. Ulcerations appear on the septum and conchae and as the condition progresses the hard palate is invaded with large spreading perforating ulcers. Small haemorrhages are frequent and involvement of a large vessel may result in a fatal termination. Cachexia is marked as a result of secondary infection and difficulty in obtaining adequate nutrition, and the patient may die of exhaustion or bronchopneumonia or from meningitis if the meninges are invaded. The course of the disease may last for years, but often it results in death within a year.

Blood Picture in Malignant Granuloma.—There may be a hypochromic microcytic anaemia due to toxic absorption, and in some cases there is an eosinophilia. Walton (1958) reported that 45·9 per cent of his 37 cases had an eosinophilia. However, a noticeable feature of the disease is the poor white-cell response associated with the extensive tissue destruction. Mills reported that the ESR was helpful in the diagnosis of malignant granuloma and was useful in monitoring the activity and progress of the disease. The very high ESR estimations are used as evidence for classifying these conditions as collagen disorders. There is a hypergammaglobulinaemia.

Urinary Changes.—There are no urinary changes in malignant granuloma, but urinalysis is valuable to exclude kidney involvement.

Bacteriology.—No specific organism has been found in either malignant granuloma or Wegener's granulomatosis.

Histology.—In the words of Stewart (1933) the main histological features of malignant granuloma are 'a chronic inflammatory process with proliferation of the endothelial cells, lymphocytes and plasma cells, and formation of granulation tissue at first cellular, but later becoming fibrous. As the disease progressed, fibrous tissue was laid down fairly loosely, just beneath the surface and more densely in the deeper parts with small, round-celled infiltrates still present among the fibrous tissue. The blood-vessels were proliferating in the early stages, but later had enormous thickening of their walls and endarteritis with hyaline changes'.

Differential Diagnosis.—A differentiation should be made between malignant granuloma and reticulum-cell sarcoma. At first sight this should not be difficult, but in practice it can be far from easy in some cases. Reticulum-cell sarcomas of the mouth or respiratory passages frequently become ulcerated and heavily infiltrated with acute and chronic inflammatory cells. In these circumstances it may take a skilled pathologist to spot the neoplastic cells. To add to the problem some reticulum-cell sarcomas die out in the older part of the lesion while continuing to invade and proliferate in the periphery. This actually results in healing of some parts of the ulcer and, of course, a biopsy from the older parts will be negative. Repeated biopsy may be needed to establish the correct diagnosis. It is possible that the cases of so-called 'malignant granuloma' which respond to irradiation are really reticulum-cell sarcomas of this type.

Treatment.—There is no specific treatment, but irradiation of the local lesion is effective in some cases of malignant granuloma. Antibiotic therapy is used to control secondary infection, but has no effect on the progress of the disease. More widespread disease is treated with cortisone, and to keep the disease in check the patient must be kept on a maintenance dose of steroids. The prognosis is very poor.

REFERENCES

BHASKAR, S. N., and LILLY, G. E. (1964), 'Traumatic Granuloma of the Tongue (Human and Experimental)', *Oral Surg.*, **18,** 206.
BLEVINS, C., DAHLIN, D., LOVESTEDT, S., and KENNEDY, R. (1959), 'Oral and Dental Manifestations of Histiocytosis "X" ', *Ibid.*, **12,** 473.
BROOKE, R. I. (1969), 'Wegener's Granulomatosis involving the Gingivae', *Br. dent. J.*, **127,** 34.
CLARKE, P. B. (1964), 'Wegener's Granulomatosis', *Br. J. oral Surg.*, **1,** 205.

LICHENSTEIN, L. (1953), 'Histiocytosis "X" Integration of Eosinophilic Granuloma of Bone, Letterer-Siwi Disease and Schüller-Christian Disease as Related Manifestations of a Single Nosolytic Entity', *Archs Path.*, **56,** 84.
MILLS, C. P. (1958), 'Malignant Granulomas', *J. Lar. Otol.*, **72,** 849.
— — (1967), 'Malignant Granulomas and Wegener's Granulomatosis', *Hospital Med.*, **2,** 183.
MORGAN, A. D., and O'NEIL, R. (1956), 'Oral Complications of Polyarteritis, and Giant-cell Granulomatosis', *Oral Surg.*, **9,** 845.
SCHWARTZ, S. (1965), 'Bilateral Lesions of Eosinophilic Granuloma', *J. oral Surg.*, **23,** 172.
SCOTT, R. BODLEY (1966), *Price's Textbook of the Practice of Medicine.* London: Oxford University Press.
STEWART, J. P. (1933), 'Progressive Lethal Granulomatous Ulceration of the Nose', *J. Lar. Otol.*, **48,** 657.
WALTON, E. W. (1958), 'Giant-cell Granuloma of the Respiratory Tract (Wegener's Granulomatosis)', *Br. med. J.*, **2,** 265.
WILLIAMS, H. L. (1949), 'Lethal Granulomatous Ulceration involving the Midline Facial Tissues', *Ann. Otol. Rhinol. Lar.*, **58,** 1013.

Chapter XII

SOME PREMALIGNANT CONDITIONS OF THE ORAL CAVITY

Leucoplakia

LEUCOPLAKIA is regarded as a premalignant disease, but some care is required in defining exactly what is meant by the term. By definition, 'leucoplakia' means 'a white patch', but all chronic white lesions in the mouth are by no means premalignant. Pindborg, Renstrup, and others (1963) defined leucoplakia as a white patch that cannot be rubbed off, cannot be reversed by removing obvious irritants, and cannot be assigned to any other diagnostic category on the basis of clinical or microscopic features. This may be a satisfactory academic definition, but it is not particularly helpful to the clinically orientated oral surgeon, for not only is some difficulty experienced in differentiating the various white patches in the mouth clinically but similar difficulty is also found by the pathologists when the material is examined microscopically. In addition, some other white lesions not normally included under the term 'leucoplakia', such as lichen planus, can also undergo malignant change. Even when the pathologist can make a definite diagnosis in the case of a white patch, there is not, at present, any simple means of assessing whether it is likely to become malignant, though Kramer (1969) has suggested a most ingenious method of predicting a malignancy by computer analysis of a number of histological features of the lesion.

Incidence of Leucoplakia.—Pindborg and others (1965a) screened 10,000 patients in India and found 328 or 3·28 per cent had oral leucoplakia. Bruszt (1962), of Hungary, found a 3·6 per cent incidence in 5613 patients. In India, Mehta and others (1969) examined 4734 men and found a 3·4 per cent incidence of oral leucoplakia.

Types of White Patch.—Some of the chronic white patches in the mouth which may be premalignant are:—

1. *Leucoplakia of Developmental Origin or Developmental Epithelial Naevi.*—These chronic white lesions have been termed 'congenital', but they are not usually found in children and may not appear until middle age. Clinically there are two varieties:

a. A generalized irregular oedematous thickening of the superficial epithelium of the floor of the mouth or a symmetrical folded lesion on the insides of the cheeks. In some instances there is a family history and the condition may be inherited as an autosomal dominant. This condition is usually termed 'white sponge naevus'.

b. The other type can involve either side of the undersurface of the tongue. It has well-defined margins and a soft wrinkled surface. Although these two conditions are termed 'developmental', it does not necessarily imply that they always remain benign.

2. *Frictional Keratosis.*—If the oral mucosa is abraded by a broken tooth or denture, it may become hyperkeratinized. If the source of the irritation is removed the oral mucosa will revert to normal provided the source of local trauma is the only cause of the keratosis. Chronic mechanical irritation of the oral mucosa has long been regarded as a potential cause of oral carcinoma, but there is no experimental evidence to substantiate this view.

3. *Keratosis from Smoking.*—Keratosis of the palate with inflammation and swelling of the mucous glands can occur as a result of smoking, but even when the leucoplakia is severe, the condition may regress if the patient can be induced to give up smoking. The condition is often seen in the palate as a result of pipe smoking. However, the palate is an uncommon site for oral carcinoma. Heavy smoking has been implicated as a cause of carcinoma of the bronchus and it has been shown by Moore and Catlin (1967) that the main sites of oral carcinoma are in what they term the 'drainage area' of the mouth, i.e., the sides and underside of the tongue and the floor of the mouth extending back into the pharynx. Some 75 per cent of all oral carcinomas develop in this region which forms only 20 per cent of the total area of the mouth. It has been suggested by Cawson (1969) that if there is a relationship between smoking and oral cancer it could be due to carcinogens from the cigarettes becoming dissolved in the saliva which could then leak down and affect this drainage area. There is certainly a direct relationship between smoking and cancer of the lip and lesions on the lip associated with smoking clay pipes are well substantiated in the literature as well as carcinoma as a result of leaving a lighted stub of cigarette lying on the lip. The likelihood of a second carcinoma appearing in the oral cavity after successful treatment of the original lesion is materially increased if the patient continues to smoke (Silverman and Griffith, 1972).

4. *Syphilitic Leucoplakia.*—There is a strong association between syphilis and leucoplakia and Weisberger (1957) reported 14 patients with leucoplakia and positive serology for specific infection. Syphilis and candida are responsible for the only cases in which leucoplakia occurs as a result of an infection, and once the leucoplakia has reached a certain stage of development the condition is irreversible even though the causative infection has been eradicated. Patients with syphilitic leucoplakia have a marked tendency to develop oral carcinoma and a reduction in the incidence of syphilis may be responsible for a falling off in the number of cases of oral carcinoma. Recently there has been an increase in the incidence of new cases of syphilis, and it would seem logical that there should be a corresponding increase in oral leucoplakia of syphilitic origin. However, the condition usually arises in the tertiary stage of the disease and with the efficacy and availability of modern anti-syphilitic treatment, this should not necessarily occur.

5. *Chemical Leucoplakia.*—Various chemical irritants will produce hyperkeratotic lesions, although not in all subjects. Examples of such irritants are hot spices, ginger, and the betel nut quid. Carcinoma of the mouth in betel nut chewers is well known, but the activity of the various ingredients is not properly understood.

6. *Lichen Planus.*—Lichen planus is clinically distinguishable from

leucoplakia, but in a minority of cases the clinical and histopathological differential diagnosis may be difficult. Lichen planus is a generalized dermatological condition, the skin lesions appearing as small flat papules a few millimetres in diameter which coalesce into larger plaques covered with a fine glistening scale which shows tiny white radiating lines (striae of Wickham) across its surface. Early in the disease the lesions are red, but they soon become violaceous. The disease often manifests itself in the oral cavity before the appearance of the skin lesions and it may occur alone. In the mouth lichen planus usually appears as a series of radiating white or grey lines which cross over each other forming a reticular pattern. The buccal mucosa in the molar area is most commonly affected and the lesions often have a violaceous hue. The oral condition may be asymptomatic, but the patient sometimes complains of a burning sensation at the site of the lesion. Occasionally vesicle or bulla formation occurs, and this erosive form of lichen planus usually arises *de novo* and not as a progression from the non-erosive lesion. Lichen planus used to be regarded as a benign condition, but recently reports have appeared in the literature of carcinomatous changes in the lesions. Warin (1960) has referred to an incidence of 10 per cent which become malignant, while Altman and Perry (1961) reported the incidence to be 1 per cent. Andreasen and Pindborg (1963) reviewed 46 cases of carcinoma developing in patients with oral lichen planus, 16 of which occurred in patients with the erosive variety of the disease. However, 24 of the 46 patients had an additional predisposing cause of oral carcinoma, some of them suffering from syphilis. In the authors' experience likewise, patients with lichen planus who have developed carcinomas in the oral lesions have also been heavy smokers. Eggleston (1970) has reported a case in which both leucoplakia and lichen planus were present in the mouth of a patient, and in view of the unknown aetiology of both conditions and difficulty of distinguishing them clinically, the explanation may be that they are variants of the same condition.

7. *Leucoplakia of Unknown Aetiology.*—In a large number of cases of leucoplakia there is not an obvious aetiological factor and only a small number of these cases are dyskeratotic. Cooke (1963) pointed out that the presence of dyskeratosis cannot be judged from the clinical appearance. Pindborg and others (1963) found that the so-called 'speckled' leucoplakias, in which the surface is patchy red and white, were often dyskeratotic or were found to be carcinomatous. Carcinoma in situ is an unusual finding in the mouth and neither leucoplakia, dyskeratosis, nor carcinoma in situ is an inevitable precursor of invasive carcinoma. Verrucous carcinoma forms a grossly proliferative warty plaque which may at times be one of the intermediate stages between leucoplakia and carcinoma.

Patients with the Paterson-Kelly (Plummer-Vinson) syndrome, i.e., microchromic, microcytic anaemia, dysphagia, koilonychia, and smooth red tongue, have a high incidence of oral carcinoma. The tongue lesions are essentially hyperkeratotic with areas of desquamation. (*Figs.* 18, 19.) Patients with widespread leucoplakia are particularly at risk and may develop multiple primaries either serially or at about the same time.

Keratinizing Squamous-cell Carcinoma.—Early carcinoma can appear clinically as a white lesion and is on inspection indistinguishable from leucoplakia. Later, of course, the lesion will probably become ulcerated. Such cases are not leucoplakic patches undergoing malignant changes, but are primary carcinomas.

Candidiasis as a Form of Leucoplakia.—Invasion of the epithelium with Candida may cause hyperplasia and the progressive development of plaques in patients with long-standing candidal infection. Beyond a certain point this epithelial proliferation appears to be irreversible, even after the original infection has been eradicated, and in this respect it resembles the reaction in syphilitic leucoplakia. It has been suggested that

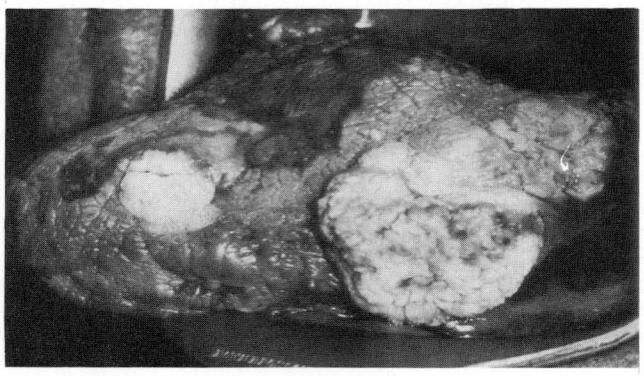

Fig. 18.—Leucoplakia of the tongue with squamous-cell carcinoma. There are two primary carcinomas; one arising in a fissure anteriorly and a fungating ulcer more posteriorly. There is also a fibro-epithelial polyp on the dorsum.

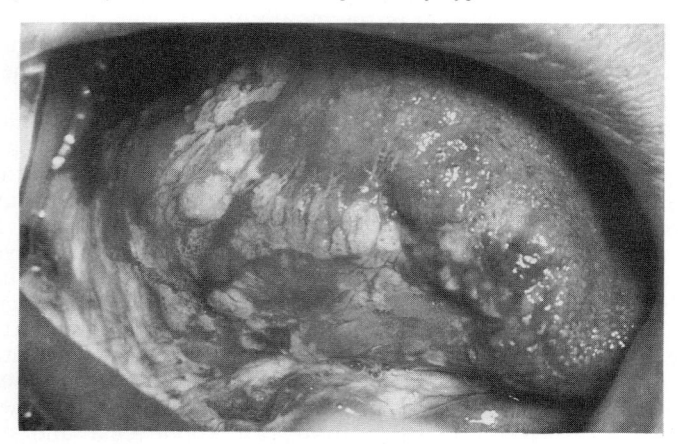

Fig. 19.—Leucoplakia of the floor of the mouth and side of the tongue with a squamous-cell carcinoma.

when candidal infection is found in association with leucoplakia it is a superimposed infection (Jepsen and Winther, 1965), but according to Cawson (1969) it is more likely that the candidal infection is itself the cause of the leucoplakia.

PREMALIGNANT CONDITIONS OF ORAL CAVITY

The Incidence of Carcinoma in Patients with Leucoplakia.—Einhorn and Wersall (1967) followed 782 patients with clinical leucoplakia for periods of 1–42 years and found that carcinoma developed in 2·4 per cent of cases within 10 years and 4 per cent in 20 years. Pindborg and others (1968), in a series of 214 patients, found malignant changes in 4·4 per cent in a period of 3·7 years. Cooke (1964) followed 50 cases of leucoplakia for varying periods of up to 10 years and reported an incidence of carcinoma of 12 per cent. This is a high figure, but the series is probably too small to be statistically significant. It is probable that about 5 per cent of cases of leucoplakia will develop malignant changes in a five-year period and this incidence is about 50–100 times the incidence in the normal mouth.

Treatment.—In view of the multiplicity of white patches which may occur in the mouth and the widely differing varieties which are clinically indistinguishable, it is essential to biopsy all white lesions in order to confirm or establish a diagnosis. If the lesion is small (i.e., up to 2 cm. across) an excision and biopsy will have the advantage of establishing the diagnosis and eliminating the lesion. It is also logical to remove leucoplakic patches which are subject to friction from dentures, etc., in view of the possible increased risk of malignancy. The problem arises as to whether all leucoplakic patches should be excised. Arguments in favour of excision are that it eradicates the disease and avoids the possible development of malignancy. However, in leucoplakia of unknown aetiology the lesion may recur and there is not, at present, any long-term follow-up of leucoplakic patches treated by excision. Indeed, Einhorn and Wersall (1967) found over a period of 15 years that the incidence of carcinoma was twice as high in those cases where excision had been carried out. In view of the available evidence that about 5 per cent of all leucoplakic patches become malignant, it follows that in 95 per cent of cases malignancy is unlikely to occur. It would therefore seem logical to adopt a more conservative approach to the treatment of leucoplakia and, therefore, after the diagnosis has been established by biopsy the condition should be kept under review at a three-month review clinic. It should, of course, be impressed upon the patient that any alteration in the lesion which occurs between visits should be reported immediately. Evidence of malignant change usually takes the form of ulceration, fissuring, or nodularity, and any suspicious area in the leucoplakic patch should be biopsied immediately. If carcinoma is found to be present, it should be treated without delay.

There are, of course, other difficulties: patients often fail to attend after a period of follow-up. This fact tends to bias the clinician towards the excision of the lesion where this is easily accomplished. It does not, of course, mean that follow-up can then be abandoned, for further white patches may appear.

Where a patient has had one malignancy of the mouth treated, the clinician may be inclined to advise the excision of any as yet non-malignant white patches in the hope of avoiding a second primary. Some lesions, of course, appear 'unstable' on clinical grounds and these will be removed and all known irritants eliminated.

The problem comes with widespread lesions. It is impracticable to replace almost all the mucosa of the mouth and pharynx and in some patients this is the extent of the disease. The areas most likely to give trouble can, of course, be excised and grafted. Repeated biopsies and surgery can cause a patient to cease to attend for follow-up and then when they do re-appear it may be with a large carcinoma. To avoid this, other methods can be used to monitor the affected areas.

Various stains such as iodine can be applied to the mucous membrane. Early carcinomas will stain darkly. A dissecting microscope can be used to examine suspicious regions and serial photographs may help the clinician to spot a shape he would otherwise overlook. Epithelial scrapings can be spread on a slide, fixed and stained, and examined for hyperkeratotic and malignant cells. Such scrapings should be taken in a way that the area from which they come can be identified. If a positive report is received a biopsy is performed. Such an examination is called an 'exfoliative cytological examination', but as the cells have not yet exfoliated, the term is more correctly used for the examination of sputum, cavity washings, etc. 'A desquamated cytological examination' is probably a better term. An excellent paper on this aspect of diagnosis of oral carcinomas has been published by Spengos (1967).

Bowen's Disease

Bowen's disease is a precancerous epithelial skin lesion consisting of firm papules covered by a keratinized layer or crust. The lesion may persist for years and in approximately one-fifth of patients with Bowen's disease the lesions undergo malignant transformation. The lesions of Bowen's disease occur on the extremities, abdomen, and buttocks, but they may also occur in the oral cavity and in this situation they are usually multicentric. Bowen's disease represents a carcinoma in situ.

Queyrat's Erythroplasia

Queyrat's erythroplasia is a rare precancerous lesion of unknown aetiology which takes the form of a bright red, velvety plaque and occurs on mucous membranes particularly the glans penis, prepuce, and vulva. Oral manifestations have been described on the buccal mucosa, tongue, and lips and histologically it appears as a squamous carcinoma in situ.

Submucous Fibrosis

Submucous fibrosis is a disease usually confined to patients of Asiatic descent and the majority of the reported cases have occurred in Indians. A few Europeans living in India have developed the disease and a recent case of an English woman married to a Pakistani, but living in Manchester, was reported by Simpson (1969). The condition arises only in the mouth and there is at first a progressive stiffening of the cheeks due to a proliferation of fibrous tissue and the fibrous replacement of muscle. As a result, fibrous bands are readily palpable in the cheeks and the condition may progress to involve the tongue, lips, faucial pillars, palate, and pharynx and all these structures become hard and lose their mobility. This leads to inability to open the mouth and dysphagia, and if the tongue or soft palate are affected there may be interference with speech. The mucosa tends to be pale in colour. Experimentally betel nut has failed to produce the lesion and it has been speculated that the consumption of chillies may play a part in the aetiology. Vesicles may appear at an early stage but are later followed by hypopigmentation or patches of irregularly mottled pigmentation. A burning sensation in the mouth is sometimes complained of.

Pindborg (1965b) and Pindborg and others (1967) found the incidence in India to be less than 1 per cent, but in 100 Indian patients with oral carcinoma the incidence of submucous fibrosis was 40 per cent. Of 50 cases of submucous fibrosis in Bombay, 2 per cent had oral carcinoma and of 51 cases seen in Lucknow, 9·8 per cent were affected. Lemmer and Shear (1968) reported 6 cases of submucous fibrosis which they examined histologically and one of these showed dyskeratosis with atypism.

Treatment.—None of the suggested treatments are very effective, but eradication of forms of chronic irritation, e.g., sharp, jagged teeth, should be carried out. Cutting of the fibrous bands only seems to lead to the production of more fibrous tissue, and the use of topical, local, or systemic corticosteroids is equally ineffective.

REFERENCES

ALTMAN, J., and PERRY, H. O. (1961), 'The Variations of the Cause of Lichen Planus', *Archs Derm.*, **84**, 179.

ANDREASEN, J. O., and PINDBORG, J. J. (1963), 'Development of Cancer in Oral Lichen Planus', *Nord. Med.*, **70**, 861.

BRUSZT, P. (1962), 'Stomato-oncological Screening Tests in 7 Villages of the Baja and Bacsalmas District', *Magy. Onkol.*, **6**, 28.

CAWSON, R. A. (1969), 'Leucoplakia and Oral Cancer', *Proc. R. Soc. Med.*, **62**, 610.

COOKE, B. E. D. (1963), 'Exfoliative Cytology in evaluating Oral Lesions', *J. dent. Res.*, **42**, 343.

— — (1964), 'Leucoplakia Buccalis', *Ann. R. Coll. Surg.*, **34**, 370.

EGGLESTON, D. J. (1970), 'Lichen Planus or Leukoplakia', *Oral Surg.*, **29**, 845.

EINHORN, J., and WERSALL, J. (1967), 'Incidence of Oral Carcinoma in Patients with Leukoplakia of the Oral Mucosa', *Cancer, N.Y.*, **20**, 2189.

JEPSEN, A., and WINTHER, J. E. (1965), 'Mycotic Infection in Oral Leukoplakia', *Acta odont. scand.*, **23**, 239.

KRAMER, I. R. H. (1969), 'Precancerous Conditions of the Oral Mucosa', *Ann. R. Coll. Surg.*, **45**, 340.

LEMMER, J., and SHEAR, M. (1968), 'Precancerous and Cancerous Lesions of the Mouth', *J. dent. Ass. S. Afr.*, **23**, 274.

MEHTA, E. S., PINDBORG, J. J., DAFTARY, D. K., and GUPTA, P. C. (1969), 'Oral Leukoplakia among Indian Villagers, the Association with Smoking Habits', *Br. dent. J.*, **127**, 73.

MOORE, C., and CATLIN, D. (1967), 'Anatomic Origins and Locations of Oral Cancer', *Am. J. Surg.*, **114**, 510

PINDBORG, J. J., RENSTRUP, G., POULSEN, H. E., and SILVERMAN, S., jun. (1963), ' Studies in Oral Leukoplakias', *Acta odont. scand.*, **21**, 407.

— — and others (1965a), 'Frequency of Oral Leukoplakia and Related Conditions among 10,000 Bombayites', *J. all-India dent. Ass.*, **37**, 228.

— — and others (1965b), 'Clinical Aspects of Oral Submucous Fibrosis', *Acta odont. scand.*, **22**, 679.

— — and others (1967), 'Oral Epithelial Changes in Thirty Indians with Oral Cancer and Submucous Fibrosis', *Cancer, N.Y.*, **20**, 1141.

— — and others (1968), 'Studies in Oral Leucoplakia', *J. Am. dent. Ass.*, **76**, 767.

— — POULSEN, H. E., and ZACHARIAH, J. (1967), 'Oral Epithelial Changes in Thirty Indians with Oral Cancer and Submucous Fibrosis', *Cancer, N.Y.*, **20**, 1141.

SILVERMAN, S., and GRIFFITH, M. (1972), 'Smoking Characteristics of Patients with Oral Carcinoma and the Risk of Second Oral Primary Carcinoma', *J. Am. dent. Ass.*, **85**, 637.

SIMPSON, W. (1969), 'Submucous Fibrosis', *Br. J. oral Surg.*, **6**, 196.

SPENGOS, M. N. (1967), 'Dental Diagnosis of Oral Carcinoma. Early Detection Cytology' *Dent. Radiogr. Photogr.*, **40,** 51.
WARIN, R. P. (1960), 'Epithelioma following Lichen Planus of the Mouth', *Br. J. Derm.*, **72,** 288.
WEISBERGER, D. (1957), 'Precancerous Lesions' *.J. Am. dent. Ass.*, **54,** 507.

Chapter XIII
THE CLINICAL DIAGNOSIS OF ORAL MALIGNANCY

THE clinical diagnosis of malignancy of the oral cavity, an area which includes the lips, tongue, floor of the mouth, cheeks, and pillars of the fauces, presents few diagnostic difficulties and, provided that the clinician carries out a systematic examination of the oral cavity, there is little chance of a malignant lesion being overlooked. Difficulty can only arise if the lesion is exceptionally small or if it lies in an anatomically inaccessible area. However, the diagnosis of malignant neoplasm arising within the mandible or the maxillae is more difficult in the early stages of the disease.

Table I.—MALIGNANT NEOPLASMS AFFECTING ORAL CAVITY

Primary Carcinomas:—	Of a surface.
	Of a gland—usually a salivary gland.
	The rare intra-bony of the jaws:—
	1. Arising in a cyst lining.
	2. *Krompecher* carcinoma arising from residual odontogenic epithelium.
Secondary Carcinomas:—	Centrally in the medullary cavity of the jaw bones.
	On the surface of the mucosa—malignant cell from sputum grafted on to raw area.
	In lymph-nodes from a head and neck primary.
Primary Sarcoma:—	Centrally in the tissues:—
	1. In the jaws osteogenic sarcoma, reticulum-cell sarcoma, Ewing's tumour, Lymphosarcoma.
	2. In the muscles Fibrosarcoma, Leiomyosarcoma, Rhabdomyosarcoma.
Reticuloses:—	Usually in the cheeks, sometimes centrally in the jaws Hodgkin's disease Leukaemic deposits, etc.

Symptoms of Carcinoma of the Oral Cavity.—The general symptoms vary according to the site of the carcinoma and as the lesions are always painless in the early stages they may be overlooked, especially when they are sited towards the back of the oral cavity. Carcinoma of the lip is usually noticed by the patient as a painless lump or ulcer on the lip, while carcinoma of the anterior part of the mouth may first be discovered by the patient's tongue probing the lesion. In the posterior part of the mouth symptoms are usually slight until the lesion has reached a diameter of 2–3 cm. or until it becomes infected, when pain and swelling supervene, which may cause difficulty in deglutition.

Pain and tenderness only develop when a malignant ulcer becomes secondarily infected or if the lesion involves a sensory nerve. Occasionally symptoms are absent until the tumour has metastasized to the regional lymph-nodes and the patient notices a hard lump in the neck. In such cases the primary growth may be merely a minute crack in the lip or in the region of the fauces and carcinoma of the nasopharynx often presents in this fashion.

Late Symptoms.—Late symptoms of carcinoma of the oral cavity are pain due to secondary infection or involvement of the nerves in the region, excessive salivation, difficulty in deglutition and speech and haemorrhage which usually manifests itself as blood-stained saliva.

Neoplasms arising within the Bone.—The early symptom of a neoplasm arising within the bone of the mandible or maxilla is a painless swelling which characteristically involves both the buccal and lingual or buccal and palatal sulci. If teeth are present they may become loose and painful and often the patient seeks aid because he thinks he has an acute alveolar abscess. If the patient is edentulous a previously satisfactory denture may no longer fit and may be displaced or it may cut into the soft tissues and produce a localized denture hyperplasia or granuloma. Anaesthesia of the upper or lower lip is quite common. The malignant conditions which may affect the mouth are classified in *Table I*.

Carcinoma of the Lip.—Carcinoma of the vermilion border is most common between the ages of 50 and 70 years and the majority of the patients are male. According to Aird (1957) it is most common among unskilled labourers and is a disease of the lower classes. The patients tend to have dirty, jagged, stained teeth and, indeed, sometimes the malignancy does arise at a site irritated by a jagged tooth. Common precipitating factors may be some form of irritation and leucoplakic change due to hot tobacco smoke caused by leaving a lighted cigarette stub lying on the lip. There is an increased incidence of carcinoma of the lip in occupations and countries where the patient is subjected to intense solar radiation. According to Rains and Capper (1969) 40 per cent of patients with carcinoma of the lip give a history of blistering cheilitis due to sunlight. Carcinoma of the lip is therefore more common in countries where there is protracted sunshine and among patients whose occupation causes them to be unduly exposed to the elements. The condition is known colloquially as 'countryman's lip'. The lower lip is affected in 93 per cent of cases and the upper lip in 5 per cent, while 2 per cent occur at the angle of the mouth. Sometimes a growth occurs on the upper lip at a point opposite the lower lip lesion, possibly due to direct implantation of cells. The tumour begins as a small, painless scabbing ulcer, which arises in the substance of the lip and if untreated spreads to the cheek, gum, and jaw. According to Aird (1957) 10 per cent of the patients with carcinoma of the lip develop metastases within a year and 36 per cent within two years and the lymph-nodes affected are the submental, submandibular, and upper jugular groups. Death eventually occurs from infection or aspiration pneumonia.

Differential Diagnosis.—Carcinoma of the lip must be distinguished from molluscum pseudo-carcinomatosum which also has a predilection for the lower lip and is clinically indistinguishable from carcinoma.

Carcinoma of the Tongue.—Carcinoma of the anterior two-thirds of the tongue affects males nine times more frequently than females. Cancer of the posterior third affects the sexes equally, and most of the patients are over 60 years of age. Females with cancer of the anterior two-thirds of the tongue are often found to be suffering from a Paterson-Kelly or Plummer-Vinson syndrome. The oral hygiene is usually bad in patients with carcinoma of the tongue. The disease is often associated with heavy drinking of alcohol and this may be correlated with a deficiency of vitamin B_1 which is known to produce a precancerous mucosal atrophy. Alcohol contains an adequate number of calories to sustain life without the necessity of eating an adequate diet, but unfortunately it does not contain vitamins. Twenty-five per cent of the patients have suffered from syphilis and 5 per cent have had leucoplakia. Other precancerous lesions include superficial glossitis, papilloma, fissures, and non-specific ulcers. The tumours lie near the lateral edge of the tongue in 58 per cent of cases and the dorsum of the tongue is involved in 2-4 per cent, the tip in 7-15 per cent, and the posterior third in 21-33 per cent. Carcinoma of the posterior third of the tongue is often overlooked by the patient and even the clinician. Alteration of the voice is often a presenting symptom in these cases. According to Aird (1957) there are five naked eye appearances of carcinoma of the tongue: (1) The ulcerative type, (2) Papillary, (3) The flat nodule, (4) A malignant fissure which is often a sequel of syphilitic fissuring, (5) Scirrhous or atrophic.

Clinical Features.—The earliest symptom is a painless swelling or an ulcer. Once the ulcer is established, pain is continuous and severe and may radiate to the ear. This is due to involvement of the lingual nerve and referred pain to auriculo-temporal region may occur. It is accompanied by excessive salivation and there is marked foetor oris, haemorrhage, and finally immobility of the tongue as it becomes fixed to the floor of the mouth. Before this stage is reached, the tongue becomes fixed on one side and when the patient protrudes the tongue it deviates towards the affected side. Dysarthria and dysphagia may also occur. The life expectancy of an untreated carcinoma of the tongue is about 16 months. Carcinoma of the tongue presents as an induration, ulceration, or fungation which spreads directly to the floor of the mouth and from there to the alveolar process. From the posterior third of the tongue the spread is to the fauces, valleculae, and epiglottis. Metastases are restricted to the regional glands. In the anterior two-thirds of the tongue metastases are ipsilateral and bilateral metastases only occur if the tumour extends to the midline of the tongue. The metastases from growths in the posterior third of the tongue are bilateral. In the untreated case death is inevitable and can occur as a result of inhalation bronchopneumonia, cachexia and starvation, haemorrhage (usually from a metastasis eroding a major artery), and asphyxia.

Carcinoma of the Mouth.—Carcinoma occurs in the floor of the mouth, cheek, palate, and faucial pillar. In the floor of the mouth it is usually a typical malignant ulcer extending to the alveolar process and tongue. The cheek lesion is often warty and proliferative. On the alveolar process the tumour may be warty, nodular, or proliferating. (*Fig.* 20.) Such neoplasms must be distinguished from the results of denture irritation and, where teeth are present, from a periodontal abscess. Carcinoma of the palate is often papillary or ulcerative and usually spreads extensively before it affects the bone. It is difficult to distinguish it from a carcinoma of the maxillary sinus which has spread to the palate.

Carcinomas of the soft palate and fauces are proliferative, fungating tumours, and carry a particularly poor prognosis. They spread to the base of the tongue and there is early involvement of the lymph-nodes bilaterally. Secondary infection causes pain and dysphagia, and death frequently occurs following erosion of the carotid artery.

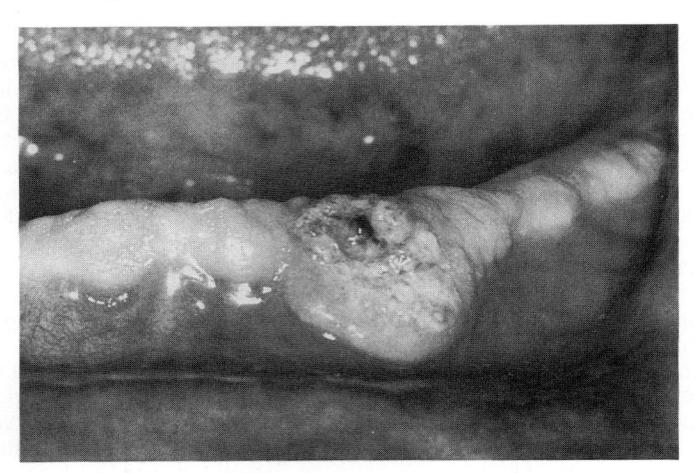

Fig. 20.—Proliferating squamous-cell carcinoma of the alveolus.

Malignant Neoplasms of the Maxillary Antrum.—The squamous-cell carcinoma accounts for between 90 and 95 per cent of antral malignancies. All degrees of differentiation are found, but many are anaplastic. The tumour infiltrates the soft tissues, destroys bone, and can ulcerate into the mouth, pharynx, and skin of the face. Lymphatic metastasis to the upper deep cervical nodes occurs and rarely lymphatic spread may take place to the retropharyngeal group of nodes. Other malignant growths arise in the maxillary sinus such as adenocarcinoma, lympho-epithelioma, and sarcoma, but their incidence is obviously small.

While confined to the bony walls of the antrum the neoplasm does not produce definite symptoms, but with extension certain clinical features develop and these specific signs and symptoms should be known to every dental surgeon to ensure prompt recognition of the disease.

The earliest presenting symptom is often a unilateral sero-sanguineous discharge or frank epistaxis. The possibility of a carcinoma of the maxillary sinus should always be considered when an elderly patient presents with epistaxis of recent origin. The established carcinoma of the maxillary sinus may produce unilateral swelling of the cheek, buccal sulcus, or palate. Intra-oral swelling may dislodge a denture which has up to that time fitted satisfactorily and, where the edge of the denture cuts into the soft tissue mass, there may be a denture hyperplasia or granuloma. If teeth are present in relation to the floor of the maxillary sinus they may become loose, painful, and periostitic. The patient may sometimes, in fact, present with an acute alveolar abscess. There may be anaesthesia of the cheek in the distribution of the infra-orbital nerve, or anaesthesia or paraesthesia of the palate due to involvement of the sphenopalatine ganglion. If the nasolacrimal duct is occluded due to medial spread, epiphora will ensue. The eye on the affected side may be proptosed and if the tumour has invaded the orbit and interfered with one or more of the orbital muscles or the nerves which innervate them, there will be strabismus, limitation of ocular movements and the patient will complain of diplopia. The pupillary level may be raised on the affected side and in very

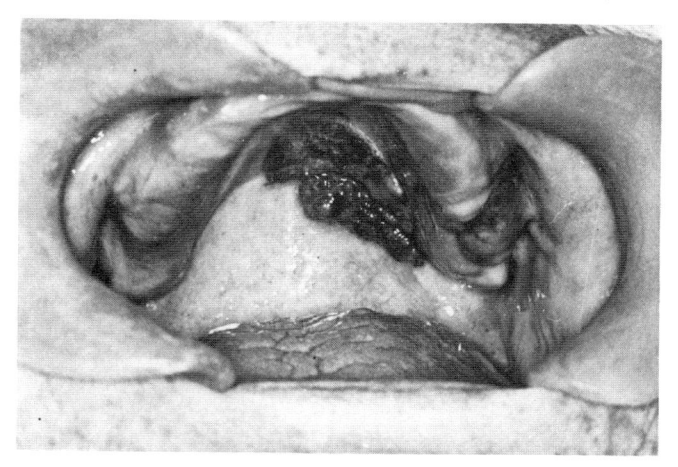

Fig. 21.—Malignant melanoma of the palate.

advanced cases there may be amblyopia. The nostril on the affected side may be blocked and on inspection with a nasal speculum the tumour mass can often be seen growing down the nostril. There is frequently a bloodstained discharge of pus from the nostril. Pain is sometimes due to secondary infection of the maxillary sinus and in extreme cases the swelling on the face bursts through the cheek and fungates. Trismus may occur due to encroachment upon the medial pterygoid.

The importance of the dental surgeon as a diagnostician in antral neoplasia is evident from the improved five-year cure rate prognosis for those with oral symptoms alone (Kay, 1970), but generally the outlook is poor, since at least 70 per cent of patients with malignancies occurring in or affecting the maxillary sinus will die from their disease (Harrison, 1971). It should be realized, however, that the characteristic radiographic changes of antral mucosal malignancy, i.e., destruction of bony walls, do not appear early, so the fact that an occipitomental view may show normal antral bony contours in a case which is suspicious on clinical grounds does not exclude the existence of serious disease.

Further Management.—A biopsy is essential to confirm the diagnosis and so that treatment is based on a proper knowledge of the nature of the lesion. Chest X-rays and/or radiographs of other bones and a careful general inquiry and physical examination are necessary, both to uncover any overt secondaries and to establish the degree of physical fitness of the patient. A haemoglobin estimation, blood-film examination, white-cell count, and blood group determination are other essential preliminary investigations.

More than in the treatment of most oral diseases, a careful social history and a discussion with relatives are necessary to understand fully the implication of the various forms of treatment.

Malignant Melanoma (*Fig.* 21).—Primary malignant melanoma of the oral cavity was first reported by Weber in 1859. It is a rare condition and Chaudhry, Hampel, and Gorlin (1958) reviewed 105 cases from the literature between 1859 and 1957. It is seen more frequently in men than in women and 75 per cent of the patients are 40 years of age or over. It presents as a raised, soft, vascular, dark brown or black mass, and bleeding and ulcerations are common. When it occurs in the mouth it destroys adjacent bone and loosens teeth in its vicinity. It has a tendency to invade blood-vessels and lymph channels and some 50 per cent of cases show involvement of the lymph-nodes when first seen. For this reason, a search of the body for a possible primary lesion should always be made when a melanoma is seen in the oral cavity. Cade (1961) believes that in many cases diagnosis can be made on clinical grounds alone and that biopsy is unnecessary. However, in view of the mutilating surgery required to treat the condition, histological evidence is usually required before embarking on treatment. Cade advocates a frozen section if biopsy is considered necessary. The prognosis of intra-oral melanoma is very poor.

REFERENCES

AIRD, I. (1957), *A Companion to Surgical Studies*, 2nd ed. Edinburgh: Livingstone.
CADE, S. (1961), 'Malignant Melanoma', *Ann. R. Coll. Surg.*, **28**, 331.
CHAUDHRY, A. P., HAMPEL, A., and GORLIN, R. (1958), 'Primary Malignant Melanoma of the Oral Cavity. A Review of 105 Cases', *Cancer, N.Y.*, **11**, 923.
HARRISON, D. F. N. (1971), Paper given at the 4th International Conference on Oral Surgery, held in Amsterdam, 17–21 May.
RAINS, A. J. H., and CAPPER, W. M., ed. (1968), *Bailey and Love's Short Practice of Surgery*, 14th ed. London: Lewis.
WEBER, C. O. (1859), *Chirurgische erfahrungen und untersuchungen reimer*. Berlin.

Chapter XIV
THE TREATMENT OF MALIGNANT NEOPLASMS

THE treatment of patients with malignant neoplasms involves a type of medicine which has been made almost redundant in many other fields by potent, effective, therapeutic agents which, by and large, have few, or tolerable, side effects. The treatment of malignant neoplasms means responsibility for the patient for the rest of his or her life. It means the making of judgements which affect the patient's survival, livelihood and social contacts. It involves a relationship with the patient and the relatives which is more emotionally charged than that experienced by oral surgeons in most other aspects of their work.

Treatment of oral malignant neoplasms starts properly with the general dental practitioner and the avoidance of premalignant conditions. Patients' mouths should be maintained in a healthy state, free from chronic sepsis and chronic irritation. Natural teeth and appliances should be kept smooth and in good repair. While there is no proper statistical evidence linking irritation from rough teeth and carcinoma, occasional highly-suggestive cases are seen and the fact remains, whatever the reason, that more lingual carcinomas are seen on the lateral borders of the tongue than on the tip or centre (unless the patient has leucoplakia of the tongue). Smoking, strong spices, strong spirits and the betel-nut quid, particularly if indulged in regularly and in excessive amounts, are known to produce premalignant lesions in a proportion of those who use them. Patients should be advised against such potentially harmful habits. The effective treatment of syphilis is important to avoid the precarcinomatous, leucoplakic tongue which is a late sequela of this infection. Benign neoplasms or granulomatous swelling should be excised, particularly if they are subject to repeated trauma. Chapter XII deals more fully with premalignant conditions.

The successful treatment of malignant neoplasms depends much on early diagnosis and again the general dental practitioner has an important role to play with regular and careful examinations of the patient. The dental surgeon should have a healthy suspicion of the slightly unusual— for example, a deep 'periodontal pocket' with florid granulations and bone destruction in an otherwise healthy mouth, or a chronic ulcer, or fissure with no apparent cause.

Features which demand careful consideration are:

a. Chronic ulcers or fissures with no apparent cause or ones which do not respond promptly to simple treatment.

b. Swellings with no apparent cause, especially if there are dilated small vessels over the surface, but no marked oedema or redness.

c. Rapid and unexpected loosening of a group of teeth, irregular bone destruction seen radiographically, or unexpected fracture following minimal trauma.

d. Signs of infiltration, such as tethering of an organ or lump, or limitation of the normal movement of the part.

e. Signs of involvement of adjacent nerves producing persistent pain, anaesthesia of the part, or paralysis of muscles.

f. Signs of obstruction of related ducts such as salivary ducts, or obstruction of related veins with vascular engorgement.

g. Repeated, small haemorrhages from a particular location.

h. Enlarged lymph-nodes without surrounding oedema and no obvious simple cause.

i. An 'abscess' with no apparent cause which may be a necrotic neoplasm.

j. Anaemia with no obvious cause.

k. Sweating, malaise and toxicity not due to an obvious infection.

The clinician should not rely solely on the biopsy report for information about the type of neoplasm. The length of history, mode of presentation and clinical and radiographic appearances may give clues as to the type of tumour which is present. If a decision is made in this way on clinical ground the validity of the biopsy report can be better assessed, particularly where there is an element of doubt.

If a malignant neoplasm is discovered in the oral cavity, the next step is to consider whether it is the primary lesion, or a secondary deposit. An inquiry into the patient's general health may reveal symptoms suggestive of another lesion elsewhere. A careful, full, physical examination likewise may reveal a primary in another organ. Careful probing of the person's past history may uncover treatment of a previous malignancy, an incident which the patient is perhaps reluctant to recall, but which may be highly relevant under the circumstances. Patients sometimes 'censor' information about a system outside the field of the specialist they are consulting and regard it as no concern of his! X-rays of the chest may reveal a bronchial primary, or secondary deposits and films of the skull may reveal further metastatic lesions. The biopsy report may contain the clue to the organ of origin.

In general, no lesion should be treated as a malignant neoplasm until histological proof has been obtained by means of a biopsy. With few exceptions it is neither legally nor morally right to treat the patient for a malignant neoplasm until proper evidence of its nature has been obtained. Nor may proper advice be given to the patient and a prognosis to the relatives unless a histological diagnosis is forthcoming. Mostly malignant neoplasms in the region of the oral cavity and its associated parts are easily accessible for removal of a specimen for biopsy. Masses in some organs like the major salivary glands or in relatively inaccessible sites present special problems (*see* p. 229) and a primary exploratory operation may be proper. Should the tumour be judged benign beyond reasonable doubt and amenable to treatment which does not leave the patient with a major deficit, definitive surgery can be undertaken at the same time. Where there is any doubt as to the nature of the mass and particularly where a more aggressive neoplasm is suspected, then a specimen for frozen section should be taken, and the report seen before surgery is continued, assuming that this is the appropriate form of treatment. Should there still be a doubt as to the diagnosis, or the right course of action, then the wound should be closed and treatment delayed until paraffin sections are available. Precautions against spillage of cells into the wound may be necessary.

Once the clinician is sure he is dealing with a primary neoplasm the extent of its spread must be determined. Local spread is assessed by physical and radiological examination and lymphatic spread by careful palpation of the regional lymph-nodes. In the neck, displacement of the relaxed sternomastoid muscle first forwards and then backwards so that the palpating fingers can seek underneath is an important manoeuvre. A search for evidence of generalized spread involves radiographs of chest and bones, for example the cranial vault and spine, a blood film for evidence of leuco-erythroblastic anaemia and a general examination for other abnormal masses, or an enlarged liver and spleen, etc.

At this stage it is proper that an explanation should be given to the patient. How frank this is depends upon any direct questions that the patient asks, an assessment of the patient's personality, and an understanding of his or her responsibilities in the home and at work (Cade, 1963). No direct lies are permissible, but what is said and the way in which it is said should carry hope and increase the patient's confidence in his adviser. If possible the patient's morale should be increased and certainly not destroyed by what is said. Phrases such as 'a tumour', 'an ulcer' or 'a lump which needs treatment' can be used without recourse to emotive words like 'cancer'. However, patients know that extensive resections, or radiotherapy, are usually used for malignant lesions and hence come to understand the nature of their disease.

Few men have the breadth of skill and experience to advise properly on all aspects of the treatment of malignant neoplasms affecting the oral cavity and a consultation at a joint appointment is advisable at this point. If such cases are handled regularly a special combined clinic should be set up. A radiotherapist and a surgeon form the basic unit for such a consultation. The surgeon should be one who has a special interest in the pathology, natural history and management of neoplastic disease of this region. Because these tumours may well transgress the anatomical boundaries or skills of more than one surgical speciality, several surgeons with appropriate abilities may need on occasion to meet over the problem. Since anaesthetic difficulties and general disease are commonly met with in these patients, the advice of an anaesthetist, or a physician, may also be appropriate. Most radiotherapists include the use of cytotoxic drugs in their armamentarium, but for some conditions, such as the leukaemias, a physician such as a haematologist may be the local expert in this field.

When the nature of the treatment is explained, the clinician should say that with prompt and proper treatment there is every chance of a cure. The patient should then be given the opportunity to ask further questions, if he or she so wishes, and honest, but kindly, answers should be given.

The patient's relatives will usually wish an opportunity for a private interview. A clear, simple statement of what has been found, what must be done, and what may be the final outcome should be given. Frequently relatives, and indeed patients, misunderstood and any misinterpretations must be cleared up as soon as they are recognized. Their co-operation and support must be mobilized and are important for the patient's well-being. A letter giving full details of the results of the investigations, consultations and proposed treatment must be sent to the medical G.P. as well as the referring dental surgeon, for the patient's doctor must play a large part in the subsequent long-term care of the patient.

Treatment may be either curative or palliative. Curative treatment can be considered for primary tumours with no evidence of spread other than local spread, and for those tumours which have metastasized to the regional lymph-nodes, but where these are still moveable on adjacent vital structures or are amenable to radiotherapy, as in the case of a reticulosis. The means available for hopefully curative treatment are radiotherapy and/or surgery and the treatment for a particular patient is best decided by discussion at the joint clinic between surgeon and radiotherapist. Certain factors need to be borne in mind when such decisions are being made. Without doubt radiotherapy, if successful, will give far better functional and aesthetic results than radical surgery and for the common squamous-cell carcinoma in many sites there is little difference in success rates between the two methods of treatment. The only major disadvantages of radiotherapy are:

a. The loss of teeth which may be necessary as a prophylaxis against post-irradiation osteomyelitis.

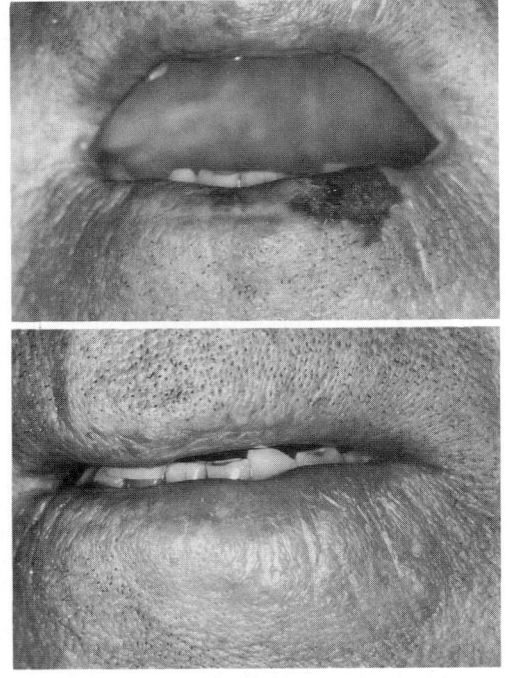

Fig. 22.—A small carcinoma of the lower lip (upper photograph) at the site where the patient habitually held a self-rolled cigarette. Lower photograph after treatment by radium needle implant; 4-year follow-up.

TREATMENT OF MALIGNANT NEOPLASMS

 b. The risk of post-irradiation osteomyelitis itself.
 c. A more remote risk of necrosis of the soft tissues, cartilage or bone due to local overdose.
 d. Damage to the salivary glands and dryness of the mouth, which together with atrophy of the mucous membrane can make the wearing of dentures difficult.
 e. Radiation cataract in the case of tumours which are close to, or involve, the eye although the latter is often excised at a subsequent operation.
 f. And, occasionally, temporary depilation, or radiation fibrosis of muscles.
With modern treatment methods the risk that the patient will suffer any of these complications is materially smaller than in the past.

 Small squamous-cell carcinomas of the anterior two-thirds of the tongue do at least as well with a radium or caesium needle implant as after surgery and the patient retains an intact tongue. Squamous carcinoma of the lower lip similarly may be treated with a substantial percentage of

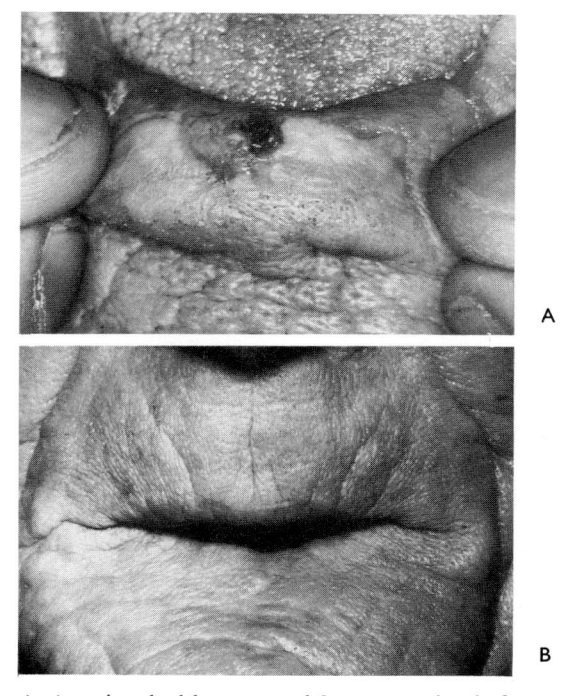

Fig. 23.—A, A patient had been treated 3 years previously for a squamous-cell carcinoma of the lower right alveolar process which had arisen in a zone of leucoplakia involving the inside of both cheeks and the floor of the mouth. Treatment 6,500r by cobalt 60 irradiation. B, He then developed a squamous-cell carcinoma of the lip. He was a heavy smoker and an outdoor worker with solar keratosis of the lower lip. Treatment: a lip shave and wedge excision of the lower lip, closing with a Z-plasty to prevent a notched lower lip.

successful results by either method, but mostly is treated by radiotherapy using radioactive gold seeds, needles, or external DXT avoiding the wide, full-thickness resection necessary for surgical treatment (*Figs.* 22 and 23). Carcinoma of the cheek near the commissure does less well than carcinoma of this site more posteriorly situated, but again the alternative is wide, often full-thickness, surgical removal and repair (*Figs.* 24 and 25). Since many such patients have extensive premalignant changes of the oral mucous membrane on both sides of the mouth radiotherapy may be the first choice. Advanced carcinoma of the anterior two-thirds of the tongue can be treated by total glossectomy, but primary treatment by megavoltage radiotherapy gives a similar, even if poor, chance of survival without the difficulties created by complete loss of the tongue.

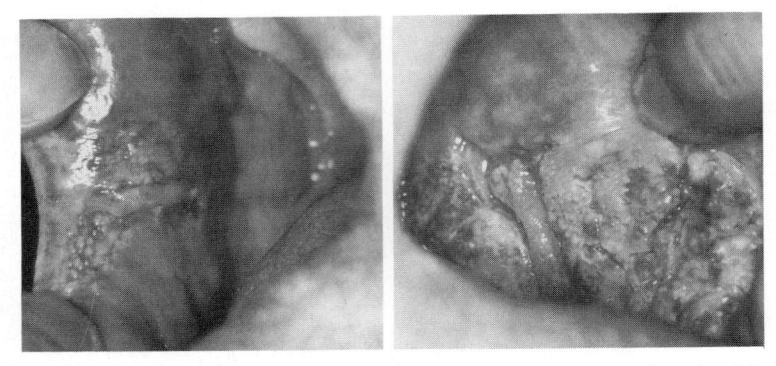

Fig. 24.—Bilateral carcinomas of the cheek, the left more extensive than the right. Treated by cobalt 60 external irradiation.

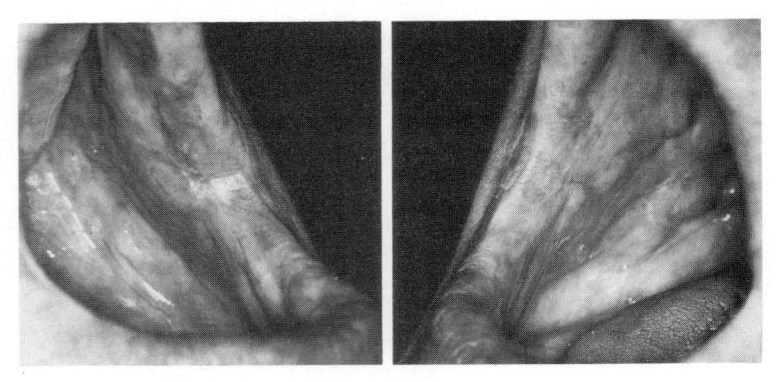

Fig. 25.—The same case as in *Fig.* 24: post-irradiation appearance at 3 years after treatment.

Where there is a choice of treatment, radiotherapy is usually employed first (Easson, 1963). If the blood-supply to the part is materially damaged by previous surgery, radiotherapy is less successful because the effectiveness of treatment is related to proper oxygenation of the tumour tissue. Again treatment planning for radiotherapy can be complicated by injudicious operative treatment. On the other hand, if radiotherapy appears not to be controlling the disease, there must be no delay in turning to surgical treatment. The treatable must not be permitted to become untreatable. There is unfortunately no way of predicting which patients will do well and which badly by a particular technique. Apart from the radiosensitivity of the neoplasm the immune response and resistance of the patient are important. Indeed, where a case does badly with radiotherapy the latter may be the reason, in which case surgery also will have a poor prognosis.

Both the histological type of neoplasm and its site affect its likely response to radiotherapy. Thus squamous-cell carcinomas tend to do well particularly if small and well differentiated—leastways, well in the context of malignant disease. Adenocarcinomas respond less well and sarcomas may melt away only to recur. Melanomas are usually unresponsive. Most authorities are now agreed that once a neoplasm involves the bone of the jaws, the chances of success with radiotherapy alone are reduced, so that subsequent surgery will be required.

Surgery is always mutilating in that sizeable blocks of tissue must be removed. Margins of apparently normal tissue of between 1 and 3 cm., depending on the type of neoplasm, must be removed, *en bloc*, from all aspects of the visible, radiographic and palpable limits of the lesion. This margin must be increased where spread is known to be facilitated in a particular direction. For example, if the posterior part of the mandible is involved the bone from anterior to the mental foramen to posterior to the mandibular foramen must be removed, irrespective of the size of the neoplasm, because of the risk of spread along the inferior dental canal.

Adenocystic carcinomas of salivary glands tend to permeate in the perineural tissues, some believe along the perineural lymphatics, so that the spread along adjacent nerves may be to a much greater distance than elsewhere. Some neoplasms will spread through medullary bone without inciting resorption of the adjacent trabeculae. The advancing edge may then be far removed from the radiographic limits of the disease. Again adenocystic carcinomas are notorious in this respect and the extent of the resection must be increased accordingly.

For some neoplasms and particularly where unpredictable, extensive, infiltration is a feature of their behaviour, experience teaches that surgical resection to the maximum extent feasible to reduce the volume of the neoplasm together with irradiation of the periphery of the surgical field gives the best chance of control of the disease. It should be stressed that such an excision should include a proper margin of tissue around the known limits of the disease. In other circumstances similar tactics will be dictated because the anatomical situation precludes the excision of an adequate margin, uniformly on all aspects.

Normally, when irradiation is used for the treatment of the primary tumour a radical neck dissection is performed only when suspicious mobile nodes are palpated. Since it is of the utmost importance that involved nodes should be detected promptly, regular follow-up visits *must* be maintained and a system of recall set up which checks on missed appointments. Initially, follow-up examinations will be at monthly intervals and this time will be extended only when the risk of the appearance of regional lymph-node metastases seems to be past—for example, after 1 year. Three-monthly and, later, 6-monthly appointments are then instituted. Since the primary neoplasm must be eradicated at the same time as, or before, a neck dissection is undertaken, radiotherapeutic treatment of the primary normally precedes neck dissection. To remove the filtering lymph-nodes before the primary has been dealt with, so permitting cells to pass further afield more readily, is obviously bad tactics. If lymph-node enlargement is noted before regression of the primary has been achieved then excision of the primary is combined with the neck dissection. In some cases a holding dose of irradiation can be delivered to the nodes to reduce the risk of further spread before the surgery is performed or to give the primary a chance to complete its resolution.

When surgical treatment is the method of choice there is greater divergence of opinion about the place of a simultaneous neck dissection (Freund, 1967). Several factors influence the decision. Adequate local surgery often involves the detachment of relevant muscles from the hyoid bone and clearance of the submandibular region, including the submandibular salivary gland and the adjacent lymph-nodes. Adhesions from such a dissection may make more difficult a subsequent neck dissection in the region of the upper deep cervical nodes—a point where adequate clearance is often most important. There is therefore good reason for doing the neck dissection as part of the initial procedure. Further, the main venous drainage is controlled before the primary tumour is handled, so reducing the systemic shower of cells. On the other hand the addition of a radical neck dissection adds to the amount of surgical trauma. Many patients with oral malignant neoplasms are elderly and may be in quite poor general condition as a result of chronic cardiovascular and pulmonary disease. Their ability to withstand the additional surgery must be considered. Furthermore, there is no convincing evidence that prophylactic block dissection improves the prognosis.

Primary neoplasms in some situations may metastasize to either or both sides of the neck (*Fig.* 26). Bilateral neck dissections have a materially more gloomy outlook in terms of survival and morbidity than the unilateral operation. Indeed the unilateral procedure occasions surprisingly little inconvenience to the patient once healing is complete.

For patients who have a primary at one of the sites susceptible to bilateral metastasis, such as lower lip and midline of floor of mouth, it is reasonable to delay a neck dissection until involved nodes are felt. If bilateral neck dissection becomes necessary, this may be performed as a staged procedure—performing the second side 3 weeks after the first. Even so, venous engorgement of the head may be seen and this is of course the major disability resulting from this treatment. Raised intracranial pressure due to venous engorgement may be treated by intravenous mannitol (Stell and Maran, 1972). Some surgeons suggest bilateral neck dissection with preservation of the internal jugular vein on one side, and this may be done. However, the fact that such a manoeuvre contravenes the principle of block removal of the tissues containing the lymph-nodes and lymphatics and takes the operator close to the malignant deposits must be recognized.

Suprahyoid block procedures are generally deprecated. However, a suprahyoid clearance almost inevitably forms a part of the local removal of neoplasms affecting the lower jaw, tongue or floor of mouth and may occasionally have a place where there is simultaneous involvement of submandibular nodes on both sides *without* detectable trouble in other groups of nodes (*Fig.* 26). By this means a bilateral full block may be avoided since if further metastatic nodes become apparent they may be on one side only.

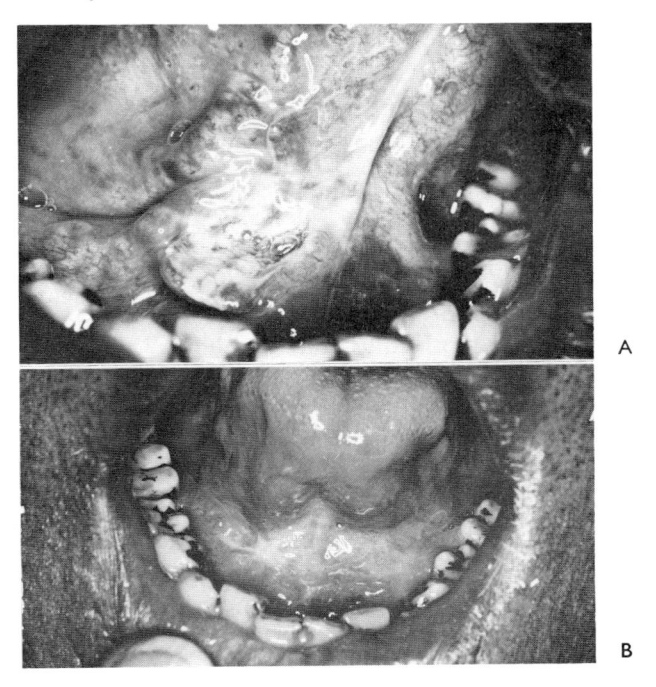

Fig. 26.—A, A small squamous-cell carcinoma in the floor of the mouth in a man of 28. Treated by a gold grain implant. B, The healed primary lesion.
He subsequently developed bilateral simultaneously-enlarged submandibular lymph-nodes which were adherent to the mandible. These were removed by a bilateral suprahyoid block which included the adjacent lower borders of the mandible. Four months postoperatively enlarged upper deep cervical nodes were noted on the right, and a right-side full neck dissection carried out. Since then (2 years) he has been free of further recurrence.

The seeding of viable cells into the operation wound from ulcerating surfaces or from accidental incisions closer than was intended to the tumour mass has given surgeons a good deal of food for thought. Thorough irrigation of the wound after resection is an important prophylaxis against local recurrence. Seeding by injudicious biopsy technique should be avoided, and the precept to remove part of the surrounding normal tissue to provide histological evidence of invasion is less strongly preached than in the past. Inadequate removal as a result of an attempted 'excision' biopsy is to be deprecated. The dissemination of cells via lymphatics or veins following the handling of the tumour also causes concern and severance of the venous drainage and lymphatic field before operative mobilization of the primary is good practice.

More recently an appreciation of the important role played by the patient's own immune mechanisms have tended to revise attitudes to accepted methods of treatment of malignancies. Most agents which attack malignant cells also damage the patient's immunological defences and the question of the degree to which these methods harm rather than help the patient is under debate. Thus cytotoxic drugs have fallen out of favour as a prophylaxis against metastatic spread as a result of cells shed at operation, because trials showed no benefit from this use of these agents. There are arguments against preoperative irradiation on the grounds that damage may be done to immune defences and spread of the neoplasm facilitated. Others (Lee and Wilson, 1973) advocate the use of preoperative radiotherapy so as to reduce the chance of successful growth of any cells shed at the operation.

Full therapeutic doses of irradiation undoubtedly reduce the vitality of the tissues in the treatment area. During the early post-irradiation period, haemorrhage at operation is increased and postoperative ooze is more persistent. Later, both soft tissues and bone withstand the trauma of surgery less well and the incidence of trouble with wound healing is increased. This particularly applies to the skin flaps over the neck. Four to 6 weeks after the completion of a full course of radiotherapy is the optimum time for surgery.

Palliative treatment covers a number of measures. Palliative radiotherapy alone is probably the best course of action. The primary neoplasm may be excised and pre- or post-operative irradiation given for a lesion where there is little hope of cure in the long term, but where such measures have been shown to give the patient a prolonged period of freedom from symptoms of his disease. Tumours which progress slowly, but which have already spread, or metastasized beyond the bounds of effective curative treatment, may be treated in this way. Pulmonary metastasis from muco-epidermoid or adenocystic carcinomas of salivary glands may increase in size very slowly and the patient may live for 3 to 6 years or more largely in ignorance of their presence.

Other primary neoplasms may be excised because their ultimate enlargement, fungation and necrosis would cause the patient great distress before death supervened. If this is done the surgeon must be reasonably sure that the risk of local recurrence following his operation is small and that the surgically-created defect and deformity is less unpleasant for the patient than the anticipated course of the disease. The cryo-probe also may be used to destroy fungating masses and so improve patient comfort.

Radiotherapy to the primary, to involved lymph-nodes and to distant metastases may be used. Such treatment may reduce pain, cause tumour masses to disappear—or at least result in a reduction in their size, or may restrain for a while their further growth—and pathological fractures may be encouraged to heal. Radiotherapy is the principle palliative measure for oral malignancies.

TREATMENT OF MALIGNANT NEOPLASMS

Cytotoxic agents have had a chequered career. In the case of Burkitt's Lymphoma, and leukaemias, progress has been made towards their curative treatment by cytotoxic drugs, often by the use of several such agents at the same time. For most solid tumours they can play only a palliative role and their side effects can be quite unpleasant. Examples of such side effects are marrow depression, gastro-intestinal disturbances, alopecia and oral ulceration. However, new drugs are constantly being produced and this is a fruitful field of research. Bleomycin is currently used in the palliation of squamous cell carcinoma.

Techniques of hormonal control of metastases are now part of standard treatment, particularly for carcinoma of breast and prostate. On occasions the first metastases from these neoplasms to manifest themselves are in the jaws.

Attempts to improve the patient's own immune response are being made, particularly as some aspects of the patient's immune defences can be quantified (Cannell, 1973). By vaccinating patients and other manoeuvres, attempts have been made to affect the course of metastatic malignant melanoma and with some limited improvements in some patients. Unfortunately the presence of large tumour masses overwhelms the patient's immunity so presenting a major stumbling-block to this form of treatment.

In the oral cavity, general dental surgeons can do much to keep the mouth and any neoplastic masses reasonably clean and inoffensive. All carious lesions need treatment, for further extractions should be avoided in case intra-bony neoplasm fungates through the socket, or in case post-irradiation osteomyelitis should be precipitated.

Pain from infection should be controlled by treating the infection, but pain due to infiltration of peripheral nerves needs effective control to prevent demoralization of the patient. Alcohol nerve blocks or peripheral nerve section can have a part to play, and the dentists' skills in giving a local anaesthetic, or the oral surgeon's skill in finding a peripheral nerve, may be required.

Analgesics, narcotics and tranquillizers may be needed to relieve chronic intractable pain and depression. Adequate control in this way of pain which cannot be relieved by other means is essential (Saunders, 1963). By the more central division of pain pathways the neurosurgeon may be able to help at times.

The management of the dying patient is not a skill which most dental surgeons have, fortunately, to employ very often. Medical general practitioners, radiotherapists and general surgeons and physicians are more skilled in this art. District nurses, social workers and the patient's religious minister are all people whose help and advice can be enlisted in the case of the terminal patient. Not least, of course, is the family necessary at this time, but relatives may in their turn seek support from the clinician. The booklet *People and Cancer* by The British Cancer Council (Bennette, 1970) is recommended reading on this subject.

Once progress of the disease has been halted and if possible when a reasonable likelihood of a cure has been achieved, reconstruction and rehabilitation become important. If surgical excision has been undertaken substantial reconstruction should be attempted at the same operation. Broadly speaking primary reconstruction can lay emphasis on either the hard or the soft tissues. Repair of both at the same time is not easily possible with current techniques. Clear advice on the repair of the soft tissues is given by Lee and Wilson (1973) and by Conley (1970). Use of the forehead flap and the deltopectoral flap to reconstruct the oral cavity and the face and neck respectively provides a standard method of repair which gives first-class results in expert hands. An adequate bulk of vascular soft tissue and a sufficient surface of epithelium is thus made available to avoid the displacement of the remaining tissues which adds to the patient's disability. The contour of the face can be restored also by this technique. However, since a seal of the wound is not achieved where the pedicles of these flaps enter the defect, simultaneous bone grafting carries a risk of infection of the graft.

Subsequent reopening of the operation area is not easy and re-establishment of space for a bone-graft at any site, once healing has occurred, can be quite difficult.

Function even without a bone-graft can be good, but too much must not be expected of such a repair. The crippling distortion of the remaining lips, cheek and part of the tongue may be avoided but the connective and adipose tissues of the flaps can never replace the functioning muscles and nerves of the original tissues.

Prefabricated metal prostheses can have a part to play where extensive resection of the mandible is necessary (Bowerman and Conroy, 1969; Cook, 1969), but allografts can be more demanding than bone-grafts in their requirements in terms of a suitable soft-tissue bed. They save the patient additional surgery at a time when extensive surgery is already necessary, but remain a buried foreign body and their eventual loss remains a permanent risk. Immediate bone-grafts too may fail since the conditions for their insertion are far from ideal, but once a successful take is achieved the chances of complications decrease and in this way they differ from allografts.

Various temporary allografts have been tried to provide stability of widely separated bone fragments. In particular prefabricated metal prostheses and temporary allografts have a place where extensive removal of tissues and mandible from the centre of the lower jaw is necessary. The use of temporary allografts may enable the best possible soft-tissue repair to be performed. Subsequently the prosthesis is removed through skin incisions, the graft bed enlarged and a bone-graft inserted, again with more favourable circumstances for survival of the graft. However, enlarging the channel for the graft and detaching the allograft from the bone ends in the face of dense postoperative fibrosis and without entering the mouth can be difficult. A bone-graft placed immediately after the resection and at the same operation occupies the maximum space and produces the best possible contour that can be achieved. The problem is soft-tissue coverage. The wound must be closed in layers and local flaps may produce difficulties with feeding, speech and saliva control, particularly if tongue flaps are used, until such time as secondary soft-tissue repair is possible. The choice therefore is between primary skeletal repair and secondary soft-tissue repair on the one hand and primary soft-tissue repair and secondary bone replacement on the other.

It must be emphasized once more that careful follow-up of the patients for the rest of their life is important, to detect recurrences, to look for evidence of metastases, or for evidence of fresh malignant neoplasms in adjacent or other sites and to record accurately the results of treatment so that rational patient management can evolve.

Following treatment of the malignancy and any necessary surgical reconstruction, the patient frequently needs prosthetic treatment, speech therapy and rehabilitation into normal social life. The construction of dentures raises a problem, for frequently the denture bearing area is abnormal and offers little scope for a retentive appliance. Thin, atrophic mucous membrane which is easily ulcerated, and a dry mouth, add to the difficulties. For some patients with widespread premalignant mucosal changes it is advisable that dentures are withheld. Both speech therapy and support of friends and relatives during the patient's return to work and during the re-establishment of social contacts is important if life is to take on a worthwhile quality.

In the case of the upper jaw the skeletal replacement is by means of an obturator with replacement of cheek only by means of suitable flaps. Provided the cavity can be maintained as a pyramidal shape the obturator will be retained in place. The inner surface of the wound is lined with a split-skin-graft on a gutta-percha bung supported on a temporary obturator.

Details of operative procedures are outside the scope of this book but can be found in standard reference works and papers. References to a few helpful publications are included in the bibliography at the end of this chapter (Conley, 1970; Stell and Maran, 1972; Lee and Wilson, 1973; Lore, 1973).

While general advice on treatment is to be found in published work, more than in any field a special assessment must be made of each patient's problem. An open mind, a willingness to try the unorthodox, if this seems in the patient's best interest, and a willingness to debate the patient's problem with colleagues and with the patient himself are necessary ingredients for a proper decision.

REFERENCES

BENNETTE, G. (ed.) (1970), *People and Cancer*. London: The British Cancer Council.
BOWERMAN, J. E., and CONROY, B. (1969), 'A Universal Kit in Titanium for Immediate Replacement of the Resected Mandible', *Br. J. oral Surg.*, **6**, 223.
CADE, SIR S. (1963), 'Cancer: the Patients' Viewpoint and the Clinicians' Problem', *Proc. R. Soc. Med.*, **56**, 1.
CANNELL, H. (1973), 'Oral Cancer and Immunity', *Br. J. Oral Surg.*, **11**, 171.
COOK, H. P. (1969), 'Titanium in Mandibular Replacement', *Ibid.*, **7**, 108.
CONLEY, J. (1970), *Concepts in Head and Neck Surgery*, p. 139. Stuttgart: Georg Thieme Verlag.
EASSON, E. C. (1963), 'Radiotherapy in Oral Cancer 1932–62', *Br. dent. J.*, **115**, 139.
FREUND, H. R. (1967), *Principles of Head and Neck Surgery*, p. 94. London: Butterworth.
LEE, S., and WILSON, J. S. P. (1973), 'Carcinoma involving the Lower Alveolus', *Br. J. Surg.*, **60**, 7.
LORE, J. M. (1973), *An Atlas of Head and Neck Surgery*, Vols. I and II. Philadelphia: Saunders.
SAUNDERS, C. (1963), 'The Treatment of Intractable Pain in Terminal Cancer', *Proc. R. Soc. Med.*, **56**, 195.
STELL, P. M., and MARAN, A. G. D. (1972), *Head and Neck Surgery*, p. 107. London: Heinemann Medical.

Chapter XV
SOME METHODS USED IN THE SURGICAL CORRECTION OF THE JAWS IN CASES OF FACIAL DEFORMITY

THE anomalies of the upper and lower jaws which constitute an unacceptable facial deformity in the patient's opinion and cause him or her to seek a surgical solution to the problem may be divided into the following categories:—
1. Patients with a receding chin.
2. Patients in whom there is a true or relative mandibular retrusion.
3. Patients in whom there is a true or relative mandibular protrusion.
4. Patients in whom the mandible deviates to one side or is otherwise asymmetrical.
5. Patients with a malocclusion unassociated with a gross skeletal malrelationship of the upper or lower jaw.

These abnormalities, the majority of which are simple growth aberrations, can be corrected surgically by means of onlays, inlays, osteotomies, and ostectomies with or without bone-grafts.

It should be appreciated that although the principal reason for an individual seeking corrective treatment is ugliness there are other problems which favour a surgical solution, such as masticatory difficulties, difficulty or the impossibility of providing prosthetic replacements for the natural teeth, speech defects, and soft-tissue trauma due to the malalinement of the teeth.

Age at which Operation should be performed.—It would seem logical in most cases to defer the operation for a jaw deformity until maturity is reached and maximum bone growth is achieved. If, however, a gross deformity of the jaws in a young patient is causing severe mental distress, a surgical correction should be performed, although the parents must be advised that a further operation may be necessary when facial growth is complete.

In cases of unilateral hyperplasia of the condyle leading to unilateral overgrowth of the mandible, operation at an early age will not only correct the deformity, but prevent further growth of the mandible. Condylectomy for this condition was first performed by Humphrey (1856) and has since become a recognized procedure (Rushton, 1946; Hovell, 1956; Taylor and Cook, 1958).

In cases of unilateral undergrowth of the mandible due to congenital causes, e.g., a first arch or other developmental defect or interference with the condylar growth centre from trauma or infection, the lack of mandibular growth gives rise to a secondary deformity of the maxilla on the affected side. In such cases serial bone-grafts between the bone-ends in the ramus following a vertical subsigmoid osteotomy will compensate for the lack of growth in the mandible and prevent the occurrence of secondary deformity of the maxilla. Possibly, in such a patient, two bone inlays may be required during the growth period of the facial skeleton.

1. The Receding Chin

Recession of the chin unassociated with micrognathia or retrognathism is uncommon, but moderate recession of the chin may occur as a hereditary characteristic in some families. It can also occur as a result of severe trauma to the chin, such as a comminuted fracture or where there has been bone loss, as in gunshot wounds of the lower jaw. It may also be the main complaint in patients who have a relative mandibular retrognathism and a small chin and in whom the dental abnormality has been treated orthodontically. The receding chin can be remedied surgically by: (*a*) Onlays on the mental prominence. (*b*) A sliding genioplasty. (*c*) A buccal inlay and prosthesis. (*d*) Bilateral osteotomy of the mandible followed by advancement of the anterior part of the mandible and bilateral bone-grafts to fill the resulting gaps.

a. Onlays to the chin may be in the form of: (i) Autografts, (ii) Homografts, (iii) Allelografts.

i. *Autograft Onlays.*—Onlay bone-grafts to the chin may be inserted from a submental or an intra-oral surgical approach (*Fig.* 27A). The submental approach has the disadvantage of leaving a scar beneath the chin, but by careful siting of the incision and closure of the wound, this scar can be made aesthetically acceptable. The intra-oral approach is made through an incision around the buccal side of the gingival margin of the anterior teeth or through an incision in the buccal sulcus. There is more risk of postoperative infection when the intra-oral route is used, but this risk is minimal when adequate doses of a suitable antibiotic are administered postoperatively. One of the problems of all onlay grafts of bone is that the graft may become resorbed in accordance with Wolf's law, through pressure of the overlying skin and tissue over the bone-graft. A chin which is built up with bone chips rapidly resumes its original contour through this mechanism and in order to overcome this tendency the tissue overlying the graft should have its tension on the graft reduced. This can be achieved by extensive undermining of the overlying skin and possibly the insertion of additional skin in the form of a graft beneath the chin. A slightly curved incision is made from one side of the mandible to the other beneath the chin with the convex aspect of the curve facing forward. The skin is undermined forwards over the chin so that tension over a graft will be relieved and then the defect beneath the mandible is grafted. This procedure has the disadvantage of leaving a skin deformity beneath the jaw.

A more simple and acceptable method is to use a block of iliac crest bone contoured with compact bone facing outwards against the overlying tissues. At operation a suitable bed is made in the bone of the mental prominence by removing cortical plate and exposing a cancellous bed. The cancellous underside of the bone onlay graft will then lie against cancellous tissue in the mandible. The compact bone of the outer aspect of the graft will resist the tissue pressures more satisfactorily than the chip grafts and will do this for a protracted period of time. Onlay blocks of bone-graft on the mental prominence are held in position by transosseous wiring at either end of the graft or with vitallium bone screws.

ii. *Homograft Onlays.*—Homograft onlays can be used to restore the mental prominence in a similar manner to the autograft onlays, but they

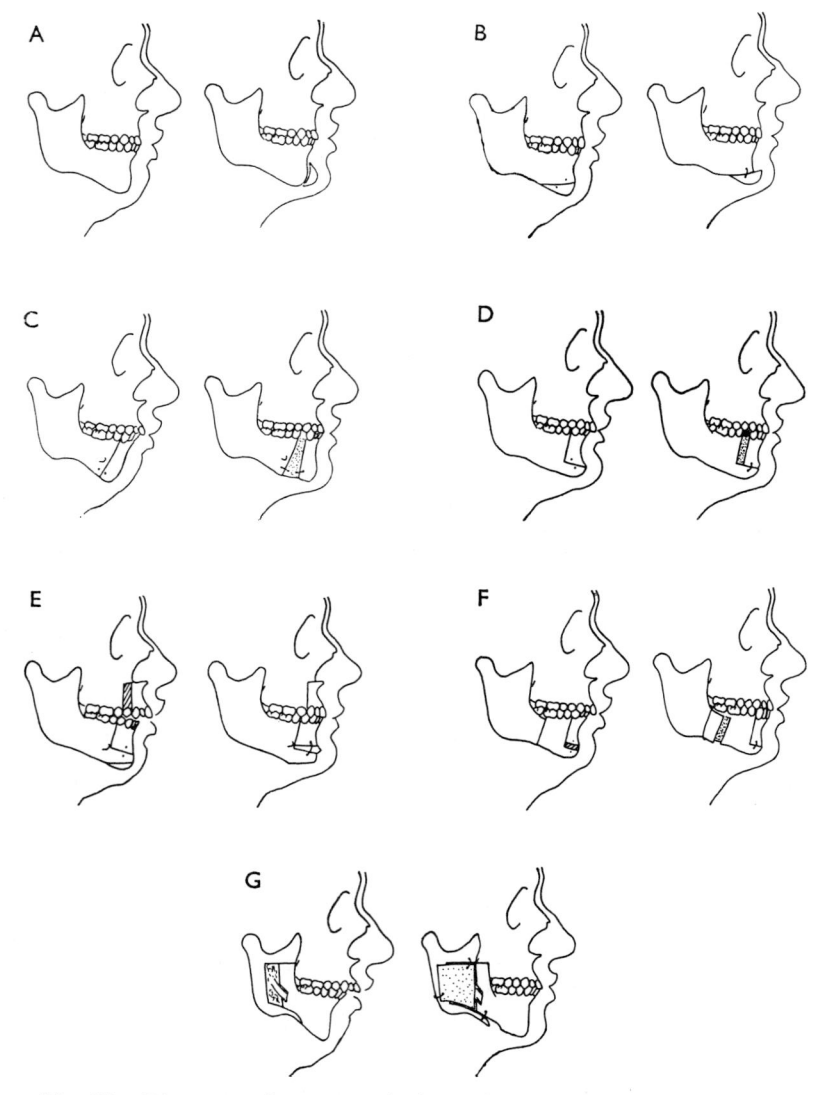

Fig. 27.—Diagrams of some methods used to treat relative mandibular retrognathism.
 A, The chin onlay. B, The sliding genioplasty. C, Body osteotomy and block graft. D, Advancement of the lower incisor segment with the placement of a graft and bridge. E, The Wassmund procedure on the premaxilla combined with the Köle procedure on the mandible. F, Advancement of the mandible using a sagittal splitting procedure combined with lowering of the lower incisor region. G, Seward's modification of the Caldwell procedure whereby a vertical osteotomy is combined with a block graft to advance the mandible.

have the added disadvantage of being less reliable than the autograft and more liable to be lost through infection.

iii. *Allelograft Onlays.*—The restoration of the mental prominence by means of allelografts is most unsatisfactory in the long term. Various allelografts, such as tantalum, stainless-steel, chrome cobalt, acrylic, nylon, teflon, terylene, wool, silastic, etc., have been tried and they may be inserted from an extra-oral or intra-oral route and fixed in position when applicable with transosseous wires or screws. They all have the disadvantage that sooner or later the allelograft either becomes a focus of infection or the patient receives a knock on the chin and the graft becomes partially extruded. Should the patient become edentulous there is the added risk that infection may reach the implant via ulceration under the denture. Infection supervenes, the graft has to be removed, and there is a sudden change for the worse in the patient's appearance. As a general rule allelografts, to be successful, must be deeply buried in the tissues as in the hip-joint, or the overlying skin must be relatively immobile as in the case of the scalp. Neither of these conditions obtain at the chin and on the whole results with allelografts are extremely disappointing in the long term. This is unfortunate, for their insertion is simple and the immediate improvement in the patient's appearance is excellent. Even where successful implantation is achieved, resorption of the bone under the graft tends to occur with a regression towards the original contour of the chin (Robinson and Shuken, 1969).

b. The Sliding Genioplasty.—Obwegeser (1957, 1969a, b) and others have described a sliding osteotomy where the bone is sectioned backwards from the chin and the lower fragment advanced to create a mental prominence (*Fig.* 27B).

An incision is made from 1st molar round to 1st molar. The junction of attached and sulcus mucosa is followed in the premolar region, but the incision passes on to the lip side of the sulcus anteriorly. In this latter part a submucosal flap is raised towards the jaw, and then the muscle penetrated down on to the periosteum. After the mandible has been 'de-gloved' the periosteum is divided around the mental nerves and vessels and these structures released, outwards towards the lip. Any double chin is mobilized by dissection deep to the platysma, well into the neck, and a wrinkled chin smoothed out by cross-hatching the periosteum beneath it. The proposed bone cut is outlined with a bur and should extend from 1st molar to 1st molar region. It may be angled to adjust the final height of the chin and the section made with a Stryker saw. If necessary a median vertical cut is made and the advancement achieved by wiring the buccal cortex of the upper fragment to the lingual of the lower. The wound is closed in two layers with vacuum drainage and a pressure dressing applied.

c. The Buccal Inlay.—The buccal inlay is a relatively simple surgical procedure which, used in conjunction with a mandibular prosthesis, enables a very acceptable restoration of the chin to be achieved. This procedure is particularly useful where there has been gross loss of genial bone. First, a surgical pocket is created in the buccal sulcus. An incision is made in the buccal sulcus about $\frac{1}{4}$ in. from the gingival margin and is extended parallel to the gingival margin from about the 1st molar region on the one side to a similar position on the opposite side of the jaw. The incision is made down to but not through the periosteum, and then deepened towards the lower border of the mandible superficial to the periosteum. This creates a large pocket in the sulcus which is maintained by filling the pocket with a black gutta-percha mould which is held in place with a perforated German silver plate on its upper surface, the plate being in turn secured either to a silver copper alloy cap splint on the teeth or, if the patient is edentulous, to a lower plate held in position by two circumferential wires in the canine region. The raw area over the periosteum is grafted with a split skin-graft taken from the inside of the patient's arm or thigh, two areas which are not normally hair-bearing. The split skin-graft is draped over the gutta-percha bung with its raw surface, of course, facing the raw area over the periosteum and the gutta-percha mould, which is in turn fixed by the prosthesis, holds the skin-graft in place until it has healed over the raw periosteum. This part of the healing process takes about seven days, and at the end of this time the gutta-percha bung is removed and cleaned with soap and water and the graft is inspected. The buccal pocket is then gently irrigated with saline and the gutta-percha mould is replaced. For convenience, a screw device is attached to the splint or plate to enable the German silver plate which holds the bung in position to be removed and replaced easily. Skin-grafts in the mouth have a great tendency to shrink and only become stable after some months. In the early days after grafting, therefore, the gutta-percha bung should only be left out for short periods. After a few weeks the graft becomes more firmly established and the gutta-percha bung can then be replaced with an acrylic prosthesis.

Meticulous attention to oral hygiene must be paid in the first weeks after grafting, for infection can rapidly destroy the graft. Infection, when present, is usually caused by coliform-type organisms, and irrigation of the buccal pocket with warm 1 per cent eusol solution is most efficacious. Small areas of sprouting granulation tissue appearing in the graft should be touched with a silver nitrate stick. The patient should be taught to change the bung every three or four days once the graft has begun to settle. If the graft is of a considerable size, it may be desirable to carry out the first change under a short general anaesthetic. The gutta-percha bung is resilient and will not cause a pressure sore on the graft, provided that it has an even surface. To provide a uniformly smooth surface and create a bung without crevices which might harbour bacteria, the appliance should be made with sealed edges. This is achieved by taking a sheet of gutta-percha, which has been softened in boiling water and then folded in half. The free edges are then trimmed with a large pair of scissors. Cutting along the edges in this manner produces a perfect seal. The gutta-percha is then folded again and the process repeated with the scissors. When a bung of roughly the correct size is achieved final trimming is carried out with scissors and again a perfect seal is attained, so that the final mould has no crevices. As gutta-percha is impervious to fluids the temporary appliance will remain sanitary even after it has been in the mouth for several weeks. This is certainly not the case if crevices exist in the mould such as those which occur when the material is trimmed with a hot knife.

It is important to remember that as acrylic is hard and unresilient, if the final prosthesis to restore the chin is fitted too early, i.e., when the skin-graft still has a tendency to contract, it will cause pressure ulcers on the surface of the graft. This inevitably leads on to infection and partial or total loss of the graft. When the skin-graft is completely stable a prosthesis is constructed which restores the normal contour of the chin. If the patient is edentulous this can be incorporated in the lower denture, and takes the form of a downward projection of the anterior part of the lower denture, into the newly created 'pocket'. The buccal inlay and prosthesis is a most satisfactory method of restoring chin contour.

d. Bilateral Osteotomy of the Body of the Mandible with Advancement of the Anterior Fragment and Bilateral Bone-grafts to fill the Defect.—A vertical body osteotomy is made bilaterally at some convenient point between the canines and the 1st molars, if necessary after liberation of the inferior dental nerve. The soft tissues are widely undermined beneath the platysma, the periosteum divided along the line of the bone cuts, and the anterior fragment tilted to put the chin into its correct position. Carefully cut block iliac crest bone-grafts are inserted into the gaps so created and wired in place. The fragments are further supported by firm inter-maxillary fixation and this should be maintained for six weeks. Some trimming of the anterior fragment may be necessary to avoid a step in the lower border of the mandible. The technique lacks the bone-to-bone contact of the original jaw fragments which is achieved by other techniques and is technically weak on this account. It is essential, therefore, that the pull of the muscles attached to the anterior fragment should be resisted until firm union has been achieved (*Fig.* 27C).

2. Patients in whom there is a True or Relative Mandibular Retrusion

Micrognathia is seen in an extreme form in the Pierre-Robin syndrome, but moderate recession of the chin is found as a hereditary characteristic in some families. Marked micrognathia is also present in the rare phenomenon of a bilateral 'first arch' defect and in such cases there is an associated deformity of the tragus of the ear with the presence of accessory auricles together with an anomaly of the malleus and incus on each side. In more severe cases there is almost complete absence of the middle and inner ears, hypoplasia of the soft tissues, skin scarring, hypoplasia of the nerves, macrostomia, and other disturbances suggesting a more widespread deficiency, possibly vascular in origin. Failure of growth of the mandible may also be caused by interference with the condylar growth centre of the mandible following trauma, infection, or irradiation. The more usual types of patient seeking correction of relative mandibular retrusion are those with an Angle's Class II malocclusion for whom orthodontic treatment has not been successful.

Bilateral osteotomy of the ramus above the level of the lingula for the correction of mandibular retrusion was originally described by Blair (1907), but experience has shown that following this operation there is a great tendency for the anterior fragment to relapse owing to muscular pull. A sliding step-like osteotomy was described by Nicolsky in which an L-shaped cut was made with the short arm of the L passing down vertically from the upper border in the 3rd molar region, and the long arm horizontally backwards. The anterior fragment was displaced forwards, the posterior border of the angle wired to the front of the posterior fragment. A Z-shaped osteotomy of the body of the mandible with the long arm passing horizontally forwards and the short arms passing up to the alveolar margin at the back and down to the lower border at the front was described by Eiselsberg in 1907. He wired the fragments end to end, but Pehrgadd (1965), who made the posterior vertical cut behind the last molar, wired the fragments after displacement across the long horizontal cut. The operation can be improved by working the horizontal cut through the bed of the inferior dental canal and thence vertically down to the lower border below the premolars (Dingman, 1948). Pichler (1948) makes a similar cut but with the vertical limbs at the opposite ends of the horizontal ones. After the mandible is sectioned, the anterior fragment is made to slide forwards to correct the mandibular recession. Owing to the slope of the long arm of the L osteotomy, bone contact is maintained. Firm, exact splinting is essential to ensure bony union with the anterior fragment in its new position since the muscle forces on the chin exert a strong downwards and backwards pull.

A bilateral body osteotomy with advancement of the anterior fragments and bone-grafting of the gap was advocated by Limberg (1928) and Axhausen (1939). In extreme cases it may be necessary to insert skin beneath the mandible by pedicle grafting in order to relieve the skin tension on the mental prominence in its new position. Correction of micrognathia by this procedure is an extensive surgical exercise, but can give a good cosmetic result when successfully completed, apart from submandibular scarring and some degree of residual anaesthesia of the lower lip.

Trauner and Obwegeser (1957) devised an L-shaped division of the ramus and inserted a bilateral bone-graft between the bone-ends. This operation is, of course, carried out through a submandibular incision. Caldwell and Amaral (1960) have described an operation for the correction of mandibular retrognathism which is a modification of a vertical sub-sigmoid osteotomy in the rami. The technique follows the usual pattern of vertical section of the rami. The bone-ends are decorticated, the body of the mandible is advanced to a predetermined functional relationship with the maxilla. An autogenous iliac bone-graft is cut and inserted so that it is inlayed both into the decorticated areas and into the gap created in the rami. Obwegeser (1964) has used his sagittal splitting osteotomy of the ramus to elongate the mandible and this technique has the advantage that neither skin incisions nor bone-grafts are required.

After discussing in general terms the treatment of retrognathism, it is important to mention the guiding principles used in selecting the treatment for individual types of cases.

1. Patients with a receding or small chin, but with a relatively normal articulation of the teeth as a result of orthodontic treatment. This condition is corrected by chin augmentation using one of the following alternatives: (*a*) Onlay graft, (*b*) Allelograft, (*c*) Sliding genioplasty (*Fig.* 27 A, B).

2. Patients with a post-normal occlusion. The two types are treated as follows:—

   a. Angle's Class II, division 1:—

      i. Where the mandible and chin are well formed (e.g., true maxillary protrusion); by a Wassmund procedure reducing the prominence of the premaxilla (*Fig. 27E*).

  ii. Where the mandible is sizeable, but the chin small; by a Wassmund procedure on the premaxilla and a sliding genioplasty.

  iii. Where the mandible is sizeable and the chin prominent, by advancement of the canine and incisor alveolar segment only. Bone-grafts and bridges or a denture are used to fill the gaps in the alveolar process and dental arch (*Fig.* 27D).

  iv. Where there is obvious mandibular retrognathism, by an Obwegeser sagittal splitting osteotomy with advancement of the mandible. The lower incisor segment may be lowered and chin contour improved as necessary by a Köle procedure.

  b. Developmental.—Treatment often has a poor chance of success because soft-tissue deficiency and lack of muscle may accentuate the deformity particularly during movement.

  i. Serial bone-grafts in a ramus osteotomy.

  ii. Köle and oblique body slide and graft.

  iii. Grafts of growing bone-end, either fibula, rib, or clavicle.

Receding Chin (*Fig.* 27).—For some patients with mandibular retrognathism the complaint is mainly of a lack of chin prominence. It is frequently the case that orthodontics has been undertaken in childhood and an acceptable arrangement of the teeth achieved. Thus, not only would any alteration of jaw position need reversal of the orthodontic treatment, since without an incisal overjet mandibular advancement is impossible, but clearly such a course is unnecessary. A genioplasty is all that is required. Of the three types of procedure available for this, the sliding genioplasty is the one which is most successful, probably because the bone is mainly cortical bone and because the bulk of the mandible remains unaltered, merely changed in shape.

Maxillary Protrusion.—Certain cases of relative mandibular retrognathism due to such factors as maxillary protrusion, or a lower dental arch which is more posteriorly placed than usual on the mandible, may be successfully corrected, or disguised by procedures devised by Wassmund, Wunderer, and Köle. These techniques mobilize the premaxilla or the lower anterior alveolar segments. Where the patient has a mandible of normal or near normal size and a good chin prominence, a premaxillary osteotomy is indicated.

The original operation was described by Wassmund (1935), and variations of this procedure have been reported by Schuchardt (1954), Wunderer (1962), Murphy and Walker (1963), Cradock-Henry (1966), Straith and Lawson (1967), Matras (1967), and Markwell (1967). The operation should be considered in patients with marked maxillary protrusion and sound anterior teeth. An osteotomy is carried out in the upper 1st premolar area, after which the anterior fragment is repositioned. Sometimes a similar procedure has to be carried out in the lower incisor region if there is an associated deep overbite.

Operative Technique.—The upper 1st premolars, or other suitable teeth, are extracted and a slice of bone of predetermined width cut from the palate and the buccal sides of the maxillary alveolar process so as to include their sockets. Both the buccal and palatal bone cuts are made with suitable burs working from the buccal side; the soft tissues of the palate being tunnelled to a minimal extent sufficient to allow the insertion of a protective retractor. If better access to the middle of the palate is required a median incision can be made. In some cases a nasal re-fracture saw is suitable for making the palatal cuts. The buccal cuts are carried forwards horizontally above the apices of the teeth to the lateral margin of the anterior bony aperture of the nose. The anterior part of the nasal septum is approached through a vertical midline incision into the labial frenum. If it is necessary for the upper anterior segment to be widened to accommodate the lower arch after it has been repositioned, a vertical midline cut is made between the upper central incisors using thin burs and special small osteotomes. Alternatively, the inter-canine width can be increased preoperatively by orthodontic means. If the premaxilla is to be split this must be completed before the nasal septum is divided. The latter manœuvre is accomplished with an osteotome introduced above the anterior nasal spine. After the anterior fragment has been freed it is repositioned and held in its new position with splints or orthodontic bands and arch bars until bony union occurs. Both the height and angulation of the upper incisors can also be adjusted during the operation. One point which must be noted is the size of the nose. These patients may well have a large one, with an obvious hump, and the reduction in size of the maxilla will increase its prominence.

Alveolar ostectomy for maxillary protrusion may be performed as a two-stage procedure and this has been recommended by Schuchardt (1954), Cradock-Henry (1966) and Mohnac (1966), but according to Barton and Rayne (1969) the single stage operation does not prejudice the blood-supply to the anterior fragment. Indeed, the two-stage procedure is illogical since the blood-supply from the greater palatine artery is damaged during the first operation and the healed wound will not compensate for this before the second stage must be performed.

Choice of Operation for Maxillary Protrusion.—If the patient's upper incisors and canines are carious, heavily filled, root filled, crowned, or in other ways unsightly, it may be more satisfactory to extract them and carry out an intra-septal alveolotomy so that they may be replaced by a denture. If the patient has an excellent set of anterior teeth the alveolar ostectomy is usually the treatment of choice, but as with other osteotomies there should be a full discussion with the patient about what is involved.

Retrusion of the Lower Dental Arch.—If the patient has a mandible of normal length and a good chin, but the lower dental arch is too far back, advancement of the lower anterior segment of the mandible will produce the required result (*Fig.* 27D). Sometimes a concurrent operation on the premaxilla will be necessary to adjust the angulation of the upper incisors.

Mandibular Retrognathism.—Treatment of the Angle's Class II, division 1 malocclusion with mandibular retrognathism requires a more elaborate sequence of treatment. In the preparatory phase the inter-canine and inter-premolar width of the maxillary arch is expanded orthodontically if this is necessary to accommodate the mandible in the new position. At the same time the inclination of the upper incisors is reduced, the spaces between them closed, and the lower incisors slightly depressed. It is useful to over-expand the inter-premolar and canine width a little, but excessive retraction of the incisors must be avoided, or adequate advancement of the mandible will be impossible. Some further reduction in the height of the lower incisors can be achieved by the grinding of their incisal edges. Finally, at operation the lower incisor alveolar process is separated, and a strip removed from below it so that the whole segment can be lowered. The excised strip can be added to the chin, if desired, to increase its prominence. Alternatively, if the overeruption of the lower incisors is not too marked the mandible may be placed so that the lower incisors contact the palatal surfaces of the uppers and the molar occlusal surfaces are in contact. Provided the open bite in the pre-molar region is not too great the teeth will come into contact within a year to 18 months as a result of various tooth movements (Hovell, 1970). Bilateral sagittal splitting procedures of the ramus permit the jaw to be advanced to the new position. Localization and immobilization of the lower incisor segment is by pre-localized and soldered locking plates and intermaxillary fixation by sectioned-tube quick-release locking plates Seward and Foreman (1972) (*Fig.* 27F).

Class II, division 2 patients are less often concerned about the distal position of the mandible since the retroclination of the upper central incisors is an effective disguise. Even so, the deep overbite can result in damage to the periodontal attachment of both upper and lower incisors and surgical rearrangement of the position of the appropriate alveolar segments can be used to overcome the problem.

Extreme Retrognathia.—Provided that the agent which resulted in the extreme retrognathia did not also damage the soft tissues unduly, advancement of the mandible may be successful. Considerable forward movement of the mandible using an Obwegeser sagittal splitting osteotomy results in lateral displacement of the posterior fragments by the anterior one. Moderate advancement, therefore, should be used together with a sliding genioplasty to increase the chin prominence.

The Trauner inverted L osteotomy of the ramus may be used, with a bone-graft, but to gain stable bone-to-bone contact a long additional cut is made forwards just short of the lower border (Seward, 1970) (*Fig.* 27G). In other cases Eiselsberg's and Pichler's Z-shaped body osteotomy is used with bone-grafts at the upper border distal to the 3rd molar and at the lower border below the premolars. To retain sensation in the lower lip the mental nerve is dissected out in continuity with the inferior dental and freed from the bone by cutting the incisive branch. Even so the nerve may be stretched and lip sensation reduced.

If developmental deficiencies are tackled, the chances of relapse must be understood by all concerned. Care must be taken to assess the part played by soft-tissue deficiencies for these may require additional procedures such as epithelial inlays, padding, and onlay grafting to disguise them. Serial grafting in the ramus is the usual procedure, but a Köle operation may be used to reduce the height of the lower incisors and alter the chin shape, combined with an oblique body slice to elongate the mandible. Grafts of growing bone ends are not yet out of the experimental stage.

3. Patients in whom there is a True or Relative Mandibular Protrusion

Mandibular protrusion is one of the most common anomalies of the jaw requiring surgical correction. The symmetrically prognathous patient may have this jaw relationship because the mandible is too long or too far forward in relation to a normal maxilla. In some patients the lower dental arch is too far forward, but the remainder of the mandible, including the point of the chin, is not. Most prognathic patients have some degree of underdevelopment of the maxilla, but in a few the mandible is entirely normal in position and shape, and is opposed by a maxilla which is noticeably too far back.

Of course, the deformity may be familial, as in the case of the Habsburgs, but often no other members of the family are affected. The condition may vary from a simple Class III malocclusion without an obvious external deformity to gross mandibular protrusion which interferes with eating and speaking and results in extreme ugliness. In its pronounced form the patient's facies have the heavy coarse appearance of the acromegalic. Mandibular protrusion, except in its most mild form, is usually disfiguring in females, but so far as men are concerned much depends upon the size of the man. A small man with a protruding jaw tends to look abnormal, but a similar degree of mandibular protrusion in a very tall, heavily-built man appears perfectly natural and there is, therefore, no necessity to operate on such a patient merely because the lower teeth bite in front of the uppers. It is also unjustifiable to advise an operation for a patient who has not experienced any difficulty with eating or speaking and has no worries about his appearance.

The operation of bilateral osteotomy or ostectomy is a sizeable surgical procedure and should not be undertaken lightly, especially since the selected procedure is often for cosmetic improvement rather than function and is not without risk, including even mortality.

Preoperative Assessment

In all cases where there is gross mandibular protrusion the possibility of a diagnosis of acromegaly must be considered. This is a comparatively rare disease in which there is hypersecretion by the anterior lobe of the pituitary due to an eosinophil adenoma, the influence being effective after ossification is complete. The patient may complain of temporal headaches, photophobia, and reduction of the lateral visual fields (bitemporal optic hemianopia), and eventual optic atrophy. The terminal phalanges of the feet and hands become large, the lips become thick, and enlargement of the tongue leads to indentations or crenations on its sides from pressure against the teeth. Overgrowth of the lower jaw together with the thickening of the lips gives rise to a very characteristic facies. The hands eventually become spade-like and a lateral radiograph of the skull shows uniform expansion of the sella turcica. There is also enlargement of the nose, supra-orbital ridges, frontal sinus, and superior nuchal line. Should the adenoma occur before the epiphyses have fused, gigantism will result and this possibility must be considered whenever mandibular protrusion is associated with excessive general growth of the patient.

Many diverse methods of preoperative evaluation of mandibular protrusion have been described, many of which are unnecessarily complex. This is especially true if too much emphasis is given to a purely orthodontic assessment of the case, for a satisfactory profile achieved by operation sometimes bears little relationship to a purely theoretical normal occlusion. In this respect the study of soft-tissue true lateral radiographs of the jaws with the teeth in a closed position is most helpful.

A relatively simple method of selecting the most appropriate type of operation in any particular case of mandibular protrusion is to begin by taking an accurate true lateral radiograph of the jaws with the teeth in occlusion. This is laid on an X-ray viewing screen and a tracing of the outline of the upper and lower jaws is made with tracing paper. The tracing must include the upper and lower teeth in occlusion. Several patterns in thick brown paper are then cut from the tracing of the lower jaw and these should, of course, include the lower teeth. With a pair of scissors it is then possible to section the brown paper patterns through various parts of the ramus, angle, or body. That portion of the paper pattern representing the condyle, coronoid process, and upper end of the ramus is then laid over the appropriate marking on the original tracing paper and the anterior fragment of pattern is positioned so that the lower teeth are in a corrected position in relation to the upper jaw. It will be immediately apparent that certain types of osteotomy or ostectomy would be useless in achieving the required result. For instance, a trial horizontal section through the ramus may be seen to result in lack of bony contact between the severed ends of the ramus after the body of the mandible has been displaced backwards for the appropriate distance. This method also allows the extent of a body ostectomy to be visualized. To do this the paper pattern is sectioned vertically in the lower 1st molar area after which the anterior part of the pattern is moved forwards on the tracing to its original position. The gap between the two parts of the pattern will represent the amount of bone which will have to be removed to correct the mandibular prognathism. By playing with several patterns and observing the probable results of the various operation sections, the most suitable operation can be selected for any particular case. Impressions should then be taken of the upper and lower teeth and plaster-of-Paris casts mounted on an articulator, the bite having been taken with a squash wax bite. The routine after this depends on the operator's experience and the complexity of the case.

If the section is to be made through the ramus or angle, duplicate plaster-of-Paris models are mounted on a backslab of plaster with the teeth in the proposed postoperative occlusion. Sometimes this occlusion is not satisfactory and in order to achieve an acceptable occlusion one or more teeth must be trimmed. Before operation this will, of course, necessitate the grinding or even extraction of these teeth so that a similar postoperative position can be attained. If a section of the body of the mandible is contemplated, duplicate models are again positioned using a backslab of plaster but this time in the preoperative occlusion. The central part of the lower model is cut out with a pad saw, leaving only the plaster teeth and alveolar process in the form of a U. This lower model is positioned at its base with another detachable slab of plaster fixed at right angles to the backslab. The lower model is then sectioned vertically through the lower 1st molar area and the posterior part of the model is correctly positioned in relation to the upper model and secured in position with the back and lower plaster slabs. The anterior part of the lower model is cut back at either end using a saw or an emery wheel until the incisor teeth can be made to occlude with the teeth on the upper model in a satisfactory position, while the distal end of the anterior part of the lower model touches the anterior ends of the posterior portions of the lower model. If the anterior fragment is then brought forwards to its original position on the lower plaster slab, the gap between the two ends of the plaster model will represent the amount to be removed from the body of the mandible in order to complete a satisfactory ostectomy. A template should be made from metal and a German silver wire handle is attached. This is used to measure the exact area to be removed at operation.

Where the case is complex or where the operator is comparatively inexperienced, full stone models of the mandible should be constructed with the aid of impressions, tracing from radiographs, and clinical measurements. This is because what happens in three dimensions cannot always be judged from consideration in two dimensions. If this precaution is not taken, an impasse may be reached at the time of the operation.

Choice of Operation

Shortening of the mandible is by far the most common procedure undertaken to correct facial deformity. A multiplicity of osteotomies (simple section through the bone) and ostectomies (excision of a portion of the bone) have been advocated for the surgical correction of mandibular protrusion since Hullihen (1849) reported the correction of a case of anterior open bite by a partial resection of the alveolar process. Since that time, osteotomies and ostectomies of every part of the ramus and body of the mandible have been described. In other aspects of medicine or surgery, whenever an excessive number of different methods of treatment are advocated, it usually means that there is no absolutely satisfactory form of treatment and this is also the case with the operations for surgical correction of prognathism.

In view of the wide variety of operations which can be used to correct mandibular prognathism, difficulty may be experienced in selecting the ideal operation for any particular patient. Many surgeons may have a personal preference for a particular operation or find that they obtain more satisfactory results from a certain technique. For example, the subsigmoid or oblique ramus osteotomy or the Obwegeser sagittal split operation can be adapted for use in most cases of mandibular protrusion. However, certain operations are more suitable for certain types of mandibular prognathism, and in order to ascertain the most suitable operation in any particular case a careful study must be made of the radiographs, tracings, and study models.

In certain cases it will be found after study of the radiographs, tracings, and models that several different types of operation would achieve the desired result, while in other cases only one particular type of section will have any chance of success. Much time and thought should be devoted to this preliminary study of all available data before coming to a decision about the type of operation to be performed. Other important considerations are:—

1. Should the Section be made Blind or under Direct Vision through an Open Wound?—The blind section of the mandible was popularized by

Kostecka (1931). In his technique, a Gigli saw is passed through the skin and around the ramus with a special introducer and a horizontal section is made above the lingula. The operation is rapid and relatively easy to perform, but it is difficult to control the position of the upper fragment which tends to be lifted anteriorly by the pull of the temporalis muscle and the subsequent lack of bony contact between the bone-ends leads in some cases to a prolonged period before union occurs. In some instances union never occurs. Carelessly used, the Gigli saw may damage branches of the facial nerve and there have been instances in which the maxillary artery was severed. As a result of its high relapse rate, this surgical technique has gone out of fashion and has been replaced by section under direct vision through an open operation.

2. If an Open Operation is to be used should an Extra-oral or Intra-oral Surgical Approach be made to the Mandible?—Extra-oral incisions give an excellent view of the mandible, but inevitably leave an external scar no matter how carefully the incision is sited and the wound repaired. In a keloid former the result could be disastrous and it would seem illogical to produce a cosmetic deformity in the performance of an essentially cosmetic operation.

The approach to the ramus is made through a submandibular incision at the angle, after which the masseter muscle is detached from its insertion to the lower end of the ramus which is then exposed in its entirety. The body of the mandible is approached by a submandibular incision of varying length depending upon the nature of the operation, but it is seldom less than 5 cm. long. Both the incisions to expose the ramus and the body must be made a finger's breadth or 2 cm. beneath the lower border of the mandible and the mandibular branch of the facial nerve preserved and retracted if it crosses the field of operation. Inadvertent neurotmesis of this branch leads to an ugly postoperative drooping of the corner of the lower lip. Careful suturing of the incisions by making use of skin creases will help to disguise the resultant scars beneath the jaws. One solution to this problem was suggested by the late Sir Harold Gillies (1955), who approached the mandible surgically through a long 'face lift' type incision sited mainly in the hairline and only coming on to the face immediately anterior to the external ear. This technique provides good surgical access and leaves minimal scarring, but is technically difficult and time-consuming.

The intra-oral approach to the mandible is certainly very simple, as the bone lies immediately beneath the mucoperiosteum. The ramus can be approached by a vertical incision down the anterior aspect of the ramus from just below the tip of the coronoid process across the retromolar fossa into the buccal sulcus. The body of the mandible is exposed through an incision of suitable length along the crest of the ridge in the edentulous jaw and around the buccal and lingual gingival margins when teeth are standing. Such an incision will give excellent exposure of the body of the mandible. A buccal incision around the gingival margin from $\overline{6\text{--}1|1\text{--}6}$ will enable the entire chin to be exposed. The arguments against this surgical approach are:—

a. Risk of Infection.—However, provided bone fragments are removed from the wound and haematoma formation is avoided, there is little risk of infection, particularly if the mouth is clean and suitable antibiotic cover is given.

b. There is Limited Access.—The access from an intra-oral approach is quite adequate for an experienced oral surgeon, but would be more difficult for a surgeon more familiar with surgery in some other regions. Advantages of the intra-oral route are:—

i. Lack of visible scars. Some patients find such scars as aesthetically embarrassing as the original mandibular protrusion.

ii. The operation is carried out within the periosteal sheath with a reduced risk to certain anatomical structures.

iii. Both the occlusal relationship of the jaws and the bone-ends are visible at the same time and a satisfactory arrangement of both more readily achieved.

It is obvious that the size of the oral cavity and rima oris greatly affect the access by this route and must be taken into account.

3. Should the Bone-ends be wired together following Section?—If the mandible is sectioned by an osteotomy or an ostectomy and the anterior fragment is repositioned, the sectioned bone-ends seldom lie naturally in such a position that rapid bony union is encouraged. Following a horizontal section of the ramus, the anterior aspect of the superior fragment tends to be pulled upwards by the temporalis muscle leaving little contact between the bone-ends. Oblique section or subsigmoid osteotomy tends to leave compact bone in contact with compact bone, and a similar condition occurs with the horizontal osteotomy of the ramus in many instances. Osteotomy through the neck of the mandibular condyle usually results in little bony contact and greatly delayed bony union occurs. For this reason this method has been largely discarded as a treatment for mandibular prognathism.

Vertical ostectomies of the body of the mandible usually result in the anterior portion of the mandible being sited within and below the posterior portions of the body of the mandible. This results in inadequate bony contact between the bone-ends with resulting protracted healing or even fibrous or non-union. Some authorities (Fickling and Fordyce, 1955) advocate grafting with bone chips to accelerate healing in such cases. However, if adequate contact between the bone-ends is obtained, the surgical fracture of the mandible produced by an ostectomy heals just as rapidly and firmly as any other traumatic fracture of the mandible. Satisfactory union should occur in six weeks.

Delayed healing can even occur in the sagittal split type operations if there is separation of the cancellous surfaces by soft tissue. It has been suggested that transosseous wiring carries a risk of infection, but with good operative technique no such trouble is experienced. In all cases of osteotomy or ostectomy, therefore, it is advantageous to achieve and maintain bony contact of the opposing bone ends by transosseous wiring with stainless-steel wire.

4. Sacrifice of Teeth in Body Ostectomy.—It should be remembered that if an operation is performed on the body of the mandible some teeth (usually the 2nd premolars or 1st molars) will have to be sacrificed in order that an ostectomy can be carried out. When working from an intra-oral approach, the teeth to be extracted may be removed at the time the ostectomy is performed, but in most other cases it is preferable to remove the teeth in question and then allow the area to heal before performing the ostectomy.

If a ramus osteotomy or ostectomy is to be performed, any unerupted lower 3rd molars must be removed first, for when the body of the mandible is pushed backwards such teeth would be sited well beneath the ramus and their subsequent extraction would be rendered difficult.

Types and Sites of Operations

Over the years a multiplicity of operations has been described for the surgical correction of mandibular prognathism and few sites in the mandible have escaped the attention of the surgeon. For example, bilateral resection of the condyle was suggested by Berger (1897) and Jaboulay and Berard (1898) and by Dufourmentel (1921). Osteotomy of the condylar neck was used by Kostecka (1931) (*Fig.* 28A), while Smith and Johnson (1940) suggested the removal of a small rectangle of bone from the sigmoid notch (*Fig.* 28B). Bilateral osteotomy of the ramus above the lingula was originally described by Blair (1907) for correction of mandibular retrusion, but was used for the correction of mandibular protrusion by Babcock (1909) (*Fig.* 28C, D). Since this time numerous variations of this operation have been carried out from a 'blind' extra-oral route by Henry (1946) and Clarkson (1955), while Kazanzian (1951) suggested an angulated cut in the anteroposterior direction made obliquely from the medial to the lateral aspect in order to obtain a wider area of bone contact.

Subperiosteal osteotomy via the intra-oral route was advocated originally by Ernst (1927). Skaloud (1951) advocated an extra-oral and intra-oral approach to the section by passing a Gigli saw from the skin behind the jaw into the mouth. He also wired the bone-ends together by passing a wire over the sigmoid notch to a hole drilled through the lower end of the ramus. Obwegeser (1957) has devised an intra-oral subperiosteal operation whereby a sagittal split of the ramus is performed. At the suggestion of Dal Pont he moved the buccal cortical cut from the ramus to the body of the mandible, increasing the area of the part which is split (Obwegeser, 1964; Dal Pont, 1958, 1961). This operation not only enables the body of the mandible to be advanced or retropositioned, but also an anterior open bite can be corrected. In all cases a considerable area of raw bone is in apposition to a similar area on the opposing fragment and healing is therefore expedited. (*Fig.* 29G.)

Body ostectomy is the procedure used to shorten the mandible in the region of the dental arch. (*Fig.* 29B.) The operation, done from an extra-oral approach was described by Angle (1898) and Blair (1907). The latter originally performed the operation as long ago as 1897 and the method has since been adopted by numerous oral surgeons. As this operation inevitably resulted in an intra-oral wound continuous with the extra-oral tissues, Ballin (1908) suggested removing the tooth or teeth at the site of the proposed ostectomy some weeks before section from an extra-oral approach of the remainder of the mandible. In this way contamination of the external wound from the mouth is avoided.

In 1917 Aller suggested an intra-oral approach in order to avoid external scarring. There was the obvious inherent danger of contamination of the wound from the mouth at the time of operation and this may have

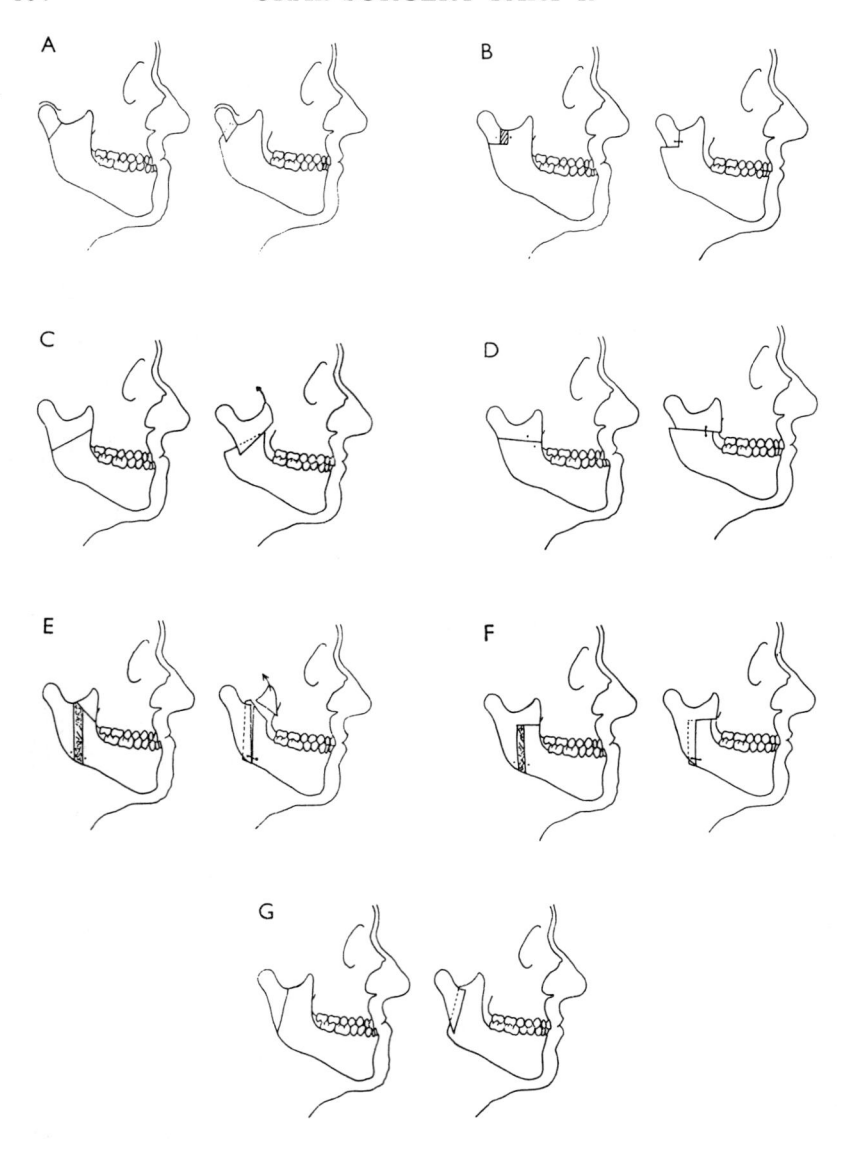

Fig. 28.—Diagrams illustrating some ramus procedures used in the treatment of mandibular prognathism.

A, Section of the condyle neck. B, Section of the condyle neck with removal of bone from below the sigmoid notch (Smith and Johnson). C, Blind section of the ramus (Kostecka). D, Horizontal ramus section. E, The vertical subsigmoid (Caldwell and Lettermann). F, The inverted L (Trauner). G, Oblique osteotomy (Thoma).

led to some lack of popularity of the procedure, but the technique was revived post-war by Thoma (1948), Dingman and Van Alstine (1952), Huebsch (1954), and Converse (1954) in view of the availability of antibiotic prophylaxis to control any infection. Advantages of the procedure are that it can be safely planned from models of the dental arch only, with or without additional help from cephalometric radiographs. Satisfactory results are achieved, particularly in terms of stability, with few operative risks to the patient. The indications for this type of operation are elongation of the body of the mandible, preferably when the tongue is of normal size and where there is an excess of space to accommodate it. An anterior open bite and low chin may also be corrected by this method, provided that there is a normal articulation as far as the premolar region.

Many operators have found that the healing of the mandible was prolonged following ostectomy and some (Fickling and Fordyce, 1955) have attempted to overcome this problem of delayed or fibrous union of the fragments by chip grafting the operation site. However, it is not always necessary to take iliac crest bone for the graft. Cancellous bone from the excised segment can be used. One way to do this is to remove only the cortex from the unwanted area, permitting the cancellous tissue to crush as the fragments are approximated. However, the main reason for protracted healing of the bone-ends is inadequate bony contact and if the bone-ends are accurately fitted together and united by a transosseous stainless-steel wire, so that maximum bony apposition is obtained, healing occurs as rapidly as with any other mandibular fracture.

A useful variant of the body ostectomy stems from the Y-shaped osteotomy of Trauner (1929) and Rosenthal (1934). Sowray and Haskell (1968) and then Obwegeser (1969a) have developed this method into a versatile and useful procedure. The mandible is reduced in length by the excision of a tooth socket on either side and reduced in both length and width by the excision of a vertical segment from the midline of the chin. The three ostectomy sites are connected by a horizontal cut below the apices of the anterior teeth. This procedure is of value where the jaw is excessively wide in proportion to its length, where the chin in a woman is square and masculine in shape, or where there are other deformities affecting the anterior part of the jaw. For example, the operation can be combined with the Köle procedure to correct an anterior open bite and a low chin point, so avoiding cuts at several sites in the mandible. The median alveolar segment is raised to close the anterior open bite, and a slice is cut off the lower border of the chin and wedged into the gap below the incisor segment, both to support it and to fashion a new chin prominence at a higher level. (*Fig. 29.*)

Disadvantages of the body procedures are: a marked diminution in tongue space (in some cases a lateral as well as an anteroposterior reduction) and a reduction in the distance between chin and angle producing a dumpy-faced appearance with a tendency to produce a double chin. However, the latter disfigurement tends to regress within nine months to a year after operation. From the foregoing it is obvious that body ostectomy will not be the preferred manœuvre if there is a large Frankfort mandibular plane angle with an obtuse angle to the mandible, or where the patient is plump with a thick subcutaneous layer.

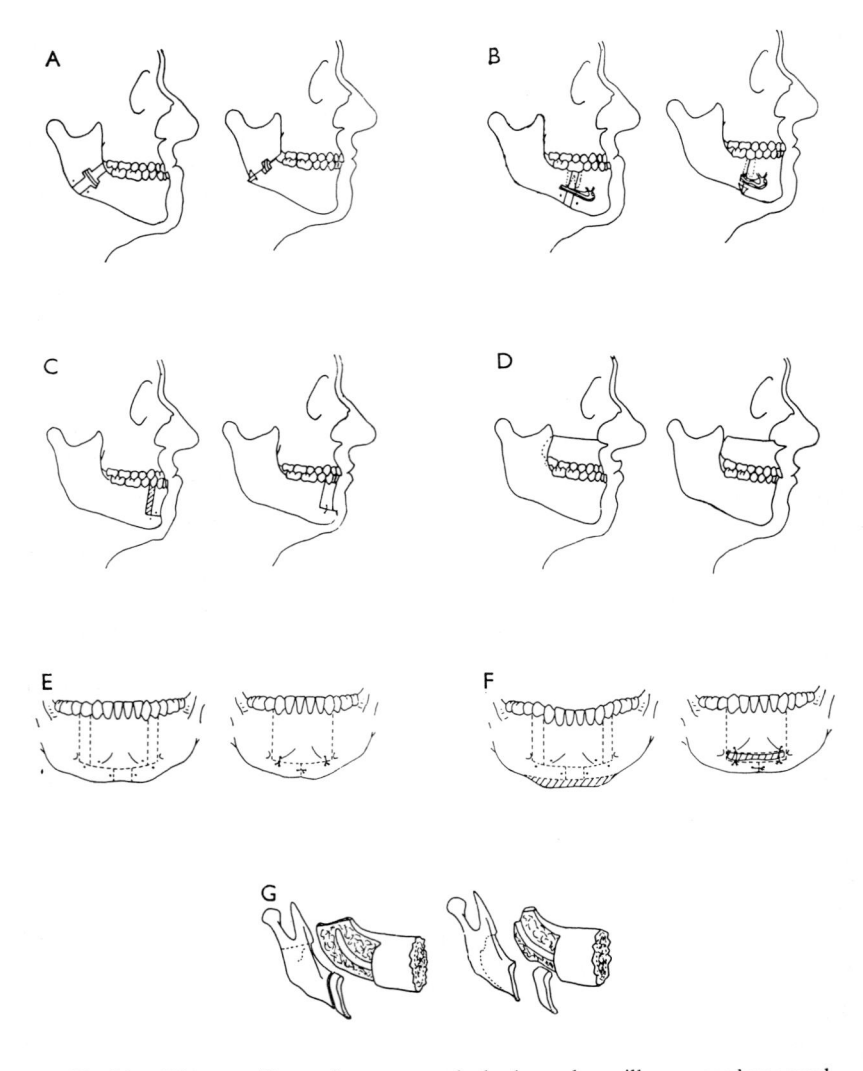

Fig. 29.—Diagrams illustrating some angle, body, and maxillary procedures used in the treatment of mandibular prognathism.

A, The angle ostectomy. B, The body ostectomy. C, Regression of the lower incisor segment. D, Maxillary osteotomy (Wassmund). E, The Y body ostectomy (Sowray and Haskell). F, The Y body ostectomy combined with the Köle procedure whereby the anterior alveolar segment is raised to close on anterior open bite, the height of the chin is reduced, and the point of the chin raised into the chin pad by wedging the chin fragment into the gap (Obwegeser). G, The Obwegeser-Dal Pont peration (left) and the Dal Pont-Hunsuck variant of the sagittal split (right).

Horizontal Osteotomy of the Ramus.—Horizontal osteotomy of the ramus above the level of the inferior dental foramen is one of the oldest and, formerly, most widely used forms of osteotomy for both mandibular protrusion and retrusion. It is the level at which section is carried out in the technique advocated by Kostecka via a blind extra-oral approach, but for reasons already discussed the osteotomy is best effected under direct vision through an open wound and bony healing is expedited by postoperative transosseous wiring of the bone-ends.

Exposure of the site is obtained by an intra-oral incision from the tip of the coronoid process down the anterior border of the ramus across the retromolar fossa and down into the buccal sulcus. The incision is made down to bone and with a Howarth's periosteal elevator the periosteum is raised from the buccal aspect of the ramus. The soft tissues are then retracted by passing the curved end of a Lack's retractor around the posterior border of the mandible. The tissues are raised from the lingual aspect of the ramus to identify the level of the inferior dental foramen so that the cut on the buccal aspect of the ramus can be sited above it. The section of the ramus is best effected with a tapered Meisinger fissure bur used in a straight handpiece. It is a simple matter to gauge the depth of the cut, but as an additional precaution a thin copper strip can be passed on the lingual side of the ramus to act as a guard. Great care must be taken when cutting through the posterior border of the mandible to ensure that the retractor is protecting the soft tissues for the maxillary artery and posterior facial vein are sited just behind the jaw in this area. After the bur cut has been deepened sufficiently the final section can be effected by a light tap with an osteotome on the anterior end of the ramus cut. Alternatively, the cut can be made from the medial to the lateral in the same way as the medial cortical cut of the Obwegeser operation. Various types of saws and drills have been suggested for use in this horizontal section and a Gigli saw can also be passed along the lingual side of the mandible and out behind the jaw to saw the mandible under direct vision. As soon as the section is complete the anterior aspect of the upper fragment will be pulled upwards by the action of the temporalis muscle. It is therefore essential to position the transosseous wire before the section is complete. Holes are drilled through the anterior aspect of the lower fragment about 1 cm. beneath the line of section and a similar hole is drilled in the upper section in a situation appropriate to the position to be taken up by the retroposed mandible. A wire is passed through the holes and the two ends of the wire are left slack. The presence of a wire through the upper fragment enables the operator to maintain control of it after the ramus is sectioned. Skaloud (1951) carried out transosseous wiring by passing the wire through a hole in the lower fragment and then over the sigmoid notch using a Reverdin needle. The wire can also be passed over the notch with a small right-angle aneurysm needle on a handle. Many operators prefer to make their section from the lingual to the buccal aspect of the mandible and this is possibly easier if a Gigli saw or orthopaedic saw is used.

When the ramus is sectioned a similar operation is carried out on the opposite side of the mandible after which the body of the mandible is repositioned and the position of the ramus fragments in relation to the mandible in its new position is checked. If they lie in end-to-end apposition the transosseous wires are tightened, but if there is an overlap on one or both sides either additional bone must be removed from one or the other end of the ramus to obtain end-to-end apposition or an overlap must be accepted. This entails compact bone facing compact bone and healing is much prolonged. When a satisfactory bone apposition is obtained the transosseous wires are tightened and the twisted end is cut short and turned into one of the holes in the ramus. The lower jaw is gently opened and closed to see that the position is maintained with the new occlusion. The wounds are then closed with interrupted black silk sutures.

Mandibular/maxillary fixation has to be maintained for about three months, for the area of bony contact between the fragments of ramus is not very great. It will be obvious that, if the lower fragment is pushed back for about half the total width of the ramus, there will be the equivalent of only half the width of the ramus in contact with half the width of the upper fragment. In fact, of the many jaw sections devised posterior to the dental arch, only the oblique (vertical subsigmoid) and sagittal splitting osteotomies with overlapping of the fragments seem likely to remain in current use. The other techniques practised result in narrow areas of bone contact and slow or unstable bone union unless cancellous bone-grafting of the approximated fragments is practised.

Oblique and Vertical Subsigmoid Osteotomy in Ascending Ramus.—These techniques were described by Thoma in 1948 and Hinds (1958) and Robinson (1958) also reported cases treated by this method in the same year. Strictly speaking, in the oblique osteotomy the lower end of the cut comes to a point on the posterior border of the angle, while in the vertical subsigmoid the cut passes through the lower border of the angle. The differences between the techniques are small however and they will be considered as together in this account. The osteotomy cut is oblique to the posterior border of the mandible and extends from the base of the sigmoid notch to the angle. Thoma regards this operation as useful in cases of mandibular protrusion and retrusion as well as in asymmetry and also valuable in some cases of open bite. It has the advantage that when the mandible is moved posteriorly the gonial angle is improved although such improvement may be temporary. (*Fig.* 28G.)

When a considerable posterior displacement of the anterior fragment has to be effected by this type of osteotomy the coronoid process must be separated or it will impinge on the medial root of the zygoma (*Fig.* 28A). Since complete separation of the coronoid results in gross contraction of the temporalis and elevation of the fragment, the inverted L osteotomy of Trauner seems a more satisfactory approach to this difficulty. (*Fig.* 28F.)

Operative Technique

Thoma (1969) performs the operation from a submandibular approach. A 5 cm. curved incision is made in the skin around and 1·5 cm. below the bony border of the angle on each side. The ramus is exposed by dividing the subcutaneous tissues and raising the masseter from the ramus. A right-angled retractor is used to retract the cheek upwards until the sigmoid notch is in view. The outline of the section is then made with Bonney's blue, and the bone is divided with a bur from the sigmoid notch either to the posterior border of the mandible at the level of the attachment of the stylomandibular ligament (oblique osteotomy), or the section passes vertically downwards to the angle (vertical subsigmoid). The simple vertical cut must be positioned behind the mandibular foramen, but for safety's sake only the buccal cortex is divided over the region of the nerve. The remaining lingual cortex is fractured by wedging the cut open from below. The condylar fragment is freed from its soft-tissue attachments on its inner surface with a Howarth's periosteal elevator and the fragment is allowed to overlap the main mandibular fragment. A sterile swab is then placed over the wound and the operation is repeated on the opposite side. After the bilateral section has been completed the loose mandible is manipulated into its new position and mandibular/maxillary fixation is effected. The external wounds are then inspected and transosseous wiring is carried out between the fragments at the posterior border of the mandible. Thoma regards the transosseous wiring as advantageous but not absolutely essential. Some surgeons advocate decortication of a matching area of the anterior fragment to the overlapping posterior fragment. This ensures a better fit, but it is not essential. If decortication is practised, it is important not to compress the inferior dental bundle for protracted nerve damage can result. If the anterior fragment is not decorticated the upper part of the lingual surface of the posterior fragment may need trimming to ensure that it lies flat against the lateral surface of the anterior fragment.

The masseter muscle is then repositioned and sutured to the lower border of the mandible. For this purpose either a stump of masseter is left at the time of exposing the outer surface of the ramus or the masseter can be sutured to the attachment of the medial pterygoid. The wound is then closed in layers.

This osteotomy can also be carried out through an intra-oral incision as has been described by Winstanley (1968). An incision is made down the anterior border of the ramus from the tip of the coronoid process to the retromolar fossa and is then extended into the buccal sulcus. A Howarth's periosteal elevator is used to separate the soft tissue from the bone on the lateral aspect of the ramus. The sigmoid notch is identified and a Moule retractor is placed around the posterior border of the mandible at the level of the stylomandibular ligament. The ramus is then sectioned obliquely from the sigmoid notch to the posterior border of the mandible using a tapered Meisinger fissure bur in a straight handpiece. Winstanley states that the access is not as good as in the external operation, but the internal operation has the great advantage of avoiding scarring on the face. Following the bilateral osteotomy the mandible is repositioned and the two intra-oral wounds are closed with interrupted black silk sutures.

Mandibular/maxillary fixation is carried out following closure of the wounds at the osteotomy sites, and it should be maintained, according to Thoma, for 6–8 weeks to ensure sound union.

The Sagittal Splitting Technique.—Sagittal splitting of the ramus of the mandible in order to correct mandibular deformity was first described by Obwegeser in 1957, who was the first to appreciate that a halving joint could be constructed by dividing the medial and lateral cortices of the ramus at different levels and then splitting the medullary bone between the cuts. A number of variants of the procedure exist. Two seem to stand out as having particular merit, namely the modification suggested by Dal Pont (1961) and Hunsuck's (1968) operation (*Fig.* 29G). The operation is carried out through an intra-oral surgical approach and so avoids facial scarring and possible damage to anatomical structures such as the mandibular branch of the facial nerve. The full width split permits apposition between a broad surface of cancellous bone in the two fragments and therefore avoids the relapse which occurs following inadequate bony contact.

The sagittal split technique also allows the main fragment to be moved in several directions, but still maintain bony contact over a wide area with the lesser fragment. This enables more than one type of mandibular deformity to be corrected for the technique can be used in cases of mandibular protrusion, mandibular retrusion and in some cases of open bite.

Operative Details

The outer surface of the mandible is exposed through an intra-oral incision from the level of the upper molar occlusal surface down along the external oblique line, across the retromolar fossa, and along the buccal aspect between the gingival margin and the external oblique ridge as far as the 1st molar. The periosteum on the lingual aspect of the mandible is raised between the lingula and the sigmoid notch, and the internal oblique line is drilled away with a large pear-shaped bur to enable the operator to visualize the bone below the sigmoid notch as far back as the posterior border of the mandible. A horizontal cut is made through the inner cortex with a tapered Meisinger bur. The outer cortex of the mandible is then cut vertically in the molar region after which the two cuts are connected by a third linking cut along the anterior border of the ramus. While the cortex is being cut the soft tissues are protected with a retractor which is gutter-shaped in cross-section. A large, thick osteotome is used to start the split and the advancing edge of the instrument must follow the inner surface of the outer cortex. The split is completed by boldly twisting the instrument in the cut in an anticlockwise direction on the right side and with a clockwise motion on the left. Some operators prefer to drive into the line of cut two thick osteotomes which tend to split some mandibles through to the lingual side just short of the angle.

Hunsuck's osteotomy, which Barton (1968) has developed, seeks deliberately to encourage this type of split. When this procedure has been carried out on each side of the mandible, the main fragment can be moved in several directions while the condylar fragment maintains its position. In cases where mandibular protrusion has been corrected, it will be found after mandibular/maxillary reposition that the cortex of the posterior fragment will overlap that of the anterior fragment and this surplus is carefully removed with a surgical bur or bone-cutting forceps. The anterior border of the ramus and the alveolar border of the posterior fragment are also trimmed. Close adaptation of the cortical surfaces of the two fragments is achieved by transosseous wiring in the retromolar area or by looping a circumferential wire around the apposed parts. Bony union should be satisfactory in six weeks.

A problem with almost all mandibular osteotomies is the avoidance of damage to the inferior dental nerve. In the sagittal splitting procedure it is necessary to avoid damage to the nerve at three stages:—

  a. When the soft tissues are elevated from the medial side of the ramus, particularly if an attempt is made to elevate the attachment of the medial pterygoid.
  b. When the vertical cut is made on the lateral side, since it must be made clean through into the medulla.
  c. When the final split is executed.

With regard to the last of the specified risk situations, the nerve is particularly in jeopardy in those patients in whom the canal lies laterally and is just beneath the buccal cortex.

One prerequisite for the sagittal split is that there should be cancellous bone between the two cortical plates. Some surgeons for preference use the submento-vertical projection for the radiographic assessment of the thickness of the cancellous tissue, but others rely on the study of good quality oblique lateral radiographs of the mandible. With reference to the latter, if a cancellous bone tracery can be seen then a medullary space exists. If the image is featureless, then it is likely that the two cortices are fused. Fortunately, most mandibles have a medullary cavity in the requisite parts, but the medial cut should be placed low down by the lingula, to be certain that it is entered.

The full width split with the Obwegeser manœuvre provides a large area of bone contact. It is appropriate for moderate degrees of prognathism and anterior open bite, and for forward slides unless the advancement is extreme. (*Figs.* 30, 31.)

Ramus procedures appear to have a number of advantages. The area of bone contact is greater than in body operations and union of the fragments faster and more certain. The attachment of the mylohyoid as well as the genial muscles is moved backwards, so that the tongue is displaced further posteriorly than is the case with body procedures. Furthermore, the size of the lower dental arch is not altered. Thus, size of tongue is less critical than with the body osteotomy.

The length of the body of the mandible is retained and the shape of the angle is initially improved. Unfortunately, the improvement of the angle is not permanent since the bone behind the new insertions of the masseters and medial pterygoids is resorbed during the first two years after the operation.

One of the disadvantages of ramus procedures is the tendency to post-operative swelling of the lateral wall of the pharynx and pillars of the fauces. This is due to oedema of the tissues and/or haematoma at the operation site, but the latter complication can be mitigated by the use of vacuum drains and careful haemostasis. The lips and cheeks should be protected from rubbing by instruments and this measure, coupled with a gentle surgical technique, should reduce the amount of postoperative oedema. The combined use of hypotensive anaesthesia and local vaso-constriction should be avoided since this results in excessive local tissue cyanosis and predisposes to excessive postoperative oedema.

Body Ostectomy.—Ostectomy of the body of the mandible is usually carried out in the $\overline{65|56}$ area and it can be performed through either a submandibular or an intra-oral incision, but for the reasons already emphasized the intra-oral operation is preferable in most cases. If a submandibular approach is adopted, it is essential to remove the specified tooth or teeth prior to performing the ostectomy. In the case of the intra-oral procedure extraction of the selected tooth or teeth prior to

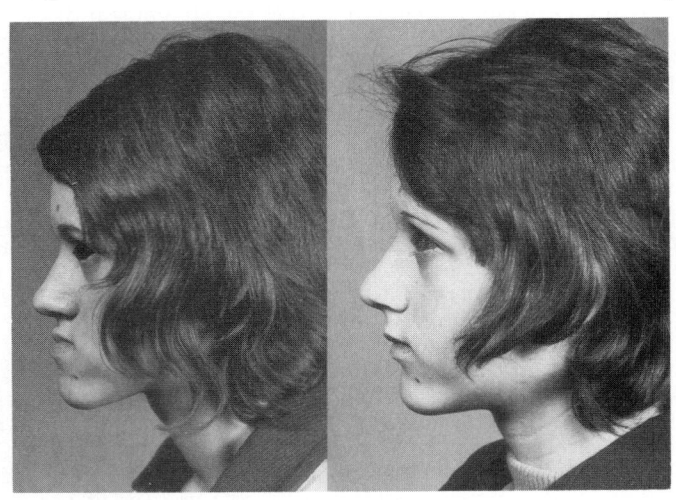

Fig. 30.—Marked prognathism treated by Hunsuck's modification of the sagittal splitting procedure: pre- and postoperative photographs.

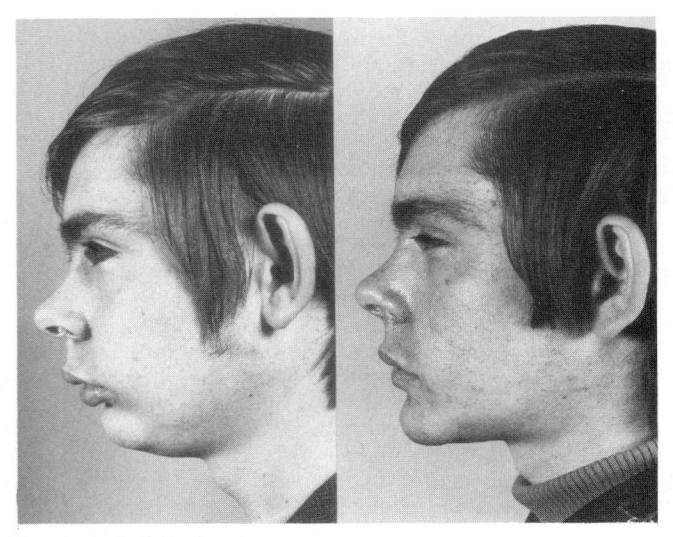

Fig. 31.—A marked degree of retrognathism (Angle's Class II, division 1) treated by the advancement of the mandible using bilateral Obwegeser-Dal Pont procedures concurrently with a lowering of the lower anterior alveolar segment: pre- and postoperative photographs.

operation is helpful, but this measure can be deferred till the time of the ostectomy without much added inconvenience. Preoperative extractions should be carried out at least six weeks prior to the ostectomy in order to allow the extraction site to heal fully and eliminate the possibility of residual infection.

Intra-oral Operation.—A local analgesic solution containing a vaso-constrictor (Xylocaine and 1 : 80,000 adrenaline) is injected buccally and lingually in the operation area to control local bleeding, and then an incision is made around the gingival margins buccally and lingually from the retromolar area to the lower canine and on the buccal side, anteriorly, taken into the sulcus for a distance of half an inch. Buccal and lingual flaps are raised with a Howarth's periosteal elevator to expose the body of the mandible down as far as the lower border of the mandible at the operation site. Retraction is obtained either with 2·5-cm. copper strips bent at one end to pass underneath the lower border of the mandible or preferably by the use of two Lack's retractors. The retractor's handle is bent in the opposite direction so that the blade with the slight curve on the end can be passed under the lower border of the mandible on each side.

When adequate exposure of the operative site is obtained the template pattern of the area to be removed is laid on the buccal aspect of the mandible, care being taken to see that the edges are well clear of the roots of adjacent teeth. Two parallel vertical cuts are then marked out either side of the marker plate using the point of a Meisinger tapered fissure bur. The template pattern is then removed and the cuts are deepened with the tapered fissure bur to penetrate the buccal cortex. Study of the oblique lateral radiographs will show the approximate level of the neurovascular canal and the cuts can be deepened at the lower border so that they penetrate through to the lingual side for a distance of about 0·5–1 cm. and still avoid the neurovascular bundle. Care must be taken to ensure that the lingual retractor is in its correct place while these cuts are made. At the upper end of the body of the mandible the two cuts are also deepened through to the lingual side until the approximate site of the neurovascular bundle is reached. A gentle tap with a chisel on the buccal plate between the bur cuts first at the lower border and then at the upper end of the mandible will remove the lower border of the mandible and upper bone almost to the site of the mandibular canal. The buccal plate covering the neurovascular canal is then knocked off by positioning a chisel on its lingual side and tapping it buccally. This manœuvre exposes the neurovascular canal.

While the mandible is still intact, holes are drilled diagonally through the buccal plate of the mandible on each side of the defect and just above the neurovascular bundle. A 0·5-mm. soft stainless-steel wire is threaded loosely between the bone-ends. It is easier to put the transosseous wire in place before finally sectioning the mandible because difficulty may be experienced when working on two mobile bone-ends. The neurovascular bundle is then exposed and identified and a Howarth's periosteal elevator is placed first above and then below the bundle to act as a guard while the Meisinger bur is used to deepen the parallel cuts through to the lingual side of the mandible. The lingual plate is knocked off with a chisel and the section is complete.

The neurovascular bundle is allowed to take up a position between the bone-ends and the transosseous wire is loosely tightened across the fracture line. The opposite side of the mandible is sectioned in a similar manner and the predetermined amount of bone removed, after which both transosseous wires are adjusted until the bone-ends are seen to be in apposition. The transosseous wires should not be too tight or they will damage the neurovascular bundle which has been allowed to curl up between the bony interfaces. It is not necessary to cut out a special recess in one of the two bone-ends to receive the slightly coiled nerve and vessels, for if the bundle is permitted to take up its own place between the sliced bone-ends and the transosseous wires are fairly slack, nerve damage will be negligible and mental anaesthesia avoided. Indeed, transosseous wires are used merely to hold the alined bone-ends in apposition to facilitate healing, and they do not need to be twisted tightly. The ends of the twisted transosseous wires are cut short and the free end is turned neatly into one of the holes.

With the fragments fixed, the soft-tissue wounds are then closed with interrupted silk sutures. When teeth are present in the lower jaw, on the anterior and posterior fragments, fixation is best effected in the following manner: a silver copper alloy cap splint which has a locking plate on each side in the lower premolar area is cemented to the lower anterior teeth, and soldered to the locking plate is a perforated arch bar which can be wired to the adjacent molar tooth or teeth on the posterior fragments. The centre part of an 20-cm. length of wire is placed over individual teeth, (8 and/or 7|7 and/or 8) on the posterior fragment in the form of a clove-hitch knot and secured to each tooth with a couple of twists on the free ends. These free ends are then threaded through the holes in the arch bars, crossed and tightened. This method provides a very effective and rigid fixation between the anterior and posterior fragments. The use of the arch bar in conjunction with a cap splint allows some flexibility when immobilizing the parts, for it is difficult to calculate exactly the final correct position of the stabilized fragments and their relation to any oral fixation. If posterior teeth are also splinted and pre-arranged localizing bars are constructed, there is the possibility that when the prefabricated connecting bars are fitted there will be a gap between the bone-ends. The other problem with silver copper alloy cap splints fitted to single teeth is that they have a tendency to become detached no matter how well the splint is constructed or how carefully it is cemented in position.

After the surgical fractures in the mandible have been immobilized, mandibular/maxillary fixation is effected with elastic bands between the hooks on the upper and lower teeth. Postoperatively a suitable antibiotic should be administered to the patient for seven days. The sutures are removed at the end of the first week and clinical union should have occurred after a six-week period of immobilization. If so, the fixation is dismantled and it is then important to balance the occlusion by the provision of a suitable partial denture to fill any gaps in the dentition. This prevents the patient from adopting a bite of convenience which might place a strain on the newly healed fracture sites. Sensory function in the mental region should be unaffected.

Symphysial Alveolar Osteotomy.—With patients in whom the dental arch only is too far forward, a backwards movement of the jaw as a whole will produce a 'weak chin'. Extraction of a first premolar tooth on each side followed by movement of the sectioned lower anterior alveolar segment to a more posterior position should produce the desired result. (*Fig.* 29C.)

Patients with a Retrusion of the Upper Jaw

A mild degree of retrusion of the upper jaw can be corrected cosmetically by fitting an upper denture which comes into correct occlusal relationship with the lower incisors and pushes the upper lip into an aesthetically satisfactory position. When the patient is edentulous the procedure is simple, but if maxillary anterior teeth are present these should be extracted if they are decayed or unsightly. If the upper teeth are sound the denture can be designed to cover them, or, alternatively, the natural teeth are allowed to protrude through the denture behind the artificial incisors. If the maxillary retrusion is more pronounced, such a solution is impossible, for if the incisor teeth of the denture are pushed forwards too far off the ridge the denture will, of course, become unstable. In such an eventuality there are three possible alternative procedures: (1) A buccal inlay and prosthesis, (2) Alveolar osteotomy, (3) Maxillary osteotomy.

1. Buccal Inlay and Prosthesis.—In cases of extreme retrusion of the upper jaw the buccal inlay and prosthesis achieves an excellent cosmetic result.

Preliminary Treatment.—Before operation a silver copper alloy cap splint is cemented to the upper teeth with Ames black copper cement. To the anterior aspect of the splint a square post is soldered and over this post a square tube is fitted to which is attached a small perforated German silver tray which projects out horizontally over the upper buccal sulcus. The square tube can be attached to the square post by a grub screw so that when the screw is undone the German silver plate can be removed.

Operation.—An incision is made around the upper buccal sulcus from approximately 6|6. The incision is taken through the mucous membrane and is then deepened vertically upwards, the cut lying just superficial to the periosteum. In this manner a large surgical pocket is made in the upper buccal sulcus and the periosteum covering the bone on the anterior aspect of the premaxillary area is exposed over a wide area. A large gutta-percha mould is then constructed to fill this pocket and correct the maxillary retrusion and the mould is held in position by the German silver tray. After the mould and tray are satisfactorily adjusted, a split skin-graft is taken from some non-hair-bearing area of the patient (inner aspect of the arm or thigh) and this graft is draped over the mould with its raw surface outwards so that when the mould is in position the skin-graft will cover the raw area of the periosteum. Complete haemostasis of the wound must be achieved before positioning the graft because haematoma formation beneath the graft may lead to its destruction. The mould is secured in place by screwing the German silver plate to the square post on the splint.

The skin-graft will take in about seven days, but the mould can be left in position for about fourteen days in the upper jaw. After this time the mould should be removed by unscrewing the grub screw and lifting out the plate and mould. The graft is inspected and the gutta-percha washed, after which the mould is replaced quickly to prevent contracture of the skin-graft. The mould should be changed daily and the patient can be trained to perform this task.

After a few weeks, the actual time depending on the area covered by graft, the gutta-percha mould can be replaced by an upper prosthesis which corrects the profile of the upper part of the patient's face. The gutta-percha mould should overcorrect the maxillary retrusion to allow for any subsequent contracture of the graft before the prosthesis is fitted.

2. Alveolar Osteotomy.—The upper incisors and canines can be advanced by carrying out an alveolar osteotomy as described for cases of maxillary protrusion, after which the anterior fragment is brought forward. To prevent the fragment relapsing, a bone-graft is placed on each side in the osteotomy gap created in the bone in the bucccal culcus. This is an extensive surgical procedure and owing to the limitations imposed by the palatal mucoperiosteum and its attendant blood-supply from the greater palatine arteries, any advance of the anterior fragment is of necessity limited in extent, unless the palatal mucosa is divided behind the greater palatine vessels and advanced as an island flap. Bilateral bridges may be placed to help to prevent relapse.

3. Maxillary Osteotomy.—A maxillary osteotomy is an extensive surgical procedure in which a Guerin- or Le-Fort-I-type fracture is created surgically and the entire tooth-bearing portion of the upper jaw is advanced. This procedure is usually undertaken when the upper occlusion has not only to be advanced, but also brought down to correct a gross open bite. The techniques employed stem from the work of Wassmund, Axhausen, and Gillies. Unfortunately, even though maxillary osteotomy has been practised for over 40 years it has not been used by so many operators as the mandibular procedures and the number of cases in which it is indicated are far fewer. Hence, there is not the same solid body of experience to help in planning and management. (*Fig.* 29D.)

Wassmund effects an osteotomy at a Le Fort I level. Through an incision in the upper buccal sulcus from the 1st molar region around to 1st molar region, the nasal septum and the medial and lateral walls of the maxillary sinuses are sectioned. A curved osteotome is directed behind the tuberosities to separate the maxilla from the pterygoid plates. Any nasal mucoperiosteum which resists movement of the fragments into the desired position with dissecting forceps is also divided (Obwegeser, 1969b). Thus, the maxilla is pedicled on the soft palate, the greater palatine vessels, and the molar sulcus mucosa.

Some operators feel this bold approach puts the blood-supply to the fragment in jeopardy since the greater palatine vessels can be damaged in the palatine canal when the maxilla is separated from the pterygoid plates. These operators prefer to keep a second strip of sulcus mucosa intact in the premolar-canine-incisor region.

Obwegeser maintains that the insertion of a block of bone between the maxilla and the pterygoid plates and flakes of bone over the lateral bony

CORRECTION OF JAWS IN FACIAL DEFORMITY

cuts are essential to the achievement of a stable bony union. Even so, there seems to be a greater tendency to relapse than with certain mandibular procedures.

More recently adventurous attempts have been made to deal with retrusion of the mid-face and even malposition of the orbits and hyperteliorism have been tackled (Tessier and others, 1967; Obwegeser, 1969b).

Henderson and Jackson (1973) have used oblique incisions below the medial corners of the orbits to effect a Le Fort II level osteotomy. Where the nasal complex also needs advancement or lengthening the incisions are joined into an inverted 'V' over the bridge of the nose.

A Le Fort II osteotomy may be carried out in the following fashion (Seward, 1973). Bilateral incisions are made over the infra-orbital margins opposite the medial two-thirds of the margin. Through these the periosteum is stripped from the orbital floor back to the inferior orbital fissure, laterally to the lateral side of the orbital floor and medially as far as the lacrimal duct. The nasal soft tissues are elevated subperiosteally over the frontal processes of the maxilla and nasal bones until the undermining from one side reaches that on the other. The anterior margins of the frontal processes and nasal bones can be visualized at this stage through the wounds by careful retraction.

By tunnelling upwards along the orbital rim the periosteum is raised between the medial canthal ligament and the lacrimal sac and a bur cut made from the point at which the anterior end of the nasal bone joins the frontal process of the maxilla back to the orbital rim between the ligament and the lacrimal sac (above the inferior concha). The cut is carried backwards medial to the sac and then with small osteotomes laterally behind the sac.

The orbital contents are retracted upwards and the cut carried laterally through the thin roof of the orbit with a rose head bur. When the infraorbital nerve is reached it is mobilized and the bone cut carried above and below it. At the lateral end of the orbital floor the bone is divided in a forward direction in a line which diverges laterally until the orbital rim is reached. The periosteum may be raised from the lateral rim of the orbit to permit onlay grafting if this is desired. The tissues are next raised from the bone vertically down the body of the zygomatic bone until the zygomatico-alveolar crest is reached. With a long-shank taper-fissure bur the bone is sectioned from the zygomatico-alveolar crest upwards, into the zygomatic extension of the antrum and to join the lateral cut in the orbital rim.

The mouth is entered and incisions made in the sulcus from the zygomatico-alveolar crest backwards. The lower ends of the bone cuts are identified and continued horizontally backwards above the apices of the teeth with a No. 8 rose head bur. Through this cut and using a smaller long-shank rose head bur the cut is carried along the posterior and medial wall of the antrum. On the medial wall the cut slopes upwards, above the inferior concha, to the region of the hiatus semilunaris. With a rose head bur there is less risk of damage to the anterior palatine artery than with an osteotome.

Separation of the tuberosity from the pterygoid plates is with a curved Obwegeser chisel. The nasal septum must be divided with care right to the back, or the maxilla will not move. This is best done through short vertical incisions just behind the columella. Where the nose needs to be advanced Henderson and Jackson's (1973) method is advocated.

If a mandibular osteotomy is to be combined with the maxillary one the mandibular sites are prepared short of final section before the maxilla is mobilized. Then the maxilla is mobilized with Rowe forceps and advanced, using the mandibular arch as a reference point, and fixed to a halo frame. The mandibular cuts are completed and the jaws fixed together.

A block of iliac crest bone-graft is wedged between the pterygoid plates and the back of the tuberosity on both sides. Thin curved flakes are used to cover the defects in the oribital floors and blocks and chips used to fill all other defects. Onlay grafts may be inserted over the lateral orbital rims to smooth their contour into the displaced infra-orbital rims.

Provided Barton and Harris's (1970) method of fixation with the jaws apart is used, Le Fort II osteotomies can be completed using nasal intubation and bilateral nasopharyngeal airways postoperatively. If both mandibular and maxillary osteotomies are performed, or Henderson and Jackson's (1973) nasal procedures, a tracheostomy will be required.

4. Asymmetrical Mandibular Deformity

In broad terms, mandibular asymmetry can be the result of overgrowth or undergrowth of one side. Condylar hyperplasia is the most common cause of mandibular overgrowth. Two main types seem to occur and have been given a variety of names. In one type the condyle head is not greatly enlarged and often moves normally in the fossa. The condyle neck is elongated and angulated downwards and forwards, displacing that side of the mandible forwards. The angle of the mandible comes to lie more anteriorly than on the other side. There is no open bite, no tilting of the occlusal plane, or increase in depth of the mandible. The condition, therefore, produces asymmetrical prognathism.

In the other type the condyle head is greatly enlarged and may simply rotate when the mouth is opened. The condyle neck is considerably elongated and leaves the condyle either vertically or even in a downwards and backwards direction. The midline of the mandible is usually centrally placed in the face, but the lower border may be tilted towards the opposite side and the lower incisors tilted towards the same side as the deformity. There is a marked downward and inward bowing of the mandible and separation of the posterior teeth. A compensatory downgrowth of the maxillary alveolar process attempts to close the gap. This increases the vertical height of the maxilla on this side. However, it seems probable that some patients have a degree of unilateral gigantism since the appropriate nostril may be enlarged and the ipsilateral supra-orbital ridge may slope upwards. The degree of orbital asymmetry may even be sufficient to require the patient to tilt the head to bring the visual axes horizontal. At operation an enlarged parotid gland and a complex of facial nerve branches may be encountered. The opposite side of the mandible may be either of normal size, or smaller than average.

Minor degrees of this deformity which do not require treatment are not uncommon, but gross examples are far less frequent than in the case of the first type. Asymmetrical prognathism can be managed by the procedures for shortening the mandible outlined previously. In some cases one side only needs to be sectioned, but in many both sides will have to be sectioned to permit a proper interdigitation of the teeth. Since the patient has a near normal joint movement condylectomy should *never* be performed in these cases.

The second type is more difficult. Hovell (1956) has shown dramatically that a condylectomy at the right age will produce a normal facial appearance. However, it seems a pity to sacrifice a joint even if the function is imperfect and a subcondylar procedure to shorten the ramus should be considered, particularly in the adult. More recently Hovell (1970) has used a condyle shave only.

An intra-oral approach to the condyle is described by Sear (1972) who showed that provided a subperiosteal resection of the condyle was effected a new condyle of more reasonable proportions developed. A satisfactory correction of the occlusion and appearance was achieved by this technique. It should be emphasized that this method is for the experienced oral surgeon as potentially marked haemorrhage in a confined wound could be produced by incautious surgery.

Some of the deformity in the lower border of the mandible appears to be secondary to the condylar deformity and condylectomy results in its resorption. Where the mental tubercle is involved, however, this part does not remodel.

A vertical movement of the ramus can only be achieved if an open bite exists or can be created on that side. Trimming of the lower border and onlay grafting of the other side if it is underdeveloped may also be needed.

As in the case of severe degrees of retrognathism, unilateral underdevelopment of the mandible may be the result of a congenital or developmental defect or the result of damage to the condylar growth centre.

The major problem in these patients is that the normal side of the mandible is bent round to meet the abnormal, producing a jaw which is shorter than average, flattened on the abnormal side, and with the central incisor region bent round to the abnormal side. The upper arch adjusts itself to fit the lower. Thus, correction requires expansion of the upper arch and remodelling of the lower incisor region. In many cases a choice lies between serial bone-grafts, which attempt to prevent some of the compensatory changes, and a disguising procedure. Neither are entirely satisfactory. Serial grafting means multiple operations during the patient's childhood and schooldays. Disguising procedures tend to relapse.

In recent years experiments have been tried with the grafting of growing epiphysial bone-ends. The results of these operations are not yet certain. A further complication where the deficiency is due to a congenital malformation is that there is often hypoplasia of the skin, muscle, and other soft tissues and delayed tooth eruption or absent teeth. The soft-tissue defects materially increase the asymmetry and accentuate it in function.

5. Patients with Malocclusion not associated with a Gross Skeletal Anomaly of the Upper or Lower Jaw

The correction of gross malocclusion is achieved to a greater or lesser extent following all the osteotomy and ostectomy operations performed upon the upper and lower jaws. In the mandible these operations involve, of course, a complete section of the jaw. Surgical correction of occlusal anomalies can also be achieved by alveolar surgery whereby a portion of the upper or lower alveolar process is detached from the underlying bone and repositioned *en bloc*.

One such procedure (alveolar ostectomy and osteotomy) has already been described for the correction of maxillary protrusion and retrusion. This type of alveolar surgery has also been termed 'subapical osteotomy', dento-alveolar surgery, and surgery of the labial segments. The technique can also be used in the lower jaw to reposition the lower incisor segment in an Angle's Class II, division 1 type of malocclusion to correct a deep overbite. This is achieved surgically by detaching the $\overline{321|123}$ by an osteotomy in which both the teeth and their investing bone are separated from the body of the mandible. A section of the body of the mandible is then removed from below these teeth so that the segment containing the teeth can be lowered, so restoring a normal occlusal plane to the mandible. Following a similar mobilization of the lower anterior segment the fragment can be raised to close an anterior open bite (Köle procedure). A slice of chin is removed and wedged into the gap below the fragment to bring the chin eminence up behind the chin pad. The blood-supply to the lower teeth is maintained through the soft tissue attached to its lingual aspect.

Maxillary ostectomy for the correction of protruding upper teeth has already been described (p. 155). A similar technique for repositioning upper buccal segments can also be carried out and was described by Schuchardt (1954) for the correction of anterior open bite. The procedure was carried out in two stages in order to preserve an adequate blood-supply to the segments. The palatal cuts are completed at the first operation and the buccal cuts are made four weeks later when an adequate blood-supply has been established through the reattached palatal mucoperiosteal flap. By means of an ostectomy on the buccal aspect, the vertical depth in molar region can be reduced. In all alveolar osteotomy and ostectomy procedures a very exact diagnostic plan must be made preoperatively with a full evaluation of the soft-tissue morphology. Careful sectioning of plaster-of-Paris models will enable the operator to calculate the exact site of the osteotomy cuts and the amount of bone to be removed in the case of an ostectomy.

Alveolar osteotomy and ostectomy procedures can, of course, be carried out in conjunction with osteotomy and ostectomy procedures which involve a complete section of the mandible. It should be remembered that alveolar osteotomy and ostectomy operations must be time-consuming otherwise there is the possibility of postoperative loss of teeth or alveolar process through inadequate blood-supply to the fragment. This should not occur in an adequately planned and skilfully performed operation, but there is always a risk.

Immobilization of Fragments following Osteotomy or Ostectomy.—Immobilization of the fragments following osteotomy or ostectomy can be effected by any of the methods used in the immobilization of jaw fractures. The fixation of choice must vary from case to case and much depends upon whether teeth are present in the fragments.

Patients with Teeth on all Fragments.—

Cap Splints.—When teeth are present the method of choice in Great Britain is the provision of silver-copper alloy cap splints on all fragments, with either prearranged localizing bars or with localization carried out postoperatively. In the case of mandibular operations when only one tooth is present on the posterior fragment, some difficulty may be experienced in cementing securely the cap splint on a single tooth and a safer fixation is to have an arch bar attached to each side of the anterior splint and secured to the tooth on the posterior fragment by means of direct wiring. If there is an edentulous posterior fragment in the lower jaw, upper border transosseous wiring (above the mandibular canal) forms a secure fixation.

Arch Bar.—Some operators prefer to use arch bars in place of cap splints and this is, of course, the method of choice when facilities for the construction of cap splints are not available.

Orthodontic Bands.—Orthodontic banding of the teeth tends to be a time-consuming procedure and requires the expert co-operation of a skilled orthodontist.

The Edentulous Patient.—

Transosseous Wires.—Transosseous wires above the mandibular canal may be used following mandibular operations and the fixation can be reinforced with Gunning-type splints fixed with peralveolar and circumferential wiring.

Bone Plating.—Bone plates may be used following mandibular operations and they provide a more rigid fixation, although more difficult to fit during the intra-oral type of operations.

The Edentulous Upper Jaw.—Alveolar osteotomy and ostectomy would not be considered in the edentulous upper jaw, for adequate adjustments to the ridge and occlusion can be effected by suitable alveolectomies and the provision of dentures.

REFERENCES

ALLER, T. G. (1917), 'Operative Treatment for Prognathism', *Dent. Cosmos*, **59**, 394.
ANGLE, E. H. (1898), 'Double Resection of the Lower Maxilla', *Ibid.*, **40**, 635.
AXHAUSEN, E. (1939), '*Die operative orthopädie bei den fehlbildungen der kiefer*', *Dt. Zahn- Mund- u. Kieferheilk.*, **6**, 582.
BABCOCK, W. W. (1909), 'The Surgical Treatment of Certain Deformities of the Jaw associated with Malocclusion of the Teeth', *J. Am. med. Ass.*, **53**, 833.
BALLIN, M. (1908), 'Double Resection for Treatment of Mandibular Protrusion', *Dent. Items*, **30**, 422.
BARTON, P. (1968), Paper read to the Autumn Meeting of the British Association of Oral Surgeons. Royal College of Surgeons, England, London, 26th Oct.
— — and HARRIS, A. N. (1970), 'An Investigation into the Efficiency of the Oral Airway and a Technique for improving the Airway in the Early Post-operative Period following Mandibular Osteotomy', *Br. J. oral Surg.*, **8**, 16–20.
— — and RAYNE, J. (1969), 'The Role of Alveolar Surgery in the Treatment of Malocclusion', *Br. dent. J.*, **126**, 11.
BERGER, P. (1897), *Du traitement chirurgical du prognathisme*. Thesis, Lyons University.
BLAIR, V. P. (1907), 'Operations on the Jaw Bone and Face', *Surgery Gynec. Obstet.*, **4**, 67.
CALDWELL, J. B., and AMARAL, W. J. (1960), 'Mandibular Micrognathia corrected by Vertical Osteotomy in the Rami and Iliac Bone Graft', *J. oral Surg.*, **18**, 3.
CLARKSON, P. (1955), 'Late Result of Kostecka's Operation for Prognathism', *Proc. R. Soc. Med.*, **48**, 984.

CONVERSE, J. M. (1954), 'Bone Grafting Malformations of the Jaws', *Am. J. Surg.*, **88**, 858.
CRADOCK-HENRY, T. (1966), in *Oral Surgery* (ed. W. H. ARCHER), 4th ed., p. 984. Philadelphia: Saunders.
DAL PONT, G. (1958), 'Die retromolare osteotomie zur korrection der retrogenic und der morden apertus', *Osterr. z. stomat.*, **58**, 8.
—— (1961), 'Retromolar Osteotomy for the Correction of Prognathism', *J. oral Surg.*, **19**, 42.
DINGMAN, R. O. (1948), 'Surgical Correction of Developmental Deformities of the Mandible', *Plastic reconstr. Surg.*, **3**, 124.
—— and VAN ALSTINE, R. S. (1952), 'Correction of Mandibular Protrusion in the Edentulous Patient', *J. oral Surg.*, **11**, 273.
DUFOURMENTEL, L. (1921), 'Surgical Treatment of Prognathism', *Presse méd.*, **29**, 235.
EISELSBERG, A. (1906), 'Plastik bei ektopium der unterkiefers', *Wien. klin. Wschr.*, **51**, 1505.
—— (1907), 'Über plastik bei ektopium der unterkiefers', *Munch. med. Wschr.*, **54**, 36.
ERNST, F. (1927), 'Progenie', in *Die Chirurgie* (ed. KIRSCHNER, M., and MORDMANN), vol. 4, part 1, p. 802. Munich: Urban.
FICKLING, B. W., and FORDYCE, G. L. (1955), 'Mandibular Osteotomy for Facial Asymmetry', *Proc. R. Soc. Med.*, **48**, 989.
GILLIES, H. (1955), personal communication.
HENDERSON, D., and JACKSON, I. T. (1973), 'Nasomaxillary Hypoplasia: The Le Fort II Osteotomy', *Br. J. oral Surg.*, **11**, 77–93.
HENRY, C. B. (1946), 'Case of Kostecka's Operation of Prognathous Mandible', *Proc. R. Soc. Med.*, **39**, 646.
HINDS, E. C. (1958), 'Correction of Prognathism by Subcondylar Osteotomy', *J. oral Surg.*, **16**, 209.
HOVELL, J. H. (1956), 'The Surgical Correction of Variations in the Facial Skeletal Pattern', *Proc. R. Soc. Med.*, **49**, 546.
—— (1970), 'Surgical Correction of Facial Deformity', *Ann. R. Coll. Surg.*, **46**, 92.
HUEBSCH, R. F. (1954), 'Correction of Mandibular Prognathism by Intra-oral Ostectomy', *J. oral Surg.*, **12**, 214.
HULLIHEN, S. P. (1849), quoted by HOGEMAN, K. E. (1951), *Acta chir. scand.*, Suppl. 159, *Am. J. dent. Sci.*, **9**, 157.
HUMPHREY, A. (1856), quoted by RUSHTON, M. A. (1946), *Proc. R. Soc. Med.*, **39**, 431.
HUNSUCK, E. E. (1968), 'A Modified Intra-oral Sagittal Splitting Technique for Correction of Mandibular Prognathism', *J. oral Surg.*, **26**, 249.
JABOULAY, M., and BERARD, L. (1898), 'Traitement chirurgical de prognathisme', *Presse méd.*, **6**, 173.
KAZANZIAN, V. H. (1951), 'The Treatment of Mandibular Prognathism', *Oral Surg.*, **4**, 680.
KOSTECKA, F. (1931), 'Die chirurgische therapie der progenie', *Zahnärztl. Rdsch.*, **40**, 780.
LIMBERG, A. A. (1928), 'A New Method of Plastic Lengthening of the Mandible in Unilateral Micrognathia and Asymmetry of the Face', *J. Am. dent. Ass.*, **15**, 851.
MARKWELL, B. D. (1967), 'The Correction of Maxillary Prognathism by One Stage Ostectomy', *Br. J. plast. Surg.*, **20**, 179.
MATRAS, H. (1967), 'Observations in Connection with the Maxillary Protrusion by Method of the Frontal Pedicle Maxillary Fragment', *Trans. int. Ass. oral Surg.*, p. 103.
MOHNAC, A. M. (1966), 'Maxillary Osteotomy in the Management of Oral Deformities', *J. oral Surg.*, **24**, 305.
MURPHY, P. J., and WALKER, R. V. (1963), 'Correction of Maxillary Protrusion by Ostectomy and Orthodontic Therapy, *Ibid.*, **21**, 275.
NICOLSKY and PEHRGADD. Quoted by REICHERBAD, E., KOLE, H., and BRUCHL, H. (1965), *Chirurgische kieferorthopädie*, p. 208. Leipzig: Barth.
OBWEGESER, H. (1957), 'The Surgical Correction of Mandibular Prognathism and Retrognathia with Consideration of Genioplasty', *Oral Surg.*, **10**, 677.
—— (1964), 'The Indications for Surgical Correction of Mandibular Deformity by the Sagittal Splitting Technique', *Br. J. oral Surg.*, **1**, 157.
—— (1969a), 'Die bewegung des unteren alveolarfortsatzes zur korrektur von kieferstellungsanomallen', *Dt. zahnärztl. Z.*, **24**, 5.
—— (1969b), 'The Surgical Correction of Small or Retrodisplaced Maxillae—Dish-faced Deformity', *Plastic reconstr. Surg.*, **43**, 351.

PICHLER, H. (1912), 'Über progenie-operationen', *Wien. klin. Wschr.*, **41**, 1333.
— — (1948), in *Mund-und Kieferchirurgie* (PICHLER, H., and TRAUNER, R.), vol. 2, part 2, p. 621. Munich: Urban.
ROBINSON, M. (1958), 'Prognathism Corrected by Open Vertical Sub-Condylectomy', *J. oral Surg.*, **16**, 215.
— — and SHUKEN, R. (1969), 'Bone Resorption under Plastic Surgery Implants', *Ibid.*, **27**, 116.
ROSENTHAL, W. (1931), 'Chirurgische Fragen in der Zahnheilkunde', *Dt. Zahnärztl. Wschr.*, **34**, 655.
RUSHTON, M. A. (1946), 'Unilateral Hyperplasia of the Mandibular Condyle', *Proc. R. Soc. Med.*, **39**, 430.
SCHUCHARDT, K. (1954), 'Die chirurgie als helferin der kieferorthopädie', *Fortschr. Kieferorthop.*, **15**, 1.
SEAR, A. J. (1972), 'Intra-oral Condylectomy applied to Unilateral Condylar Hyperplasia', *Br. J. oral Surg.*, **10**, 143–153.
SEWARD, G. R. (1970), personal communication.
— — (1973), personal communication.
— — and FOREMAN, B. C. (1972), 'Quick-release Locking Plates', *Br. Dent. J.*, **132**, 366–368.
SKALOUD, F. (1951), 'A New Surgical Method for Correcting Prognathism of the Mandible', *Oral Surg.*, **4**, 689.
SMITH, A. E., and JOHNSON, J. B. (1940), 'Surgical Treatment of Mandibular Deformities', *J. Am. dent. Ass. dent. Cosmos*, **27**, 689.
SOWRAY, J. H., and HASKELL, R. (1968), 'Ostectomy at the Mandibular Symphysis', *Br. J. oral Surg.*, **6**, 97.
STRAITH, R. E., and LAWSON, J. M. (1967), 'Surgical Orthodontia: A New Horizon for Plastic Surgery', *Plastic reconstr. Surg.*, **39**, 366.
TAYLOR, R. S., and COOK, H. P. (1958), 'The Surgical Correction of Skeletal Deformities of the Mandible', *Br. dent. J.*, **105**, 349.
TESSIER, P., and others (1967), 'Osteotomies Cranio-naso-orbito-faciales. Hypertelorisme', *Annls Chir. plastic.*, **12**, 103.
THOMA, K. H. (1948), *Oral Surgery*, vol. 2. St Louis: Mosby.
— — (1969), *Ibid.*, 5th ed.
TRAUNER, F. (1929), 'Unterkieferplastik nach Verlast beider Gelenkköpfchen', *Zbl. Chir.*, **56**, 1986.
TRAUNER, R., and OBWEGESER, H. (1957), 'The Surgical Correction of Mandibular Prognathism and Retrognathia with Consideration of Genioplasty', *Oral Surg.*, **10**, 787.
WASSMUND, M. (1935), *Lehrbuch der praktischen chirurgie des mundes und der kiefer*, vol. 1. Leipzig: Meuser.
WINSTANLEY, R. P. (1968), 'One Stage Maxillary Ostectomy for Correction of Class II, Division I Malocclusion', *Br. J. oral Surg.*, **2**, 173.
WUNDERER, S. (1962), 'Die prognathie operation mittels frontal gesticltem maxilla fragment', *Ost. Z. Stomat.*, **59**, 98.

Chapter XVI

THE REPLACEMENT OF BONE

BONE which has been destroyed by accident, disease, or surgery in any quantity must be replaced, for there are limits to the degree to which such bone will regenerate. Bone can be replaced by bone-grafts or by allelografts. Bone-grafts can be taken from the host himself (autograft), from a donor of the same species (homograft), or from a donor of another species (heterograft). Cortical bone, cancellous bone, or mixed cortical cancellous slabs may be used. Such grafts can be applied as chips, flakes, or shaped blocks. The bone can be used when freshly cut or after storage. Heterogenous material is usually prepared for use in ways which remove the soft tissues, or attempt to destroy their antigenicity. Allelografts can be of metal, plastic, or silastic.

It is, perhaps, worth while considering the circumstances in which new bone will successfully regenerate before considering the indications for grafts. For example, new bone will be produced to unite the fragments of a fractured bone. Ideally the bone-ends should be held firmly together without movement until union occurs, the tissues, of course, being free from infection, healthy, and vascular. However, fractures will unite in spite of movement, though the time required may be considerable. Movement, of course, implies movement of one fragment relative to the other. Considerable movement will have little effect if the fragments move together with little relative movement of the bone-ends. Thus, one should not be too dogmatic about the prognosis for an un-united fracture of the mandible with rounded and eburnated bone-ends. Even without fixation, freshening of the bone-ends, or grafting it will be found that some such fractures are united if the patient is seen 2–3 years later.

A gap between the bone-ends will delay union, but again a significant gap can be bridged. Provided the gap width is less than the cross-section of the bone-ends, there can be reasonable hope of success if immobilization is continued for an adequate time.

Even following full-thickness resection of part of the mandible, there can be a surprising amount of new bone deposited, particularly if the periosteum has been retained and especially during childhood and adolescence. Indeed, where a metallic implant has been placed within the periosteum in a child to replace part of the mandible which has been resected, a layer of bone will often be deposited over the surface. A surprising regeneration of bone can occur after a marginal or partial-thickness resection of the mandible. In fact, restitution of the full width of the basal bone can be hoped for. In the maxilla a similar state of affairs exists. Quite sizeable bony perforations penetrating into the nose or maxillary sinus will be repaired if the soft-tissue covering is lined by periosteum.

Because of the difficulty which was experienced in the past with the reduction and fixation of maxillary fractures, the story grew up that bony union did not occur in this bone and that bone regeneration was poor. In fact, fractured maxillae do unite; indeed impacted fractures become solid with considerable speed, and full-thickness defects in the flat bones heal provided that periosteum covers them. On the other hand, there seems a greater likelihood of cyst cavities in the maxilla filling slowly, or incompletely, after marsupialization than in the mandible, particularly where the lining has reached the palatal, nasal, or maxillary sinus mucoperiosteum.

Bone-grafts are used in oral surgery in the following situations:—
1. In the treatment of un-united fractures.
2. To speed the union of the fragments after certain osteotomies.
3. To replace excised segments of mandible or to repair large defects in the maxilla.
4. To restore continuity in the bone where osteotomies have been performed to lengthen the mandible or radically displace the maxilla.
5. As onlay grafts to improve the contour of a bone.
6. To increase the height of the alveolar process so as to improve the foundation for a denture.
7. To fill bony cavities left after the enucleation of cysts or benign neoplasms and hasten healing, or to maintain the normal contour of the bone.

The Fate of Fresh Bone-grafts

If all the cells of a bone-graft were to die and osteogenetic activity spread into the mass only from the site of contact with the adjacent bone, then the process of incorporation would take a considerable time, far longer than is found in practice. That, at best, the vast majority of the original cells within the graft die, even with autografts, can be confirmed by histological section. However, shortly after the invasion of the cancellous spaces by granulation tissue, both osteoclastic resorption of the graft trabeculae and deposition of new bone upon the graft trabeculae is evident throughout the mass. While there is considerable circumstantial evidence that a few of the superficial osteoblasts survive in autografts, much of this activity must result from inductive changes brought about by the bony mass on the cells of the invading granulation tissue. Some believe that a chemical substance, which Lacroix (1951) terms 'osteogenin', is present in the graft and brings about this inductive change.

It is obvious that porous cancellous bone is more easily invaded and incorporated than cortical bone; thus within six weeks most cancellous bone-grafts will be firmly united to the recipient bone.

The Fate of Stored Bone

If grafting between twins and between individuals of an inbred population is excluded, then whenever tissue is transferred from one individual to another an immunological reaction is induced, unless, of course, immunosuppression has been used, as when organ transplantation is attempted. Following a first transfer of tissue there is initial acceptance of the transplant, followed by rejection after about 10–14 days. If tissue is transferred between the same two individuals a second time, the rejection process starts immediately and is more severe. In the process of homografting of bone, there is no practical reason for transferring tissue a second time, so that only the first type of reaction is relevant.

Homografts are invaded by granulation tissue in the same way as autografts, and necrotic soft tissue is removed. Because an immune response must be elicited by the graft, almost certainly no donor cells survive. Unlike the situation with other tissues, with bone homografts there is a calcified matrix which is not destroyed by the host's response. Furthermore, this calcified matrix seems to be capable of exerting an inductive influence on the invading granulation tissue resulting in osteogenesis. Thus, by twelve weeks there is little difference between an autograft and a homograft. However, clinically, there is a somewhat smaller chance of a successful 'take' with homograft bone compared with autograft bone.

The attraction of homo- and heterograft bone is that a second and often debilitating surgical procedure is not necessary in order to obtain the bone. It is rare that suitable homograft bone is available in the fresh state at the right time for a grafting procedure. The bone has therefore to be stored. Healthy sterile bone may be obtained when ribs are resected during thoracotomy or nephrectomy operations. In some countries it is possible to obtain suitable bone from cadavers. Any flesh is carefully removed and the bone freeze-dried.

There is a considerable attraction in the concept of having available for use regular supplies of bone suitable for grafting and of a convenient size. A number of attempts have been made to satisfy this need. One of the earliest was to take the excised diseased segment of bone and to boil it. This destroyed any neoplastic cells or infection. The boiled and defleshed bone was replaced in its original site. As such a graft is composed of cortical bone on the outside so invasion by granulation tissue is difficult and slow and success proportionately low. Os purum, or bone from which some of the organic elements had been removed, was advocated by Orell in 1937. More recently a number of other materials have become available: anorganic bone, Kiel bone, and Boplant bone.

Anorganic bone is prepared by boiling the bone in ethylenediamine for several days. At the end of this time the ethylenediamine is washed out. The anorganic bone can be stored indefinitely without refrigeration. Although brittle it can be trimmed with a scalpel and cut up into chips.

Kiel bone is bovine bone treated with hydrogen peroxide and a de-fatting agent. Boplant is similar save that the bovine bone is treated with β-propiolactone to sterilize it and detergents and organic solvents to remove the fat. They are freeze-dried for storage. Killey, Kramer, and Wright have investigated these substances with the object of determining their possible usefulness for grafting procedures in oral surgery (Killey, Kramer, and Wright, 1966, 1970; Kramer, Killey and Wright, 1968 a, b, c.

Unfortunately these materials appear to be of limited usefulness in this field. Anorganic bone is largely inert. It is neither subject to osteoclastic resorption, except very slowly, nor does it induce osteoblastic activity. Indeed, it impedes the normal repair of a bony defect. Once incorporated in the part, it remains virtually unchanged for many months. Its only place would appear to be as a cavity filler where contour of the bone is of more importance than strength, or as a subperiosteal onlay graft, when it can be placed reasonably deep in the tissues, and where its inertness might prove an advantage. Other forms of onlay graft tend eventually to be resorbed.

Both Kiel bone and Boplant are treated by the host in a similar manner. Initially the graft is invaded rapidly by granulation tissue and trabeculae adjacent to the host bone are covered by new bone. Then giant cells appear on the surface of the uncoated graft bone trabeculae and they are surrounded by lymphocytes, plasma cells, macrophages, and even a few polymorphs. This reaction appears to be immunological in type and induced by the considerable amount of bone matrix and dead osteocytes which remain after the chemical preparation. Fragmentation and destruction of all the uncovered trabeculae follows, but the activity of the giant cells differs from that seen in normal osteoclasis. The inflammatory cell infiltration does not disappear until all the exposed graft bone has been destroyed.

It would appear that these products can only be used with success where rapid coating of the graft bone with new host bone can occur. That is, where the graft can be protected from the immunological response.

The Conditions for Success in Bone-grafting

In the rest of this chapter only autogenous bone-grafting will be described, since this is in general the most successful type of procedure. The conditions for success in bone-grafting are as follows:—

1. Absence of Infection.—It is obviously desirable that there should be an absence of infection, for should the graft become infected before it has been revascularized it will constitute a sequestrum. Even if the infection should not become established until after the graft has been revascularized, then the situation would be the same as an infected fracture.

Ideally, therefore, bone-grafts are inserted through skin incisions since the skin can be more thoroughly cleaned and disinfected on the surface than the more delicate mucous membranes of the mouth. Further, the wound edges can be covered with adhesive drapes or wound towels. Nevertheless, after careful preparation of the oral cavity bone-grafts can be successfully placed through oral incisions (Obwegeser, 1966 and 1968), even where a sizeable opening into the mouth exists. Meticulous multilayer closure and the postoperative use of antibiotics are necessary aids to a good result.

It is even possible to replace parts of the mandible affected by chronic osteomyelitis by an immediate bone-graft, but it is important to ensure that wound contamination is reduced to a minimum by the technique of excision. Thorough irrigation of the wound, the local instillation of an antibiotic to which the organisms are sensitive, and the postoperative administration of systemic antibiotics increase the chances of success.

The reason for attempting immediate grafting in these circumstances is that once the space for the segment of jaw has been allowed to collapse it is difficult to re-open it since the area becomes considerably scarred. Should the attempt fail, however, the graft will have to be removed and the infection cleared up before a further attempt can be made. Also the first donor site will have been operated on in vain.

Chip grafts are in general more rapidly vascularized and therefore more resistant to infection than block grafts. In fact, if infection does supervene only some of the chips may be lost. Curiously, there is a minimum size below which cancellous bone chips cease to act as grafts and are treated as foreign bodies (Hey Groves, 1917; Anderson, 1961).

2. A Vascular, Unscarred Bed.—Unless the recipient site has an adequate blood-supply to ensure rapid invasion of the graft by granulation tissue and its adequate nourishment, the graft will fail. The greater the proportion of cortical to cancellous bone, the more vascular must be the graft bed to ensure success. In general, rib grafts require a more vascular bed than iliac crest grafts (Gillies and Millard, 1957).

3. An Adequate Area of Contact between Graft and the Bone-end.—A good broad contact between the graft and the medullary bone of the recipient bone is essential for union of the graft.

4. Immobilization.—As in the case of union of a fracture, firm contact of the parts with complete immobility produces the best environment for the early stages of union of the graft to the recipient site. Even when chips are used, the fragments should be packed tightly together so that the necessary degree of contact and lack of movement is obtained.

Once new bone unites the graft to the host bone, a degree of functional stress leads to the most rapid consolidation of the graft (Steinhäuser, 1967). Radiographic density increases as new bone is deposited throughout the graft. A layer of bone appears over the whole surface of the mass to form a new cortex, but while there is some remodelling of the inner architecture, only in the young does the graft completely loose the trabecular characteristics of the donor bone.

It is important that all parts of the graft function. For example, a nicely shaped angle on a graft replacing part of the mandible will not be retained unless the masseter and medial pterygoid can be reattached to it. Indeed, in the long term, that is over twenty to thirty years, there seems to be a tendency for all mandibular grafts to be reduced in bulk. Particularly is it true of those replacing the ramus and condyle. Indeed, if it is possible without prejudice to the procedure, the condyle and condyle neck should be conserved and attached to the graft.

CHIP AND FLAKE GRAFTS

In the adult, bone for grafting is usually taken from the iliac crest. Iliac crest bone has a large bulk of cancellous tissue compared with cortex and grafts of a uniform porous texture can be cut from it.

The assistant places his hand on the skin above the iliac crest and depresses it towards the abdomen. This draws the skin upwards so that the scar will lie in the 'bikini' line and not over the crest where it will be subject to friction. The incision follows the line of the outer lip of the crest and is deepened to the muscles. The periosteum is incised between the external oblique origin and the gluteus medius. About 2·5 cm. of the gluteus medius origin is elevated from the bone and a strip of cortex of adequate length and about 2 cm. in width removed from just below the crest. Flakes of cancellous bone can now be removed with a chisel, or blocks separated through as far as the inner cortex. The blocks can be cut up into chips of a size suitable for the procedure.

Where larger amounts of cancellous bone are required, the crest is divided across through the muscle with an osteotome and then separated by a cut parallel with the crest, so that it hinges upwards on the oblique muscles and periosteum. Osteotomes are then driven in to separate a length of ilium about 2 cm. shorter than the crest 'lid'. The crest can be reattached either with braided wire suture or No. 1 chromic cat gut. A disadvantage of this approach is that comfortable walking is delayed until the crest has united to the rest of the bone—about 3–4 weeks. Where it is necessary to take grafts in children or young adolescents, however, it is necessary to conserve the crestal epiphysis and this approach may be required.

Ooze from the bone is controlled by crushing bleeding points and by the use of bone wax and Surgicel. The wound is closed in layers with vacuum drainage.

If a small amount of chips is required, as in the grafting of an un-united fracture or an osteotomy site, a 5-cm. incision only is made. A 1–2-cm. square of cortex is lifted off from just below the crest and a straight curette used to remove the cancellous bone. It can be swept laterally between the cortical plates and surprising amounts removed. The technique was described by Scott, Petersen, and Grant (1949) and by Flint (1964).

Block Grafts

Block grafts are used to replace full thickness segments of a bone, since they are mechanically stronger and easier to handle for this purpose than chips. Chips can be packed into a relatively short gap between bone-ends, but some form of strut must be used to give the mass cohesiveness over a long stretch. In addition, block grafts can be contoured more accurately than an aggregate of chips and are used where this aspect is important.

The end or ends of the bone to which the graft is to be fixed are recessed by removing the cortex. This not only forms a lap joint, but exposes medullary bone against which the graft can be fixed.

After applying an adhesive skin drape the iliac crest is exposed as before. The periosteum and muscles are elevated from the crest of the ridge and the medial surface of the ilium is exposed. The iliacus is not as tightly attached to the medial surface of the ilium as the gluteus medius to the lateral and its elevation causes less disturbance to the gait.

A template cut from a thin sheet of malleable metal, such as relief chamber metal, is applied to the bone. Where a replacement for one-half of the mandible is to be cut, the ilium on the same side is exposed and the template inverted. The lower border follows the crest, the angle lies just posterior to the anterior superior spine and the anterior end lies towards the sacro-iliac joint.

An outline of the proposed graft is traced on the bone either with the corner of a narrow osteotome or a No. 10 rose head bur. The outline should be somewhat oversize to allow for trimming. It is particularly important to have some excess in length to ensure an accurate joint with the bone-end. The outline is deepened either with osteotomes or drill up to the outer cortex. This cortex should be penetrated in the region of the condyle but not elsewhere. Only in some thin male pelves is it necessary to take the full thickness of the bone.

With a thin-bladed osteotome the graft is separated from the outer cortex. This should be done with patience, deepening the cut a little at a time, or either the graft or the osteotome will be fractured. Haemostasis is achieved and the wound is closed as before. To avoid a haematoma a tube drain connected via a bottle to a pump is used.

Careful contouring with sharp osteotomes, bone nibblers, and vulcanite burs will produce a suitable replica of the missing part. The graft is fitted into place and wired securely to the bone-end. The inner cortex of the

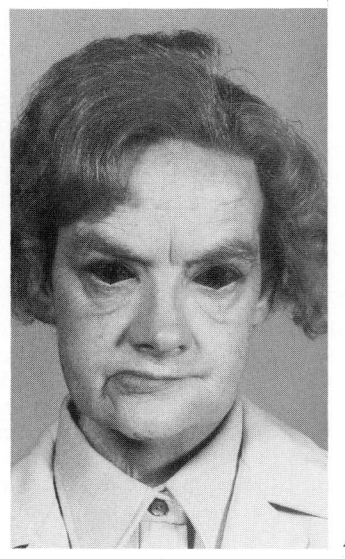

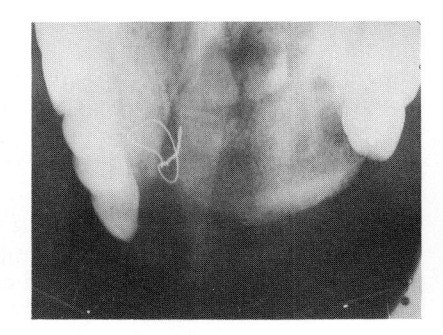

Fig. 33.

Fig. 32.

Fig. 32.—This patient had a primary carcinoma of the right side of the tongue treated by radiotherapy and a block dissection of neck. There has been no recurrence. A fresh primary has arisen in the left lingual sulcus and the new neoplasm has been excised together with the left mandible, left half of tongue, and contents of the left submandibular region. An immediate bone-graft was placed giving good function and a good aesthetic result.

Fig. 33.—A 0·5 cm. squamous carcinoma of the palate has been excised with a block of maxillary bone. An immediate iliac crest bone-graft has been inserted to replace ridge and palate and chips packed in to restore the contour of the floor of the nose. Bilateral sulcus and cheek flaps were used to cover the graft. The X-ray shows good union and acceptance of the graft.

ilium gives the graft reasonable strength and the cancellous surface aids early vascularization.

There has been considerable improvement in the aesthetics of bone-grafts to the mandible. (*Fig.* 32.) Manchester emphasizes how it is possible to provide a graft which closely mimics the original in appearance and function (Manchester, 1965), and Obwegeser (1966) has encouraged the intra-oral excision of the part and its immediate replacement through the same incision. (*Fig.* 33.) Provided an adequate margin of tissue can be removed without trespassing on the lesion, this approach has advantages. Great care must be taken to avoid a haematoma forming, as this will put tension on the suture line. Vacuum drains, circumferential sutures, and careful closure in layers are all aids to this end.

CURVED BONE-GRAFTS

From time to time it will be necessary to replace segments of bone of such a curvature that part of the iliac crest will not do, for example, in the replacement of the anterior part of the mandible. (*Fig.* 34.) Several approaches can be made to this problem. Sizeable chips of ilium can be threaded on a stout wire (Kirschner wire) which has been bent to the

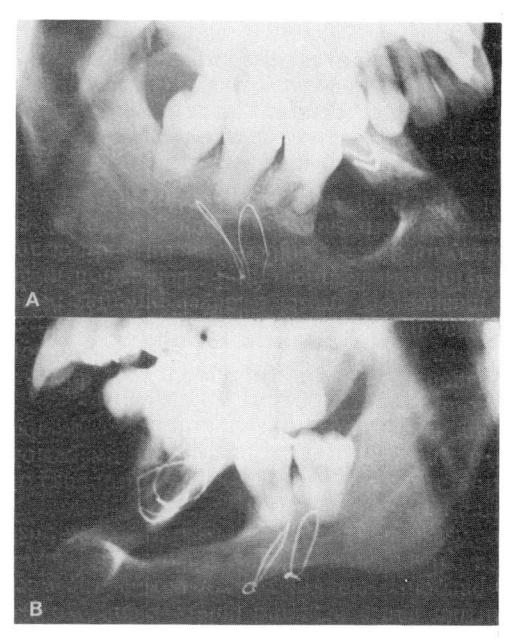

Fig. 34.—Right and left oblique lateral jaw radiographs showing replacement of the anterior part of the mandible by a single horseshoe-shaped piece of bone. A, A radiograph of the left side at three months postoperative and, B, a radiograph of the right side at one year.

desired shape. The ends of the wire are thrust into the medullary cavities of the bone-ends and more chips built up around the strut as the wound is closed.

Another technique (Albee, 1919; Dingman, 1950; Seward, 1967) utilizes a 'U' of bone cut from the surface of the ilium. A graft from molar region to molar region can be managed in this manner. A further alternative uses a length of rib which is notched with a saw so that it can be bent with a series of green-stick fractures (Steiss, 1949; Gillies and Millard, 1957). Finally, where all or almost all of the mandible has been removed the two sides are replaced by cortico-cancellous blocks cut as already described. The front ends of the blocks are cut to form a step. A third piece cut to include the tubercle from one iliac crest is fixed across between the bone-ends. It is shaped at each end to complement the steps cut in the lateral pieces and fixed to them with two wires on each side.

Rib Grafts

Because it is denser bone and not of a size that favours contouring, rib is not generally used to replace parts of the jaws, though there are special circumstances where it is used.

Ribs removed by subperiosteal dissection are replaced. Indeed, in a child the replacement may defy detection in a radiograph. Thus, rib is used in infants for grafting alveolar clefts and in young children in preference to iliac bone. An incision is made over the 7th rib and deepened to its surface. The periosteum is raised and divided at right angles to the line of the rib at each end. A Doyen periosteal elevator is used to separate the periosteum on the inner surface. This must be done with care, since the parietal pleura is close below and a tear in the rib bed will almost certainly open the chest cavity. A cuffed tube should be used by the anaesthetist so that if necessary the lungs can be inflated and, if the chest is accidentally opened, an underwater drain must be inserted.

The required length of rib is resected and the wound closed in layers. It is common practice to split the rib lengthwise so that medullary bone is exposed in the graft.

Cartilage Grafts

These may be cut for onlay grafting from the costo-chondral junction region of the 8th, 9th, and 10th ribs. Full-thickness removal of cartilage should be avoided. Where sizeable quantities are required freeze-dried, bank cartilage should be used if it is available.

Allelografts

The concept of tailor-made or ready-made allelografts which can be screwed, or bolted into place is one which holds great attractions for those doing radical surgery for malignant neoplasms. Acrylic resin, silastic, teflon, tantalum, stainless steel, and various chrome-cobalt alloys have been used in this way.

Such appliances can be used in several ways: one way in which allelografts are used is as a temporary replacement for a segment of jaw until bone-grafting can be undertaken at a second operation. Such a use prevents the collapse and scar contracture which otherwise occurs and impedes the establishment of a bed for the graft at the next procedure. The simplest appliance of this type is a Kirschner wire which has been threaded at each end to take a nut. Henny and McClelland (1959) have used such an appliance by impacting the wire into the bone-ends so that the nuts prevent the wire from working farther into the bone-ends. Provided that full intermaxillary fixation is used, such appliances do not become displaced and work well.

Others (*see* Henny and McClelland, 1959) use the appliance as an aid to immobilization during the actual grafting. A stout wire or a tray screwed to the lower borders of the bone-ends may be used in this manner.

Finally, permanent implants may be used. These may be either made for the individual occasion or system-built commercial appliances assembled to meet the operator's requirements. They are usually bolted to the remaining bone fragment. Dewey and Moore (1962), Mallet (1963),

Cooke (1969), and Bowerman and Conroy (1969) have described examples of these systems.

It is perhaps unfortunate that the long-term success of these prostheses is poor. Even in the hands of experts the soft tissues seem ultimately to break down over some prominence. Perhaps the depth to which it is possible to bury them in these regions is too little. Alternatively, the fixation of the implant to the jaw works loose. Initially, all are agreed, the fixation must be very strong indeed but, even so, should the slightest movement start to occur, osteoclastic resorption will result in rapid loosening. Neither does it seem easier to get the wound to heal over these materials. Indeed, bone-grafts are far less demanding in terms of environment. For example, if the flaps are thin, or the tissues have been irradiated, an allelograft will not be a success.

In the authors' opinion, in spite of the additional operative trauma, an immediate, but not elaborate, iliac crest bone-graft is preferable in many cases where an implant would be used.

ELECTIVE TRACHEOSTOMY

After resection of large segments of the mandible and adjacent tissues, and the insertion of bone-grafts, the patency of the airway is of concern. In certain patients a tracheostomy is necessary to safeguard the airway during the early postoperative days.

The head is extended on the neck by means of a small sandbag between the shoulders. A collar incision about 5 cm. long is made a finger's breadth above the medial ends of the clavicles. It is deepened through the platysma and flaps raised mainly upwards, but also downwards.

The midline is carefully identified and the strap muscles separated to expose the thyroid gland. The upper edge of the thyroid isthmus is separated from the front of the trachea. Blunt dissection with an artery forceps releases the rest of the isthmus and the forceps emerge below its lower border. Any adjacent inferior thyroid veins are gently picked up and a retractor inserted under the lower border of the isthmus. This both exposes the second, third, and fourth rings of the trachea and lifts the trachea up into the wound. Cautiously the trachea is incised, so that neither the anaesthetist's tube nor the vulnerable posterior wall of the trachea are damaged. With cartilage shears an oval window, of suitable size and with its long axis vertical, is cut in the front of the second and third rings. The fragment is grasped before it is finally cut off so that it is not dropped into the lumen of the trachea. Tracheal dilators are inserted and a cuffed, plastic tracheostomy tube is inserted as the anaesthetist withdraws the endotracheal tube.

The strap muscles, platysma, and the skin are closed in layers about the tube, but not too tightly. The wound is sprayed with a plastic dressing, a dry dressing applied, and the tapes of the tube tied behind the neck.

REFERENCES

ALBEE, F. H. (1915), *Bone Graft Surgery*, p.35. Philadelphia: Saunders.
— — (1919), *Orthopedic and Reconstructive Surgery*, p. 1062. Philadelphia: Saunders.
ANDERSON, K. (1961), 'A Histological Study of the Effect of Size of the Implant', *J. Bone Jt Surg.*, **43A**, 980.

BOWERMAN, J. E., and CONROY, B. (1969), 'A Universal Kit in Titanium for Immediate Replacement of the Resected Mandible', *Br. J. oral Surg.*, **6**, 223.
COOK, H. P. (1969), 'Titanium in Mandibular Replacement', *Ibid.*, **7**, 108.
DEWEY, A. R., and MOORE, J. W. (1962), 'Mandibular Repair after Radical Resection, *J. oral Surg.*, **20**, 34.
DINGMAN, R. O. (1950), The Use of Iliac Bone in the Repair of Facial and Cranial Defects', *Plastic reconstr. Surg.*, **6**, 174.
FLINT, M. (1964), 'Chip Bone Grafting of the Mandible', *Br. J. plast. Surg.*, **17**, 184.
GILLIES, Sir H., and MILLARD, D. R. (1957), *The Principles and Art of Plastic Surgery*, vol. 2, p. 527. London: Butterworths.
GROVES, E. HEY (1917), 'Methods and Results of Transplantation of Bone in the Repair of Defects caused by Injury or Disease'. *Br. J. Surg.*, **5**, 185.
HENNY, F. A., and MCCLELLAND, W. D. (1959), 'Methods of Fixation in Mandibular Bone Grafts', *J. oral Surg.*, **17**, 34.
KILLEY, H. C., KRAMER, I. R. H., and WRIGHT, H. C. (1966), 'The Effects of Implanting Heterogenous Compact and Cancellous Anorganic Bone into Long Bones of Rabbits', *Archs oral Biol.*, **11**, 1117.
— — — — — — (1970), 'The Response of the Rabbit to Implants of Processed Bovine (Kiel Bone) and the Effects of Varying the Relationship between Implant and Host Bone', *Ibid.*, **15**, 33.
KRAMER, I. R. H., KILLEY, H. C., and WRIGHT, H. C. (1968a), 'The Replacement of Bone', *Aust. dent. J.*, **13**, 17.
— — — — — — (1968b), 'A Histological and Radiological Comparison of the Healing of Defects in the Rabbit Calvarium with and without Implanted Heterogenous Anorganic Bone', *Archs oral Biol.*, **13**, 1095.
— — — — — — (1968c), 'The Response of the Rabbit to Implants of Processed Calf Bone (Boplant)', *Ibid.*, **13**, 1263.
LACROIX, P. (1951), *The Organisation of Bones*. London: Churchill. Translation of 1949 French edition.
MALLET, S. P. (1963), 'A Method of Preparing and Using Stainless Steel in Oral Surgery', *Oral Surg.*, **16**, 1160.
MANCHESTER, W. M. (1965), 'Immediate Reconstruction of the Mandible and Temporomandibular Joint', *Br. J. plast. Surg.*, **8**, 291.
OBWEGESER, H. L. (1966), 'Simultaneous Resection and Reconstruction of Parts of the Mandible via the Intra-oral Route in Patients with and without Gross Infections', *Oral Surg.*, **21**, 693.
— — (1968), 'Primary Repair of the Mandible by the Intra-oral Route after Partial Resection in Cases with and without Preoperative Infection', *Br. J. plastic Surg.*, **21**, 282.
ORELL, S. (1937), 'Surgical Bone Grafting with Os Purium, Os Novum and Boiled Bone', *J. Bone Jt Surg.*, **19**, 873.
SCOTT, W., PETERSEN, R. C., and GRANT, S. (1949), 'A Method of procuring Iliac Bone by Trephine Curettage', *J. Bone Jt Surg.*, **31A**, 860.
SEWARD, G. R. (1967), 'A Method of Replacing the Anterior Part of the Mandible by Bone Graft', *Br. J. oral Surg.*, **5**, 99.
STEINHÄUSER, E. (1967), 'Influence of Function on Bone Grafts reconstructing the Mandible—An Experimental Study', *Excerpta Medica*, **174**, 137. 4th International Congress of Plastic and Reconstructive Surgery, Rome, 1967.
STEISS, C. F. (1949), 'Utilization of the Tube Pedicle in the Reconstruction of Facial Defects', *Plastic reconstr. Surg.*, **4**, 545.

Chapter XVII
SOME SKELETAL DISEASES OF INTEREST TO THE ORAL SURGEON

Fibrous Dysplasia of Bone

Much of the confusion in the literature surrounding fibrous dysplasia stems from the multiplicity of titles under which cases have been described, for Lichtenstein and Jaffe (1942) reported no fewer than 37 such synonyms. In order to understand this aspect of the problem more clearly, it is necessary to consider a chronological history of the condition.

In 1891 Von Recklinghausen published a monograph in which he described several cases of bony dysplasia which appeared to fall into one group but which, in fact, represented several different conditions. Two of the cases in this series were generalized osteitis fibrosa and his name is still attached to this condition.

In 1904 Askanazy reported a case of osteitis fibrosa in which a parathyroid tumour was discovered after death, and in 1926 Mandl successfully performed a parathyroidectomy for a case with the characteristic bone changes. Hunter and Turnbull (1931) pointed out that there was a large group of dysplasias which were obviously not due to hyperparathyoidism and called them 'diffuse osteitis fibrosa' in contradistinction to the lesions associated with hyperparathyroidism, which were known as 'osteitis fibrosa cystica generalisata'. The non-hormonal group continued to be classified as varieties of osteitis fibrosa until it was observed that some of the lesions were associated with extraneous pigmentation and other extra-skeletal manifestations. The first of these cases was described by Weil in 1922, but subsequently cases were reviewed by McCune and Bruch (1937) and by Albright, Butler, Hampton, and Smith (1937). The condition is now referred to as Albright's syndrome. The subjects are usually children and the classic triad consists of:—

1. Polyostotic fibrous dysplasia with a tendency to a unilateral distribution.
2. Abnormal pigmentation of the skin and occasionally of the mucous membrane.
3. Sexual precocity especially in females due to endocrine dysfunction.

Skin Pigmentation.—The pigmentation is of the *café-au-lait* type and is usually scattered over the back, thighs, and buttocks. Cases have been reported with oral pigmentation.

Endocrine System.—The most common feature is precocious puberty with the menarche at from 1 to 5 years of age in 50 per cent of cases and from 6 to 10 years in another 33 per cent. Breast development and pubic and axillary hair appear after the menarche. Occasionally precocious puberty occurs in males and it may be accompanied by gynaecomastia.

In 1938 Lichtenstein observed that the bone lesions which were the essential feature of the disease could occur in the absence of the extra-skeletal manifestations and suggested the term 'polyostotic fibrous dysplasia'. In 1942 Lichtenstein and Jaffe made the further observation that the condition could be confined to a single bone and, therefore, suggested the term 'fibrous dysplasia' to describe the entire group, but stipulated that monostotic or polyostotic varieties could occur.

Aetiology.—The aetiology of fibrous dysplasia is unknown, but most workers now regard it as a developmental defect. The disease is neither familial nor hereditary, and where an identical twin is affected it is usual for the other to be entirely normal.

Jaffe (1958a) suggested that it may have its basis in some deep-rooted defect. Caffey (1956) considered that the dystrophy was of neurogenic origin. Tannhauser (1944) related it to neurofibromatosis. Snapper (1949) considered fibrous dysplasia should be linked with lipoid histiocytosis, a view discarded by Falconer, Cope, and Robb Smith (1942) and Fairbank (1950). Schlumberger (1946) attributed the lesion to injury.

Incidence.—The Memorial Sloan-Kettering Cancer Centre found 47 cases of craniofacial fibrous dysplasias in the period 1930–65. The classic Albright's syndrome is rare and only occurs once for every 20 to 30 cases of monostotic or polyostotic fibrous dysplasia without extra-skeletal manifestations. In a series reported by Zimmerman, Stafne, and Dahlin (1958) from the Mayo Clinic, only 1 out of 69 patients with jaw lesions had polyostotic fibrous dysplasia and of 13 patients with polyostotic fibrous dysplasia only 2 had jaw involvement.

Stewart, Gilmer, and Edmonson (1962), at the Campbell Clinic, Memphis, Tennessee, found 20 cases of fibrous dysplasia in a 30-year period. Reviewing the world literature in 1951, Pritchard found 256 cases. He found an equal distribution between male and female. However, Stewart and others (1962) who reviewed 20 cases found 15 males and 5 females.

Sex and Race.—Ramsey, Strong, and Frazell (1968), in their series of 47 patients, found 26 female and 21 male. Most authorities consider the condition more common in females.

Age.—Age of onset of symptoms in Ramsey and others' (1968) series varied from one and a half years to 73 years of age and 83 per cent noted symptoms within the first two decades of life.

Bones Involved.—Any bone may be involved, but the long bones are most frequently affected, especially the upper end of the femur, and this may result in bowing of the leg.

The condition may be asymptomatic, but pain and even fracture may occur, the fractures being multiple and recurrent. Facial asymmetry may develop due to involvement of one or more facial bones, and occasionally there may be proptosis of the eye with associated visual disturbance. The calvarium may be involved and thickened with frontal bulging. The bossing may be asymmetrical and sometimes there is unilateral or bilateral obliteration of the sinuses. The facial bones are involved in about half of the cases. Lesions of the skull are found in about one-half of the cases with a moderate degree of skeletal involvement, and in severe cases the skull is almost always affected (Lucas, 1962).

Oral Manifestations.—The jaws may be enlarged, expanded, and distorted. Radiographs show a dense mass often 'ground glass' in appearance which in the upper jaw expands into and can obliterate the sinuses. In the mandible the jaw may be expanded and distorted and occasionally radiographs reveal a radiolucent area similar to that seen in the long bones. In a few instances there is oral pigmentation. The mandible was the bone most frequently involved in Ramsey's series of 47 cases (Ramsey and others, 1968), but Lucas (1962) states that the lesion is more commonly found in the maxilla. The lesions tend to become inactive after the normal period of bodily growth has terminated, but cases have been reported where the lesion continued to enlarge after this time (Seward, 1970).

The monostotic type of fibrous dysplasia of the craniofacial bones is rarely accompanied by extra-skeletal manifestations, although it is identical histologically to the polyostotic form. The cranial bones are often involved, particularly the base of the skull.

Signs and Symptoms.—The presenting symptom in most instances is swelling and this occurred in 80 per cent of Ramsey's series.

Pain is a less common symptom in jaw cases (Lucas, 1962). Pathological fracture of long bones may occur, but there is no reported case of fracture of the mandible. Harris, Dudley, and Barry (1962), in a series of 50 cases, reported that 85 per cent sustained a fracture of a long bone.

There is little disturbance of function, though teeth may be displaced and occlusion upset. In children, teeth in the affected part may fail to erupt (Lucas, 1962).

Radiology.—The radiological picture of fibrous dysplasia depends on the proportions of fibrous and osseous tissue in the lesion. When the bone in the affected area is predominantly replaced by fibrous tissue an area of radiolucency results and the cortex is thinned and expanded. As ossification occurs in the fibrous tissue, the radiograph becomes more opaque.

With regard to the facial bones the area affected by fibrous dysplasia may vary from a minimal lesion in a single bone, often the maxilla, to the most extensive involvement of both mandible and maxillae with further lesions in the skull. Often the fibrous dysplasia is confined to one side of the face and the deformity may assume bizarre shapes. In the mandible the lesion is usually confined to one side and results in considerable bony expansion. Not infrequently in young patients there is a cyst-like area in the involved bone (Stafne, 1964). In the upper jaw the lesion is usually confined to one maxilla and its neighbouring bones and the maxillary sinus is reduced in size by the dysplasia.

Fibrous dysplasia can be demonstrated on radiographs from a very early age, but in the very young patient the affected area appears almost translucent. As the patient grows the area affected increases in size and becomes more opaque as the fibrous tissue becomes more calcified. At this stage the area involved has a uniform density and assumes the radiographic appearance of ground glass. (*Fig.* 35.) Sometimes the affected bone has the appearance of orange peel. If the lesion involves the teeth the lamina dura may sometimes be lost (Worth, 1963).

When the skull is involved, unusual radiographic appearances may result and often there is an irregular radiolucent area similar to that seen in osteoporosis circumscripta of Paget's disease. There is often an increased density and thickening of the base of the skull.

With the passage of time there is a change in structure of the lesion (Worth, 1963). Serial radiographs have shown that in some cases the lesion becomes more calcified with increasing age of the patient, but exceptions to this are not uncommon (Stafne, 1964).

When such changes occur, the uniform ground-glass appearance of the radiograph gives way to patchy areas of sclerosis until eventually the radiographic appearance is similar to the cotton-wool effects seen in Paget's disease. (*Fig.* 36.) At operation such bone is found to be extremely hard and avascular.

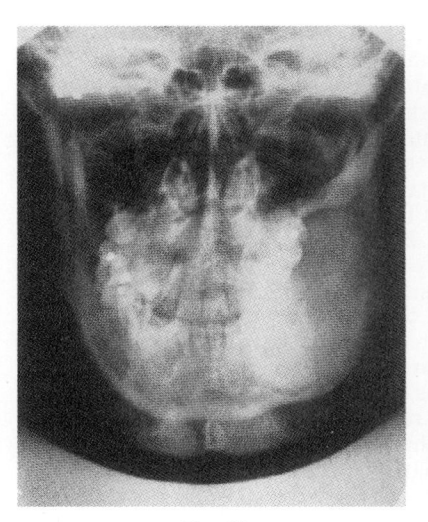

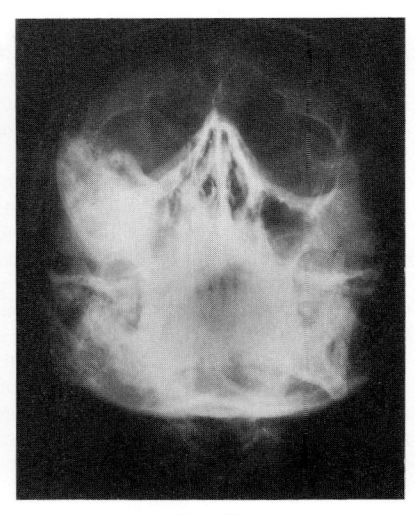

Fig. 35

Fig. 36

Fig. 35.—Postero-anterior radiograph showing fibrous dysplasia of the mandible. The patient is 20 years of age and the lesion has the ground-glass appearance.

Fig. 36.—Occipitomental radiograph in a patient of 40 years of age showing patchy areas of sclerosis in the region of the zygomatic bone which is affected with fibrous dysplasia.

Worth has pointed out that there is no correlation between the radiographs and the histological appearances of the bone involved. A diagnosis of fibrous dysplasia can usually be made on the radiographic appearances alone, but occasionally the lesion may assume most unusual appearances. However, whenever a long-standing bony lesion is seen, the possibility of the diagnosis of fibrous dysplasia must always be considered irrespective of its radiographic appearance.

Histopathology.—Most authorities agree that the lesions in the polyostotic and monostotic types are histologically identical. However, some workers consider that while polyostotic fibrous dysplasia is a developmental anomaly, the monostotic lesions are reparative reactions to trauma (Schlumberger, 1946).

In the area affected there is replacement of normal bone with greyish white tissue which imparts a gritty sensation to the knife due to the newly formed bony trabeculae it contains. Microscopically the cancellous spaces of the marrow are seen to be occupied by cellular fibrous tissue arranged in whorls and interlacing bundles. In this fibrous tissue newly formed woven bone is seen, the trabeculae being irregularly arranged. The original trabeculae are absent and osteoclasts are very few in number. Groups of foam cells may be seen and there is an abrupt demarcation between the affected and the adjacent normal bone, and the lesions are more vascular than normal bone. The proportion of bone in the replacement tissue is variable; in some only scattered trabeculae are seen while others contain a sponge-like arrangement of woven bone which can become quite dense.

Malignant Changes in Fibrous Dysplasia.—Although fibrous dysplasia is regarded as a relatively benign lesion, malignant changes have been recorded by numerous authorities. In 1914 Emslie reported giant-celled sarcoma in a femur with fibrous dysplasia, and further cases have been recorded by Coley and Stewart (1945), Dustin and Ley (1950), Sutro (1951), Perkinson and Higginbotham (1955), Vahkurkina (1958), Jaffe (1958a), Seth, Climie, and Tuttle (1962), and Riddell (1964).

Probably the greatest risk occurs when areas of fibrous dysplasia are irradiated and Sabanas, Dahlin, Childs, and Nins (1956) reported post-irradiation sarcoma in bone affected by fibrous dysplasia, and Van Horn, Johnson, and Dahlin (1963) reported a post-irradiation sarcoma of the maxilla which was affected by monostotic fibrous dysplasia. In a series of 50 cases of fibrous dysplasia, Harris, Dudley, and Barry (1962) reported 2 cases where sarcoma occurred in lesions that had been irradiated.

Cases in which fibrous dysplasia of the jaws have undergone malignant change have also been reported. De Marchi (1956) recorded osteogenic sarcoma occurring in the mandible which was affected by monostotic fibrous dysplasia. Tanner and others (1961) found 4 cases of sarcoma arising in lesions of fibrous dysplasia in the facial bones and in all cases the lesions had been subjected to radiation. Jäger (1962) reported osteogenic sarcoma of the maxilla in a case of Albright's syndrome. Bruckner and others (1967) reported osteogenic sarcoma arising at a site of fibrous dysplasia in the mandible, and Pilheu and Soldato (1966) reported a particularly large fibro-osteosarcoma of the jaw in a case of polyostotic fibrous dysplasia.

Treatment.—Because there is little disturbance of function in cases of craniofacial fibrous dysplasia, most patients seek treatment for cosmetic reasons. In view of the fact that areas of fibrous dysplasia·continue to enlarge during the period of general skeletal growth it is advisable to defer surgery until growth has ceased. It is best to avoid operations designed to reduce the size and contour of the jaws affected by fibrous dysplasia before skeletal growth has ceased since, particularly during adolescence, extremely rapid growth of the remaining part may be induced. However, once growth has ceased contouring operations produce a pleasing and reasonably permanent result. It would appear logical, therefore, to postulate that such surgery should be deferred until the patient is about 21 years of age. However, occasionally the deformity may be so cosmetically unacceptable that earlier operation is indicated, but in such cases the patient should be warned that some relapse is to be anticipated and that a secondary operation may be necessary when general skeletal growth has ceased.

Operations on the upper and lower jaws can usually be satisfactorily effected through an intra-oral incision along the crest of the ridge in the edentulous case and round the buccal aspect of the gingival margin when teeth are present. The operation consists of exposing the affected bone and trimming the excess with chisels or Jansen-Middleton bone gouges. It is not necessary or desirable to excise all the affected bone.

In the young patient the affected bone is quite soft and feels gritty as it is cut. Surgical trimming is a simple matter in such cases, but with increasing age the bone in fibrous dysplasia becomes more sclerotic and great difficulty may be encountered in cutting it. The bone involved by fibrous dysplasia in the young is highly vascularized and haemorrhage may be brisk. It is important to achieve complete haemostasis before closing the wound or large haematoma formation may occur. Bony organization of such a haematoma may contribute to residual bony enlargement in the area. Where possible, a postoperative pressure dressing should be applied.

Elderly patients with fibrous dysplasia not only have hard sclerotic bone, but the area is relatively avascular and liable to postoperative infection. Chronic low-grade osteomyelitis may occur postoperatively in such individuals. All patients with fibrous dysplasia should be reviewed at regular intervals in view of the possible risk of malignant changes developing in the lesion.

Hyperparathyroidism

As long ago as 1877, Langedorff described a patient with cystic disease of the bones and was able to demonstrate evidence which pointed towards an upset in calcium metabolism, and in 1884 Davies-Colley described a 13-year-old girl who had generalized skeletal disease, a tumour of the jaw, and renal stones with an increased renal excretion of calcium.

When Jung reviewed Von Recklinghausen's autopsy material he felt certain that in 2 cases what had been described as a 'lymph-node' was, in fact, a parathyroid adenoma. Askanazy (1904) was the first to relate the bone disease to parathyroid disease and Mandl (1926) was the first to excise the gland for a patient.

Hyperparathyroidism may be due to the presence of one or more parathyroid adenomas, a parathyroid carcinoma, or parathyroid hyperplasia. Parathyroid hyperplasia may be primary or secondary to renal disease or occasionally steatorrhoea. Tertiary hyperparathyroidism occurs when autonomous adenomas arise in a hyperplastic gland. In children the sexes are equally affected, but in adults females are twice as common as males.

The clinical picture exhibited by these people may be presented under three headings: skeletal signs and symptoms, urinary tract signs and symptoms, and signs and symptoms of hypercalcaemia.

Skeletal Signs and Symptoms.—The patient may suffer from aches and pains in the bones which may be tender to pressure. Often such complaints are dismissed initially as muscular rheumatism. Later the bones bend, the skeleton becomes deformed, and pathological fractures occur. The ends of the terminal phalanges are resorbed so that the tips of the fingers and toes fall in, giving an appearance of clubbing. A curious, dull, wooden note may be elicited if the skull is percussed. Giant-cell tumours may develop in the bones, causing expansion of the bone. On occasions they may grow with surprising speed and may be mistaken for a sarcoma.

Finally, in advanced cases the skull may exhibit basilar inversion which carries a danger of medullary compression and death if the neck is extended during parathyroidectomy.

Urinary Tract Signs, Symptoms, and Complications.—A high serum calcium results in a high urinary calcium. This together with the increased phosphorus excretion induced by parathormone leads to calcium diabetes with polyuria and polydipsia.

Renal stones may form and migrate into the ureter, stimulating ureteric colic. Ascending infection, renal damage, and renal failure can follow. Calcification of the renal tissues or nephrocalcinosis will also disturb renal function.

Symptoms and Signs of Hypercalcaemia.—The patient may suffer from anorexia, nausea, and vomiting with abdominal cramps, weakness, wasting, and drowsiness. A parathyroid crisis can resemble an acute abdominal catastrophy. Although the reason for the relationship is unknown, duodenal ulcers and amenorrhoea are common.

Calcium salts may be deposited in the conjunctiva and, when renal impairment produces retention of phosphorus and hyperphosphataemia is added to hypercalcaemia, calcium salts are deposited in the cornea, lungs, blood-vessels, and gastric mucosa.

Curiously, even though some adenomas reach an inch or more in diameter, it is exceptional to be able to palpate them. Perhaps this is because 84 per cent develop in the inferior parathyroid gland.

Pathology.—Osteoclastic resorption of bone takes place under the stimulus of parathormone with progressive destruction of the normal bone. Much woven bone is deposited to replace the lamellar bone and zones of cellular fibrous tissue and giant-cell tissue appear.

Radiology.—Radiographically there is thinning and disappearance of the cancellous trabeculae with resultant widening of the medullary spaces. The cortex initially develops a streaky appearance as Haversian canals are widened, then it, too, is reduced in thickness. Clouds of woven bone spicules are formed and the bone takes on a 'moth-eaten' appearance. Once the cortex has been completely destroyed radiolucency may be extreme, particularly in the jaws where the bone assumes a uniform cloudy or granular pattern.

Giant-cell lesions may form before, or after, obvious generalized bone changes have occurred. They are usually similar in appearance to giant-cell granulomas and are of particular significance if multiple, or if they recur after local surgery. Sometimes giant-cell epulides are formed. In some patients a localized zone of cortex is destroyed which, when viewed from the surface, produces an oval radiolucency. This is the appearance which is loosely described as 'cystic change'.

In all such cases screening tests for hyperparathyroidism should be performed. Although investigation of this condition is now quite sophisticated, the best test for this purpose is still the serum calcium estimation. To be of value, this test should be done properly. The specimen should be taken before the first food in the morning and the vein from which the blood is to be drawn should not be occluded for sufficient time for cyanosis to occur. The tourniquet should be released before the blood is aspirated. Further, the patient must not be taking alkali even if he has a peptic ulcer.

In doubtful cases the test should be repeated at weekly or fortnightly intervals for some months.

The lamina dura will be reduced in thickness as the cancellous trabeculae are thinned, but this change is difficult to spot in the early stages. Any cause of bone atrophy will produce a similar change. A readily detectable loss of lamina dura coincides with the appearance of other obvious bony changes.

The hands are a useful part to radiograph, since detailed pictures can be made. Some even employ macroradiography, whereby an enlarged image is produced by deliberately increasing the object–film distance. The tube must, of course, have an ultra-small focal spot if resolution of detail in the image is to be maintained. Alternatively, fine grain, single emulsion film and magnification of the image can be used. The particular changes which are looked for in these films are loss of the terminal feathering of the distal phalanges and subperiosteal resorption at the junction of the base and the shaft of the phalanges. Such resorption is seen as a roughening of the surface of the bone and small hemispherical cavities.

Another site where subperiosteal resorption is seen is below the medial condyle of the tibia. A sizeable indentation in the surface results and this appearance is called 'Pugh's sign'.

For TREATMENT, *see* p. 96.

RENAL OSTEODYSTROPHY

There are basically two renal conditions which produce bone changes. The first of these is renal rickets in which as a result of a developmental error there is a renal leak of phosphorus and amino-acids. Such patients develop vitamin-D resistance, rickets in childhood, and osteomalacia in adult life. They tend to develop chronic pyelonephritis and the resulting renal damage eventually results in uraemia.

The second condition is azotaemic bone disease or renal osteodystrophy. The uraemic state appears to exert an anti-vitamin D effect and also to reduce the absorption of calcium and phosphorus from the gastro-intestinal tract. These patients have a low serum calcium and develop rickets in childhood and osteomalacia in adult life. Azotaemic bone disease can be added to the osteomalacia due to the renal leak of phosphorus of the first group as uraemia supervenes.

When renal damage becomes severe phosphorus retention tends to occur. This stimulates parathyroid hyperplasia since parathormone controls phosphorus excretion. Thus, secondary hyperparathyroidism is added to osteomalacia, though in renal rickets the rise in serum phosphorus may improve the bone disease.

In some patients certain parathyroid nodules may exhibit autonomous growth converting the secondary hyperparathyroidism into tertiary hyperparathyroidism. Management of these patients involves large doses of vitamin D and, where appropriate, parathyroidectomy.

At one time the problem of renal osteodystrophy was self-limiting since the patients ultimately died from their renal disease. Now with renal dialysis and transplantation the problem has been enhanced and, indeed, dialysis has added to the complexity of the bone disease. It is easy to wash calcium out of the dialysed patient over a period, so it is important to have the correct amount of calcium in the dialysate. Too low a calcium will result in the removal of calcium from the patient and a stimulation of parathyroid hyperplasia. In such patients a return to a normal serum calcium may be an indication of hyperparathyroidism and the need for parathyroidectomy rather than the assumption that all is well with the dialysis. On the other hand, too high a dialysate calcium can result in metastatic calcification.

In practice, because of the large volumes of solution involved, it is not easy to prevent dialysis bone disease. In many centres most patients have bone pain in the feet, knees, and shoulders by the time they have been on regular dialysis for 4–5 years.

For the reasons indicated above, patients with renal rickets and azotaemic osteodystrophy exhibit a mixed picture of bone disease; namely osteomalacia and hyperparathyroidism. In the jaws the appearances of the latter condition dominate the picture as shown in the radiograph. Cawson (1964) described hypoplastic defects in such patients' teeth. Because the hyperparathyroidism is a response to a low serum calcium, the result of the original disease, renal stones are not a feature of secondary hyperparathyroidism.

In dialysate bone disease the appearance more resembles osteoporosis and differs histologically in that there is the resorption of hyperparathyroidism, but no bone deposition and hence no wide osteoid seams. Parathyroidectomy in these patients halts the bone resorption, but does not result in bone deposition and without osteoid vitamin D is useless.

Osteitis Deformans: Paget's Disease of Bone

In 1891 Von Recklinghausen published a paper on generalized osteitis fibrosa. His cases included 2 which today would be classed as polyostotic fibrous dysplasia of bone, but the remainder were either cases of hyperparathyroidism or Paget's disease of bone. While our understanding of polyostotic fibrous dysplasia and hyperparathyroidism has increased greatly since the end of the 19th century, our understanding of Paget's disease is only a little better than that of Paget himself when he wrote his classic paper in 1877.

Aetiology.—The aetiology of osteitis deformans remains obscure and none of the many suggestions as to its cause stands careful scrutiny.

Sex Incidence.—If the skeleton as a whole is considered the sex incidence is about equal, though it is often said that males are somewhat more commonly affected than females. Schmorl (1932) found 80 cases of Paget's disease in 2279 autopsies on male patients and 58 cases among 2235 female cadavers. Barry (1969), in a series of 2630 cases of Paget's disease, found that 1420 were men and 1210 were women.

Incidence.—According to Schmorl (1932) and Collins (1956) some evidence of Paget's disease is present in 3–4 per cent of patients over 40 years of age. In a series of 4614 necropsies performed on unselected persons over the age of 40 years Schmorl (1932), of Dresden, found 138 cases of Paget's disease. Similarly selected post-mortem examinations on 650 persons by Collins (1956) in Leeds and Sheffield showed an incidence of 3·7 per cent cases of Paget's disease.

Figures published by Barry (1969) revealed that in Australia 2630 patients were admitted to hospital with Paget's disease out of a total of 1,769,664 admissions, an incidence of 1:673. All statistics of the disease show that Paget's disease is essentially a disease of old age.

Although the incidence of the disease increases in age-groups above 40, rare cases are known to have been affected from their late teens or early twenties. A point of importance is that usually the condition develops quite slowly. For example, it may take 20 years for the evolution of the typical thickened, cranial vault with cotton-wool radio-opacities, from the time at which osteitis circumscripta appears. Indeed, the slow progress of the disease and lack of obvious physical signs in the early stages probably lead to misunderstandings concerning the age incidence.

Racial and Geographical Distribution.—According to Barry (1969), Paget's disease is fairly common in the United Kingdom, France, and Germany, but rare in Scandinavia. The incidence also appears to be low in Spain, Italy, Central Europe, and Russia. The disease is also less common in North and South America than in England. As yet only occasional cases have been reported from Africa, the Middle East, India, Japan, and China.

Family History.—While in many cases there is no family history, this is not invariably so and periodically papers are published describing families in which several members are affected. According to Barry (1969) the evidence that the disease may have a genetic basis is by no means conclusive.

Signs and Symptoms.—Patients may complain of aching in the diseased bone, pain on weight-bearing, or headaches. When it involves the jaws the pain of the disease during periods of activity may be attributed to the teeth and demands made for their removal. As the affected bones enlarge the pressures to which the teeth are subjected by the soft tissues are altered and they tend to tilt. Their articulation changes and temporomandibular joint dysfunction can follow.

When the condition is widespread there may be stiffness of the joints, muscular weakness, and fatigue. Affected bones increase in thickness and become bent. Dilated blood-vessels are observed in the overlying soft tissues which may feel warm to the touch. Some of the thickened areas of bone are highly vascularized and on auscultation the arteriovenous shunt produces a marked bruit.

Hypercementosis makes the removal of teeth from an affected jaw difficult. (*Fig.* 37.) When they are extracted the sensation is like the pulling of a screw from rotten wood. A brisk haemorrhage follows, but usually ceases spontaneously. Following the extractions, patches of dense bone near the socket may become infected, leading to septic sockets or even to localized osteomyelitis. Other dental complications of this condition are resorption of the roots of teeth and ankylosis. Where a tooth affected by hypercementosis is adjacent to a mass of sclerosed bone, union of the two tissues tends to occur. Ankylosis then leads to submersion of the tooth as the alveolar process continues to enlarge.

Histology.—Histologically in Paget's disease there is resorption of existing bone and deposition of new. There is destruction of the cortex with widening of the Haversian canals until large, vascular, Haversian lakes are formed. The normal fatty marrow is replaced by a cellular connective tissue, the so-called 'fibrosis of the marrow', and new bone is deposited both endosteally and subperiosteally. Resorption and deposition of bone continue at an abnormal rate, leading to the formation of the classic mosaic pattern. Fluorescent marker studies suggest that the turnover of bone is ten times the normal.

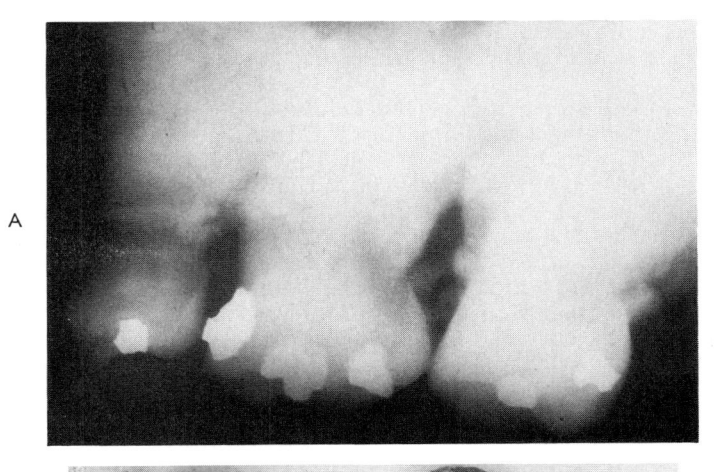

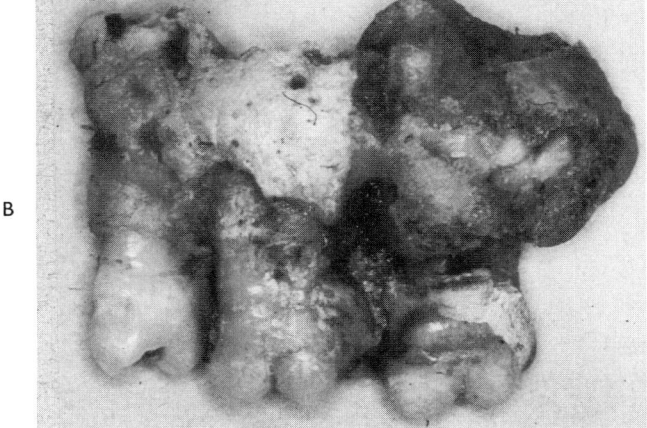

Fig. 37.—A, Intra-oral radiograph of |678 showing marked hypercementosis in a patient suffering from Paget's disease. B, The |678 removed in one block from patient shown in A.

In early cases much of the new bone which is laid down is woven bone. Later, lamellar bone is deposited and patchy sclerosis appears. In the denser bone osteones resembling Haversian systems may be formed, but true cortical bone is not produced.

Subperiosteal deposition of bone results in enlargement while minute, incomplete fractures lead to bending and bowing. Both factors produce accentuation of the natural curvatures of the bone.

At first sight Paget's disease appears to be without pattern but this is not entirely so. Some bones are affected more commonly than others; the maxilla more frequently than the mandible, and the mandible alone more often than both mandible and maxilla together.

Paget's disease of the tibia always starts near the upper end and progresses downwards. Similarly if Paget's affects the maxilla it does so before it affects the cranial vault and it enters the calvarium via the frontal bone.

What is the basic error in osteitis deformans? Is the turnover of bone increased so that there is no time for the formation of complex Haversian systems and proper cortical bone? In which case is it a result of abnormal osteoclasis? Are more osteoclasts formed or do they persist longer than the usual 48 hours? Or is the ability to lay down Haversian systems lost so that as the cortical bone is resorbed in the normal way it is not replaced and an increased surface area of bone is exposed to osteoclastic activity? Either way, the deposition of new bone both subperiosteally and endosteally can be explained as an attempt to compensate for the loss of the mechanically efficient cortex. That the bone so deposited should be woven bone in the early stages of the process is in accord with the deposition of this type of bone anywhere where rapid bone production is necessary.

The Radiology of Paget's Disease.—In long bones, the earliest lesion as seen in radiographs is a fusiform zone of cortical radiolucency. A similar appearance is to be seen in the mandible before the whole of the bone has been involved. The affected area of cortex slowly spreads round the bone, but maintains a pointed extremity in its long axis. Where it is seen tangentially the lesion again forms a fusiform radiolucent patch, outlined by a thin layer of bone on both endosteal and periosteal surfaces.

In the jaws the normal lamellar bone is at first largely replaced by woven bone and the normal cortex is destroyed. Radiographically the bone takes on a granular pattern of low radiographic density. A striated pattern may be seen in the maxillary premolar region and in the mandible. This pattern is produced by the persistence of a few of the normal trabeculae on which new bone is deposited, so increasing their thickness and radiopacity. The lamina dura is reduced in thickness and may be difficult to detect. As the disease progresses the typical cotton-wool clumps of sclerotic, mosaic patterned bone appear and they tend to form first near the apices of the teeth.

Enlargement of the affected jaw occurs. In the maxilla, the extra bone has the same texture as the rest of the jaw and is covered by a thin sheet of subperiosteal bone. In the mandible successive layers of subperiosteal bone are deposited, giving the new bone an onion-skin appearance.

As the condition spreads from the maxilla it involves the walls of the orbits and the sphenoid. It extends into the frontal bone as an advancing front of cortical bone destruction. Thus, osteoporosis circumscripta is produced which spreads backwards to involve the whole vault. Thickening occurs mainly on the outer surface since the shape of the inner surface is controlled by contact with the dura and brain. The classic cotton-wool pattern spreads in by the same route until the whole vault is involved. Finally, the heavy, structurally weak calvarium sags over the cervical spine to produce basilar inversion and a 'tam-o-shanter' skull.

In some patients enormous enlargement of the maxilla can occur. This highlights two matters of radiological interpretation. One is that where there is a considerable thickness of bone the mass is radio-opaque. But, of course, the radio-opacity does not mean that the bone is sclerotic. Indeed, per unit volume the bone may still be more radiolucent than normal except for the cotton-wool patches. Furthermore, just because the outlines of the maxillary sinuses cannot be visualized it does not mean they have been obliterated. It is far more likely that they are present, even if reduced in size, and that their image is overshadowed by the masses of bone on the surface. Moreover, with the loss of cortex any linear image from the margins of the sinuses is lost.

Differentiation of Paget's disease from fibrous dysplasia of bone involves a consideration of the clinical as well as the radiographic features. Advanced cases are rarely a difficulty, but early cases in which enlargement of the jaw is localized can be a problem. Two factors are a help: the first is that radiographic involvement of the whole jaw is usually present by the time enlargement occurs in Paget's disease, whereas in fibrous dysplasia the radiographic changes remain more localized to the changes in contour. Secondly, hypercementosis of involved teeth is usual in Paget's disease and uncommon in fibrous dysplasia.

Complications.—There are many complications which may befall the patient with Paget's disease. Deformity of individual bones can lead to postural deformity and osteoarthritis of the joints. Curious transverse fractures, both complete and incomplete, may occur. If, for any reason, patients with this condition are confined to bed there is a risk that rapid resorption of bone will take place, leading to a rise in serum calcium and renal stone formation. The foramina of the skull may be narrowed, producing cranial nerve palsies and optical field defects or deafness.

The bone of osteitis deformans is unusually vascular and blood-flow may be up to 20 times the normal. Intra-bony vessels form numerous arteriovenous shunts so that the cardiac output is raised and may reach three times the normal value. Cardiac hypertrophy follows and eventually cardiac failure. In advanced cases the thoracic cage becomes deformed with an increased liability to bronchitis and bronchopneumonia. Thus, patients with Paget's disease can present an increased anaesthetic risk.

Malignant change in the form of osteogenic sarcoma or malignant osteoclastoma is an uncommon but well recognized risk. Hutter and others (1963) describe benign osteoclastomas in Paget's disease, some of which were in the jaws. Whether they were true neoplasms, or more of the nature of giant-cell granulomas, it is difficult to say. Barry (1969) describes 2 examples of benign giant-celled tumours from Australia—one seen in the tibia and one in the sacrum. Hutter and others (1963) reported 5 cases of benign giant-cell tumour at the Memorial Center for Cancer, New York. McKenna and others (1964), from the same hospital, found 12 cases of benign giant-cell tumour in patients with Paget's disease: 5 were in the calvaria and 2 each in the mandible and maxilla. In a case reported by Cones (1953) a giant-cell tumour in a patient with generalized Paget's disease was irradiated, after which the tumour rapidly recurred as a chondrosarcoma causing death in six months.

Sarcoma.—Paget's original case developed sarcoma at the elbow, and of the 23 cases reported by Paget 5 died from a malignant change in the lesion. Barry (1969) reported 116 patients with sarcoma developing in this way in Australia. Coley and Sharp (1931) reported 72 cases of sarcoma from the records of the Memorial Hospital, New York, and the American Tumour Registry. In 20 of these cases (28 per cent), the tumour had developed in patients suffering from Paget's disease.

Porretta, Dahlin, and Janes (1957) found 16 cases of bone sarcoma among 1753 patients with Paget's disease in the records of the Mayo Clinic. Coley (1960) and Lichtenstein (1959) considered the incidence of bone sarcoma in Paget's disease to be 10 per cent. Barry (1961), however, considered the incidence to be less than 1 per cent in Australia, a figure which agrees with Porretta and others' (1957) figures from the Mayo Clinic.

Aspects of Paget's Disease which affect the Oral Surgeon.—

Extractions.—Marked hypercementosis of the teeth causes considerable difficulty during their extraction with forceps and this may lead to fracture of the tooth. It is preferable to extract the teeth surgically, after which the wound should be carefully closed and sutured to prevent chronic infection in the underlying sclerotic bone which might lead to a protracted osteomyelitis of the jaw. In this respect, it is important that all fractured roots should be removed. Sometimes several upper teeth are united by masses of hypercementosis and surgical removal of the teeth and attached bone is required. Excessive force exerted on such teeth with forceps leads to fracture of the teeth concerned and also fracture of the underlying sclerotic masses which eventually sequestrate.

Bone Pain.—Pain due to Paget's disease of the jaws must be differentiated from other causes of facial pain. By and large, bone pain in the jaws is uncommon and care should be taken to exclude all other causes. In particular osteomyelitis of the Paget bone as a cause of the pain, or malignant change, should be considered. Where bone pain is severe, consideration should be given to the use of porcine serocalcitonin and the advice of a physician specializing in metabolic disease should be sought to this end. Injections of 1 unit per kg. of body-weight of serocalcitonin are given daily. Following this alkaline phosphatase levels in the blood fall, the urinary output of hydroxyproline also falls, the bone remodels and pain is relieved. Currently such treatment is expensive and hence not widely available.

Prosthetic Considerations.—When Paget's disease affects the jaws, it is usually the maxilla which is involved. Clinically the disease manifests itself by a great widening of the palate, especially in the tuberosity region, but sometimes a series of bony bumps are present in the sulcus. Such bony projections, particularly in the tuberosity region, cause difficulty in the construction of satisfactory dentures and should therefore be removed surgically. When the condition is of recent origin the bony masses can be removed fairly easily as the bone is soft, though haemorrhage may be profuse. However, in the elderly patient where the condition has been present for many years, the bone becomes exceedingly hard and resists most cutting instruments. Such bone is also very sclerotic and avascular and the introduction of infection into such an area may result in a protracted chronic osteomyelitis. Following surgery in such cases careful soft-tissue closure and suturing is necessary in order to avoid the introduction of infection. The patient should, of course, have antibiotic therapy until the area is healed. It is also a wise precaution to support the soft tissues against the bone with acrylic base plates lined with black gutta-percha. For the upper jaw circumzygomatic wires may be safely used to hold such a plate in place and circumferential wires are suitable for the lower jaw.

Osteomyelitis.—Patients with Paget's disease may also be referred with a chronic osteomyelitis, usually of the upper jaw. This has often developed following an unsuccessful extraction. At one time this condition was a cause of mortality of patients with Paget's disease who died of anaemia, septicaemia, pyaemic abscesses, or amyloid disease. However, the condition can be controlled by antibiotic therapy and the affected area of bone should be removed surgically as soon as a line of separation is established. Spontaneous sequestration may take many years and to wait for this event leaves the patient with a painful and suppurating area in the mouth (McGowan, 1974).

ACROMEGALY

Aetiology.—Acromegaly is caused by an adenoma of the eosinophil cells of the anterior lobe of the pituitary gland. When the adenoma develops after the epiphyses have closed, acromegaly occurs but prior to epiphysial closure the glandular dysfunction results in gigantism.

Clinical Features.—Acromegaly is most commonly found in males. The hands are enlarged and spade-like and the feet are similarly affected. There is an overgrowth of the nasal cartilage which results in a thick, enlarged nose. The substance of the subcutaneous tissues is also affected and this gives a coarse appearance to the skin. The lips are grossly thickened. The frontal sinuses are enlarged and this gives increased prominence to the supra-orbital ridges. Closure of the epiphyses prevents any increase in the patient's height, but periosteal appositional bone growth is not prevented and the bones increase in thickness due to surface deposition. In the mandibular condyle, however, the fibroblasts deep in the fibrous covering of the condylar head differentiate into chondroblasts and then to chondrocytes. Therefore, an anteroposterior increase in the length of the mandible is possible and an extreme mandibular protrusion occurs. The muscles attached to the angle of the mandible (masseter and medial pterygoid) cannot elongate and, therefore, resorption of bone occurs at the angle producing a more or less straight gonial angle. Because the condylar growth centre faces downwards as well as forwards, the ramus lengthens and the mandibular teeth are carried down away from the maxilla. As the freeway space is increased the prognathism is not so obvious in the resting position of the mandible as when the teeth are brought together.

The enlarging adenoma of the pituitary presses on the optic chiasma and the decussating fibres of the nasal half of the retina are affected. This results in bitemporal optic hemianopia. The patient often suffers from severe headaches and the voice becomes deep due to enlargement of the laryngeal cartilages. There may be diabetes insipidus.

Radiology.—The marked mandibular protrusion and the configuration of the lower jaw can be demonstrated by the true lateral radiograph and this film will also demonstrate the enlargement of the pituitary fossa and the destruction of the posterior clinoid process. Appositional bone growth produces an increased density of bone and osteophytic outgrowths may be seen on the vertebrae and the phalanges.

Treatment.—Successful removal of the adenoma is difficult and carries a relatively high mortality, but radiotherapy can often control the disease.

Oral Surgical Aspects of Acromegaly.—Cases of acromegaly are sometimes referred to the oral surgeon with a view to mandibular osteotomy or ostectomy. It is, of course, important to diagnose the condition, for any surgical interference would at best produce only a temporary improvement in the condition, for the mandible would continue to grow. More important, valuable time would be lost in instituting therapy for the acromegaly. The oral surgeon should always consider the possibility of acromegaly when confronted by a case of extreme mandibular protrusion and institute the appropriate investigations. Jaw surgery should not be contemplated until the mandibular growth has been arrested.

OSTEOPETROSIS, ALBERS-SCHÖNBERG, OR MARBLE BONE DISEASE

Osteopetrosis, first described by Albers-Schönberg in 1904, is a rare disease of unknown aetiology which is characterized by a generalized and extreme density of the bone. The medullary cavities tend to become obliterated due to failure of bone resorption and the continued deposition of bone. This renders the bone highly susceptible to infection since its vascular supply is decreased, and it also gives rise to a secondary anaemia.

It has been suggested (Weinmann and Sicher, 1955) that there is a delay in the appearance of osteoclasts so that remodelling resorption is out of phase with deposition and overtaken by the next wave of osteoblastic activity in the region.

Involvement of the skull leads to a reduction in the diameter of the foramina with consequent pressure on the cranial nerves. This may eventually lead to deafness and amblyopia. The disease is hereditary (McPeake, 1936) and is transmitted through both males and females as a Mendelian recessive (Hurscher and Stein, 1940). The condition is usually congenital, but occasionally the diagnosis is not made until later in life. Despite the density and thickening of the bones, they are very fragile and fractures often occur following minimal trauma. According to Thompson and others (1969) radiographic diffractions and microradiography have shown that the molecular structure is similar to that of normal bone. However, the distribution of mineral salts has an abnormal characteristic pattern and the arrangement of the collagen is irregular. This may account for the extreme fragility of the bone.

Incidence.—Gomez (1966) found 200 cases during a survey of the literature and Thompson and others (1969) reported 270.

Clinical Features.—Osteopetrosis may be characterized by either a severe or a relatively mild systemic disturbance and is usually divided into two types. The extreme or malignant form of the condition occurs early in life and may be present in utero. Such children seldom survive much beyond puberty (McPeake, 1936; Zawisch-Ossenitz, 1947) and they have marked anaemia, deafness, mental retardation, and often suffer from hydrocephalus. Their limbs are deformed as a result of multiple fractures. According to Winter (1945) they have a characteristic facies with a broad face, snub nose, hypertelorism, and frontal bossing. There is a hepatosplenomegaly due to the compensatory extramedullary haemopoiesis. According to Gomez (1966) and Thoma (1969) delayed eruption and impaction of teeth are common. The teeth are also said to be of defective quality and prone to caries.

The less extreme or benign variety is often not diagnosed until late in life, and a case reported by Dyson (1970) was first detected at the age of 74 years. Such patients tend to be asymptomatic, but they may suffer from a modified form of any of the symptoms associated with the more extreme variety of the disease.

Radiology.—Radiological examination shows extreme density of the entire skeleton with no differentiation between the cortex and marrow. In the skull views there is gross thickening at the base of the skull with increased density of the remainder of the calvarium. Long bones are club-shaped and have transverse bands at their ends, and bossing of the ribs occurs at the costo-chondral junctions. It would, of course, be incompatible with life for all the bones to have complete obliteration of their medullary cavities and, therefore, on radiological survey some bones will appear within the range of normal.

Haematological Investigations.—In the mild variety of the disease there may be a moderate iron deficiency anaemia, but in the more severe disease there may be a leuco-erythroblastic or aplastic type of anaemia. The serum calcium and phosphorus are normal (Thompson and others, 1969).

Treatment.—No effective treatment has been discovered for osteopetrosis and the various complications are treated as they arise.

The main complications from an oral surgical point of view are fracture of the jaw and osteomyelitis, and either of these complications can arise as a result of dental extractions. The removal of teeth should therefore be effected with minimal trauma and the operation is best carried out under general anaesthesia. The raising of mucoperiosteal flaps is unwise and should be avoided whenever possible. Following extractions, accurate soft-tissue closure and suturing of the socket wounds should be carried out and an antibiotic should be used until the wounds have healed. In spite of such treatment, Radden (1949) reported a case which developed osteomyelitis.

Fractures of the jaws tend to heal provided that they do not become infected, but in view of the risk of introducing infection to the avascular bone, the types of fixation available for treatment are of necessity limited. For example, it would be most imprudent to employ bone plating, transosseous wiring, or extra-skeletal fixation. Osteomyelitis usually occurs in the mandible, but Wallace and Kemp (1945) reported a case from the literature of maxillary involvement. Chronic osteomyelitis of the jaws in osteopetrosis is an extremely difficult condition to eradicate, for surgical removal of the affected area only results in further areas of sound bone becoming necrotic. Surgery is, therefore, contra-indicated except to effect drainage during an acute episode. Rowe (1970) attempted to treat a case with hyperbaric oxygen in the belief that local oxygenation of the tissues would help, but the results were not especially encouraging.

The established osteomyelitis of the jaws in a case of osteopetrosis should therefore be treated conservatively, but suitable antibiotics are prescribed should an acute exacerbation occur. Probably the only effective method of curing the condition is by mandibulectomy.

Cleidocranial Dysostosis

Cleidocranial dysostosis is a disease of unknown aetiology which is probably hereditary and when it occurs is inherited as a dominant Mendelian characteristic which can be transmitted by either sex. However, many sporadic cases occur and the sexes are equally affected.

The most striking features of the condition are the defects in ossification of the cranium and clavicles and the persistence of the primary dentition with delay or failure of eruption of the permanent dentition.

Clinical Appearances.—

1. *The head:* The head appears to be large and there is a marked median furrow in the centre of the forehead which runs vertically downwards towards the bridge of the nose. The frontal bone tends to bulge either side of the furrow. There is a depression in the region of the anterior fontanelle which may be palpable and similar depressions may be felt over the anterolateral and posterior and posterolateral fontanelle sites. The nasal bridge may be depressed and there is a hypoplasia of the middle third of the facial skeleton with a relative mandibular protrusion.

2. The deciduous teeth erupt normally, but are retained and fail to show normal osteoclastic resorption of their roots. The permanent teeth are largely unerupted and their roots are stunted and deformed. Rushton (1937) reported on the deformity of the roots of teeth in patients with cleidocranial dysostosis. Supernumerary teeth are common. Owing to pseudo-anodontia dentures are required from an early age.

3. *The thorax:* The shoulders appear to droop and the clavicles may be completely or partially absent. The absence of clavicles imparts an extreme mobility to the shoulders and enables the patient to approximate the shoulders towards the midline until they meet. Absence of the clavicles does not appear to cause the patient any inconvenience, but occasionally they may develop the scalenus syndrome.

4. *The pelvis:* There is often a defect in the ossification of the pubic symphysis which may be detected on palpation. A coxa vara or valga deformity of the hip is present in some cases.

5. A variety of other skeletal abnormalities are reported from time to time.

Radiographic Appearances.—

1. *The skull:* Defects in ossification are seen and the anterior, anterolateral, and posterolateral fontanelles remain patent. Small Wormian bones may be seen in their vicinity. In some cases part or all of the zygomatic bone is missing and the mastoid bone may fail to pneumatize. The middle third of the facial skeleton is hypoplastic and there is a relative mandibular protrusion. Very rarely the suture line at the mandibular symphysis may persist (Fleischer-Peters, 1967).

2. *The clavicles:* Usually the acromial end of the clavicle is absent or deficient, but the clavicle may be in two portions joined by a fibrous band. Sometimes only the sternal end is absent and occasionally the clavicle is entirely absent.

3. *The spine:* Scoliosis and kyphosis may be present as well as spina bifida occulta.

4. *The pelvis:* There may be an increase in width of the pubic symphysis and coxa vara and valga deformities of the hip may be present.

5. *The jaws:* Radiographs will demonstrate the presence of numerous unerupted and supernumerary teeth. According to Thoma (1969), if supernumerary teeth are present they are present in the incisor and premolar regions.

Oral Surgical Aspects of Cleidocranial Dysostosis.—The oral surgeon is primarily concerned with the problem of the unerupted teeth. Some success may be obtained by surgically uncovering the unerupted teeth provided the patient is operated upon during the erupting phase, and the chances of success decrease considerably with patients over 16 years of age. Thoma (1969) recommends the removal of all supernumerary teeth, but he states that good results are not obtained due to lack of erupting force. The mere presence of numerous unerupted teeth is unlikely to cause the patient any inconvenience, but due to normal alveolar atrophy with age the crowns of some of the teeth become exposed to the mouth and infection may occur, leading in some instances to osteomyelitis. At this stage extraction of the teeth presents additional difficulties. To avoid such a situation developing, it is prudent to remove the unerupted teeth earlier in life when the mandible is more substantial and infection is not present. One of the complications of removing a large number of unerupted teeth in the mandible is the possibility of jaw fracture.

REFERENCES

ALBERS-SCHÖNBERG, H. (1904), 'Röntgenbildung einer selteren knochererkrankung', *Munch. med. Wschr.*, **51**, 365.
— — (1907), 'Eine bisher nicht beschriebene allgemeinerkrankung des skelletes im röntgenbild', *Fortschr. Geb. Röntg Strahl.*, **11**, 261.
ALBRIGHT, F., BUTLER, A. M., HAMPTON, A. O., and SMITH, P. (1937), 'Syndrome Characterised by Osteitis Fibrosa Disseminata', *New Engl. med. J.*, **216**, 727.
ASKANAZY, M. (1904), 'Arbeiten auf dem gebiet der pathologischen anatomie und bakteriologie aus dem pathologisch-anatomischen', *Institut zu Tubingen*, **4**, 398.
BARRY, H. C. (1961), 'Sarcoma in Paget's Disease of Bone in Australia', *J. Bone Jt Surg.*, **43A**, 1122.
— — (1969), *Paget's Disease of Bone*. London: Churchill-Livingstone.
BRUCKNER, R., and others (1967), 'Osteogenic Sarcoma arising at a Site of Fibrous Dysplasia', *Oral Surg.*, **24**, 377.
CAFFEY, J. (1956), *Pediatric X-ray Diagnosis*, 3rd ed., p. 814. Chicago: Year Book.
CAWSON, R. (1964), 'Defects of Enamel Structure in a Case of Renal Osteodystrophy', *Br. dent. J.*, **117**, 141.
COLEY, B. L. (1960), *Neoplasms of Bone*, 2nd ed., p. 753. New York: Hoeber.
— — and SHARP, G. S. (1931), 'Paget's Disease a Predisposing Factor to Osteogenic Sarcoma', *Archs Surg.*, *Chicago*, **23**, 918.
— — and STEWART, F. W. (1945), 'Bone Sarcoma in Polyostotic Fibrous Dysplasia', *Ann. Surg.*, **121**, 872.
COLLINS, D. H. (1956), 'Paget's Disease of Bone', *Lancet*, **2**, 51.
CONES, D. M. T. (1953), 'Unusual Bone Tumour complicating Paget's Disease', *J. Bone Jt Surg.*, **35B**, 101.
DAVIES-COLLEY, N. (1884), 'Bones and Kidneys in a Girl Aged 13', *Trans. Path. Soc. Lond.*, **35**, 285.
DUSTIN, P., and LEY, D. A. (1950), 'Contribution à l'étude des dysplasies osseuses', *Revue belge. Path. Méd. exp.*, **20**, 52.

Dyson, D. P. (1970), 'Osteomyelitis of the Jaws in Albers-Schönberg Disease', *Br. J. oral Surg.*, **7**, 178.
Emslie, R. C. (1914), 'Fibrocystic Diseases of Bones', *Br. J. Surg.*, **2**, 17.
Fairbank, H. (1950), 'Fibrocystic Disease of Bone', *J. Bone Jt Surg.*, **32B**, 403.
Falconer, M. A., Cope, C. L., and Smith, A. H. T. Robb (1942), 'Fibrous Dysplasia of Bone with Endocrine Disorders', *Q. Jl Med.*, **11**, 121.
Fleischer-Peters, A. (1967), 'Therapeutische Möglichkeiten bei der clyostosis Cleidocranialis', *Dt. zahnarztl. Z.*, **22**, 80.
Gomez, L. S. A. (1966), 'The Jaws in Osteopetrosis', *J. oral Surg.*, **24**, 67.
Harris, W. H., Dudley, R., and Barry, R. J. (1962), 'The Natural History of Fibrous Dysplasia', *J. Bone Jt Surg.*, **44A**, 207.
Hunter, D., and Turnbull, H. M. (1931), 'Hyperparathyroidism', *Br. J. Surg.*, **19**, 203.
Hurscher, H., and Stein, J. J. (1940), 'Osteopetrosis associated with Hodgkin's Disease', *Am. J. Roentg.*, **43**, 74.
Hutter, R. V. P., and others (1963), 'Giant Cell Tumours complicating Paget's Disease of Bone', *Cancer, N.Y.*, **16**, 1044.
Jaffe, H. L. (1958a), *Tumerous Conditions of Bone and Joints*. London: Kimpton.
— — (1958b), *Desmoplastic Fibroma in Tumours and Tumerous Conditions of Bone and Joints*, p. 298. Philadelphia: Lea & Febiger.
Jäger, M. (1962), quoted by Riddell, D. M. (1964), 'Osteoidsarkom auf dem Boden einer fibrös-polyostotischen dysplasiel (Jaffe-Lichtenstein)', *Zentbl. allg. Path. path. Anat.*, **103**, 291.
Langedorff, X. (1877), *Br. med. J.*, **1**, 667.
Lichtenstein, L. (1938), 'Polyostotic Fibrous Dysplasia', *Archs Surg., Chicago*, **36**, 874.
— — (1959), *Bone Tumours*, 2nd ed. St. Louis: Mosby.
— — and Jaffe, H. L. (1942), 'Fibrous Dysplasia of Bone', *Archs Path.*, **33**, 777.
Lucas, R. B. (1962), 'Fibrous Dysplasia in the Jaws', *J. R. Coll. Surg. Edinb.*, **7**, 255.
McCune, D. J., and Bruch, H. (1937), 'Osteodystrophia Fibrosa', *Am. J. Dis. Child.*, **54**, 806.
McGowan, D. A., (1974), 'Clinical Problems in Paget's Disease affecting the Jaws', *Br. J. oral Surg.*, **11**, 230–235.
McKenna, R. J., and others (1964), 'Osteogenic Sarcoma arising in Paget's Disease', *Cancer, N.Y.*, **17**, 42.
McPeake, C. N. (1936), 'Osteopetrosis: Report of Eight Cases in Three Generations in One Family', *Am. J. Roentg.*, **36**, 816.
Mandl, F. (1926), 'Die behandlung der lokalisierten und generalisierten osteitis fibrosa', *Wien. klin. Wschr.*, **39**, 1046.
de Marchi, R. (1956), Sulla trasformazione sarcomatosa della displasia fibrosa monostotica', *Friuli med.*, **11**, 639.
Paget, J. (1877), 'On a Form of Chronic Inflammation of Bones (Osteitis Deformans)', *Med. chir. Trans.*, **60**, 37.
Perkinson, N. C., and Higginbotham, N. L. (1955), 'Osteogenic Sarcoma arising in Polyostotic Fibrous Dysplasia', *Cancer, N.Y.*, **8**, 396.
Pilheu, F., and Soldato, G. (1966), 'Fibro-osteosarcoma of Jaw in a Case of Polyostotic Fibrous Dysplasia', *oral Surg.*, **21**, 778.
Porretta, G. A., Dahlin, D. C., and Janes, J. M. (1957), 'Sarcoma in Paget's Disease of Bone', *J. Bone Jt Surg.*, **39A**, 1314.
Pritchard, J. E. (1951), 'Fibrous Dysplasia of Bone', *Am. J. med. Sci.*, **222**, 313.
Radden, H. G. (1949), 'Albers-Schönberg's Disease', *Aust. J. Dent.*, **53**, 353.
Ramsey, H., Strong, E., and Frazell, E. (1968), 'Fibrous Dysplasia of the Cranial Bones', *Am. J. Surg.*, **116**, 542.
Rowe, N. L. (1970), quoted by Dyson, D. P. (1970), 'Osteomyelitis of the Jaws in Albers-Schönberg Disease ', *Br. J. oral Surg.*, **7**, 178.
Riddell, D. M. (1964), 'Malignant Change in Fibrous Dysplasia', *J. Bone Jt Surg.*, **46B**, 251.
Rushton, M. A. (1937), 'Partial Gigantism of Face and Teeth', *Br. dent. J.*, **63**, 65.
Sabanas, A. O., Dahlin, D. C., Childs, D. S., and Nins, J. C. (1956), 'Post-radiation Sarcoma of Bone', *Cancer, N.Y.*, **9**, 528.
Schlumberger, H. G. (1946), 'Fibrous Dysplasia of Single Bones', *Milit. Surg.*, **99**, 504.

SCHMORL, G. (1932), 'Über ostitis deformans Paget', *Virchows Arch. path. Anat. Physiol.*, **283**, 694.
SETH, R. S., CLIMIE, A. R. W., and TUTTLE, W. M. (1962), 'Fibrous Dysplasia of the Rib with Sarcomatous Change', *J. Bone Jt Surg.*, **44A**, 183.
SEWARD, G. R. (1970), personal communication.
SNAPPER, I. (1949), *Medical Clinics on Bone Diseases*, 2nd ed., p. 223. New York: Interscience.
STAFNE, E. C. (1964), *Oral Roentgenographic Diagnosis*. Philadelphia: Saunders.
STEWART, M., GILMER, S., and EDMONSON, A. (1962), 'Fibrous Dysplasia of Bone', *J. Bone Jt Surg.*, **44B**, 302.
SUTRO, C. J. (1951), 'Osteogenic Sarcoma of the Tibia in a Limb affected with Fibrous Dysplasia', *Bull. Hosp. Jt Dis.*, **12**, 217.
TANNER, H. C., DAHLIN, D. C., and CHILDS, D. S. (1961), 'Sarcoma Complicating Fibrous Dysplasia', *Oral Surg.*, **14**, 837.
TANNHAUSER, S. J. (1944), 'Neurofibromatosis and Osteitis Fibrosa Cystica Localisata et Disseminata', *Medicine, Baltimore*, **23**, 105.
THOMA, K. H. (1969), *Oral Surgery*, 5th ed., Vol. 1. St. Louis: Mosby.
THOMPSON, R. D., HALE, M. L., MONTGOMERY, J. C., and MONTANA-VILLAMIZAR, E. (1969), 'Manifestations of Osteopetrosis', *J. Oral Surg.*, **27**, 63.
TRUBNIKOV, V. F., and SKOBLIN, A. P. (1956), 'Transformation of the Local Fibrous Osteodystrophy into a Sarcoma', *Ortop. Traumat. Protez.*, **17**, 53.
VAHKURKINA, A. M. (1958), 'Malignant Osteoblastoclastoma developing on the Background of Fibrous Osteodysplasia', *Arkh. Patol.*, **20**, 18.
VAN HORN, P. E., JOHNSON, E. W., and DAHLIN, D. C. (1963), 'Fibrous Dysplasia of the Femur with Sarcomatous Change', *Am. J. Orthop.*, **5**, 6.
VON RECKLINGHAUSEN, F. (1891), *Die fibrose oder deformirende ostitis die osteomalacie carcinose in ihren gegenseitigen beziehungen*. Berlin: Reimer.
WALLACE, E. S., and KEMP, H. R. (1945), 'Marble Bone Disease', *Dent. J. Aust.*, **17**, 81.
WEIL, P. (1922), 'Jähriges Mädchen mit pubertas praecox und Knochenbrüchigkeit', *Klin. Wschr.*, **1**, 2114.
WEINMANN, J. P., and SICHER, H. (1955), *Bone and Bones: Fundamentals of Bone Biology*, 2nd ed., p. 151. London: Kimpton.
WINTER, G. R. (1945), 'Albers-Schönberg Disease', *Am. J. Orthod.*, **31**, 637.
WORTH, H. M. (1963), *Principles and Practice of Oral Radiologic Interpretation*. Chicago: Year Book.
ZAWISCH-OSSENITZ, C. (1947), 'Marble Bone Disease: Study of Osteogenesis', *Archs Path.*, **43**, 55.
ZIMMERMAN, D. C., STAFNE, E. C., and DAHLIN, D. C. (1958), 'Fibrous Dysplasia of the Maxilla and Mandible', *Oral Surg.*, **11**, 55.

Chapter XVIII

THE MAJOR SALIVARY GLANDS

ACUTE sialo-adenitis, recurrent swelling, and a persistent swelling are the three most common conditions of the major salivary glands with which patients present to the dental surgeon.

A. ACUTE SIALO-ADENITIS

The most frequent cause of an acute sialo-adenitis is infection of secretions retained behind an obstruction to the main duct. Indeed, such an episode may be the first intimation of the presence of such an obstruction.

Far less common in these days is an ascending infection, usually of a parotid gland, occurring in a dehydrated and debilitated patient. The affected gland becomes swollen, tender, and very painful. There is considerable oedema of the surrounding soft tissues or even a frank cellulitis. There may be some difficulty in distinguishing between an acute infection of the parotid gland and a submasseteric abscess and between an acute infection of the submandibular gland and a sublingual or submandibular cellulitis due to other causes. In the case of salivary gland infections the duct is also inflamed and, if the clinician is gentle, pus can be expressed from it. Furthermore, the maximum swelling in acute parotitis is rather more posterior than that produced by a submasseteric infection and it involves the tissues beneath the lobe of the ear.

Fortunately, in these days most infections can be controlled by vigorous antibiotic treatment with drainage occurring via the duct. In a few instances, a considerable abscess may form either in the gland or within the associated lymph-nodes. There is no problem with the submandibular gland since drainage by Hilton's method can be effected in the usual manner. With the parotid, however, the site of the abscess can be difficult to detect on clinical grounds and, indeed, one occurring in the deep part of the gland may burst into the external auditory canal before its presence is suspected.

Most sizeable parotid abscesses form in the lower pole. An incision is made in the crease in front of the pinna and curved downwards behind the angle of the mandible. The anterior flap is reflected a short distance over the deep fascia and the gland explored with a pair of fine sinus forceps or straight mosquito artery forceps. If the fascia is tough it may be incised parallel to the branches of the facial nerve. A corrugated rubber drain is placed in situ and the skin closed above and below its point of exit.

B. RECURRENT SWELLING

Recurrent swellings occur with two types of periodicity. The first type appears only when a flow of saliva is stimulated. This is usually due to the thought, sight, or taste of food, but the smoking of tobacco can produce a profuse salivary flow. The second type comes up at intervals of weeks, months, or even years and lasts for periods of days or weeks. These swellings are due to attacks of ascending infection.

The Causes of Recurrent Salivary Gland Swellings
1. *Sialo-angiectasis* or punctate sialectasis.
2. *Papillary Obstruction:*—
   a. Acute (ulcerative) papillary obstruction.
   b. Chronic (fibrotic) papillary stenosis.
   c. Relative papillary obstruction.
3. *Duct Obstruction* due to:—
   a. Causes in the lumen.
   b. Causes in the wall.
   c. Causes outside the wall.
4. *Gland Distension* due to:—
   a. The effect of drugs.
   b. An allergic reaction.

Sialo-angiectasis:—The characteristic sialographic appearance in this condition is of multiple small cavities occurring proximally in the duct tree. Patey and Thackray (1955) attribute these cavities to rupture of the diseased intralobular ducts under the pressure of the sialographic injection. However, the cavities start to fill quite early on during the injection, before any quantity of fluid has been introduced. Moreover, from time to time cases are seen in which multiple calculi have formed in the periphery of the gland, each one in a sialographic cavity, suggesting that the cavities existed before the injection and are not the result of duct rupture.

The aetiology is obscure. Rose (1954) suggests a developmental cause. Maynard (1965) considers that a reduction in salivary flow is the first change, with sialectasis, large duct dilatation and stricture formation, ascending infection, the production of abnormal mucous saliva, and calculi all playing a part in different cases. Patey (1965) appears to view the condition as an aspect of Sjögren's syndrome. Infection by an unknown virus or an auto-immune condition separate from Sjögren's syndrome have also been suggested as possible causes. In fact, there seem to be two varieties of sialo-angiectasis: primary sialo-angiectasis, which is the condition seen in childhood, and secondary sialo-angiectasis.

Primary sialo-angiectasis manifests itself in childhood as recurrent subacute infections of a parotid gland. Both sides may be affected, but rarely at the same time. Attacks of pain and swelling last for 3 to 14 days at intervals of 3 or more months. During these episodes the spontaneously discharged saliva is clear, but massage of the gland produces streaks and flakes of pus. Children as young as 3 months or as old as 12 years may suffer the first attack, but the commonest age of onset is 4–6 years. Occasionally brothers and sisters and even aunts and uncles have been similarly affected. Katzen (1969), in a longitudinal study of 45 patients, found that most cases spontaneously remitted by 15 years of age.

Patey and Thackray (1955) and Katzen (1969) examined histological material and found duct epithelial hypoplasia, periductal lymphocytic infiltration, acinar atrophy, and fibrosis. Katzen (1969) records that the basement membrane of the acini was absent or fragmentary.

Acute attacks should be treated with systemic penicillin since the causal organisms are usually *Streptococcus viridans*, staphylococci or pneumococci sensitive to this drug. Treatment is important as a few cases progress to a chronically infected state with severe gland destruction.

Sialography frequently produces a remission, perhaps because some of the contrast medium remains in the cavities and is antiseptic. The use of sugar-free chewing gum between meals can be tried to maintain a flow of saliva, so discouraging ascending infection.

Secondary sialo-angiectasis is the occurrence of similar cavities in a gland affected by a number of conditions: chronic infection, Sjögren's disease, and the effects of irradiation. These changes do not occur in all such cases nor do they appear early in the disease, but when present they are accompanied by changes in the diameter of the large ducts. If anything, the cavities are rather larger and more irregular in shape than those seen in primary sialo-angiectasis.

Papillary Obstruction.—Papillary obstruction may be acute and due to an ulcer affecting the papilla, or chronic when fibrosis follows repeated trauma to the papilla.

Swelling is of the obstructive type, although attacks of ascending infection may occur once the stage of papillary stenosis is reached. If the obstruction is due to the oedematous swelling caused by an acute ulcer, then the symptoms last only for the time that the ulcer is present and are of comparatively sudden onset. If, on the other hand, obstruction is caused by steadily increasing fibrosis, then the onset of mealtime swelling will be insidious and only when it becomes severe, or when an ascending infection occurs, will the patient complain.

The commonest cause of both types of papillary obstruction is trauma, from such things as a sharp tooth, a cross-bite on a denture, a denture with a high occlusal plane, a projecting clasp, or the large lingual flange of a lower denture.

If the condition is chronic the opening to the duct will be difficult to find and will feel rigid when a probe is inserted into it. Milking the gland may fill the dilated duct behind the papilla with saliva, thereby producing a bluish swelling.

Sialography will demonstrate the narrowed papillary segment and the dilated duct behind. Treatment involves removal of the source of the irritation and, if there is stenosis, a papillotomy with careful suture of the duct lining to the mucosa of the mouth.

Relative papillary stenosis occurs when the saliva is unusually viscous. In some patients it resembles a clear jelly and will only pass the duct orifice if the gland is massaged. Chronic obstruction, chronic infection, and auto-immune disease can produce this change and mucous gland metaplasia of the duct epithelium is said to account for it. Papillotomy may permit the material to pass with symptomatic relief.

Duct Obstruction.—

Duct Obstruction due to Causes in the Lumen.—Calculi are the commonest intraluminal cause of recurrent salivary gland swelling. Submandibular calculi are the most common, but parotid stones occur more often than is frequently believed. Sublingual calculi may occasionally be seen. If the calculus becomes impacted at the papilla or enlarges to fill the lumen of the duct, then obstructive symptoms follow. Alternatively, an acute infection behind the calculus may make the patient seek aid. Should the inflamed duct wall clamp down upon the stone, then distension of the gland at mealtimes will add to the discomforts of the acute infection. In such cases temporary relief can be obtained by treatment with antibiotics. As the oedema subsides duct obstruction will be reduced.

Calculi in the submandibular duct are often visible or palpable through the floor of the mouth. Those in the parotid papilla may likewise be seen or felt.

Inspection of the face when the gland is swollen may give an indication of the situation of a parotid calculus, since, if it is well within the gland, only the lower pole will become enlarged. Palpation of calculi in the upper pole of the submandibular gland is performed bimanually with the intraoral finger facing downwards and outwards in the lingual sulcus and with the other hand displacing the lower pole of the gland upwards. A small, hard, submandibular gland is probably chronically infected and should be considered for excision.

Radio-opaque calculi can be demonstrated by plain radiographs. A central true occlusal view of the floor of the mouth, together with a posterior oblique occlusal and an oblique lateral jaw film, will be required for the detection of submandibular stones. A periapical film inside the cheek, a maxillary posterior oblique occlusal, a tangential film with the cheek blown out (Stafne, 1958), or an off-centred P.A. projection can be used to demonstrate parotid calculi.

A sialogram is required when a radiolucent calculus is suspected, where the calculus is close to or within the gland, or where considerable damage to the gland may have occurred.

The removal of anterior submandibular calculi is performed under local anaesthesia. A suture is passed around the duct behind the calculus and tied once, not too tightly. An incision in the floor of the mouth is deepened with scissors until the duct is identified. The duct is mobilized and a silk thread passed around it and clamped with artery forceps. This steadies the duct while a longitudinal incision is made over the calculus. Should the calculus be adherent to the duct a stitch is passed through one edge of the incision in the duct wall before it is levered out. The lumen is irrigated and sucked out, the posterior stitch removed and the gland squeezed to express any tiny calculi which might have formed behind the major one, and then the stay sutures removed. Only the mucosal wound should be closed. Indeed, attempts to suture the incision in the duct can lead to formation of a stricture.

Posterior submandibular calculi are surgically approached under endotracheal anaesthesia. The floor of the mouth is infiltrated with 1:100,000 adrenaline solution and the submandibular duct isolated towards its anterior end. By following the duct backwards the lingual nerve is identified and a tape passed around it to draw it laterally. Once the lingual nerve is safe the duct is traced back to the upper pole of the gland. A calculus in the posterior duct can be released at this point. One just inside the upper pole may be attempted by raising the duct upwards and incising into the anterior part of the gland just beneath the duct. On no account should the posterior part of the upper pole be incised lest the facial artery be divided. Control of bleeding from the vessel in this situation could be most difficult.

Where the length of history, number of inflammatory episodes, consistency of the gland, and appearance in the sialogram suggest gross gland damage the whole gland should be excised. Calculi which lie below the junction with Wharton's duct of the most distal intralobular duct should not be tackled from the mouth and again the gland should be excised. A gland with dilatation of the intra- and interlobular ducts seems able to recover. Irregular cavitation represents frank intraglandular abscess formation, and once this stage is reached permanent freedom from infection is unlikely.

Excision of the submandibular gland is accomplished through a 5-cm. long submandibular incision. The incision should be placed in, or parallel to, a skin crease at the junction of the upper two-thirds and lower one-third of the palpable part of the gland. The wound is deepened through platysma

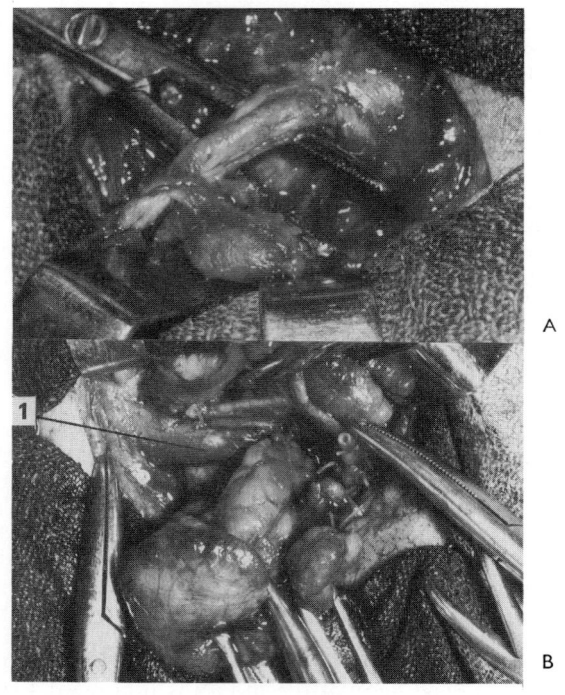

Fig. 38.—A, The gland has been separated from the lower border of the mandible and the facial artery is exposed where it emerges from the outside of the mandible. It is divided again at this point.

B, The anterior border of the gland has been freed from the mylohyoid muscle which is shown at 1. The groove between the superficial and deep parts of the gland is clearly seen now that it has been separated from the muscle. The submandibular branch of the facial artery runs forward just above the muscle.

and deep fascia and the local branches of the facial nerve identified. With care they can be mobilized and retracted. After the anterior facial vein has been taken, the lower pole of the gland is separated, grasped with Allis' forceps and turned upwards and forwards. The posterior belly of the digastric and the stylohyoid muscles are retracted downwards and backwards to expose the facial artery deep to the gland. It is doubly ligated and divided at this point.

Separation of the gland from the lower border of the mandible reveals the facial artery lateral to the gland where it is divided and ligated again. (*Fig.* 38.) The Allis' forceps are transferred to the front of the lower pole and the gland turned backwards so that the attachment to the posterior

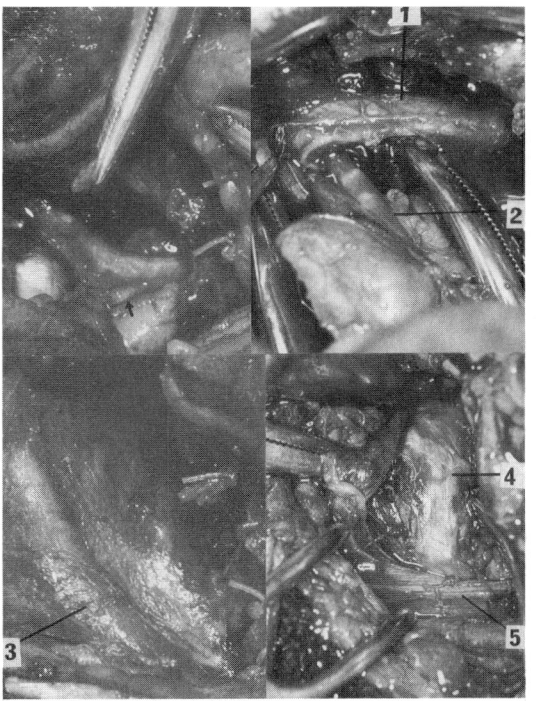

Fig. 39.—A, The gland has been mobilized sufficiently to draw it downward, bringing the lingual nerve into view. The arrow points to the sublingual ganglion. Right, the lingual nerve (1) has been separated from the upper pole of the gland and has been displaced upward so as to expose the duct of the submandibular gland (2). The duct contains two calculi which can be seen shining through its wall. The posterior root of the sublingual ganglion is seen leaving the nerve where it crosses the duct, but the ganglion itself is now hidden by the deep part of the gland which is passing anterolateral to, and parallel with, the duct.

B, The gland bed as it is normally seen, with the muscles covered by a thin layer of connective tissue. 3, The tendon of the digastric muscle. Right, the connective tissue has been removed from part of the gland bed so that a small vein which passed from the deep surface of the gland through the hyoglossus could be controlled. It is seen clamped by the artery forceps. The hypoglossal nerve (4) has been uncovered where it passes upwards and forwards over the hyoglossus. The stylohyoid tendon (5) divides at this point to embrace the digastric.

border of the mylohyoid can be uncovered. Once this has been separated the gland can be mobilized and drawn down to display the lingual nerve. (*Fig.* 39.) The latter is attached to the upper pole of the gland lateral to the point from which the duct emerges. Careful scissor dissection is usually necessary. Sometimes the nerve is most adherent, due to scarring induced by inflammation around an adjacent calculus.

Once the lingual nerve has been freed, the deep part of the gland can be enucleated and the duct ligated and divided. The wound is closed in layers with vacuum drainage.

Parotid calculi anterior to the accessory parotid may be removed through the mouth. A Y-shaped incision encloses the parotid papilla and the submucosal part of the duct is raised on the underside of a V-shaped flap. The duct is traced through the buccinator and a loop from lateral to

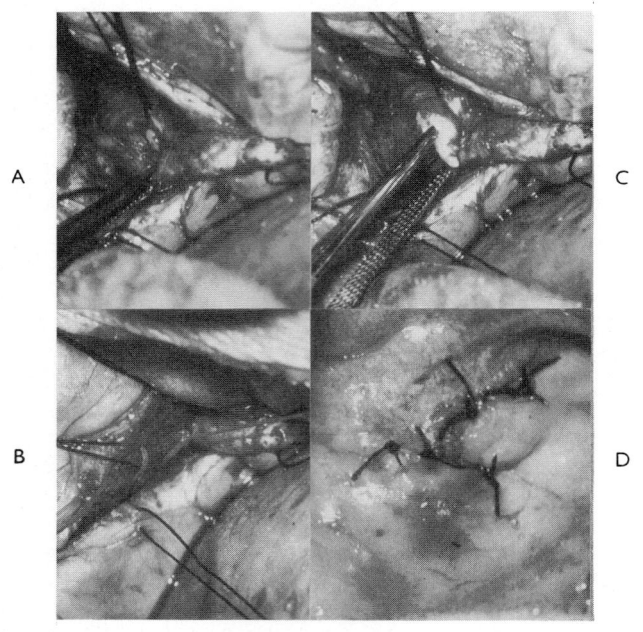

Fig. 40.—Removal of an extraglandular parotid calculus. A triangular flap has been raised from the inner surface of the buccinator which contains the parotid duct and a loop of duct from external to the buccinator is mobilized.

A, Shows an incision in the loop of duct over the calculus and a stay suture inserted.

B, The calculus is withdrawn.

C, The opening in the buccinator is approximated with a continuous 5/0 plain catgut suture.

D, The flap is sutured with black waxed silk.

this muscle drawn into the mouth. A longitudinal slit is made over the calculus and a silk suture passed through one edge to steady the duct while the stone is removed. Closure of the buccinator with plain catgut is necessary to prevent herniation of the buccal pad of fat. The mucosa is closed with silk in the usual manner. (*Fig.* 40.)

Calculi more posterior than this in the parotid duct should be tackled through a parotidectomy incision. A flap is raised from the surface of the gland and the duct identified at the anterior border. From this point it can be followed backwards through the substance of the gland until the calculus is uncovered. Due attention is given to the preservation of branches of the facial nerve, particularly the lower zygomatic branch which lies on the surface of the duct just below the accessory parotid.

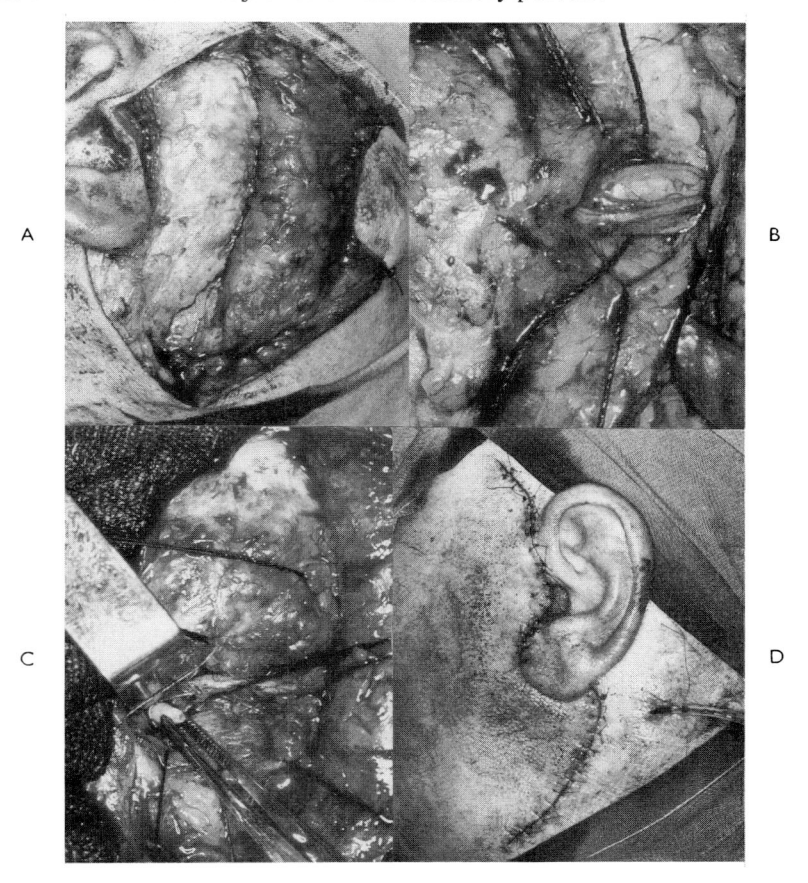

Fig. 41.—The removal of an intraglandular parotid calculus.
A, A flap is raised from over the parotid gland and sutured forward.
B, The deep fascia is incised in line with the duct and the duct isolated. A branch of the facial nerve lies on the surface of the duct.
C, By tracing the duct backwards through the gland, the calculus is uncovered.
D, The wound is closed in layers and vacuum drainage instituted. A pressure dressing is applied to keep the flap firmly in contact with the underlying tissues.

The fascial sheath of the gland is closed with care to prevent a leak of saliva into the tissues and the wound closed in layers with vacuum drainage. (*Fig.* 41.) Further details of these procedures can be found in papers by Seward (1968).

Obstruction due to Causes in the Wall.—Strictures are the most important cause of duct obstruction in this group and ulceration around a calculus the most common cause of stricture of the submandibular duct. Parotid calculi may present at the duct orifice and may be discharged spontaneously if small. The orifice of the submandibular duct, however, is small compared with the lumen of the duct and it is exceptional for calculi to pass through it. Instead, even quite small ones will ulcerate through into the mouth. A characteristic short stricture can be a sequel to such a happening, particularly if the resulting fistula closes. Traumatic injury to the ducts is another cause of strictures. Where the stricture is reasonably well forwards, the dilated duct behind the narrowing can be anastomosed to the mucosa of the mouth. This should be by an 'end to side' procedure for a 'side to side' procedure will narrow down and become ineffective.

Certain parotid duct strictures are less easy to explain. Some occur bilaterally either opposite the anterior border of the coronoid or opposite the posterior border of the mandible. Perhaps friction from the movement of the ramus is a factor in these cases. Perhaps auto-immune processes play a part, for in a few instances duct dilatation precedes the appearance of the stricture. The retromandibular strictures are of special interest since the patient's complaint may closely mimic temporomandibular joint arthrosis. Diagnosis may be difficult as there is no visible swelling because only the deep part of the parotid is involved.

Dilatation of these strictures with graduated sizes of gum-elastic urethral bougies is the safest form of treatment. The bougies are lubricated with lignocaine urethral gel and this will often give symptomatic relief for up to three years.

In order to avoid the formation of strictures or external salivary fistulae, the correct management of traumatic injuries to ducts needs to be mentioned. If a duct is transected by a facial laceration or during the course of an operation anastomosis of the two ends should be attempted. To prevent narrowing of the healed suture line each duct end is slit longitudinally for a short distance. Where it is difficult to repair the duct the proximal end may be implanted in the mucosa of the mouth. A tube pedicle of oral mucosa as advised by Anderson and Byers (1965) may help repair of a damaged parotid duct.

Duct Obstruction due to Causes Outside the Wall.—Both benign and malignant neoplasms can compress one of the salivary gland ducts. Benign neoplasms simply compress the duct, inducing dilatation proximal to the point of compression. Removal of the neoplasm cures the obstruction.

Malignant neoplasms may also produce simple compression but, alternatively, they may invade the duct wall. If the latter event occurs, a stricture may be produced with dilatation proximally, or the neoplasm may ulcerate into the lumen of the duct. Sialographically, such ulceration produces an irregular enlargement of the lumen of the duct.

Sjögren's syndrome may be discussed under this heading. Patients with this condition suffer from a dry mouth, dry eyes, difficulty in swallowing, and rheumatoid arthritis, or varying combinations of these complaints. The damage to the lacrimal and salivary glands is thought to be auto-immune in nature. In well-established cases there is a positive latex test for rheumatoid factor, a positive antinuclear factor test and salivary duct antibody test. There may be an increase in serum globulin, and where the eyes are affected by kerato-conjunctivitis sicca this can be demonstrated by Rose-Bengal staining. Labial salivary gland biopsy can provide a specimen of salivary gland for study which is relatively unaffected by ascending infection.

Histologically, destruction of gland acini and their replacement by a lymphocytic and plasma-cell infiltration is seen; features which account for the decreased salivary secretion. Epithelial hyperplasia leads to obstruction of the smaller ducts, the formation of 'casts' in the larger ducts, and possibly predisposes to calculus formation. The jelly-like saliva mentioned previously may be formed in some cases.

In the early stages there are no sialographic changes. Then, by comparison with normal glands, the intralobular ducts are seen to be more sparse than usual. Finally many changes occur: the ducts may be grossly dilated, strictures may be found or re-duplication of the lumen suggestive of the presence of epithelial casts. The periphery of the gland becomes difficult to demonstrate and gross, irregular cavitation of the gland occurs. A coarse sialectasis may appear in some patients.

Apart from a progressive dryness of the mouth the patient may suffer from attacks of infection of the salivary glands or distension of the gland with jelly-like material. In some patients a nodular enlargement of a gland occurs resembling neoplastic disease. Where a more uniform, symmetrical enlargement of the salivary and lacrimal glands is found the condition is described as 'Mikulicz's disease'.

Treatment is difficult. Nothing can be done to restore the glandular tissue which has been destroyed, so that the dryness of the mouth cannot be cured. Demulcent mouthwashes and tablets, sips of water with the food, and cream on the lips are all that can be tried. Because the progress of the condition is so variable the effect of steroid therapy is difficult to assess. The well-known hazards of long-term systemic steroid therapy need to be balanced against the possibilities of slowing the progress of the disease. The risk that the exhibition of steroids will increase the susceptibility to secondary infection has also to be considered. Chronic or subacute attacks of infection of the parotids add to the patient's discomfort and further damage the glandular substance. Such infections must, of course, be treated with systemic antibiotics.

Single glands which are enlarged or show nodular enlargement may require exploration and biopsy to exclude the presence of a neoplasm. Where the enlargement of Mikulicz's disease is embarrassing, surgical reduction may be considered. However, it is obvious that superficial parotidectomy with conservation of the facial nerve may be far from easy as the gland may well be adherent, inflamed, and fibrosed. Furthermore, the operation may increase the dryness of the mouth. These are factors which must be weighed carefully in individual cases.

Swelling due to Gland Distension and Infiltration.—Certain drugs can cause enlargement of the salivary glands. Iodine, thiouracil, and thiocyanates used in the treatment of thyrotoxicosis may occasionally have this effect. The minor as well as the major glands may enlarge and interfere with mastication.

Phenyl and oxyphenbutazone can cause water and salt retention with parotid enlargement and certain curious dietary habits, like the eating of clay, which can produce the same effect.

In some people fat is deposited in the gland causing it to enlarge, although such enlargement is progressive rather than recurrent. Allergic parotitis is a further cause of gland enlargement. An association of the swelling with a particular time of year or part of the week's routine may suggest this as a cause. Other allergic phenomena such as hay fever or asthma may coexist, and it may be possible to establish a cause-effect relationship with a particular antigen.

A normal sialogram, a sterile saliva, plugs of mucus containing eosinophils in the saliva, or a high eosinophil count in the peripheral blood may support the diagnosis. Antihistamine preparations frequently reduce the swelling and discomfort.

Differential Diagnosis.—A number of calcified objects must be distinguished from salivary calculi. These are calcified tuberculous lymph-nodes, phleboliths in a haemangioma, tonsilloliths, calcified parasites in cysticercosis in the masticatory muscles, developmental bone islands in the hyoid and the stylohyoid ligament, and calcification in an atheromatous facial artery. Many of these calcified structures differ in detail in their appearance compared with salivary calculi. Two-plane radiography and sialography will show that they are in a position outside the salivary glands.

Recurrent subacute infection of pre-auricular lymph-nodes or those in the lower pole of the parotid can simulate lobular parotid infection. The difference is that lobular parotid infection is usually secondary to duct obstruction, the cause of which can be demonstrated by sialography.

Finally, it must be remembered that mumps and a number of other virus infections cause salivary gland swelling, though not recurrent enlargement. In particular, not all such patients are obviously ill and, in some, one or both submandibular glands may be affected rather than the parotids. Determination of S and V antibody titres in the patient's serum on two occasions two to three weeks apart will confirm or refute a diagnosis of mumps in difficult cases.

C. Persistent Swellings of the Salivary Glands

Where a patient has a persistent, localized swelling of a salivary gland the likelihood of its being a neoplasm springs to mind. Other possibilities are chronic enlargement of the associated lymph-nodes, for example as a result of chronic infection, sarcoid, Hodgkin's disease, or (rarely these days) tuberculosis. Occasionally auto-immune disease may produce a nodular rather than a diffuse enlargement. Neoplasms of associated tissues such as neurofibromas, haemangiomas, lipomas, or even simple cysts may be encountered. Sialography can help to distinguish the salivary from the non-salivary masses, although difficulties exist. A peripheral neoplastic mass cannot be distinguished from an extra-salivary mass indenting the gland. Furthermore, lymph-nodes adjacent to the parotid can contain salivary tissue, and neoplasms have been known to arise in these enclaves. Such neoplasms may then be outside the parotid capsule but do *not* represent metastases.

Neoplasms of the Major Salivary Glands.—Both the histopathology and the surgery of these neoplasms have their difficulties. As a result, the responsibility for the care and treatment of these cases tends to gravitate into the hands of those with special knowledge and experience in the field.

The parotid gland is more commonly the site of neoplastic change, the submandibular gland next, and the sublingual last.

The Pleomorphic Adenoma (*Fig.* 42).—Pleomorphic adenomas are the most common salivary gland neoplasms and usually they are benign.

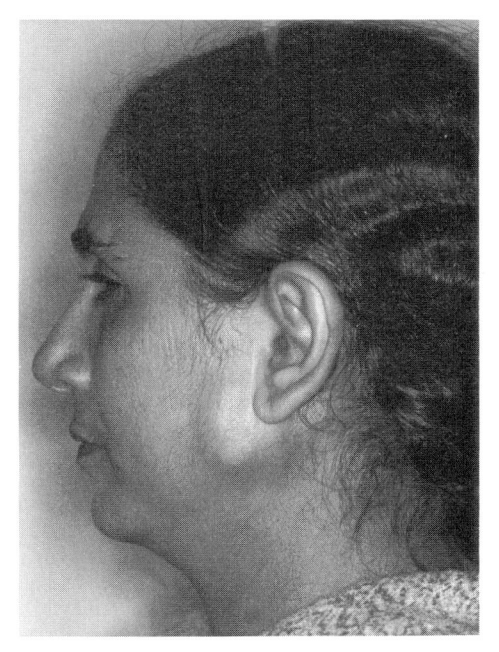

Fig. 42.—Pleomorphic adenoma of the left parotid region.

That is, they neither invade the facial nerve nor do they metastasize. Indeed, because they are slow-growing and cause the patient little trouble, they may be permitted to remain for many years and to attain a considerable size. Their benign behaviour, however, is deceptive and their periphery is lobulated and complex and any capsule is thin and histologically penetrated in places by growth. What is more, they 'seed' readily if penetrated at operation, so that the wound is contaminated with tumour cells. Hence they require to be removed with a narrow margin of apparently normal tissue. Fortunately, the narrow sheath of connective tissue which surrounds the facial nerve branches is an adequate margin at these points. Once the position of the related branches has been established, it is not too difficult to include an adequate layer of adjacent tissue at intermediate places and separate the mass.

The pleomorphic adenoma usually presents as a firm, lobulated mass, although soft or even fluctuant areas may be demonstrated if part of the tumour contains large amounts of mucus.

As the neoplasm enlarges it displaces the normal gland and its duct system to the periphery producing the so-called 'grasping fingers' appearance in a sialogram. Many are in the part of the gland superficial to the facial nerve, but others start in the deep part of the gland. The latter may not manifest themselves until they have reached a large size. The styloid process and posterior border of the ramus of the mandible constitute a bony tunnel for these neoplasms: the deeper part bulging into the lateral wall of the pharynx and soft palate, the more superficial part ultimately pushing up to the surface between the branches of the facial nerve. Because of their shape they are described as 'dumb-bell' tumours. Adequate access to them is most difficult to achieve and an approach may be required from both a preauricular incision and one across the soft palate and pterygomandibular fold. It may be necessary to perform a vertical subsigmoid osteotomy of the mandibular ramus to permit delivery of the mass. Obviously both the internal carotid and jugular vein are in close posterior relationship to the tumour and constitute an additional surgical hazard.

Because excision of the submandibular salivary gland is a far easier surgical problem, the results of the excision of pleomorphic adenomas of this gland should be better than those of the parotid. This, however, is by no means always so. One reason is the temptation to grasp the gland with instruments during the removal, particularly during display of the lingual nerve. Unfortunately, such instrumentation can rupture the tumour, disseminating cells into the wound.

A few pleomorphic adenomas both clinically and histologically are malignant. They should be excised radically like other malignant tumours.

Papillary Cystadenoma Lymphomatosum (Warthin's Tumour).—This is a benign tumour which affects men more often than women, and the middle-aged and elderly rather than young subjects. The tumour is smooth, soft and rounded, and may well be fluctuant. There may be more than one papillary cystadenoma present so that a recurrence after the excision of one neoplasm may really represent the appearance of a new one. The cut surface has a reddish-brown appearance in contrast to the pale yellowish grey of the pleomorphic adenoma. Treatment is by excision.

Adenocystic Carcinoma (Cylindroma).—Some adenocystic carcinomas grow comparatively slowly, but this does not necessarily improve the prognosis for the patient since they are likely to be looked upon as a pleomorphic adenoma and excised in too conservative a fashion. Indeed, these neoplasms can penetrate surprising distances away from the main mass; particularly along the perineural lymphatics. This means, unfortunately, that cells may have penetrated far beyond the reach of surgery with little to show for it macroscopically.

Over-generous surgical excision combined with postoperative radiotherapy offer the best chance of control. Some advocate the use of frozen sections of related nerves at the time of operation to try to ensure that perineural extensions are removed. Although there can be a depressingly high recurrence rate with this tumour, patients may be free of symptoms of the disease for many years after such treatment. An otherwise inexplicable pain or paralysis can be the first sign of recurrence.

Muco-epidermoid Carcinoma.—This is another malignant neoplasm exhibiting a very variable degree of aggressiveness. Some examples grow very slowly indeed, and again may be mistaken for a pleomorphic adenoma on clinical grounds so that once more there is a risk of inadequate excision. Fortunately, once the correct diagnosis is understood, adequate excision presents less of a problem than with the adenocystic carcinoma.

Squamous-cell Carcinoma.—There is little clinical difference between the more rapidly progressive and invasive salivary tumours. Fixation of the tumour mass, pain, involvement of related motor nerves, radiographic evidence of invasion of the adjacent bones all point to their malignant nature. However, as elsewhere, squamous-cell carcinoma tends to feel very hard and to metastasize early to the regional lymph-nodes.

Treatment.—Radical neck dissection may be required as part of the treatment of the more aggressive malignant neoplasms.

Biopsy of Neoplasms of the Major Salivary Glands.—It is an obvious advantage for the clinician to have histological evidence of the nature of any neoplasm about which he has to advise a patient. The problem with other than superficial lesions is that biopsy carries a risk of spillage of viable cells into the tissue planes opened up by the surgery. The risk of such contamination is particularly great if fluid in cystic parts of the tumour is released and flows into the wound. Widespread dissemination of the lesion can result. Because of this risk some surgeons prefer not to biopsy salivary neoplasms, but to rely upon the clinical findings plus the general feel of the mass at operation.

Others consider that a drill biopsy carries little risk of contamination of the drill track. This is probably true if the drill penetrates only as far as the neoplasm, but there would appear to be a risk if the neoplasm were transfixed and the drill went on into sound tissue beyond. Furthermore, the sample obtained by a drill biopsy may be very small.

In some centres frozen sections made during the operation are advocated, but special experience in interpreting these is required if the report is to be relied upon.

Where the pathologist prefers to use paraffin sections for this, often difficult, corner of pathology, an incisional biopsy may be preferred. An accessible part of the mass should be approached through a short incision, the wound should not be opened laterally and should be closed carefully after the specimen has been taken. The biopsy incision should be so sited that the entire wound, with a margin, can be conveniently excised when the definitive surgery is undertaken.

Dissection of the Facial Nerve.—The main trunk of the facial nerve is found by reflecting the lower pole of the parotid gland forwards, detaching it from the mastoid process and external auditory canal. It curves round below the external auditory canal just deep to the junction of the cartilagenous and bony part. It can be found anterior to the mastoid process and above the posterior belly of the digastric, curving forwards over the origin of the stylohyoid muscle. It is quite deeply placed, but a pointed process of the cartilaginous part of the canal points to its path.

The branches of the nerve are readily picked up as they leave the gland; the lower zygomatic branch lies on Stenson's duct and the mandibular branch lies near to the posterior facial vein (retromandibular vein).

If a neoplasm is to be excised, a flap is reflected from the surface of the gland, care being taken neither to thin out the flap too much, nor to pass too close to the surface of the mass. The tumour is outlined to delineate an adequate margin. Both the main nerve-trunk and the peripheral branches should be identified as convenient and separation of the lesion started by working first along the most accessible parts of the nerve. As in all cancer surgery, the aim when removing the neoplasm is to think in three dimensions and never approach nearer to the tumour than the width of apparently normal tissue considered necessary to include all outgrowths from the periphery (*Fig.* 43).

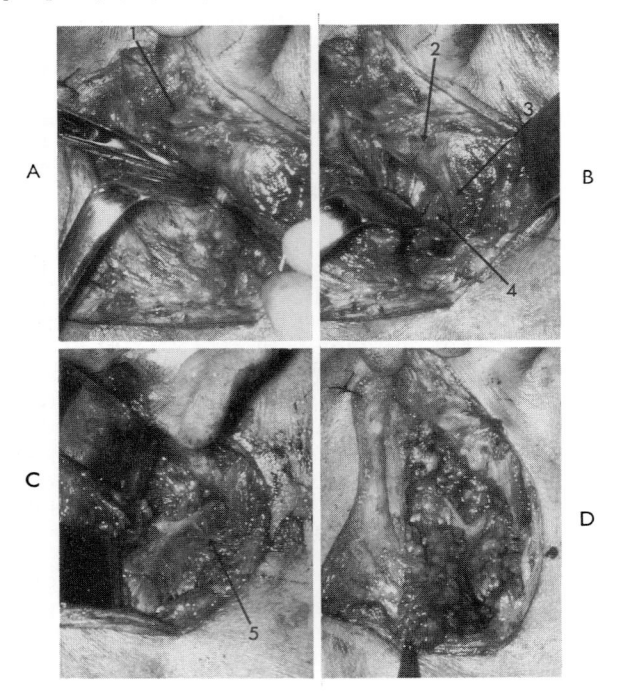

Fig. 43.—The exposure of the facial nerve during conservative parotidectomy.
A, The view of the main trunk immediately the overlying temporoparotid fascia has been divided. The pointed end of the tragal cartilage is outlined in black (1).
B, The parotid gland has been retracted anteriorly to show: the relationship of the main trunk to the temporo-mastoid fissure (2), to which the temporoparotid fascia was previously attached; the sterno-mastoid muscle (3); and the posterior belly of the digastric muscle (4).
C, The cervico-mandibular division of the nerve has been identified and branches to the stylohyoid and posterior belly of the digastric are seen arising from the main trunk of the facial nerve (5).
D, The zygomatico-facial division has now been identified and a small pleomorphic adenoma of the lower pole of the gland removed.

Stimulation with an electrical stimulator or by pinching with forceps is a wise precaution to avoid section of an unsuspected branch of the nerve, but the ability to recognize the peripheral branches on sight is perhaps the most valuable safeguard.

Where branches of the nerve must be sacrificed they can be replaced by grafts taken from the great auricular nerve.

Frey's Syndrome.—Frey's syndrome is sweating and sometimes flushing of the skin over the distribution of the auriculo-temporal nerve which is occasioned by a stimulus to salivary secretion. It is thought that as a result of damage to the auriculo-temporal nerve post-ganglionic parasympathetic fibres from the otic ganglion become united to sympathetic nerves from the superior cervical ganglion going to supply the sweat-glands of the skin.

The syndrome can follow parotid surgery, temporomandibular joint surgery, and injuries and injections in this region. Congenital cases probably follow birth injuries. The condition is rarely sufficiently severe to warrant any treatment. If this is necessary, a neurosurgeon may be asked to consider interrupting the intracranial course of the secreto-motor fibres.

REFERENCES

ANDERSON, R., and BYERS, L. T. (1965), *Surgery of the Parotid Gland*. St. Louis: Mosby.
KATZEN, M. (1969), 'Recurrent Parotitis in Children', *S. Afr. med. J.*, **7**, 37.
MAYNARD, J. D. (1965), 'Recurrent Parotid Enlargement', *Br. J. Surg.*, **52**, 784.
PATEY, D. H. (1965), 'Inflammation of the Salivary Glands with particular reference to Chronic and Recurrent Parotitis', *Ann. R. Coll. Surg.*, **36**, 26.
— — and THACKRAY, A. C. (1955), 'Chronic "Sialectatic" Parotitis in the Light of Pathological Studies on Parotidectomy Material', *Br. J. Surg.*, **43**, 43.
ROSE, S. S. (1954), 'A Clinical and Radiological Survey of 192 Cases of Recurrent Swellings of the Salivary Glands', *Ann. R. Coll. Surg.*, **15**, 374.
SEWARD, G. R. (1968), 'Anatomic Surgery for Salivary Calculi', *Oral Surg.*, **25**, 150, 287, 525, 670, 810; **26**, 1, 137.
STAFNE, E. C. (1958), *Oral Roentgenographic Diagnosis*, p.132. London: Saunders.

CHAPTER XIX

DISEASES OF THE TEMPOROMANDIBULAR JOINT

Developmental Disturbances

Hypoplasia of the Joint.—Hypoplasia of the condyle head can occur as part of unilateral or bilateral hypoplasia of the mandible. In such cases the joint is small, although the zygomatic arch is normal. In other instances, as, for example, in the case of the so-called 'first arch' syndrome, not only is the condyle head diminutive but the zygomatic process of the temporal bone also is small. This state of affairs, together with deficient zygomatic bones, is seen too as a symmetrical deformity in the genetically determined Treacher-Collins syndrome.

Hemifacial microsomia, first and second arch syndrome or otomandibular dysostosis occurs about once in 300–500 live-births and with no sex preference. The abnormalities are usually unilateral and of varying degrees of severity, with reduction in size or abnormality of the shape of the pinna and tragus, irregularities of the auditory ossicles, hypoplasia of the ramus and condyle of the mandible, deficiency of the muscles attached to the ramus and paresis of the muscles of facial expression. The external ear is also set lower on the head. In severe cases the external ear and auditory canal may be absent and the condyle and posterior part of the mandible fail to develop. Eruption of the teeth is frequently incomplete so that multiple impactions in the ramus are seen and teeth fail to reach the occlusal plane. Teeth may also be absent. Poswillo (1973a, b; 1974a) has shown that a haemorrhage occurs from the anastomosis of developing vessels which initiate the stapedial arterial stem at about the 6th week of embryonic life. The resultant haematoma produces a varying degree of tissue damage dependant on its size. Depending on the amount of destruction and the time required to resorb the debris and effect repair, so will the potential for 'catch up' differentiation be affected before the end of that phase of morphogenesis. Since the functional matrix of the face is affected in that region, so will secondary growth disturbances become manifest as growth proceeds.

In the Treacher-Collins' syndrome or mandibulofacial dysostosis the symmetrical defect is inherited as an autosomal dominant trait with equal sex incidence. There are an antimongoloid slope to the palpebral fissures, colobomas of the outer third of the lower lid, absence of cilia medial to the coloboma, deformed pinna, not uncommonly an absent external auditory canal, anomalies of the middle ear, extra ear tags, deficient malar bones, a receding chin and hypoplastic condyles and ramus. Poswillo (1973b; 1974b) suggests that there is a destruction of neural crest cells destined for the face and affecting those moving later in development rather than earlier. The severity depends on the degree of destruction. As a result of the destruction the developing otic pit moves up into first arch territory and the ear becomes located closer to the angle of the mandible. Since the genetic programme is now carried out, but with smaller amounts of material, the tissues affected are hypoplastic and to this extent a caricature of the normal part is found, rather than an absent part. Unlike the first and second arch syndrome cases, the degree of deformity is not increased as somatic growth proceeds, so that the appearance does not deteriorate as the child grows older.

Hyperplasia of the Joint.—Bony hyperplasia of all components of the joint probably only occurs with facial hemi-hypertrophy. Thus, although the cavity is increased in size to accommodate the enlarged head of unilateral condylar hyperplasia, there is no comparable enlargement of the zygomatic process of the temporal bone. This usually applies even though there may be some enlargement of other elements of the patient's face on the same side.

Basically, there are two types of unilateral condylar hyperplasia and a variety of terms are used to indicate this. One type has a not very greatly enlarged condyle head. The condyle neck, which is moderately elongated, is inclined downwards and forwards along the usual axis. Thus, the rest of the mandible on that side is pushed forwards. The angle is also farther forwards, the patient has mandibular prognathism, and the midline of the mandible is pushed to the opposite side. The point to note is that the joint functions normally, i.e., the condyle translates as well as rotates. Therefore, excision of the condyle should *never* be considered as a means of surgical correction. If this is done a normal jaw relationship may be restored together with a symmetrical face at rest, but deviation of the chin towards the side of surgery will occur as the patient opens the mouth. Instead, the Obwegeser sagittal splitting operation or the vertical subsigmoid procedure should be used. In a few patients it may be sufficient to shorten the elongated side of the mandible, rotating the jaw round the normal joint. The twisting of the condyle in its fossa produces no ill-effects. Usually, however, it is necessary to operate on both sides to produce a satisfactory occlusion. This is a further reason why simple condylectomy is unsatisfactory.

In the other form of condylar hyperplasia the condyle head is greatly enlarged, the neck elongated and directed downwards. A lateral open bite is established on that side, but the mandible is neither displaced forwards nor is the midline shifted to the other side. Many other associated changes may occur, some of them compensatory in nature. Hovell (1970) has shown that condylectomy practised at the correct time can produce a near-normal face for some of these patients. Therefore, in such cases, this method of management is acceptable since the greatly enlarged condyle only rotates in its fossa and there is no translatory movement to be lost.

Traumatic Injury to the Temporomandibular Joint

Traumatic Arthritis.—An injury which is insufficient to produce a fracture of the condyle or condyle neck, or a dislocation, may yet be sufficient to produce a traumatic arthritis.

Following the injury the patient complains of pain and limitation of movement of the joint. There is slight puffiness over the affected regions, the joint is markedly tender and the condyle head may appear more prominent than usual. This is usually due to a slight deviation of the mandible towards the opposite side, but there may be a unilateral posterior open bite without deviation. Whichever posture is adopted the patient is unwilling to close the teeth in centric occlusion because of pain. A joint radiograph will demonstrate widening of the radiographic joint space.

Immobilization of the jaw with a pair of eyelet wires on each side for a few days can give comfort, but the patient may require an occlusal wafer of acrylic resin which is inserted between the occlusal surfaces of the teeth before the intermaxillary wires are tightened. Often reassurance and analgesics are all that is required.

Acute Subluxation.—In this condition there is a sudden onset of limitation of opening, pain with movement of the affected joint, and reluctance to close in centric occlusion. Equally suddenly, and usually after some days, the patient will be aware of a jolt in the joint and normal movement is restored. Exactly what happens within the joint is not known. It is usually postulated that the condyle head manages to slip backwards over the posterior thickening of the disk. Muscle spasm leads to the other phenomena observed, including the slight deviation of the chin towards the *opposite* side seen when the patient is at rest.

Chronic Subluxation.—Some people can open their jaws to the point where the joints 'stick', then they free the joints, one at a time. The habit is a dangerous one since it can progress to recurrent subluxation of the joint. Should the latter develop, the patient should still be persuaded to try to control the situation voluntarily, for although there are many ingenious operations for this condition little is written about their long-term effectiveness.

Dislocation.—Dislocation of the condyle head upwards and forwards into the temporal fossa occurs when the masticatory muscles contract at a time when the mouth is open to its greatest extent, or when a blow is delivered to the point of the chin, again when the jaw is wide open. Cineradiography of the joint demonstrates that the condyle moves normally to a point beyond and above the lowest point on the eminentia. The jaw is controlled at this point by the balanced pull of the muscles and can be brought back smoothly under the eminentia and up into the fossa. Thus, there need only be a temporary lack of balance in the muscular pull for dislocation to occur.

Reduction is accomplished by downward pressure with the padded thumbs on the lower molars, together with an upwards and backwards force applied to the underside of the chin with the fingers. Once the patient's confidence has been gained most acute dislocations may be reduced in this manner. Rarely will it be necessary to resort to anaesthesia to produce the muscular relaxation necessary for success.

Chronic dislocation is seen almost always in edentulous patients, for where teeth are present the matter is drawn to everyone's attention by the gagged occlusion. Once the muscles are relaxed in a patient under a general anaesthetic, the condyles can be dislocated and replaced in their fossae with the greatest of ease for it is the muscles which normally prevent this occurrence. Both the operator and the anaesthetist maintain a forward displacement of the jaw to ensure a free airway. With a prop or gag between the molar teeth acting as a fulcrum, this pressure easily pushes the condyles over the eminentia. If, during the anaesthetic, the patient's teeth are extracted, all reference points between the upper and lower jaw are removed. Postoperatively the patient expects both some discomfort in the jaw and a change in appearance, so a dislocation is easily overlooked. Muscle spasm and then fibrosis and muscle-shortening prevent reduction of the dislocation.

Once such a state of affairs has persisted for some months treatment is difficult. There are several alternatives. First, the situation can be accepted, but, alternatively, condylectomy can be performed with replacement of the mandible. Open reduction has been tried, but this can prove very difficult. Hayward (1965) has had success with manipulation and muscle relaxation, and Popesca (1960) uses a roll of gauze placed between the molars to act as a fulcrum and an upward force applied to the chin.

An unusual injury to the joint is fracture of the roof of the articular fossa with dislocation of the condyle head into the middle cranial fossa. The injury is of importance because the patient may have some degree of opening of the mouth (Pirok and Merrill, 1970) and derangement of the occlusion may be the only clue to the nature of the occurrence.

Tearing of the Disk.—Campbell (1965) has shown by some beautiful arthrography and radiography that the meniscus may be torn free at one margin and crumpled up within the cavity. Movement of the condyle head is then restricted. If the disk lies behind the condyle the latter cannot return to its proper position in the fossa. Badly torn and crumpled disks should be removed. This constitutes one of the few indications for menisectomy.

A damaged meniscus used to be blamed as the cause of the painful and locking joint. It is now realized that such damage is uncommon. Further, removal of the disk gives only temporary relief in this particular type of case.

Damage to the Condyle.—Injury or disease affecting the condyle during childhood can affect the condylar growth centre and produce changes in mandibular growth. (*Fig.* 44.) Trauma to the condyle, infection, and Still's disease are the main offenders. Infection may reach the condyle by direct spread from osteomyelitis, or as a result of a suppurative arthritis, in some cases secondary to otitis media.

The mandible can be considered as composed of three elements, a bar of bone which stretches from the condyle to the mental eminence, the alveolar process, and the muscular processes of the coronoid and angle. The condylar growth centre is responsible for the growth in length of the basic bar or arch of bone. If growth ceases the distance between the condyle and the point of the chin remains the same. As the maxilla grows downwards in relation to the joint the chin end of the bar is tilted down into the neck. In an attempt to compensate, the alveolar process, particularly that in the incisor region, grows upwards and forwards towards the maxilla. Both the muscular processes achieve a near normal size, so by comparison with the condyle the coronoid is elongated and the sizeable angle accentuates the facial notch.

Ankylosis of the Temporomandibular Joint.—Ankylosis can be a sequel to an intracapsular fracture of the condyle (particularly in members of

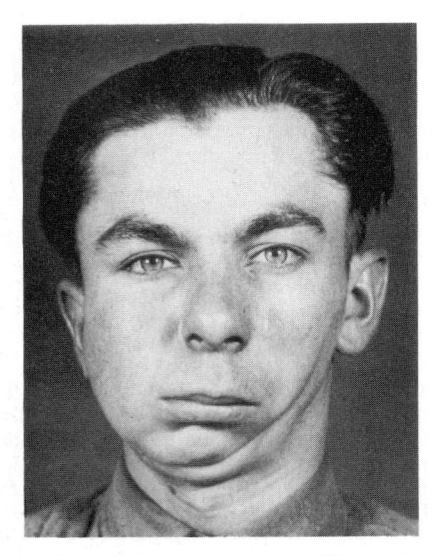

Fig. 44.—Osteomyelitis of the right ramus in childhood has resulted in damage to the condylar growth centre and deviation of the mandible to the right.

the coloured races), severe infection of the joint (particularly suppurative infections), and long-standing active rheumatoid arthritis, Still's disease, and, of course, to ankylosing spondylitis. Ankylosis may be either bony or fibrous. When the union is fibrous it may be possible to demonstrate a joint space by radiography, particularly short-distance radiography of the condyle head, or tomography. Also with fibrous ankylosis there is frequently a considerable rotational movement of the joint. (*Fig.* 45.)

Curiously, a unilateral bony ankylosis seems to be compatible with some degree of jaw movement, even when the bony union seems to be quite extensive at operation. When bony ankylosis follows a fracture the area of bony union may be considerable in extent, involving the condyle, sigmoid notch, coronoid, and lingula, on the one hand, and the joint, zygomatic arch, pterygoid plates, and the base of the skull on the other.

Operations to free an ankylosis seek to produce a pseudarthrosis. The bony or fibrous attachment is divided and the abnormal tissue removed. Three manœuvres are employed to try to prevent reattachment: the part of the mandible adjacent to the joint may be widely excised; a soft tissue, such as muscle or dermis, may be interposed between the bone-ends; alternatively, an allelograft material can be inserted in the gap or over one of the bone-ends. The disadvantage of creating a wide gap is that, subsequently, muscle pull shortens the jaw towards the joint producing a micrognathic appearance and an anterior open bite.

Ward (1961) pointed out that a direct attack on the joint region can involve the operator in a difficult dissection. He devised a curved, low ramus section which avoids these problems. His operative technique consists essentially of fitting a plate of chrome-cobalt over the bone-end to discourage bony union. A new joint made in this fashion tends to become stiff as the area of contact is too great for the length of false capsule which develops. Reducing the end of the upper fragment to a point can cure this difficulty.

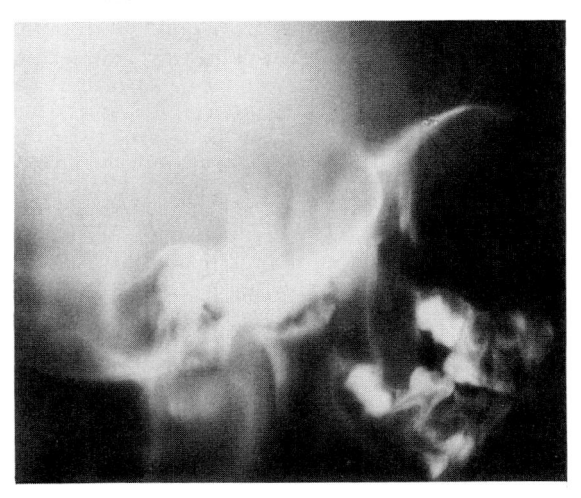

Fig. 45.—A radiograph of a congenitally ankylosed mandible. A band of radiolucent cartilage separates the condylar bone from that of the temporal like an irregular epiphysial plate.

Both muscle and dermis have been used to discourage osteogenesis. The dermal graft is cut by raising a Thiersch graft. The epidermal graft is left attached by one edge while the dermal graft is dissected off the underlying fat. The epidermis can then be replaced to cover the wound. The bone-end is rounded and holes drilled just behind the end. The dermal sheet is stretched over the bone-end and fixed by sutures which are passed through the holes.

Silastic has been used freely in recent years as a barrier between the bone-ends, but the long-term results with this material are not yet known.

Other Causes of Limited Opening

Mechanical Causes.—In some patients the tissue which prevents proper mandibular movement is outside the capsule of the joint (extracapsular ankylosis) or even at a distance from the joint. A fractured zygomatic arch, for example, can interfere with movement of the coronoid process.

Conversely, the coronoid process may be enlarged as in the condition called 'coronoid hyperplasia'. Cartilage, and as a result bone, proliferate so as to elongate the coronoid and produce a knob-like expansion. An adventitious bursa develops between the coronoid and the inside of the zygomatic arch, which may be resorbed on its inner aspect so as to accommodate the mass. Compensatory deposition of bone on the outer aspect of the zygomatic bone produces an enlargement of the cheek.

Quite often the hyperplasia affects both coronoid processes. Because an accessory cartilaginous growth centre is formed for a while in the coronoid process during development, it has been suggested that persistence of this cartilage is the cause of the hyperplasia. As the coronoid enlarges, first lateral movements of the jaw and then opening of the mouth become restricted. Excision of the coronoid process gives good results.

The operation is carried out in the following manner. Anaesthesia is induced and blind endotracheal intubation is performed. A vasoconstrictor is infiltrated into the operation site and an incision is made vertically through the mucous membrane and buccinator over the anterior border of the ramus. The deep facial vein and buccal artery have to be divided and must be ligated. At first sight, access is very limited since the patient's jaw cannot be separated very far. However, the cheek wound is distensible and only the buccal pad of fat is likely to reduce visibility. If the latter cannot be satisfactorily retracted, it should be drawn out of the wound, ligated, and excised. The masseter and temporalis insertion are elevated to clear the mandible in a line from the wound to the sigmoid notch and a hole is drilled in the base of the coronoid. A wire must be passed through this to prevent the temporalis from pulling the coronoid upwards out of sight once it has been separated. The coronoid is sectioned with a bur. Once the cut has been completed, with an osteotome if necessary, the jaws can be separated unless the other side is affected. Traction is applied to the wire and the mass separated from the temporalis and removed. A vacuum drain is threaded through the submandibular skin and the wound closed. A new coronoid forms from the periosteum, but it is of normal size.

Dense fibrous bands can develop in the muscles of mastication which limit mandibular movement. This reaction may be seen on occasions in the temporalis after the injection of alcohol into the ganglion in cases of trigeminal neuralgia. A similar response can follow the injection of dental local anaesthetic solutions suggesting that a haematoma, or possibly a low-grade infection, has been caused by the injection.

Cleft palate operations can produce fibrosis of the pterygomandibular raphe and, consequently, limitation of opening. Moderate degrees of fibrosis can be released or a coronoidectomy performed if the temporalis is involved. The jaw should be propped wide open, and although it may be removed at mealtimes the prop must be replaced afterwards for at least a fortnight.

Submucous fibrosis (*see also* p. 126) results in dense fibrous bands in the cheeks and pillars of the fauces which stretch from mandible to maxilla. While almost all the cases have been recorded in Indians and a few other Asians and Europeans living in India, a few similar cases in white people have, however, been reported outside India: one by Lemmer and Shear (1967), in South Africa, and one by Simpson (1969), in Manchester. The latter had been married to a Pakistani for 12 years and had been eating Indian food. Sirsat and Khanolkar (1962) have produced a similar response in rats' palates by painting them with capsaicin, a constituent of chillies, and it is thought that this may be the aetiological factor. Affected individuals are usually between 20 and 40 years of age, but cases from 10 to 70 years of age are seen. Dense acellular masses of collagen and strands of an elastic-like material form in the submucosa limiting movement of the mandible, tongue, and soft palate and occluding the Eustachian tube. The overlying epithelium is thin and lacks rete pegs. There is no effective treatment.

In some subjects myositis ossificans develops as a response to injury. Many cases of myositis ossificans of the masseter have now been recorded. The probable mechanism is a tear of the muscle origin or insertion such that the periosteum is also damaged. As a result, bone develops in the healing haematoma. Usually the new bone is resorbed, which is fortunate. The excision of myositis ossificans, as in the case of scar bands, can be followed in some patients by a recurrence to a greater degree than before.

Rarely the progressive, generalized myositis ossificans affects the tissues of the face, uniting mandible to maxilla. There is also a rare congenital deformity in which the upper and lower alveolar processes are conjoined on one or both sides.

Functional Causes.—The most frequent cause of limited opening is an inflammation affecting the tissues about the jaws. Usually this is described as trismus, but is not strictly so as it is not due to muscle spasm. Indeed, Moore and Greenfield (1967) have shown that inhibition of muscular activity is a reason for limited mandibular movement after 3rd molar surgery, and this seems to be a logical way for the part to be rested. Oedema of the elevators of the mandible such that they cannot lengthen to permit depression of the mandible is another cause.

Two cases of tetanus have been seen by the authors which presented as cases of limitation of opening. In both cases the patient had been referred as a suspected case of temporomandibular joint disorder. One was due to a penetration wound in the foot, the other to a similar small wound in the hand.

In an unusual neurological case true muscular spasm resulted in inability to open the mouth, or part the cords in the larynx. The patient required a permanent tracheostomy. So severe was the spasm of the masticatory muscles that a considerable dose of curare was required to abolish electromyographic evidence of activity and to permit the jaws to be separated. The remaining few teeth were sheathed in deep pits in the opposing alveolar ridge.

Occasionally there is no physical cause for the inability to open and the patient is a hysteric. Such cases can be baffling until it is realized that the patient is mentally disturbed.

ARTHRITIS AND ARTHROSIS

Infective Arthritis of the Temporomandibular Joint.—Infective arthritis of the temporomandibular joint is by no means a common complaint. Suppurative arthritis from staphylococcal infection may arise as a result of a penetrating injury of the joint or by the spread of infection from adjacent structures. Involvement of the condyle head following an osteomyelitis of the ramus is one mechanism and extension of infection from otitis media is another. The latter may develop as a complication of measles in children, but can also occur in adults where the mastoid air cells extend into the zygomatic process of the temporal bone. Rarely, a boil or an infected pre-auricular sinus is the source of the infection. Many of the older clinicians can recall cases of gonococcal arthritis of the temporomandibular joint.

Suppurative arthritis should be treated by aspiration of the joint, the instillation of an antibiotic solution, and the administration of a systemic antibiotic. A smear should be made from the aspirate and a sample sent for culture and sensitivity tests.

Even less common are non-suppurative infections such as tuberculosis, but an acutely swollen joint from Reiter's disease may be seen from time to time.

Rheumatoid Diseases.—Rheumatoid arthritis, psoriatic arthritis, and, in children, Still's disease can affect the temporomandibular joint. However, this joint is only one of many which may be affected and, in general, the patient's management will be in the hands of a rheumatologist. The manifestations of the disorder in the temporomandibular joint differ little from those in joints elsewhere. There will be pain particularly on movement, some swelling of the overlying tissues, and limitation of opening. Radiographically the condyle head and articular fossa will be less radioopaque than usual and erosion of the articular surface of the condyle may be seen.

In Still's disease there may be damage to the growth centre of the condyle and the development of both extra- and intracapsular adhesions which limit joint movement.

In addition to the general measures recommended for the patient, all local causes of joint strain should be eliminated. Courses of short-wave diathermy may give comfort, and the cautious use of intra-articular hydrocortisone can be of benefit.

One factor of importance is the effect of systemic steroids on condyles affected by rheumatoid arthritis. The bone is progressively resorbed, sometimes over quite a short period of time, until no condyle remains. The first intimation of this effect may be the development of an anterior open bite.

Gout.—Gout of the temporomandibular joint is most uncommon. One of the authors has seen a case in a child with leukaemia. The importance of the condition lies in the presentation of acute inflammation of the joint in such a way that the condition can be mistaken for a suppurative arthritis.

Osteoarthritis.—Osteoarthritis is detected mostly in the older age-groups, but can be found affecting joints which have previously suffered a fracture. The joint is painful, often has a palpable and audible grate when the mouth is opened, and is tender to palpation. Careful radiography can demonstrate localized resorption cavities in the condyle head, sclerosis of the underlying bone, osteophytic masses particularly anteriorly, and occasionally small cystic cavities.

As with other joints, there are probably many osteoarthritic ones which are symptomless, and not a few which return to a painless state after months or years of causing trouble.

The full range of conservative measures should be tried: analgesics, attention to the occlusion, the use of shortwave diathermy. Altering the mechanics of the joint with a bite-raising appliance or the provision of new dentures which restore the proper vertical dimension may both help.

The mechanism, presumably, is similar to that seen in the femur where an osteotomy which permits a slight displacement of the femoral head can improve an osteoarthritic hip. In some patients the occasional intra-articular injection of hydrocortisone will give quite long periods of relief.

Henny (1957, 1968) employs a high condylectomy for those cases in which bony changes can be demonstrated and where the patient has considerable trouble with the joint. In a large series of middle-aged women he obtained good results with this operation. Through a pre-auricular incision he uncovers the joint, incises the capsule over the condyle, and removes a thin layer of articular surface with a drill. There should be minimal occlusal changes as a result of this procedure.

Functional Derangement of the Temporomandibular Joint.—That so many young people suffer pain and disordered function of the temporomandibular joint makes it a quite unusual condition, for often it affects fit subjects in whom it is impossible to demonstrate either disease of the surfaces of that particular joint or of any other joints. In what ways then are the temporomandibular joints unusual anatomically? First, they are the only joints at each end of a bone which have to function in concert with one another, a situation which arises because of the horseshoe shape of the mandible. Secondly, the path of movement of all other joints is dictated solely by the articular surfaces of the joint and the muscles. With the temporomandibular joints the path of movement is in part imposed upon the joints from without, by the articulation of the teeth and by the movement of the opposite joint. Finally, each joint has two compartments separated by a disk, and both the condyle head and the disk are to be found balanced on the posterior sloping surface of the eminentia when the maximum masticatory force is exerted. It is in order to control the final movement of condyle head and disk from the eminentia into the fossa under this heavy load, that the lateral pterygoid has such a complex insertion into both condyle and disk. A malfunction of this muscular control by the lateral pterygoid could permit the condyle head to move separately in relation to the disk, starting the chain of events that gives rise to clinical clicking.

Much has been written about the derangements of the temporomandibular joint, but much is, of necessity, pure speculation. The condition appears to be more common in women than men. The complaint may be of pain in the joint, limitation of opening, locking of the joint, or a click. Not infrequently the pain is less clearly related to the joint and may be described as passing across the face or down the ramus and either into the neck or along the mandible. Other patients may complain of pain in the ear.

On examination the joint is usually tender to pressure. Limitation of opening may vary from the barely perceptible to the extreme. There may be deviation of the mandible as the mouth is opened: the chin coming back into the midline after the condyle has moved laterally apparently around an obstruction, or after a click or palpable thud.

Many aetiological factors have been suggested for this condition. Frequently when a patient is examined not one, but several, possible precipitants are uncovered. What causes the joint to give symptoms in one patient, but not in others with similar anomalies, remains an enigma. The main factors include abnormalities of the occlusion, particularly Angle's Class II, division 1, which require the patient to protrude in order to incise, and deep overbites which deny affected persons the facility of lateral chewing movements. Alterations and adaptations in the chewing mechanism, which a patient may have to effect because of the ravages of dental disease, can throw a considerable strain on the joints. Habitual chewing on one side of the arch and chewing on the incisors are examples of this type of disturbance. The avoidance of gaps, a sore pericoronal gum flap, or elongated unopposed teeth are other provocants. Even the insertion of a restoration with a high spot or the wrong angle of a cusp plane can precipitate symptoms.

Certain habits seem to strain the joint. Sleeping with the side of the face pressed against the pillow will displace the jaw laterally and the patient may wake with a stiff, aching joint. Nocturnal bruxism, pencil-chewing, and other habits which cause pressure on the mouth and lips can play their part.

Just as there are many aetiological factors so there are many treatments. If possible, the factor which precipitated symptoms should be identified and reversed. If this is not feasible, another factor which is amenable to alteration should be tackled. For example, if as a result of the extraction of the posterior teeth the patient is overclosing, dentures should be provided. Where there are gaps in the dental arch, these can be filled to provide more uniform use of both sides for chewing.

Advice can be given about posture during sleep, recommending that the back of the head should rest on the pillow. If a patient cannot follow this advice, a bite-locking plate can be tried. This is similar to a lower acrylic bite-raising plate, but made to fill the freeway space and with deep indentations in the upper surface for the upper teeth. Such a plate prevents lateral displacement of the jaw during sleep.

The bite-raising appliance is a standby of much temporomandibular joint treatment. In many cases the effect is probably just to alter the mechanics of joint function, at the same time providing free lateral articulation. If the patient's major complaint is of an early click, a bite-raising appliance may prevent the condyle from going back into the pre-click position.

Occlusal grinding, drugs which reduce muscle spasm, exercises, and short-wave diathermy are other forms of treatment which may prove beneficial.

Condylectomy and meniscectomy have no place in the treatment of this condition and, in general, operations of any kind should be avoided. In a few carefully selected patients the Ward condylotomy may be performed (Ward, 1961). In this procedure the condyle neck is sectioned with a Gigli saw, passed round the back of the ramus with the mouth open so that it emerges in front of the condyle neck through the sigmoid notch. When the saw is almost through, section is completed by pressure with the thumbs. Following the operation the jaw is immobilized for two weeks. Slight displacement of the condyle head occurs. As with the bite-raising appliance, it is probably the slight alteration in joint mechanics which produces the benefit.

Radiography and Radiology of the Temporomandibular Joint

Many of the techniques and interpretations of temporomandibular joint radiography in the past were based on a narrow concept of normal function and an incomplete understanding of the applied anatomy. For the most part, disturbances of joint movement are as easily observed clinically as radiographically. Thus, the place of radiography is to confirm, or refute, the presence of overt joint disease. For this purpose the orthopantomograph emerges as the best diagnostic weapon so far (Tammisalo, 1964). Where the bony structure of the condyle and condyle neck are to be recorded, Toller's variant of the short distance, transpharyngeal technique is advocated (Toller, 1969). For an A.P. view of the condyle head and neck the transorbital A.P. is advised.

While some excellent arthrograms have been produced by a number of experts in the field, this technique has its hazards. The yield in diagnostic information is probably not enough to warrant its routine use.

Surgical Exploration of the Temporomandibular Joint

Of the many surgical approaches to the temporomandibular joint that of Henny (1968) seems to have many advantages. The pre-auricular tissues are infiltrated with a vasoconstrictor and the skin incision begins in front of the pinna, runs downwards to join the crease above the tragus, and then follows the free edge of the tragus. It ends in the crease in front of the lobe of the ear. The wound is deepened by keeping the edge of a number 15 blade against the outer surface of the cartilage of the auditory canal. This separates the auriculo-temporal nerve, the superficial temporal vessels, and the upper pole of the parotid from the auditory canal. The facial nerve is safe provided that the dissection is not carried below the canal. Once the zygomatic arch is reached the temporalis fascia is divided and the tissues are swept forwards with the rounded blade of the Howarth's rugine. The middle temporal vein passes horizontally just above the zygomatic arch and this is picked up, divided, and ligated.

If the correct plane of dissection is used the tissues strip readily off the surface of the joint capsule. An L-shaped incision with one limb parallel with the floor of the articular fossa and the other vertically behind the condyle head will open the capsule.

Careful haemostasis is secured after the operative procedure has been completed and the wound closed in layers without drainage. A pressure dressing is applied for 48 hours.

REFERENCES

CAMPBELL, W. (1965), 'Clinical Radiological Investigations of the Mandibular Joint,' *Br. J. Radiol.*, **38**, 401.
HAYWARD, J. R. (1965), 'Prolonged Dislocation of the Mandible', *J. oral Surg.*, **23**, 585.
HENNY, F. A. (1957), 'Treatment of the Painful Temporomandibular Joint', *Ibid.* **15**, 214.
— — (1968), in *Textbook of Oral Surgery* 3rd ed. (ed. KRUGER, G. O.), p. 379. St Louis: Mosby.
HOVELL, J. H. (1970), 'Surgical Correction of Facial Deformity'. *Ann. R. Coll. Surg.*, **46**, 92.
LEMMER, J., and SHEAR, M. (1967), 'Oral Submucous Fibrosis', *Br. dent. J.*, **122**, 343.

MOORE, J. R., and GREENFIELD, B. E. (1967), 'Electromyographic Investigation into Postoperative Trismus'. Lecture, Meeting of the British Association of Oral Surgeons, Edinburgh, July, 1967.

PIROK, D. J., and MERRILL, R. G. (1970), 'Dislocation of the Mandibular Condyle into the Middle Cranial Fossa', *Oral Surg.*, **29**, 13.

POPESCA, V. (1960), 'A Practical Method for the Reduction of Temporomandibular Dislocation', *Stomatologia*, **4**, 87.

POSWILLO, D. E. (1973a), 'The Pathogenesis of the First and Second Branchial Arch Syndrome', *Oral Surg.*, **35**, 302–328.

— — (1973b), 'The Pathogenesis of the Treacher-Collins Syndrome', Paper presented at British Association of Oral Surgeons meeting, October 1973.

— — (1974a), 'Orofacial Malformations', *Proc. R. Soc. Med.*, **67**, 343–349.

— — (1974b), 'Otomandibular Deformity: Pathogenesis as a Guide to Reconstruction', *J. Max. fac. Surg.*, **2**, 64–72.

SIMPSON W. (1969), 'Submucous Fibrosis', *Br. J. oral Surg.*, **6**, 196.

SIRSAT, S. M. and KHANOLKAR, V. K. (1962), 'Submucous Fibrosis of the Palate and Pillars of the Fauces', *Indian J. med. Sci.*, **16**, 189.

TAMMISALO, E. H. (1964), 'Orthopantomographic Roentgenography of the Temporomandibular Joint', *Suom. Hammaslääk. Seur. Toim.*, **60**, 139.

TOLLER, P. A. (1969), 'The Transpharyngeal Radiography for Arthritis of the Mandibular Condyle', *Br. J. oral Surg.*, **7**, 47.

WARD, T. G. (1961), 'Surgery of the Mandibular Joint', *Ann. R. Coll. Surg.*, **28**, 139.

Chapter XX

NERVE INJURIES OF INTEREST TO THE ORAL SURGEON

THE nerves most likely to sustain damage as a result of an oral surgical procedure or a facial fracture are the facial, auriculo-temporal, mandibular, lingual, and infra-orbital.

THE FACIAL NERVE

Injury to the facial nerve results in facial paralysis.

Differential Diagnosis of Causes of Facial Paralysis.—Dealt with in detail, the differential diagnosis of causes of facial paralysis is a complex subject. Those interested in this degree of detail are referred to neurological texts. Briefly, facial paralysis may be supranuclear, nuclear, and infranuclear in origin or due to primary degeneration of the muscles of facial expression.

Supranuclear Paralysis.—The commonest cause of supranuclear facial nerve paralysis is a stroke. Movements of the lower part of the face are more severely affected than those of the upper. There is no reaction of degeneration when the nerve is electrically stimulated and emotional facial movements are unimpaired. Rarely the reverse state is seen and there is loss of emotional facial expression.

Nuclear and Infranuclear Paralysis.—Lesions within the pons may affect the VI nucleus because of the curvature of the facial nerve-fibres around the nucleus. More extensive lesions will involve the spinal tract of V, the motor fibres of V, and spinothalamic and pyramidal tracts destined for the upper and lower limb of the other side.

Within the posterior cranial fossa facial paralysis is associated with deafness and vestibular disturbances, due to damage to the VIII nerve. There is an associated loss of taste in the anterior two-thirds of the tongue.

Damage to the nerve within the facial canal is usually associated with damage to the taste fibres of the anterior two-thirds of the tongue, either while they are with the nerve or in the chorda tympani. Should the branch to the stapedius be involved there will be hyperacusis, but loss of salivary secretion due to damage to secreto-motor fibres is not easily appreciated. Lesions in the last part of the facial canal do not affect taste and the commonest cause here is Bell's palsy. Occasionally the lesion in Bell's palsy migrates sufficiently far proximally to affect the chorda tympani and then taste is affected.

Outside the stylomastoid foramen the nerve branches almost immediately, but loss of function in the stylohyoid muscle, the posterior belly of the digastric, and occipital belly of the occipito-frontalis, which are supplied by the first branches, is difficult to spot clinically. Damage to individual branches within, or distal to, the parotid gland is more easily distinguished.

Primary Muscular Weakness and Degeneration.—Myasthenia gravis, muscular dystrophy, and dystrophia myotonica are possible causes of facial weakness in this group. Other muscular groups elsewhere in the body will be involved.

Electrical Stimulation Tests.—Following inadvertent trauma to the facial nerve, tests with electrical stimulation are of some value in ascertaining the extent of the nerve damage.

The Reaction of Degeneration.—Normal muscles respond to stimulation by faradic and galvanic current (interrupted and constant). Faradism causes a muscular contraction which persists as long as the current is passing, but galvanism causes a muscular contraction only when the current is made or broken. In normal muscle, if the kathode is used (a kathodal closing current, KCC) a more vigorous response is obtained than when the anode (anodal closing current, ACC) is used. Following a lower motor neuron lesion a muscle ceases to respond to faradic stimulation of its motor point in 4–7 days and after 10 days a normal response to galvanism ceases, though the muscle may respond with a sluggish contraction. At this time the ACC is more effective than the KCC, a condition known as 'polar reversal'. Taken collectively these phenomena constitute the reaction of degeneration.

According to Brain (1962) electrical records obtained directly from muscles by electromyography give much more detailed and accurate information of muscular function than the test for reaction of degeneration which will be superseded by electromyography.

Oral surgical procedures may occasionally produce a temporary or a permanent facial paralysis if one or more branches of the seventh nerve are inadvertently severed (neurotmesis) or bruised (neurapraxia). The possibility of cutting the facial nerve or one or more of its branches must always be considered when incisions are made on the face, especially when carrying out surgery in the temporomandibular joint area. Nerve damage may also occur through misplaced incisions when opening facial abscesses, but the most commonly damaged branch of the facial nerve is the mandibular branch which can be inadvertently severed during a submandibular surgical approach to the mandible. This injury leaves the patient with an ugly weakness of the angle of the lower lip. All submandibular incisions must therefore be made at least 1 cm. beneath the lower border of the mandible in order to avoid this mishap. Branches of the facial nerve may also be bruised as a result of rough retraction, excessive postoperative swelling of the cheek, or by blunt dissection in the vicinity of the facial nerve. Temporary facial paralysis may also be caused through a misdirected mandibular injection in which the analgesic solution is deposited too far posteriorly and diffuses within the parotid gland. The resultant unilateral facial paralysis is complete and, though it is alarming to both patient and operator, it is a purely temporary phenomenon and normal muscle movement is gradually restored as the effect of the local analgesic wears off.

Treatment.—Facial paralysis is an ugly deformity and the management of the case depends upon whether the condition is likely to be permanent or if there is hope of recovery. Most cases of Bell's palsy tend to recover though progress is slow in the older patient. When recovery is anticipated the musculature of the cheek should be lifted by fitting an intra-oral prosthetic appliance attached to the patient's teeth or denture which is designed to lift the cheek and side of the lip. This helps to mask the facial deformity and removes tension on the cheek. The rheumatologist may suggest electrical stimulation of the muscles to improve their tone until re-innervation begins. When the nerve begins to recover, feeble muscular movement is seen and at this stage the patient should be instructed to exercise the affected side while facing a mirror. In order to prevent the overaction of the unaffected side of the face interfering with the exercise, the patient should hold one hand firmly over the normal side of the face to prevent its muscle pull interfering with muscular movements on the affected side. In most instances recovery is a slow process.

The treatment of facial paralysis where there is no hope of recovery is not particularly rewarding and none of the suggested treatments is uniformly effective. The possibilities are:—

1. *A Nerve Graft.*
2. *An Anastomosis* of the proximal section of the facial nerve to the spinal accessory.
3. *Sling Operations* where the angle of the mouth and cheek are connected by a sling within the tissues to some stable point such as a hole drilled in the zygomatic bone. The slings are made of fascia lata, kangaroo tendon, floss silk, polythene tape, stainless-steel wire, etc., which are threaded through the tissues with a straight needle. The results are not particularly impressive and many of the materials such as fascia lata stretch, so leading to a relapse of the deformity. On the other hand, materials such as stainless-steel or tantalum wire do not stretch, but they tend to become unduly prominent beneath the skin and constitute an unacceptable deformity.
4. *Re-animation Procedures.*—Various re-animation procedures have been suggested where strips of active muscle, such as the temporalis or masseter muscle, are connected to the angle of the mouth and cheek. If the operation is successful considerable training of the patient is necessary to enable the best use to be made of the new muscle connexion.
5. *Disguising Procedures.*—This treatment consists of a series of cosmetic operations to restore an appearance of normality to the affected side. The main procedures are a unilateral face-lifting procedure and a partial tarsorrhaphy to correct the droop of the lower lid. An incision is made in the nasolabial fold on the affected side and incisions are made to correspond with the creases in the normal side of the forehead. These incisions are sutured so that an inverted scar is formed and the two sides of the face are then relatively similar. If these procedures are skilfully performed the results are quite good.
6. *Selective Neurectomy.*—It has been suggested that by cutting the corresponding branches of the facial nerve on the unaffected side of the face, a harmonious muscular balance can be achieved. In practice this procedure produces a most lugubrious expression.

THE AURICULO-TEMPORAL NERVE

Gustatory Sweating and Flushing.—Frey-Baillarger syndrome. Dupuy's syndrome, auriculo-temporal and chorda tympani syndromes.

The auriculo-temporal nerve, in addition to supplying sensory fibres to the pre-auricular and temporal areas, carries parasympathetic fibres to the parotid gland and sympathetic vasomotor and pseudomotor fibres to the skin of the same area. Injury to the auriculo-temporal nerve denervates the sweat-glands and vessels of the skin over its distribution in addition to producing sensory disturbances. Both the parasympathetic and sympathetic nerves of the face are cholinergic and in the process of regeneration parasympathetic fibres become misdirected and grow along sympathetic pathways. Thus, a gustatory stimulus produces sweating and flushing. This syndrome develops about five or more weeks after injury to the auriculo-temporal nerve. The syndrome is usually permanent, but regression and even disappearance of the symptoms may occur in a very small proportion of cases. There is no effective treatment.

THE MANDIBULAR NERVE

The mandibular nerve may be inadvertently severed as a result of fracture of the mandible or it may be bruised or sectioned during surgery. The most common sites of injury are in the lower 3rd molar area and where the nerve emerges from the mental foramen. The mandibular nerve supplies a small area to one side of the lower lip and cutting or bruising the nerve results in anaesthesia of this section of the lower lip. Fortunately, this area of the lower lip has an accessory nerve-supply from C2 and C3 and some recovery of sensation can be confidently anticipated in all instances, though the patient may complain of a variation in quality of the sensation compared with the normal side. Recovery following neurapraxia may take from 6 weeks to 3 months and following neurotmesis recovery takes 18 months to 2 years. Some patients experience protracted hyperaesthesia during the recovery period, but in the course of time recovery is more or less complete. In all the long-term follow-up surveys of mandibular fractures complete recovery of sensation in the lower lip is found in almost all cases.

Since anaesthesia of the lower lip is not particularly uncommon after the removal of impacted 3rd molars, this situation can be considered further to illustrate the ways in which this nerve may be damaged. Anaesthesia may be present immediately following recovery from the effects of the anaesthetic. Such anaesthesia may be due to pressure on the nerve during elevation of the tooth or a transmitted shock wave during tooth division with an osteotome. A neurapraxia results and early and complete recovery of normal sensation will occur. Alternatively, the nerve may have been crushed, but continuity of the bundle remains. Degeneration occurs and the condition is known as 'axonotmesis'. Recovery will be delayed and will be accompanied by paraesthesia (unpleasant, abnormal sensation), but this will be short-lived and ultimate recovery will be complete.

If the nerve has been completely severed (neurotmesis) recovery will again be delayed until regeneration occurs and the paraesthesiae will persist until cortical reorientation has taken place. Ultimate recovery may not be perfect.

It may be possible with an intelligent patient to distinguish between neurapraxia and neurotmesis, even within 48 hours of the operation, since the loss of sensation is usually more profound with the latter.

In some cases lip sensation is normal immediately after recovery from the anaesthetic, but sensory impairment develops over the next 24 hours.

This is often due to a rise in pressure within the inferior dental canal as a result of postoperative oedema. The defect is a neurapraxia and resolves quite rapidly. A similar sequence may follow the handling of the nerve in circumstances which make it unlikely that there is a postoperative increase in pressure.

The Lingual Nerve

If the lingual nerve is severed loss of sensation in the anterior two-thirds of the tongue occurs. This area of the tongue has no accessory nerve supply and neurotmesis results in loss of sensation. The lingual nerve may be inadvertently severed during lower 3rd molar surgery, for the nerve runs very superficially on the lingual aspect of the mandible in this area. The nerve must be retracted and protected by an instrument such as a Howarth's periosteal elevator when operating on lower 3rd molars. Retraction should be gentle or neurapraxia may occur. The nerve may also be kinked at the pterygo-mandibular raphe or under-run with a suture, particularly if much bone has to be removed to uncover the 3rd molar. Such an injury usually recovers comparatively rapidly, but occasionally unilateral anaesthesia of the anterior two-thirds of the tongue may be protracted. Surgical exploration of the lingual nerve in patients where the nerve has been severed has shown a neuroma on the proximal end of the nerve. Muscular movements of the tongue probably preclude the possibility of regeneration of the lingual nerve following neurotmesis.

The Nerve to the Mylohyoid

Recently (Roberts and Harris, 1973) attention has been drawn to the occurrence of small patches of anaesthesia in the lower part of the chin and close to the midline as a sequel to lower 3rd molar surgery. It has been shown by these authors that selective infiltration of the nerve to the mylohyoid will produce an identical area of anaesthesia. They postulate that neurapraxia of the nerve may be caused by the retraction of the soft tissues in an attempt to protect the lingual nerve.

The Infra-orbital Nerve

Neurapraxia or neurotmesis of the infra-orbital nerve occurs as a result of fracture of the zygomatic bone and in Le Fort 2- and 3-type fractures. It results in anaesthesia of one side of the upper lip, the side of the nose, and an area of the cheek. Recovery of sensation in the affected area can be confidently expected in almost all cases, though if the nerve is severed it may take 8–12 months.

REFERENCES

Brain, R. (1962), *Diseases of the Nervous System*, 6th ed. London: Oxford University Press.
Roberts, E. D. D., and Harris, M. (1973), 'Neurapraxia of the Mylohyoid Nerve and Sub-mental Analgesia'. *Br. J. oral Surg.*, **11**, 110.

Chapter XXI

SOME NON-PYOGENIC INFECTIONS OF THE SOFT TISSUES

ALL non-pyogenic infections are of interest and importance to the oral surgeon, but it is obviously impractical in a work of this nature to discuss such infections as leprosy and yaws, etc. Even the non-pyogenic infections such as syphilis and tuberculosis are becoming rarer at the present time in countries where effective therapy is available. In any case, only limited features of these diseases are of particular concern to the oral surgeon, and discussion will be confined to the relevant aspects of these infections.

Syphilis

It is of primary importance that syphilitic lesions are recognized early in view of the risk to both operator and patient. It is therefore imperative that the possibility of a syphilitic infection should always be considered whenever an unusual ulcerative lesion is encountered and when operation sites fail to heal in the usual manner. Soft tissue manifestations of syphilis can occur anywhere in the oral cavity, but lesions are most commonly encountered on the lip and tongue and occur during the primary, secondary, or tertiary stage. Meyer and Shklar (1967) published 81 cases of oral lesions in acquired syphilis, and they concluded that oral manifestations were rare in the primary and secondary stages since 84 per cent of their cases occurred in the tertiary stage.

The Lip.—The lip is said to be the most common extragenital site for chancre. The lesion presents as a smooth elevated, painless, coppery-coloured ulcer which is about 0·5–1 cm. in diameter and is surrounded by an area of induration. The upper lip is usually affected and within a few weeks the regional lymph-nodes undergo a shotty enlargement. The condition must be distinguished from a neoplasm. However, carcinoma usually affects the lower lip and a chancre develops much more rapidly than a malignant ulcer. The diagnosis is, of course, confirmed by identification of the spirochaete on dark ground illumination from a direct smear of the ulcer or after scarification of the lesion. It should be remembered that few patients will admit to contact which would have resulted in a venereal infection and, therefore, a history of exposure is seldom obtained. It is also important to remember that the Wassermann and Kahn reactions and V.D.R.L. slide test do not become positive until infection has been present for 6 weeks to 3 months.

Mucous Patches.—Mucous patches in the mouth are sometimes seen by the oral surgeon when examining a patient suffering from the secondary stage of syphilis, and a speedy diagnosis is essential in view of the increased risk of infection to both patient and operator at this period.

The Tongue.—Primary syphilis can affect the tongue and the chancre usually occurs on or near the tip. There is a lymphadenopathy of the cervical nodes within 10 days. The secondary rash can also involve the tongue and in tertiary syphilis the tongue may be affected by a midline gumma which, on breaking down, forms a characteristic punched-out type of ulcer with a washleather slough.

Leucoplakia.—Leucoplakia of syphilitic origin has already been discussed. (*See* p. 122.)

Primary Syphilis of the Gingiva.—In 1921 Klauder reviewed the literature and found 113 reported cases of primary syphilis of the gingiva. Straith (1937) added a further 42 cases. In 1966 Steiner and Alexander reported 2 more cases. The typical primary manifestation is an erosive ulcerative lesion with a smooth red surface which may be as much as 2–3 cm. in diameter. There is a regional lymphadenopathy.

TUBERCULOSIS

It is generally agreed that oral manifestations of tuberculosis are usually secondary to lesions elsewhere in the body, especially the lungs. However, primary tubercular lesions have been reported by Boyes (1956), Brand and Ballard (1951), Miller (1953), Galloway and Horne (1953). Darlington and Salman (1937) reported 27 cases of tubercular lesions in the mouth. Tuberculous lesions may appear anywhere in the oral cavity, and according to Carmody, Appleton, and Ivy (1923) the most common site is the tongue, especially the tip. Brodsky (1942) lists the following sites for his 72 patients: pharynx, 22; tonsils, 19; tongue, 16; cheeks, gingiva, and floor of mouth, 9; lips, 6.

Tuberculosis of the Tongue.—Tuberculosis may reach the tongue from the exterior, by auto-inoculation from affected sputum, by haematogenous or lymphatic spread, and by direct spread from neighbouring structures. The infection may take the form of tubercles, tuberculoma, cold abscess, tuberculous fissures, or papillomas and ulcers.

The Tuberculoma.—The tuberculoma usually ulcerates early, but occasionally it may reach a considerable size before ulcerating and when this occurs it must be distinguished from a gumma on the tongue.

Tuberculous Fissures.—Tuberculous fissures occur at the sides or tip of the tongue and are often stellate or branched.

Tuberculous Papillomas.—Tuberculous papillomas occur as an overgrowth of epithelium at the edges of tuberculous fissures.

The Tuberculous Ulcer.—The tuberculous ulcer is the most common tuberculous lesion and usually develops as a tiny tubercle which ulcerates. The ulcers are always at the tip of the tongue and may extend backwards along its sides. They are shallow, yellowish, and are usually very painful, but not always, while their edges are sloping rather than undermined and the ulcer is deeper than it appears. Unlike tuberculous ulcers in other situations, they are usually painful and extremely tender. The tubercle bacillus may be found, but bacteriological identification is often difficult if the ulcer is secondarily infected. The patient is usually suffering from pulmonary tuberculosis and the ulcers in the mouth tend to reflect the progress of the lesion in the lungs and improve with the pulmonary disease.

However, the tongue is seldom affected until the pulmonary disease is well advanced. The oral surgeon may also encounter tuberculous ulceration on the neck and if it is associated with severe oral sepsis the patient may have been referred in the erroneous belief that the oral sepsis is responsible for the breakdown of the lymph-nodes. Tuberculous ulceration in the neck is due to breakdown of an affected lymph-node which has formed a cold abscess. Characteristically the base of the ulcer is soft and pale and it is covered with granulations. The edges of the ulcer tend to be bluish and undermined. The outline is serpigenous and there may be a watery discharge. Bacteriological examination of the ulcer reveals the characteristic acid-fast tubercle bacillus. More than one broken-down lymph-node may be present. Bailey (1933) recorded tuberculosis infection in a branchial cyst. Occasionally the oral surgeon is confronted with a cold abscess which has resulted from the breakdown of a submandibular lymph-node. It is important to diagnose the lesion by aspiration before incising the abscess for tuberculous lesions are notoriously slow to heal and the incisions tend to produce ugly keloid scarring.

Lupus Vulgaris

The dusky red, slightly elevated lesions with pale pink scarred areas interspersed have sharp margins and pale apple-jelly nodules which can be demonstrated with a glass slide. They occasionally may become ulcerative lesions of lupus vulgaris (tuberculous infection of the skin), but are virtually never seen these days, and with them has gone one cause of carcinoma of the face. Patients with destruction of the nose from old, healed lesions are still seen from time to time.

Anthrax

Anthrax is a disease caused by the *Bacillus anthracis* which occurs in both man and animals. The oral surgeon may occasionally encounter the cutaneous variety of the disease in patients who work with animal skins such as tanners, butchers, veterinary surgeons, etc. This condition is called the 'malignant pustule' which occurs as a result of the entrance of the anthrax bacillus through a cutaneous abrasion on some exposed body surface such as the face. The lesion is usually solitary and commonly on the face. The incubation period is 2 hours to 7 days, but is usually 24–48 hours. Itching is followed by pain and the appearance of a red papule. This develops a central vesicle surrounded by an area of hyperaemia and by the third day the vesicle bursts and the centre of the papule becomes a black necrotic area which is surrounded by secondary vesicles which also slough. The area is surrounded by marked oedema. Even a tiny pustule may be followed by septicaemia when it occurs on the face. The oedema may spread to the glottis. Onset of septicaemia usually leads to a fatal termination. This dangerous condition must always be considered in patients who may have been at risk due to their occupation. The condition must be distinguished from a virulent furuncle and accidental vaccinia.

Treatment: The *B. anthracis* is susceptible to penicillin which should be used in large doses.

Ecthyma Contagiosum (Orf)

This is the infection in man caused by the virus of ovine pustular dermatitis and is transmitted to man by direct contact with live or dead affected lambs and sheep or indirectly through fomites. Three to seven days after inoculation there is a macule at the portal of entry and then a papule. The papule enlarges rapidly up to 1–4 cm. in diameter and is covered with small vesicles containing clear fluid. The vesicles coalesce into a flaccid, white, umbilicated bulla which breaks down and then the lesion crusts over. Healing can take 4–8 weeks and the regional nodes are enlarged.

These rather florid lesions may be mistaken for a variety of infective and inflammatory processes about the jaws such as tuberculosis, and even for malignant neoplasms. Diagnosis depends in part on obtaining a suggestive history of contact with sheep. The topical application of Dermevan Iodophor speeds resolution of the lesions (Parnell, 1965).

REFERENCES

BAILEY, H. (1933), 'The Clinical Aspects of Branchial Fistulae', *Br. J. Surg.*, **21**, 173.
BOYES, J. (1956), 'Oral Pathology in Children', *Proc. R. Soc. Med.*, **43**, 503.
BRAND, T. A., and BALLARD, C. F. (1951), 'Oral Tuberculosis', *Archs Dis. Childh.*, **26**, 261.
BRODSKY, R. H. (1942), 'Oral Tuberculous Lesions', *Am. J. Orthod.*, **28**, 132.
CARMODY, T. E., APPLETON, J. L., and IVY, R. H. (1923), 'Diagnostic Importance of Tuberculous Lesions of Oral Cavity', *Dent. Summary*, **44**, 233.
DARLINGTON, C. G., and SALMAN, I. (1937), 'Oral Tuberculous Lesions', *Am. Revue Tuberc.*, **35**, 147.
GALLOWAY, W. J., and HORNE, N. W. (1953), 'Primary Tuberculosis Infection of the Gum', *Br. dent. J.*, **15**, 9.
KLAUDER, J. (1921), 'Wassermann Test with Secretions, Transudates and Exudates in Syphilis', *Dent. Cosmos*, **53**, 1067.
MEYER, I., and SHKLAR, G. (1967), 'The Oral Manifestations of Acquired Syphilis', *Oral Surg.*, **23**, 45.
MILLER, F. J. W. (1953), 'Recognition of Primary Tuberculous Infection of Skin and Mucosae', *Lancet*, **1**, 5.
PARNELL, A. G. (1965), 'Ecthyma contagiosum (Orf)', *Br. J. oral Surg.*, **3**, 128.
STEINER, M., and ALEXANDER, W. N. (1966), 'Primary Syphilis of the Gingiva', *Oral Surg.*, **21**, 530.
STRAITH, F. (1937), 'Chancre of the Gingiva', *Am. dent. Ass. J.*, **24**, 196.

CHAPTER XXII

THE FUNGAL DISEASES

ACTINOMYCOSIS

HUMAN cervicofacial actinomycosis is a comparatively rare disease, but even so it is one of the most common of the systemic mycoses. It is caused by an anaerobic, Gram-positive, branched filamentous organism, the *Actinomyces israeli*, which was first isolated by Wolff and Israel in 1891, though many authorities consider that it is a variant of the *Actinomyces bovis* which causes 'lumpy jaw' in cattle. However, Ajello (1968) states that *A. israeli* is an exclusively human parasite while *A. bovis* causes actinomycosis in animals and that, on biochemical and antigenic properties, they have been proved to be distinct and separate entities. At one time some confusion occurred between the human pathogen and some saprophytic varieties of the organism that were found outside the body, and this gave rise to the myth that the disease could be introduced into the mouth by sucking a straw. Even so, actinomycosis is more common in country populations (Aird, 1957).

The usual pattern of the condition is one of a chronic granulomatous infection which eventually results in abscess formation and drainage via multiple fistulae. Macroscopic examination of pus from the abscess may show small bright yellow or grey lumps known as 'sulphur granules'. Microscopic examination of these granules shows colonies of the actinomyces. Sulphur granules are not found in all cases and in a series of 32 patients with actinomycosis, sulphur granules were only seen in 5 instances (Thoma, 1969). The actinomycete has long been known to be a commensal in the oral cavity of man where it lives in competitive existence with other micro-organisms and the actinomycete israeli can be demonstrated in and cultured from carious teeth, crypts of the tonsils, and dental calculus. There are no authenticated records of the isolation of *A. israeli* from soil or any other inanimate source (Ajello, 1968).

The pathogenesis of actinomycosis is imperfectly understood, but it may occur following trauma such as the extraction of a tooth or a jaw fracture which provides a portal of entry for the organism into underlying tissues. Goldin (1945) and Rowe and Killey (1970) reported actinomycosis following a jaw fracture. Zachary Cope (1920) considered that actinomycosis would not occur in the absence of a carious cavity in a tooth, and Aird (1958) says that the disease is of low incidence in the edentulous. It has been suggested that organisms can enter the tissues via a carious cavity or a periodontal pocket, but this is not proved.

Actinomycosis is classified anatomically as: (1) Cervicofacial, (2) Pulmonary, (3) Abdominal. The cervicofacial form is the most common variety of the disease and comprises two-thirds of all cases (New and Figi, 1923). It is of prime interest to the oral surgeon, though Zachary Cope (1962) reported a case of a dental surgeon who attempted an extraction for a colleague, a general surgeon, and inadvertently displaced the fractured crown of the tooth into the surgeon's lung, a mishap which resulted in the unfortunate patient developing pulmonary actinomycosis.

Clinical Features.—Organisms which enter the underlying tissues through the oral mucosa may remain localized in the soft tissues or spread to involve the salivary glands, bone, or skin of the face and neck. The fungus has a preference for growth in the fascia and subcutaneous tissues.

Actinomycosis in the upper jaw may extend to involve the meninges and Zitka (1952) reported a case in which a fatal meningitis occurred. He also reported cases from the German literature with metastatic involvement of the lungs, liver, kidney, and brain. Once the organism gains admittance to the tissues it gives rise to an infection which results in a low-grade swelling and induration of the tissues. Eventually, abscess formation occurs and the pus is discharged extra-orally through multiple skin sinuses. (*Fig.* 46.)

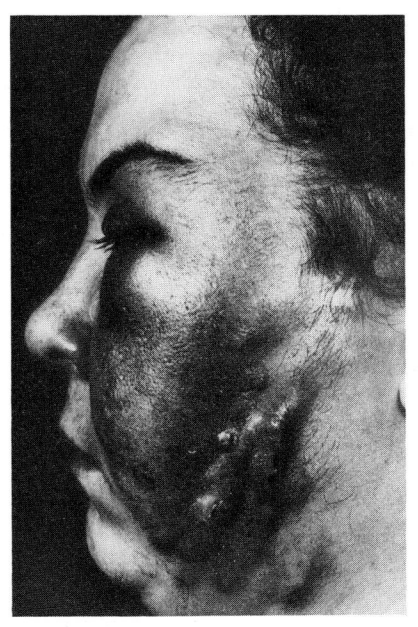

Fig. 46.—Actinomycosis of the cheek. After the cervical region this is the most common site for this infection about the jaws. The skin is a purplish-red colour and there are multiple subcutaneous hemispherical abscesses and multiple sinuses.

This results in scarring and cosmetic deformity due to puckering of the skin. The soft tissue infections may extend to involve the bone. Usually the mandible is affected, but the condition can also occur in the maxillae and it results in fungal osteomyelitis which causes extensive bone destruction. The radiological appearance of such a lesion resembles an osteitis.

On rare occasions the salivary glands are involved. In a case seen by the authors the patient presented with a hard, painless swelling of the right submandibular gland. There was no history of dental extractions on that side and the patient did not have a rise in temperature. The white-cell count and the sedimentation rate were normal. A sialogram showed an irregular space-occupying lesion and the pathological process continued to increase in size in spite of two courses of antibiotic therapy. A neoplasm was suspected and a very experienced general surgeon confirmed the diagnosis. At operation he encountered extreme difficulty in removing the gland owing to the marked induration of the tissues. The submandibular gland appeared to be the seat of a squamous-cell carcinoma when it was examined macroscopically after removal, but pathological examination proved the condition to be actinomycosis.

When the soft tissues are affected there is usually a history of extraction or fracture in the area some five weeks previously. The swelling is hard, indurated, and painless and resistant to antibiotic therapy administered empirically. Later, it may or may not break down to discharge pus through multiple sinuses and at this stage the sulphur granules may be seen. In the absence of a discharge the swelling should be aspirated to obtain pus for bacteriological examination. Actinomycosis should be suspected whenever an abscess-like swelling in the region of the jaws fails to respond to antibiotic therapy of the customary duration, 7–10 days, and which shows no signs of improvement or worsening. Routine investigations such as the white cell-count and sedimentation rate are often normal.

Treatment.—Treatment is by protracted antibiotic therapy and penicillin remains the drug of choice. Of the various preparations available, fortified procaine penicillin B.P. in 2–3 ml. doses daily or phenoxymethylpenicillin 250 mg. 6-hourly for a period of six to eight weeks are suitable. It has been demonstrated by Holm (1948) that some strains of actinomyces develop a resistance to penicillin. However, Blake (1964) demonstrated that the resistance of the colonies to antibiotics has been shown to be solely a resistance to bactericidal effect, and he found no evidence of strain variation to the bacteriostatic effect of antibiotics. Oxytetracycline 250 mg. 6-hourly is an alternative to penicillin when patients are hypersensitive to that drug, and recent work by Blake (1970) shows that lincomycin is efficacious in the treatment of actinomycosis. Occasionally a low-grade abscess-like swelling is found to contain actinomycete on bacteriological examination of the pus following aspiration or incision and drainage, and yet the lesion will resolve on minimal antibiotic therapy and in some instances incision and drainage of the area alone is sufficient to eradicate the disease. This raises the possibility that there are two varieties of the disease with organisms which appear bacteriologically similar, or that there is a variation in the pathogenicity of the organism. Hertz (1960) employed the term 'pseudoactinomycosis' for cases in which the smear shows only a few mycelia and where a tender swelling contains foul-smelling pus. Anomalies in the clinical behaviour and response to treatment of some abscesses which appear to be due to actinomycosis may result from an inability in the present state of knowledge to distinguish organisms which resemble the actinomycete israeli.

CANDIDIASIS

Candidiasis, or monilial infection, is an acute or chronic fungal disease involving the superficial tissues of skin or mucous membrane and more rarely it may disseminate haematogenously to produce systemic disease. Septicaemic candidiasis is often not diagnosed until the post mortem and according to Wright and Symmers (1966) the incidence has risen with the introduction of the corticosteroids. Chronic candidiasis can affect the skin, nails, and hair follicles, while in the lungs it may present as a pneumonia or a lung abscess.

Man can be infected with a variety of candida organisms which are commonly present in the mouth, vagina, sputum, and stools of otherwise normal persons. Monilial infection in the form of oral thrush, skin lesions, or disseminated disease can arise in patients with other diseases or under special circumstances, i.e., in infancy, old age, diabetes, debilitation, antibacterial treatment, pregnancy, etc. Barlow and Chattaway (1969) found a 45 per cent incidence of candida in 125 patients. There tends to be an exacerbation of monilial infection of the vagina before menstruation and in pregnancy. Oral thrush in infants may be the result of infection from the vagina during childbirth (Winner and Hurley, 1964). It is not uncommon to find oral thrush in one or more young children in a family when the mother is known to have severe monilial infection of the vagina. The source of the children's infection probably results from poor hygiene on the part of the mother.

Clinical Features.—The oral lesions may occur on any mucosal surface and are white or greyish-white, discrete or confluent patches which resemble curdled milk. If the patch is removed a raw bleeding area is left in the underlying membrane. Various clinical types have been described in the oral cavity. In infants the condition is referred to as thrush, but in adults the plaque-like lesions are less friable and are thicker. Atrophic candidiasis has been recognized in various conditions such as denture-sore mouth, angular cheilitis, and glossitis. Chronic lesions may become hyperkeratinized and develop pseudoepitheliomatous hyperplasia. *Candida leucoplakia* or chronic hyperplastic or hypertrophic candidiasis may show a strong tendency to undergo neoplastic change and such cases cannot be clinically differentiated from leucoplakia due to other causes. Oral candidiasis is sometimes seen during protracted antibiotic therapy especially when tetracycline is used. Angular cheilitis in edentulous patients with a markedly overclosed bite often has the commissural fissures infected with *Candida albicans*.

Systemic candidiasis with a fatal outcome has been reported in 4 patients following dental extractions and these cases have been reviewed by Lehner (1964), though in an experimental study of the blood of 50 postextraction cases candida was not cultured. According to Zegarelli and Kutschner (1964), 4 of their cases under treatment with topically applied corticosteroid developed monilial infection. Denture-sore mouth may be due to monilial infection in some instances and Cawson (1963) isolated *C. albicans* in 23 patients out of a series of 35 cases suffering from denture-sore mouth.

Treatment.—Thrush in infants is best treated with a 1 per cent aqueous solution of one of the aniline dyes such as gentian violet, brilliant green, neutral red, etc., while adults and children over 5 years of age can be treated with nystatin or amphotericin B—4 tablets or lozenges respectively should be taken daily and sucked slowly. Severe monilial infection arising as a result of protracted antibiotic therapy should be treated by stopping the antibiotic and prescribing nystatin, or by painting the area with one of the aniline dyes in a 1 per cent aqueous solution. Candidal leucoplakia is best treated by excision of the leucoplakic patch, but if this is impractical a protracted course of nystatin is often efficacious. Angular cheilitis due to monilial infection may be associated with an overclosed bite or iron deficiency, and this should be corrected. Nystatin should be used if the condition fails to improve after the correction of the bite and if this is not effective, the area should be excised and a Z-plasty performed.

Often secondary to the antifungal treatment of denture sore-mouth, one or more of the following measures may be necessary:—

1. Correct denture hygiene by using a detergent to clean it, e.g. cetrimide.
2. Correct the height of bite of the denture.
3. Correct the fit and eliminate roughness on the underside of the denture which abrades the palate as a result of:—
   a. Alginate impressions—mucus on the palate.
   b. Bubbles in models.
   c. Too much detail in the model.
4. Process new dentures against burnished foil.
5. Use vacuumed or vibrated stone model.
6. Free lateral articulation of teeth to reduce movement over the ridge.
7. Treat papillary palatal hyperplasia.
8. Correct posture of lip by placing canines in proper buccopalatal position and use of 'plumpers'.
9. Use nystatin cream under the denture, but better still leave the denture out while taking nystatin tablets, on a dosage basis of 4 daily.

It is also advisable to investigate the haemoglobin level, the serum iron concentrate, and iron absorption and utilization to exclude iron deficiency. If the condition is recurrent in a young person, the possibility of *Candida vaginitis* must be considered in women, and proctitis must also be excluded, for either of these conditions may re-infect the mouth.

Histoplasmosis

Histoplasmosis is a systemic fungal disease which is respiratory in origin and spreads via the pulmonary lymphatics and blood to mediastinal lymph-nodes, spleen, liver, kidneys, and skin. The central nervous system, heart, and other organs may also be affected. The disease may be asymptomatic, acute, or progressive and eventually fatal.

Aetiology.—The causative organism is the *Histoplasma capsulatum*. The disease usually occurs in infancy or old age and it affects the sexes equally. Man is infected by inhalation of dust contaminated with the organisms, and soil from chicken houses or bat and bird droppings are rich in the organisms. The disease can also affect animals such as dogs and cats.

Clinical Manifestations.—Primary infection is usually asymptomatic, but there is often a febrile respiratory disease, cough, shortness of breath, chest pain, and even haemoptysis. The pulmonary symptoms may resolve completely, but occasionally the disease may progress to the severe disseminated form in which there is pyrexia, weight-loss, lymphadenopathy, and anaemia. There may be local lesions in the mouth which are nodular, ulcerative or vegetative, and these are associated with a marked lymphadenopathy. The tongue, lips, and cheeks are most commonly affected and biopsy of the lesions may be suggestive of neoplastic change.

Diagnosis.—The isolation, culture, and identification of the fungus microscopically are required in order to diagnose the disease. There are also skin and complement-fixation tests available. Biopsies of mucosal lesions may be suggestive of carcinoma and the material must be cultured to confirm the disease.

Treatment.—Amphotericin B is the most effective antifungal drug available at present, but X-5079, a polypeptide drug, has been shown to have strong antifungal activity.

North American Blastomycosis

This disease, commonly known as 'North American Blastomycosis', is caused by the fungus *Blastomyces dermatitidis*. It used to be thought that the condition was confined to North America, but there have been recent reports of the condition from several African countries such as the Republics of Zaïre (formerly Congo), and of South Africa, Tanzania, Tunisia, and Uganda (Destombes and Drouhet, 1964; Emmons and others, 1964). Cases have also been reported from Latin America (Arias Luzardo, 1962). The source of the infection in human beings is unknown, but it is a chronic systemic fungal disease which is respiratory in origin that clinically disseminates to skin, subcutaneous tissue, bone, and other organs. The disease is found more commonly in men than in women.

Clinical Features.—The disease starts as an acute respiratory infection and, although the cutaneous lesions are respiratory in origin, they are often the presenting symptom. The cutaneous lesions start as small, red papules which increase in size and form tiny pustules which ulcerate and discharge pus through tiny fistulae. These coalesce and crateriform lesions with elevated borders are formed, but sometimes the lesion becomes warty. Systemic spread can occur as a result of the infection becoming disseminated through the subcutaneous tissues into the blood-stream. This results in pyrexia, weight-loss, and, if the lungs are infected, a productive cough.

When the condition occurs in the mouth a chronic granulomatous lesion arises with multiple sinuses which resembles actinomycosis.

Diagnosis.—The diagnosis is made by culture of the *B. dermatitidis* from pus or lesions.

Treatment.—Amphotericin B has been used extensively for all forms of the disease.

South American Blastomycosis

This type of blastomycosis is caused by *Paracoccidioides brasiliensis*, which affects workers in the coffee-growing regions of Brazil. The fungus is related to the North American form of the disease, the South American fungus being considerably larger, varying in size between 10 and 60 microns.

Clinical Findings.—The disease starts as a small papular lesion often on the cutaneous surface of the lip and resembles a squamous-cell carcinoma. The condition may also involve the gingiva and may begin following a

dental extraction. The regional lymph-nodes are enlarged and hard and may resemble either tubercular adenitis or those of Hodgkin's disease. The lungs may become secondarily infected.
Diagnosis.—Diagnosis is by culture of the organism.
Treatment.—Treatment is with amphotericin B.

REFERENCES

AIRD, I. (1957), *A Companion in Surgical Studies*, 2nd ed., p. 91. Edinburgh: Livingstone.
AJELLO, L. (1968), *Systemic Mycoses*, p. 130. Ciba Foundation Symposium. London: Churchill.
ARIAS LUZARDO, J. J. (1962), Doctoral Thesis, Universidad Nacional Autonoma de Mexico, Escuela National de Medicina.
BARLOW, A. J. E., and CHATTAWAY, F. W. (1969), 'Observations on the Carriage of *Candida Albicans* in Man', *Br. J. Dermat.*, **81**, 103.
BLAKE, G. C. (1964), 'Sensitivities of Colonies and Suspensions of *Actinomyces Israeli* to Penicillins, Tetracyclines and Erythromycin', *Br. med. J.*, **1**, 145.
— — (1970), personal communication.
CAWSON, R. A. (1963), 'Denture Sore Mouth and Angular Cheilitis. Oral Candidiasis in Adults', *Br. dent. J.*, **115**, 441.
COPE, V. Z. (1920), 'Actinomycosis considered specially in its Relationship to the Jaws', *Ibid.*, **41**, 649.
— — (1962), Lecture at Rooksdown House, Basingstoke.
DESTOMBES, P., and DROUHET, E. (1964), 'Mycoses d'importation', *Bull. Soc. Path. exot.*, **57**, 848.
EMMONS, C. W., and others (1964), *Sabouraudia*, **3**, 306.
GOLDIN, H. (1945), 'Case of Cervicofacial Actinomycosis following Fractured Mandible', *S. Afr. dent. J.*, **19**, 392.
HERTZ, J. (1960), 'Actinomycosis Borderline Cases', *J. int. Coll. Surg.*, **34**, 148.
HOLM, P. (1948), 'Some Investigations into Penicillin Sensitivity of Human Pathogenic Actinomycetes and some Comments on Penicillin Treatment of Actinomycosis', *Acta path. microbiol. scand.*, **25**, 376.
LEHNER, T. (1964), 'Oral Candidiasis', *Dent. Abstr.*, Chicago, **9**, 104.
NEW, G. E., and FIGI, F. A. (1923), 'Actinomycosis of the Head and Neck: A Report of 107 Cases', *Surgery Gynec. Obstet.*, **37**, 617.
ROWE, N. L., and KILLEY, H. C. (1970), *Fractures of the Facial Skeleton*. Edinburgh: Livingstone.
THOMA, K. H. (1969), *Oral Surgery*, 5th ed. St. Louis: Mosby.
WINNER, H. L., and HURLEY, R. (1964), *Candida albicans*. London: Churchill.
WOLFF, M., and ISRAEL, J. (1891), 'Ueber reinkultur des actinomyces und seine uebertragbarkeit auf tiere', *Virchows Arch. Path. Anat. Physiol.*, **126**, 11.
WRIGHT, P., and SYMMERS, W. (1966), *Systemic Pathology*, p. 828. London: Longmans.
ZEGARELLI, E. V., and KUTSCHNER, A. H. (1964), 'Oral Moniliasis following Intra-oral Topical Corticosteroid Therapy', *J. oral. Ther.*, **1**, 304.
ZITKA, E. (1952), 'Toplich verlaufene falle von cervicofacialer aktinomykose', *Wien. med. Wschr.*, **102**, 939.

Chapter XXIII

THE MANAGEMENT OF SOME OF THE FOREIGN BODIES SEEN IN AND AROUND THE JAWS

Some of the more common foreign bodies which may be lodged in the soft tissues, the paranasal sinuses, or the bony structure of the upper or lower jaw can be considered under the following headings:—

1. Broken Hypodermic Needles

The main causes of hypodermic needles being broken during an injection in the mouth are a violent movement on the part of the patient, a structural fault in the needle, or faulty technique on the part of the operator. The breaking of a hypodermic needle in the tissues, is, fortunately, an uncommon accident, but the injections most likely to result in an accident of this nature are the inferior dental nerve block and the posterior superior dental nerve block. (*Fig.* 47.) Infiltration injections round the

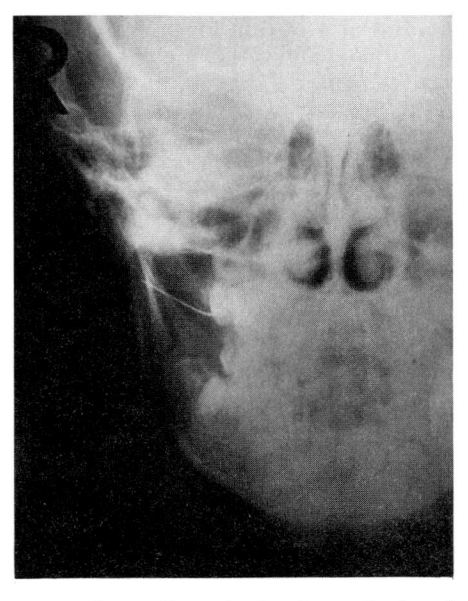

Fig. 47.—Postero-anterior radiograph showing a broken hypodermic needle lying in the soft tissue on the lingual aspect of the ramus.

teeth are so superficial that if the needle breaks the fragment can usually be recovered with little difficulty. In the case of the mandibular and posterior superior dental injections, it is easy to retrieve the broken fragment of needle if it is projecting from the tissues, and whenever an injection is being carried out an instrument such as an artery forceps should be at hand in order to grasp the needle fragment should this accident occur.

Removal of a Fragment of Needle.—The decision to remove a fragment of needle must depend upon the size of the fragment and its situation in the tissues, for there is little point in operating to remove a minute portion of needle buried under the periosteum and, therefore, unlikely to move in the tissues. Hypodermic needles broken elsewhere in the body in muscle, or even worse in veins, are liable to travel considerable distances and may come to rest in vital organs such as the heart, but most hypodermic needles broken in the mouth are firmly sited under the periosteum. Occasionally a needle broken in the oral cavity may be in thick muscle such as the medial pterygoid and the fragment may be propelled deep into the tissues by muscular action. Therefore, if a needle is considered to be lying free in the tissues, there is some urgency in arranging for its removal.

Small portions of needle in the tissues which show no tendency to move do not give rise to symptoms but, unfortunately, once a patient knows there is a needle broken in the tissues he tends to become extremely anxious about its presence. For this reason, it may be advisable to remove fractured portions of hypodermic needle provided that the operation is considered feasible.

The Surgical Removal of a Needle Medial to the Ramus.—Many techniques have been described for localizing a needle lying medial to the ramus. Most of them depend on the insertion of one or more additional needles and then taking radiographs in order to localize the broken fragment in relation to the needles inserted. Ingenious methods have also been devised to enable the guide marker needles to be held in place during radiography. A simple device can be constructed by jamming a sterile cork between the teeth and passing the guide needles through the cork and into the tissues. However, personal experience has shown that such marker needles are of little practical help in searching for a needle, and not only interfere with the operator's access but cause additional oedema in the tissues. A true lateral and a postero-anterior radiograph taken with the mouth open, since this is how the patient will be during the operation, are quite adequate to establish the presence of the needle and its approximate location.

Provided that the operator is familiar with the anatomy of the region, it is a simple matter to search the area systematically to locate the fragment. The mouth is gagged open wide and an incision is made down the anterior aspect of the ramus from almost the tip of the coronoid process to the retromolar fossa and then down into the buccal sulcus. The soft tissue is raised from the bone, exposing the subperiosteal area. Often the needle is seen sticking through the periosteum and can be grasped with mosquito forceps. If there is no sign of the needle, the medial tail of the temporalis tendon and the inferior dental neurovascular bundle should be separated so that the pterygomandibular space can be searched. If the needle is neither beneath the periosteum nor in the pterygomandibular space, it must be within the medial pterygoid muscle. In the line of the musclefibres a Howarth's periosteal elevator can be used to separate the fibres so as to systematically search the muscle.

As soon as the needle is seen, a pair of mosquito forceps is clamped on it and then the needle is worked anteriorly in its direction of insertion. As soon as the needle end is visible, it is grasped with another pair of mosquito forceps and withdrawn. No attempt should be made to pull the needle laterally through the tissues with the first mosquito forceps or the needle will bend, so making it more difficult to remove, or it may even break and it is then necessary to remove two broken fragments. The search for a needle should be carried out largely by blunt dissection in a good light, and the operative field should be as avascular as possible to facilitate the search.

Ingenious electrical devices have been advocated whereby one electrode of an electrical circuit is made with the patient and the other is connected to a probe which is passed through the tissues. When the probe touches the broken portion of needle a bell or buzzer sounds. The use of such devices poses further problems. For example, plastic retractors must be used, as metal ones are bound to be touched by the probe in such confined quarters. Also, some locators are so sensitive that they buzz when 0·5 cm. from the needle. This is a help in a limb, but in this particular instance it can be easy to predict where the needle will be within 0·5 cm., but still difficult to find it.

The only postoperative complication is limitation of opening, but if the operation is carried out carefully and the medial pterygoid muscle is not damaged, this symptom is trivial and temporary.

Needles broken during the Posterior Superior Dental Injection.—Needles broken during a posterior superior dental injection usually penetrate the periosteum and their broken end projects downwards towards the mouth in the line of the injection. To obtain adequate access an incision is made anterior to the upper 2nd molar and a soft tissue flap is raised superficial to the periosteum. The flap is retracted and the area overlying the tuberosity is inspected. If the needle is not seen, the tip of a finger is gently inserted into the wound and the fragment, which feels like a stiff bristle, is usually palpated quite easily. It is useful to remember that a needle in the tissues feels less stiff than one would expect. Care must be taken not to dislodge the needle further up into the soft tissues by milking movements with the finger, but usually the tip of the needle has penetrated the periosteum and jammed into the bone and so this is unlikely. However, every care must be taken to avoid dislodging the needle with the finger tip. Once the needle is palpated a pair of curved mosquito forceps is guided into the area with the other hand and the needle is grasped and withdrawn along its line of insertion.

2. Tooth or Root in the Soft Tissues

Teeth or roots can be inadvertently displaced into the soft tissues during exodontia or as a result of trauma such as road traffic accidents and fights. Common situations from which teeth or roots have to be extricated are as follows.

The Lingual Space.—Lower 3rd molars or their roots can be inadvertently displaced into the so-called 'lingual space' or 'pouch' during lower 3rd molar surgery. This potential space is bounded by the periosteum and the lingual aspect of the mandible, and it extends vertically down the neck.

An entire tooth may be dislodged into this area and the usual reason for the accident is that force is applied to an impacted lower 3rd molar when a gingival flap is still covering the posterior part of its crown. During delivery the crown of the tooth is impeded by the resistant gum flap and is levered over the upper border of the lingual plate and slips down the lingual side of the mandible. The apices of many lower 3rd molars actually penetrate the lingual plate of the mandible and attempts to elevate out such roots may result in their deflexion through the lingual plate into the lingual space.

When this accident occurs the operator should place a finger on the lingual side of the mandible beneath the tooth or root which can be easily palpated beneath the mucosa. The tooth is then gently pressed upwards towards the operation site. Sometimes the incision must be lengthened to enable the dislodged tooth or root to be properly visualized. When the fragment can be seen, it is grasped with a small pair of Allis forceps and lifted out of the wound. A finger must be positioned on the lingual mucosa beneath the tooth or root until the fragment is retrieved, for attempts to grasp the tooth or root without taking this precaution will only result in further displacement of the object. The passage of a conically rooted tooth through the tissues is facilitated by rotating the tooth with the fingers over the mucosa covering the lingual plate so that the conical apex is directed towards the original socket.

Tooth or Root in the Lateral Pharyngeal Space.—Occasionally during surgery in the area a lower 3rd molar or its root is inadvertently displaced backwards into the lateral pharyngeal space. This unfortunate accident causes the patient considerable pain especially on deglutition and the tooth should be removed as soon as possible, for infection in this region could have serious consequences. Following such an accident the patient has marked limitation of opening and the tooth can travel backwards and become positioned beneath the mucosa on the posterior pharyngeal wall. Usually, however, the displaced tooth can be palpated beneath the overlying mucosa reasonably near to the operation site and can then be gently pushed towards the original incision by pressure with the operator's finger through the mucosa behind the tooth or root. As soon as the fragment can be seen through the original operation incision, it should be grasped with Allis forceps. Again, no attempt should be made to grasp the tooth or root with an instrument without anchoring the fragment by finger pressure behind it or the foreign body will be pushed backwards. If the original operation wound is small, it should be enlarged by extending the incision up the ramus. Suitable antibiotic therapy should be maintained until there is no risk of a residual infection in the lateral pharyngeal space.

Tooth or Root in the Pterygoid Plexus Region.—Occasionally an upper 3rd molar or its root is displaced into the soft tissues between the coronoid process and the maxillary tuberosity. It can then pass upwards towards the pterygoid plexus. This is not only a surgically inaccessible region, but it is a very haemorrhagic area and due to the vascular anastomosis with the cavernous sinus any infection in the area must be regarded as extremely serious. The incision in the area should be widened by bringing it forwards from the tuberosity to the upper 1st molar area. The incision should be on the crest of the ridge in the edentulous case and round the gingival margins when teeth are standing. It should be deepened down to, but not through, the periosteum. Careful retraction usually allows the tooth or root to be visualized deep in the wound. Occasionally a Howarth's periosteal elevator can be inserted on either side of the tooth or root and the fragment can be gently levered down into the wound. On other occasions it can be grasped with a narrow-bladed pair of Allis forceps. Blind manipulation within the wound using a finger or an instrument usually results in the tooth or root being displaced further into the soft tissues.

Tooth Fragments in the Soft Tissues following Facial Trauma.—Teeth or tooth fragments can be displaced into any of the facial soft tissues as a result of trauma. Retrieval is usually a simple matter of palpating the object beneath the tissues and then immobilizing it by finger pressure beneath and to one side before approaching it surgically by a direct incision. The cut is made over the fragment from either an extra-oral or intra-oral approach depending whether it is nearer the outer or inner surface of the face. As soon as the tooth or tooth fragment is exposed it can be carefully dissected out of the wound. The most common area for such displaced teeth or fragments is the upper or lower lip. As a result of an accident either the maxillary or mandibular teeth may be driven into the inside of the lip and broken off. Such fragments are readily palpated and radiographs held behind the lip confirm the diagnosis. They are most easily removed before the original wound has been sutured. Mosquito artery forceps are inserted closed into the wound until the fragment is touched. When they are opened the piece will enter the gap between the blades. Once the wound has healed no attempt should be made until the scar has softened. Infected fragments can be reached by inserting a probe along the resulting sinus. Small, uninfected, impalpable fragments are best left alone.

Tooth or Root in the Maxillary Sinus.—The problem of the tooth or root in the maxillary sinus has already been discussed. (*See* AN OUTLINE OF ORAL SURGERY, PART I, revised reprint, p. 157).

Other Foreign Bodies in the Maxillary Sinus.—If a patient has a patent oro-antral fistula almost any foreign body can enter the sinus from the mouth. When these objects have been in the maxillary sinus for any considerable time they tend to become encrusted with calcific concretions. The authors have removed mummified peas, nuts, cotton-wool, and other articles from the maxillary sinus including from one patient sufficient chewing gum to fill the entire cavity. The broken blade of an upper extraction forceps has also been reported in the maxillary sinus. Probably the most common foreign body in the maxillary sinus is impression material such as an alginate impression compound or plaster-of-Paris, and these substances should not be used in the presence of an oro-antral fistula. Root canal instruments and filling materials are also easily introduced through the apices of the molar and premolar teeth.

Tooth or Root in the Floor of the Nose.—Occasionally a tooth or root is displaced either into the floor of the nose or between the undersurface of the palatal shelf and the overlying soft tissue of the floor of the nose. The deflected tooth is usually the maxillary canine, but supernumeraries and incisors can also be involved. The tooth may have developed in this position or been displaced there as a result of attempted exodontia. Most teeth which have grown in such a situation can be approached and removed through the routine intra-oral surgical approach, but as an additional precaution, to prevent the entire tooth being inadvertently displaced into the nasal passage during operation, it is helpful to have the anaesthetist position the endotracheal tube in the nostril overlying the operation site. If a tooth or root is displaced into the nasal cavity during an operation under general anaesthesia, the patient's head should be extended so that it will pass into the nasopharynx and fall on to the throat pack where it can be retrieved. If it remains stuck in the nose, it can be gently pushed back with a nasopharyngeal airway, unless it can be seen and grasped with Allis forceps pushed up the nostril.

The more usual problem is a tooth or root displaced beneath the nasal mucosa and against the upper surface of the palatal shelf. A horizontal incision is made in the upper buccal sulcus and deepened to bone. It should be of sufficient length to expose the anterior bony aperture of the nose. The nasal mucosa forming the floor of the nose is then gently retracted from the bone and the tooth or root is pulled forwards on the tip of the sucker. If the fragment is stuck and cannot be removed in this fashion, the end of a silver probe is bent to form a large hook which is gently passed round the tooth or root after which it can be pulled forwards towards the incision.

3. Rhinoliths

Rhinoliths are calcareous bodies which are occasionally found in the nose and very rarely in the maxillary sinus. Polson (1943), in a review of the literature, found 384 cases and he reported 6 personal cases. These objects are usually single and unilateral and consist chiefly of calcium carbonate and phosphate which originate mainly from inflammatory exudates. If sectioned, it is seen that they have been deposited round a nucleus which may be endogenous or exogenous in origin. The exogenous nucleus can be any small foreign body such as a fruit stone, bead, etc., while the endogenous nucleus can be nasal crusts, mucus, sequestra, etc. They are often spherical and their surface is a rough greyish-white, grey, or dark brown in colour. Symptoms of a nasal rhinolith are usually a unilateral purulent nasal discharge and/or obstruction. Cases have been reported of nasal rhinoliths which have ulcerated through the palate and presented in the mouth (Gilbert, 1952; Allen, 1967).

Treatment.—Rhinoliths are removed through either the anterior or posterior nasal aperture. Large ones are fragmented and removed in pieces.

Antroliths.—Those rhinoliths which occur in the maxillary sinus are also known as 'antral stones', 'antral calculi', 'antroliths', 'antral rhinoliths', and 'maxillary rhinoliths'. Bowerman (1969) defined them as a complete or partial encrustation of an antral foreign body usually of endogenous or occasionally of exogenous origin. They are hard calcareous bodies found within the maxillary sinus consisting of a central nucleus upon which are deposited mineral salts, especially calcium phosphate and carbonate, forming a rough surface, blackish-grey in colour. The salts are probably derived from antral secretions or inflammatory exudates and the foreign body with complete or partial encrustation may have been in situ for several years and associated with long-term chronic infection.

Clinical Features.—Usually the lesion is asymptomatic and is discovered on routine radiography as a radio-opaque mass, but it may give rise to a maxillary sinusitis, produce a foul smell, nasal discharge, an oro-antral fistula, and destroy alveolar or palatal bone.

Treatment.—Treatment is removal through a routine Caldwell-Luc incision.

4. FOREIGN BODIES IN THE TISSUES AS A RESULT OF GUNSHOT WOUNDS

Shell fragments and bullets may be lodged in the hard or soft tissues for many years without causing symptoms. Much depends on the size and the site of the fragment. The presence of a small metallic foreign body in the lip, for example, can be felt by the patient and should be removed, but a larger fragment can be deeply buried in the tissues and remain asymptomatic. Fragments of metal which project into the maxillary sinus or nose may become infected and should be removed, though this may in some instances be technically difficult. It is important to remember when searching for such foreign bodies that those which are palpable through the intact skin are *less* easily rather than more easily felt through the open wound at operation. Further, a readily palpable object can be quite impalpable once a solution of local anaesthetic or vasoconstrictor has been injected. Multiple lead shots from a shot gun injury are extremely hard to find at operation and as they are usually asymptomatic they should be left in situ.

OTHER FOREIGN BODIES IN THE TISSUES

Following severe trauma such as a road traffic accident, almost any type of object can be implanted into the tissues. Some of the more common foreign bodies of interest to the oral surgeon are:

Tar and Road Dirt.—If a patient's face has been scraped along the road the soft tissue lacerations may be ingrained with road dirt, including tar. If this is not cleaned away before the wound is sutured, it produces an ugly tattoo when it heals which is difficult to eradicate surgically even by excising all the scars. This road dirt must be cleaned out before suturing and a satisfactory method of cleaning such wounds is to use a toothbrush with 1 per cent cetrimide. Only when all tar and other road debris has been removed should the wound be closed.

Pieces of Glass.—Glass fragments may enter the soft tissues at the time of an accident. Sometimes the patient or operator can feel these fragments in the soft tissues and they should then be removed. Almost all glass in common use is sufficiently radio-opaque to produce a shadow when displaced into the soft tissues. The degree of opacity varies, of course, with the composition. The few which may not produce a shadow on radiological examination include some of the high soda translucent tubular lights of American pattern, some of the textile glass fibres (borates) and a few special glasses not likely to be met in everyday life (Cameron, 1970).

Wood.—Wood is radiolucent and if splinters enter the tissues it may be difficult to locate them on the radiographs. However, if the wood is painted, the paint usually shows up quite well (Gerry and Kopp, 1966).

Dentures.—The patient's dentures may be shattered as a result of an accident and portions of the dentures may enter the soft tissues or be impacted into the maxillary sinus or throat. Unfortunately, acrylic denture material is radiolucent and if the objects are not palpable it may be difficult to demonstrate their presence and locate them surgically. The older denture materials such as vulcanite are, however, radio-opaque. A radiolucent denture impacted in the throat can be demonstrated as a space-occupying lesion following a barium swallow. Patients engaged in bad risk occupations or sports should be fitted with special dentures made of a radio-opaque acrylic.

Rubber Base Impression Material.—This substance may be closely confined in a special impression tray in order to obtain a detailed and defect-free impression of inlay crown or bridge preparations.

Where one of the preparations includes the canal of a root-filled tooth, the situation can be hazardous because there may be an unsuspected lateral canal or other perforation in the wall of the root canal. Unrecognized, localized, deep, periodontal pockets present a similar hazard. One of us has seen a case in which rubber base material gained access to the medullary cavity of the jaw during the taking of an impression of mandibular teeth. The material infiltrated the bone from 1st premolar to 2nd molar region and provoked a severe inflammatory reaction with much oedema of the face. Fortunately, removal was easy once the mandible had been decorticated on that side as the impression material pulled out in long irregular strands.

Other Plastic Objects.—Many items such as internal trim in cars and instrument knobs are made of plastic. These again are often radiolucent or only slightly radio-opaque. Surprisingly large objects can be accommodated in the swollen tissues, in the paranasal sinuses, and in regions of thick muscle.

Grease-gun Grease.—An injury from a grease gun is similar to the wound produced by a jet injection device. Hence, if the nozzle is at right angles to the skin surface a puncture wound is formed, or if it is at an angle a cut results. The grease is forced widely into the tissue planes and is highly irritant. Enormous oedema results, and when the injury is to the face or neck a tracheostomy may be required. Vascular impairment in the part due to the pressure produced by the swelling and gross infection are other hazards. Early and thorough wound débridement and drainage are essential in treatment.

Indelible Pencil.—Laceration of the palate occurs when a child falls with a toy, stick, or pencil in the mouth. Usually such injuries are easily dealt with. However, if fragments of lead from an indelible pencil remain in the wound, a troublesome and persistent granulomatous reaction results.

REFERENCES

ALLEN, S. G. (1967), 'A Rhinolith presenting in the Palate', *Br. J. oral Surg.*, **4**, 240.
BOWERMAN, J. E. (1969), 'The Maxillary Antrolith', *J. Lar. Otol.*, **83**, 873.
CAMERON, J. D. (1970), 'The Treatment of Glass Injuries to the Hand at Work', *Hand*, **2**, 52.
GERRY, R. G., and KOPP, W. K. (1966), 'Wooden Foreign Body in the Parapharyngeal Space', *J. oral Surg.*, **24**, 545.
GILBERT, R. K. (1952), 'Case of a Rhinolith', *Br. dent. J.*, **93**, 75.
POLSON, C. J. (1943), 'Rhinolith in Palate', *J. Lar. Otol.*, **58**, 79.

INDEX

	PAGE
ABRIKOSSOFF'S tumour	68
Abscess formation in actinomycosis (*Fig.* 46)	254, 255
— pain from	6
Acid phosphatase estimation	21
Acromegaly	209
— causing mandibular protrusion	158
— oral surgical aspects	210
Actinomycosis, cervicofacial (*Fig.* 46)	254
— treatment	256
Adamantinoma	22
Adeno-ameloblastoma (*Fig.* 14)	103
Adenocarcinoma, treatment of	141
Adenocystic carcinoma of salivary gland	141, 144, 228
Adenoma, pleomorphic, of salivary glands (*Fig.* 42)	227
Adenosine diphosphate	45
Agranulocytosis	15
AHG (antihaemophilic globulin), human or animal	48
Albers-Schönberg disease	210
Albright's syndrome	195, 196
Alcohol consumption, heavy, associated with cancer of tongue	131
Alginate impression compound in antrum	265
Alkaline phosphatase estimation	20
Allelograft(s) onlays to chin	131, 154
— in replacement of bone	184, 192
— — of mandible	146
— temporary	146, 192
Allergic causes of salivary gland swelling	226
Alveolar ostectomy	180
— osteotomy	180
— — for maxillary protrusion	156
— — — retrusion	176
— — symphysial (*Fig.* 29C)	175
— process, carcinoma of (*Fig.* 20)	131
— surgery in correction of malocclusion	180
Ameloblastic fibroma	104
— fibrosarcoma	105
— odontome (*Fig.* 16)	107
Ameloblastoma	99, 100
— treatment	99
Anaesthesia, general, extraction under, causing dislocation of condyles	234
— for tooth extraction in haemophilia	47
Anaesthetic area around ulcer	11
Anaphylactoid purpura	53
Aneurysm causing swelling in neck	33
— demonstration of	19
Angiography	19
Angle ostectomy for mandibular protrusion (*Fig.* 29A)	166

	PAGE
Ankylosis of temporomandibular joint (*Fig.* 45)	235
Anorganic bone	186
Anthrax	252
'Anticoagulant rebound'	58
— reversal	52
— therapy complicating surgery	58
Anticonvulsant therapy, lymphadenopathy complicating	30
Antihaemophilic globulin (AHG), human or animal	48
Antral calculi	266
— polyp, prolapsed (*Fig.* 4)	61
Antroliths	266
Arch bar in immobilization of fragments after osteotomy	181
Arteriovenous shunt into central haemangioma	75
Arthritis of temporomandibular joint	239
— traumatic of temporomandibular joint	233
Arthrosis of temporomandibular joint	239
Articular fossa, temporomandibular, fracture of roof, with dislocation of condylar head	235
Aspiration biopsy	22
Aspirin contra-indicated in haemophilia	50
Asymmetrical mandibular deformity	148, 178
Atrial fibrillation	12
Auricular nerve, great, pain involving	7
Auticulo-temporal nerve injuries	247
Autogenous bone-grafting	187
Autograft(s) onlays to chin (*Fig.* 27A)	149
— in replacement of bone	184
Axonotmesis	248
Azotaemic bone disease	202
BARIUM swallow	19
Bence-Jones protein	16
Benign soft-tissue cysts (*Figs.* 9–11)	81–88
Biopsy	21
— of ameloblastoma	102
— dangers	22
— of neoplasms of major salivary glands	229
— in oral carcinoma	133, 136, 143
— postal regulations regarding	23
— of white patches in mouth	125
Bite wing films	18
Bite-raising appliance in temporomandibular joint treatment	240, 242
Blastomycosis, North American	259
— South American	259
Bleeding time	15
— — prolonged, in thrombocytopenia	52, 53
— vessels, securing of, with haemostats	40

ORAL SURGERY PART II

	PAGE
Bleomycin	145
Block grafts (*Figs.* 32, 33)	189
Blood clotting mechanism	45, 47
— examination in antral carcinoma	133
— picture in malignant granuloma	119
— tests	20
— transfusion, bacterially contaminated	52
— uric acid estimation	20
— in urine	16
Blood-pressure taking	12
Blood-urea estimation	20
Body ostectomy for mandibular protrusion (*Fig.* 29 B)	120, 165, 171
Bone destruction, malignant	135
— fibrous dysplasia of (*Figs.* 35, 36)	195
— fractured, re-union of, by regeneration	184
— malignant neoplasms arising within	130
— onlay graft to chin (*Fig.* 27 A)	149
— plating in immobilization of fragments after osteotomy	181
— replacement of (*Figs.* 32–34)	184–194
— resection for cancer, extent of	141
— — reconstruction after	145
— stored	185
— wax in haemostasis	41
Bone-end(s) in mandibular section, wiring	162, 165, 167, 168, 173, 174
— need for adequate area of contact between graft and	188
Bone-graft(s), curved (*Fig.* 34)	191
— fresh, fate of	185
— in replacement of bone	146, 184, 185
— serial, in correction of unilateral mandibular overgrowth	179
— vascular unscarred bed required for	188
Bone-grafting, conditions for success	187
Boplant bone	186, 187
Bowen's disease	126
Branchial (branchiogenic) carcinoma	32
— cyst (*Fig.* 2)	30, 83
Brown tumours or nodes	95
Buccal inlay in correction of receding chin	151
— — and prosthesis for maxillary retrusion	175
Burkitt's lymphoma	145
CALCIFYING odontogenic cyst	106
— — epithelium tumour (*Fig.* 15)	104
Calcium, serum, estimation	21
Calculi, antral	266
— salivary duct (*Figs.* 39, 40)	218, 226
— — gland causing mucocele	84
Campbell de Morgan spot	73
Cancellous grafts, taking of, from iliac crest	188
— osteoma	76
Candida leucoplakia	257, 258
Candidiasis	256
— as form of leucoplakia	124
— chronic hyperplastic or hypertrophic	257
— treatment	257

	PAGE
Cap splints in immobilization of fragments after osteotomy	181
Capillary abnormality, diseases in which there is	53
— haemangioma	71, 73
Carcinoma (*see also* Oral Carcinoma; Malignant Neoplasms)	
— branchial (branchiogenic)	32
— incidence of, in patients with leucoplakia	125
— keratinizing squamous-cell (*Figs.* 18, 19)	123
— Krompecher	129
— oral (*see* Oral Carcinoma)	
— secondary, in cervical lymph-node	29
— in situ	125
— squamous-cell (*see* Squamous-cell Carcinoma)	
— of thyroid gland	35
— verrucous	123
Carcinomatous deposits in left supraclavicular lymph-nodes	33
Cardiac origin of pain	7
Carotid body tumour	32
Cartilage grafts	192
Case history	1
Cat scratch fever causing cervical node enlargement	26
Cataract, radiation	139
Cavernous haemangioma (*Fig.* 8)	73
— — central	74
Cells in urine	16
Cementifying fibroma	111
Cementoma, gigantiform	111
— multiple	111
Central haemangioma	74
— medullary giant-cell granuloma of jaws	90
Cervical lymph-nodes	24
— — malignant involvement	28
— — — search for primary lesion	25
— — rib causing swelling in neck	32
Cervicofacial actinomycosis (*Fig.* 46)	254
Chancre of lip or tongue	260
Cheek, actinomycosis of (*Fig.* 46)	255
— carcinoma of, treatment of (*Figs.* 24, 25)	140
Cheilitis, angular	257, 258
Chemical leucoplakia	122
Cherubism	97
Chewing mechanisms, abnormal, causing derangement of temporomandibular joint	242
Children, scarring in	37
Chin, receding, correction (*Fig.* 27)	149, 154, 155
Chip grafting following ostectomy of mandible	165
— grafts	187, 188
Chorda tympani syndrome	247
Christmas disease	47, 51
Cineradiography	19
Cingulum invagination	113
Clavicles, abnormalities of, in cleidocranial dysotosis	212
Cleidocranial dysostosis	212
— — oral surgical aspects	213
Clicking of temporomandibular joint	241, 242

INDEX

	PAGE
Clotting time	15
Coagulation defect, diseases where there is	45
— mechanism	45
— system and fibrinolytic enzyme system	56
Collar-stud abscess	27
Colloid goitre	33
Colour index	14
Complex odontome (*Fig.* 17)	108
Compound odontome	186
Condylar hyperplasia causing mandibular overgrowth	148, 178
— — unilateral	148, 233
— hypoplasia	232
— neck, osteotomy of, for mandibular protrusion (*Fig.* 28A)	163
Condyle, damage to (*Fig.* 44)	235
— dislocation of	234
— intra-oral approach to, Sear's	179
Condylectomy in condylar hyperplasia	233
— high, in osteoarthritis of temporomandibular joint	241
— for overgrowth of mandible	148, 179
Condylotomy, Ward	242
Consistency of enlarged cervical lymph-nodes	25
— lump	8
Coronitis of 3rd molar, pain of	7
Coronoid hyperplasia	237
— process, excision	238
Cosmetic operation in craniofacial fibrous dysplasia	199
Cough restarting haemorrhage	43
Craniofacial fibrous dysplasia (*Figs.* 35, 36)	196
Cryoprecipitate in haemophilia	48, 49
Cryosurgery for haemangiomas	73
— malignant disease	144
Curettage biopsy	22
Curved bone-grafts (*Fig.* 34)	191
Cutaneous naevus	71
— neurofibromatosis	66, 67
Cylindroma	228
Cyst(s), aspiration biopsy of	22
— benign soft-tissue (*Figs.* 9–11)	81–88
— branchial (*Fig.* 2)	30, 83
— Calcifying Odontogenic	99, 106
— dermoid (*see* Dermoid Cysts)	
— elicitation of fluctuation in	9
— of jaws, differential radiographic diagnosis	101
— mucous extravasation and retention (*Fig.* 11)	84
— odontogenic	99, 106
Cystadenoma lymphomatosum, papillary	228
'Cystic' change in bone	201
— disease of jaws, familial multilocular	97
— hygroma	31
— — of mouth	88
— swellings in neck (*Fig.* 2)	30
Cytology, oral	22
Cytotoxic drugs	144, 145
Deciduous teeth, giant-cell granuloma occurring at time of loss of	92

	PAGE
Degeneration, reaction to	246
Dens in dente	113
Dental abnormalities due to cherubism	97
— anomalies associated with multiple osteomas	78
— arch, lower, retrusion of, correction (*Fig.* 27D)	155, 156
— canal, inferior, spread of cancer along	141
— complications of Paget's disease (*Fig.* 37)	204, 208
— injection, posterior superior, needles broken to	263
— nerve, inferior, avoidance of damage to, in mandibular osteotomies	171
— sepsis associated with fibrous enlargement of tuberosity	65
Dentigerous cyst and ameloblastoma	100, 101
Dentinoma	106
Dento-alveolar surgery	180
Denture(s) to correct maxillary retrusion	175
— hyperplasia (*Fig.* 6)	63
— in soft tissues	268
Denture-sore mouth	257, 258
Dermoid cyst(s) of floor of mouth and tongue (*Figs.* 9, 10)	81
— — sublingual	30
Desquamated cytological examination	126
Developmental disturbances of temporomandibular joint	232
— epithelial naevi	121
— post-normal occlusion, correction of retrognathism in (*Fig.* 27D, E)	154, 157
Dialysate bone disease in renal osteodystrophy	203
Dichotomy	112
Dilated odontome	113
Disguising procedures in facial paralysis	247
Disk, tearing of	235
Dislocation of temporomandibular joint	234
Disseminated juvenile fibrous dysplasia	97
'Drainage area' of mouth, cancer of	122
Drill biopsy	22
Drug(s) causing cervical node enlargement	29
— — enlargement of salivary glands	225
— therapy, gingival hyperplasia following	63
Duct obstruction causing recurrent salivary gland swellings	217, 218
'Dumb-bell' tumours of salivary gland	228
Dupuy's syndrome	247
Dyskeratosis	123
Dysostosis, mandibulofacial	232
Dysplasia of bone, fibrous (*Figs.* 35, 36)	195
EACA (epsilon aminocaproic acid) in haemophilia	50

	PAGE
Ear abnormalities in hemifacial microsomia	232
— — in Treacher-Collins syndrome	232
Ecthyma contagiosum	252
Ectodic oral tonsils	87
Edentulous patient, chronic dislocation of condyles in	234
— — immobilization of fragments in following osteotomy	81
Ehlers-Danlos syndrome (E.D.S.)	54
Electrical devices for locating needle fragment	263
— stimulation tests of facial nerve	246
Elephantiasis neuromatosa	67
Embryonal rhabdomyoma	68
Encephalofacial angiomatosis	72
Endocrine dysfunction in fibrous dysplasia of bone	195
Endosteal osteoma	76, 77
Endostosis	77
Eosinophilic granuloma	116
Epilepsy, drug therapy for, gingival hyperplasia following	63
Epistaxis due to antral carcinoma	132
— familial condition with	55
Epithelial naevi, developmental	121
— odontogenic tumours (*Figs.* 14–17)	99, 100
— odontome, melanotic	69
Epsilon aminocaproic acid (EACA) in haemophilia	50
Epulis, congenital	68
— — pigmented	69
— — traumatized by opposing teeth (*Fig.* 3)	61
— giant-cell or myeloid (*Fig.* 13)	93
Erythroplasia, Queyrat's	126
Essential thrombocytopenia	52
Evaginated odontome	113
Excision and biopsy	21
Exfoliative cytological examination	126
Exostosis	77
Extraction(s), Paget's disease complicating (*Fig.* 37)	204, 208
— under general anaesthesia causing dislocation of condyles	234
Extra-oral surgical approach to mandible	161, 168
Extravasation cyst, mucous (*Fig.* 11)	84
Eyelid incisions	39
FACIAL artery, haemorrhage from	44
— deformity, surgical correction of jaws in (*Figs.* 27–31)	148–181
— hemi-hypertrophy	233
— nerve, dissection of	229
— — electrical stimulation tests of	246
— — injuries	245
— paralysis, differential diagnosis of causes	245
— — treatment	246
— trauma, tooth fragments in soft tissues following	265
Factor V deficiency	47, 51
— VII deficiency	47, 51
— VIII deficiency (*see also* Haemophilia)	47, 55
— IX concentrates	51
— — deficiency	47, 51

	PAGE
Factor X deficiency	51
— XI deficiency	51
Factors, clotting	45
Family history	2, 4
Fear increasing haemorrhage	56
Fibrin monomer	45
Fibrinogen	45
Fibrinolytic enzyme system	56
— states, acute, in surgery	56
Fibro-epithelial polyp (*Fig.* 5)	61
Fibroma (*Figs.* 3–5)	60
— ameloblastic	104
— cementifying	111
— of gums, diffuse	64
— palate tuberosity	64
— symmetrica gingivalis	64
Fibromatosis gingivae	62
Fibromyxoma, diagnosis from ameloblastoma	101
— odontogenic	110
Fibrosarcoma, ameloblastic	105
Fibrosis, submucous	126
— — limiting movement at temporomandibular joint	238
Fibrous dysplasia of bone (*Figs.* 35, 36)	195
— — — diagnosis from Paget's disease	207
— — — malignant changes in	199
— — treatment	199
— — disseminated juvenile	97
— — periapical	111
— enlargement of tuberosity, bilateral	64
— — traumatized by opposing teeth (*Fig.* 3)	61
— overgrowths (*Figs.* 3–5)	60
— — following drug treatment	63
— swelling of jaws, familial	97
'First arch' defect, bilateral, micrognathia in	153
— syndrome	232, 233
Fissure, precancerous	135
Fistulae, exploration of sinuses and	19
Flake grafts	188
Fluctuation in lump	9
Fluid intake, importance of adequate	16
Foreign bodies in and around jaws, management (*Fig.* 47)	261
— — in tissues due to gunshot wounds	267
Fracture, malignant	135
Frey's syndrome	231
Frey-Baillarger syndrome	247
Frictional keratosis	122
Functional causes of limited opening of temporomandibular joint	239, 241
— derangement of temporomandibular joint	241
Fungal diseases (*Fig.* 46)	254
GENIOPLASTY, sliding (*Fig.* 27 B)	151, 154, 155
German measles causing cervical node enlargement	26
Germination	112
Ghost cell change in calcifying odontogenic cyst	106
Giant-cell epulis (*Fig.* 13)	94
— granuloma, central	89

INDEX

	PAGE
Giant-cell granuloma, central medullary	90
— — diagnosis from ameloblastoma	101
— — hyperparathyroidism and	95
— — of jaws, osteoclastoma and	93
— — — treatment	92
— — subperiosteal (*Fig.* 12)	91
— lesions of jaws (*Figs.* 12, 13)	89
— — — malignant	93
— tumours of bone in hyperparathyroidism	200, 201
Gigantiform cementoma	111
Gingiva, hyperplasia of, symmetrical	64
— primary syphilis of	251
Gingival fibromatosis, hereditary	62
— hyperplasia following drug therapy	63
Gingivitis, chronic hyperplastic	257
— pain of	7
— Vincent's acute ulcerative	44
Glanders causing cervical node enlargement	27
Glandular fever causing cervical node enlargement	26
Glanzmann's disease	53
Glass fragments in soft tissues	267
Glossopharyngeal pain	7
Glucose in blood, tests for	20
— tolerance test	20
Glycosuria	16
Goitre, inflammatory	33, 35
— non-toxic	33
— toxic	33, 34
Gout of temporomandibular joint	240
Grafting after excision of fibrous enlargement of tuberosity	65
Granular-cell myoblastoma	68
Granuloma, central giant-cell (*Fig.* 12)	89
— denture (*Fig.* 6)	63
— eosinophilic	116
— malignant	118
— subperiosteal giant-cell (*Fig.* 12)	91
Granulomatosis, Wegener's	118
Grease-gun grease in soft tissues	269
Gumma of tongue	251
Gummatous ulcer	10
Gunshot wounds, foreign bodies in tissues due to	267
Gustatory sweating and flushing	247
Gutta-percha bung, construction	152
HAEMANGIOMA(S)	71
— capillary	71, 73
— cavernous (*Fig.* 8)	73
— central	74
— simplex	71
— traumatic	74
Haematocrit value	14
Haematological investigations	13
Haematoma formation, postoperative	44
Haemoglobin content of blood	13
Haemophilia	47
— B.M.	51
— treatment	48
Haemophiliac requiring oral surgery, investigation and management	47
— undergoing oral surgery, management	49
Haemorrhage during operation	40

	PAGE
Haemorrhage, factors restarting, postoperative	43
— from tooth socket	44
— management of, in normal patient	40
— — in oral surgery	40–58
— oral, due to hereditary haemorrhagic telangiectasia	72, 73
— postoperative	43
— protracted, after extractions	54
— reactionary	44
— secondary infection causing	42, 44
— — postoperative	44
— severe, due to central haemangioma	74, 76
Haemorrhagic diseases	45
— telangiectasia, hereditary (H.H.T.)	55, (*Fig.* 7) 71, 73
— tumours	22
Haemostasis, failure to effect at end of operation	43
— through pressure with swabs	41
Haemostatic agents, use of	41
Haemostats, securing of bleeding vessels with	40
Halsted's mosquito forceps as haemostats	40
Hamartomas	99
Hand-Schüller-Christian disease	117
Hashimoto's disease	34
Hemifacial microsomia	232
Henderson and Jackson nasal operation	177, 178
Henny's approach to temporomandibular joint	243
Henoch's purpura	53
Hereditary haemorrhagic telangiectasia (H.H.T.)	55, (*Fig.* 7) 71, 73
Heterograft in replacement of bone	184, 185
H.H.T. (hereditary haemorrhagic telangiectasia)	55, (*Fig.* 7) 71, 73
Histiocytosis 'X'	116
— — chronic and acute	117
Histoplasmosis	258
History-taking	1
Hodgkin's disease causing cervical node enlargement	29, 30
Homograft onlays to chin	149
— in replacement of bone	184, 185
Horizontal osteotomy of ramus for mandibular protrusion (*Fig.* 28)	167
Hormonal control of malignant metastases	145
Horsley's bone wax in haemostasis	42
Horton's syndrome, pain of	7
Hunsuck's osteotomy for mandibular protrusion (*Figs.* 29G, 30)	170
Hygroma, cystic	31
— — of mouth	88
Hypercalcaemia, signs and symptoms in hyperparathyroidism	201
Hypercementosis complicating tooth extraction in Paget's disease (*Fig.* 37)	204, 208
Hyperparathyroidism	95, 200
— blood determinations for	95, 96
— brown tumours due to	95
— in renal osteodystrophy and renal rickets	202, 203

	PAGE
Hyperplasia, coronoid	237
— of temporomandibular joint	233
Hypertension, causing haemorrhage.	44
— significance	13
Hypertrophic scars	36
Hypodermic needles, broken, in and around jaws (*Fig.* 47)	261
Hypoplasia of temporomandibular joint	232
Hypoprothrombinaemia, conditions in which there is	51
Hypotension, significance	13
Hypotensive anaesthesia to reduce haemorrhage	42
ILIAC crest, taking block grafts from	189
— — — chip and flake grafts from	188
Immobilization, need for, in successful bone-grafting	188
Immunological factor in cervical node enlargement with hepatosplenomegaly	30
— — in malignancy	141, 145
Implants, permanent, in repair of bone	192
Impression material, rubber base	268
Incision(s), neck	38
— peri-orbital	38
— planning to avoid excessive haemorrhage	40
— pre-auricular	39
— skin	36
Incisional biopsy	21
Indelible pencil in soft tissues	269
Infancy, melanotic neuroectodermal tumour of	69
Infection(s), absence of, necessary for success in bone-grafting	187
— non-pyogenic, of soft tissues	250
— at wound site causing haemorrhage	43
Infective arthritis of temporomandibular joint	239
Infranuclear facial paralysis	245
Infra-orbital nerve injury	249
Intra-oral body ostectomy	171
— surgical approach to mandible	161, 163, 169
— swelling in cherubism	97
Invaginated odontomes	113
Inverted L osteotomy of Trauner (*Fig.* 28F)	168
Ivory osteoma	76
JAW (*see also* Mandible)	
— deformities requiring correction	148
— enlargement of, in cherubism	97
— fracture of, complicating osteopetrosis	211
— giant-cell lesions of (*Figs.* 12, 13)	89–98
— impression material in medullary cavity of	268
— lesions, radiology in diagnosis	17
— malignancy involving	141
— management of foreign bodies in and around (*Fig.* 47)	261
— non-malignant tumours in and around (*Figs.* 3–8)	60–80

	PAGE
Jaw, Paget's disease in (*Fig.* 37)	204, 206, 207
— radiolucent area in, atypical	75
— surgical correction of, in facial deformity (*Figs.* 27–31)	148–181
KAHN test	17
Keloid(s) scars	36
— symmetric gingival	64
Keratinizing squamous-cell carcinoma (*Figs.* 18, 19)	123
Keratocyst, odontogenic, diagnosis	22
Keratosis, frictional	122
— from smoking	122
Kiel bone	186, 187
Kirschner wire, use as allelograft	192
Köle procedure for anterior open bite (*Fig.* 29F)	165
Krompecher carcinoma	129
LABIAL artery, upper, haemorrhage from	44
— segments, surgery of	180
Langer's lines, incisions placed parallel to	36
Lateral displacement of jaw during sleep	242
Le Fort II osteotomy	177
Leong's odontome	113
Lesion, investigation of	12
Lethal midline granuloma	118
Letterer-Siwe's disease	117
Leucopenia	14
Leucoplakia (*Figs.* 18, 19)	121, 251
— candida	257
— candiasis as form of	124
— chemical	122
— of developmental origin	121
— incidence of	121
— — carcinoma in patients with	125, 135
— syphilitic	122, 135
— of unknown aetiology	123
Leukaemia causing cervical node enlargement	28, 30
— — haemorrhage	57
— cytotoxic agents in	145
Lichen planus	122
Lingual nerve injury	249
— space, tooth or root in	263
Lip, carcinoma of (*Fig.* 23)	122, 129, 130, 139
— incisions involving free margin	39
— lower, anaesthesia of, after removal of impacted 3rd molars	248
— syphilitic lesions of	250
Lipoma	67
— of neck	32
Localized histiocytosis 'X'	116
Locking of temporomandibular joint	241
Lower third molar surgery, lingual nerve injury during	249
Lump, examination	7
Lupus vulgaris	252
Lymph-node enlargement associated with lump	8
— — — ulcer	10
— — histological and bacteriological examination	25

INDEX

Lymph-node metastases of oral carcinoma (*Fig.* 26) 138, 141, 142
— — in neck examination . . 24
Lymphadenoma causing cervical node enlargement . . . 29
Lymphadenopathy, cervical . . 25
— pyogenic 26
— of viral origin 26
Lymphangioma of dorsum of tongue 88
Lymphatic leukaemia, chronic . . 29
— swellings of neck . . (*Fig.* 1) 24
— — — classification . (*Fig.* 1) 26
Lymphocyte count 15
Lymphosarcoma causing cervical node enlargement . . 29, 30

MACROGLOBULINAEMIA . . . 53
Macroradiography in hyperparathyroidism 202
Malignancy (*see also* Carcinoma)
— of lump 10
— oral, clinical diagnosis
 (*Figs.* 20, 21) 129
Malignant changes in bone in Paget's disease 207
— — fibrous dysplasia . . . 199
— — neurofibromatosis . . 66, 67
— disease causing cervical node enlargement 28
— — diagnosis of 135
— granuloma and Wegener's granulomatosis 118
— melanoma (*see* Melanoma, Malignant)
— neoplasms of salivary glands . 28
— — treatment of (*Figs.* 22-26) 135-147
— — — follow-up of . . 141, 146
— — — palliative 144
— pustule 252
— ulcer 10, 11, 135
Malocclusion, Angle's Class II, correction 153
— — division 1, correction
 (*Fig.* 27 D–F) 154, 156, 180
— — II 157
— — III 158
— causing derangement of temporomandibular joint . . . 242
— not associated with gross skeletal anomaly 179
Mandible (*see also* Jaw)
— abnormalities of, in hemifacial microsomia 232
— bone-graft of, long-term reduction in bulk of 188
— central haemangioma of . . 74
— changes to growth of, due to damage to condyle . (*Fig.* 44) 235
— elongation of, operation for . 154
— fracture, causing mandibular nerve injury 248
— osteomyelitis of, bone-grafting for 187
— regeneration of bone in . . 184
— replacement of by allelograft . 146
— — anterior part by bone-graft
 (*Fig.* 34) 191
— — half, by block graft . (*Fig.* 32) 189

Mandible, routine radiography of . 17
— section of, blind 160
— — in open operation . . . 161
— stone models of, in preoperative assessment of mandibular protrusion 160
— unilateral overgrowth of, operation 148, 178
— — undergrowth of operation . 148
Mandibular body osteotomy and block graft, for receding chin
 (*Fig.* 27C) 153
— deformity, asymmetrical . 148, 178
— nerve injuries 248
— osteotomy combined with maxillary osteotomy 178
— protrusion, choice of operation . 160
— — due to acromegaly . . . 209
— — preoperative assessment . . 158
— — true or relative, correction
 (*Figs.* 28-31) 157-175
— — types and sites of operation
 (*Figs.* 28, 29) 163
— retrognathia, extreme, correction
 (*Fig.* 27G) 157
— retrognathism, correction
 (*Figs.* 27, 31) 149, 154, 156
— retrusion, sagittal splitting, operation for . . . (*Fig.* 31) 170
— — true or relative, correction
 (*Fig.* 27 D–F) 153
Mandibulofacial dysostosis . . 232
Maxilla, central haemangioma of . 74
— fibroma of tuberosity . . . 64
— regeneration of bone in . . 184
— resection of, incision . . . 38
— routine radiography of . . . 17
Maxillary antrum, malignant neoplasms of 132
— carcinoma, pain of . . . 7
— ostectomy for correction of anterior open bite . . . 180
— osteotomy to correct retrusion
 (*Fig.* 29D) 176
— protrusion, choice of operation . 156
— — correction . . (*Fig.* 27E) 154
— retrusion causing prognathism . 158
— — correction . . (*Fig.* 29D) 175
— rhinoliths 266
— sinus, foreign bodies in . . 265
Mean corpuscular haemoglobin concentration (MCHC) . . . 14
— — volume (MCV) 14
Mechanical causes of limited opening of temporomandibular joint 237
Melanoma, malignant, involving cervical nodes . . . 29
— — oral . . . . (*Fig.* 21) 134
— — metastatic 145
— — treatment of 141
Melanotic neuroectodermal tumour of infancy 69
Meniscus, tearing of 235
Mesodermal odontogenic tumours 99, 110
Metallic foreign bodies in tissues . 267
Micrognathia 156
Microsomia, hemifacial . . . 232
Mikulicz's disease 225

276 ORAL SURGERY PART II

	PAGE
Monilial infection	256, 257
Mononucleosis, infective, causing cervical node enlargement	26
Monostotic fibrous dysplasia	196, 197, 198
Mouth, carcinoma of (*Fig.* 20)	131
— care of, in presence of cancer	145
— dermoid cysts of floor of (*Figs.* 9, 10)	81, 83
— dryness, post-irradiation	139
Mucocele	84
Muco-epidermoid carcinoma of salivary gland	144, 229
Mucous extravasation and retention cysts (*Fig.* 11)	84
— patches in mouth	250
Multilocular cystic disease of jaws, familial	97
Multiple osteomas	77
Muscular spasm preventing opening of temporomandibular joint	239
— weakness and degeneration, primary, affecting facial nerve	245
Mycobacterial infection, unclassified, causing cervical lymphadenitis	28
Myeloid epulis	93
— leukaemia, chronic	29
Myoblastic myoma	68
Myoblastoma, granular-cell	68
Myositis ossificans of masseter	239
Myxoma, odontogenic	110
NAEVUS(I) developmental epithelial	121
— white sponge	121
Nasal cavity, tooth or root in	265
— sinuses, 'endosteal osteoma' of	77
Neck dissection, radical	141, 142
— — bilateral	142
— — — secondary haemorrhage after	43
— incisions	38
— swellings of, differential diagnosis (*Figs.* 1, 2)	24–35
Needle(s) biopsy	22
— broken hypodermic, in and around jaws (*Fig.* 47)	261
— removal of fragment	262
Neoplasms of major salivary glands (*Fig.* 42)	226, 227
Nerve damage during oral surgery	246
— injuries of oral surgical interest	245
— involved in pain	7
Nerve-sheath tumours	66
Neurectomy, selective, in facial paralysis	247
Neurilemmoma	66
Neurinoma	66
Neuroectodermal tumour of infancy, melanotic	69
Neurofibroma causing swelling in neck	33
— solitary	67
Neurofibromatosis	65
— cutaneous	67
— plexiform	66
— Von Recklinghausen's	66
Neurofibrosarcoma	67
Neuropraxia	246, 248, 249
Neurotmesis	246, 248, 249
Neutropenia	15
Nodular goitre	33

	PAGE
Non-chromaffinparaganglioma	32
Non-malignant tumours in and around jaws (*Figs.* 3–8)	60–80
Non-pyogenic infections of soft tissues	250
North American blastomycosis	259
Nose, advancement of, Henderson and Jackson	177, 178
— malignant granuloma in	118
— tooth or root in floor of	265
Nuclear facial paralysis	245
OBLIQUE osteotomy in ascending ramus (*Fig.* 28 A, G)	168
Obturator, replacement of upper jaw by	147
Obweseger's maxillary osteotomy	176
— sagittal splitting operation in condylar hyperplasia	154, 163, 189, 233
Obwegeser-Dal Pont operation for mandibular deformity (*Figs.* 29 G, 31)	163, 167, 170
Occipital lymph-nodes, enlarged	25
Odontogenic cyst, calcifying	106
— epithelium tumour, calcifying (*Fig.* 15)	104
— myxoma or fibromyxoma	110
— tumours, classification	99
— — epithelial (*Figs.* 14–17)	99, 100
— — mesodermal	99, 110
— — and odontomes (*Figs.* 14–17)	99–115
Odontome(s)	99, 112
— ameloblastic (*Fig.* 16)	107
— complex (*Fig.* 17)	108
— compound	110
— evaginated	113
— invaginated	113
— Leong's	113
— Tratman's	113
Onlay(s) to chin (*Fig.* 27 A)	149, 154
— graft, subperiosteal, of anorganic bone	186
Oral carcinoma (*see also* Carcinoma)	
— — associated with lichen planus	122
— — — syphilitic leucoplakia	122
— — main sites	127
— — primary (*Figs.* 18, 19)	124, 129
— — secondary	129
— — symptoms	129
— cavity, bone-grafts inserted through	187
— — malignant neoplasms affecting	129
— — premalignant conditions of (*Figs,* 18, 19)	121
— cytology	22
— lesions of H.H.T.	55
— — syphilis	250
— lipoma	67
— malignancy, clinical diagnosis (*Figs.* 20, 21)	129
— manifestation of fibrous dysplasia of bone	196
— surgery producing facial paralysis	246
— tonsils, ectopic	87
Orf	252
Oro-antral fistula, foreign bodies passing into maxillary sinus through	265

INDEX

	PAGE
Orthodontic bands in immobilization of fragments after osteotomy	181
Orthopantomograph in radiography of temporomandibular joint	243
Osler-Weber-Rendu disease	55
Ostectomy, alveolar	180
— bilateral, for mandibular protrusion	158, 160
— body, for mandibular protrusion (*Fig.* 29 B)	163, 165, 171
— immobilization of fragments following	162, 180
— of mandible, wiring of bone-ends in	162
Osteitis deformans . (*Fig.* 37)	203
— fibrosa	195
Osteoarthritis of temporomandibular joint	240
Osteoclastoma of jaws	93
— long-bone and giant-cell granuloma of jaws	89
— periosteal (*Fig.* 13)	93
Osteodystrophy, renal	202
Osteogenesis, discouragement of, in production of pseudarthrosis	236, 237
Osteoma(s)	76
— endosteal	76, 77
— multiple	77
— periosteal cancellous	76, 77
Osteomalacia in osteodystrophy and renal rickets	202, 203
Osteomyelitis in childhood causing mandibular deviation (*Fig.* 44)	235
— complicating osteopetrosis	211
— — Paget's disease	208
— of mandible, bone-grafting for	187
— post-irradiation	138, 139
Osteopetrosis	210
Osteoporosis circumscripta in Paget's disease	206
Osteotomy, alveolar (*Fig.* 29 C)	156, 175, 176, 180
— bilateral, for mandibular protrusion	158, 160
— immobilization of fragments following	162, 180
— Le Fort II	177
— of mandible, wiring of bone-ends in	162
— mandibular body, and bone-graft for receding chin (*Fig.* 27 C)	153
— maxillary, to correct protrusion	156
— — — retrusion (*Fig.* 29 D)	176
— subapical	180
— symphysial alveolar (*Fig.* 29 C)	175
— vertical subsigmoid (*Fig.* 28 E)	168
Otitis media causing temporomandibular arthritis	239
Otomandibular dysostosis	232
Overbite, deep, correction of	180
PACHYDERMATOCELE	66
Pack, socket	44
— in wound to control persistent haemorrhage	41
Packed cell volume	14
Paget's disease of bone (*Fig.* 37)	203
— — — aspects affecting oral surgeons	208

	PAGE
Paget's disease of bone, complications	207
Pain, assessing severity	5
— clinical examination	5
— control of, in oral cancer	145
— phenomena associated with	5
— in temporomandibular joint	240, 241
Palate, bone-grafting of (*Fig.* 33)	190
— carcinoma of	131
— fibrous overgrowth of (*Fig.* 5)	60, 62
— keratosis of, from smoking	122
— malignant granuloma involving	118
— soft, and fauces, carcinoma of	132
— tuberosity, fibroma of	64
Pancytopaenia, drugs associated with	53
Pantomography	85
Papillary cystadenoma lymphomatosum	228
— obstruction, causing recurrent salivary gland swellings	217, 218
Papilloma	60
Paraganglioma, non-chromaffin	32
Parathyroid abnormality, brown tumours due to	95
— tumour causing hyperparathyroidism	200, 201
Parotid calculi	218, 219, 224
— — removal (*Figs.* 40, 41)	222
— infection and abscess	226
Paterson-Kelly syndrome	123
Patient, personal history	2
— — physical examination	5
— — complaint	2, 4
Paul-Bunnell test	20
Pedicle graft after excision of cancer	146
Periapical fibrous dysplasia	111
Pericoronitis of 3rd molar, pain of	7
Periodontal abscess, pain of	7
— disease, haemorrhage in extraction for	44
— pocket, deep, with granulation and bone destruction	135
Peri-orbital incisions	38
Periosteal cancellous osteoma	77
— osteoclastoma (*Fig.* 13)	93
— osteoma	76
Peripheral giant-cell tumour	93
Pharyngeal space, lateral, tooth or root in	264
Phosphatase, alkaline and acid, estimation	20, 21
Phosphates, inorganic, value of serum	21
Physiological goitre	33
Pierre-Robin syndrome	153
Pigmentation in fibrous dysplasia of bone	195
Pindborg tumour (*Fig.* 15)	104
Pituitary adenoma causing acromegaly	209, 210
Plasminogen-plasmin system	56
Plaster-of-Paris models in preoperative assessment of mandibular protrusion	159, 160
Plastic objects in soft tissues	268
Platelet abnormalities	53, 55
— aggregation	45
— deficiency	52, 53
— function	52
Pleomorphic adenoma of salivary glands (*Fig.* 42)	227

278 ORAL SURGERY PART II

	PAGE
Plexiform neurofibromatosis	66
Plummer-Vinson syndrome	123
Plunging ranula	86
Polymorphonuclear leucocyte count	15
Polyostotic fibrous dysplasia	195, 196, 198
Polyp, antral, prolapsed (*Fig.* 4)	61
— fibro-epithelial (*Fig.* 5)	61
Port-wine stain	72
Post-auricular lymph-nodes, enlarged	25
Post-extraction haemorrhage, protracted	54
— — — in leukaemia	57
Post-irradiation complications	138
Post-normal occlusion, correction of retrognathism in (*Fig.* 27 D, E)	154
Postoperative haemorrhage	43
'Potato' tumour	32
Pre-auricular incisions	39
Precocious puberty in fibrous dysplasia of bone	195
Premalignant conditions of oral cavity (*Figs.* 18, 19)	121, 135
Pressure effects of lump	9
— with swabs, haemostasis through	41
Price's precipitation reaction	17
Probe, radio-opaque	19
Prognathism, asymmetrical	178, 179
— operations for	160
— symmetrical	158
Progonoma, melanotic neuroectodermal	69
Prosthetic considerations in Paget's disease	208
Proteinuria	16
Prothrombin	45, 51
— deficiency	51
— level, measurement	57
Prothrombinase	45
Pseudarthrosis, production of, in temporomandibular ankylosis	236
Pseudoactinomycosis	256
Pseudocysts forming from ectopic oral cysts	88
Pseudohaemophilia	54
Psoriatic arthritis of temporomandibular joint	240
Psychosomatic pain, recognition	5, 6
Pterygoid plexus region, tooth or root in	264
Pterygomandibular raphe, fibrosis	238
Pugh's sign	202
Pulp disease, pain due to	7
Pulsating mass diagnosis of central haemangioma	75
Pulsation of lump	9
Pulse-taking	12
Punch biopsy	21
Purpura	52, 53
Pyogenic lymphadenopathy	26
QUEYRAT's erythroplasia	126
RADIOGRAPHIC appearances in cleidocranial dysostosis	212
— assessment for mandibular sagittal splitting operation	171
Radiography in fibrous dysplasia of bone (*Figs.* 35, 36)	196, 197
— giant-cell granuloma of jaws	90, 91

	PAGE
Radiography, preoperative assessment of mandibular protrusion	159, 160
— and radiology of temporomandibular joint	243
— routine	17
— in temporomandibular ankylosis (*Fig.* 45)	236
Radiology	17
— in ameloblastoma	101
— in central haemangioma	75
— cherubism	98
— cleidocranial dysostosis	212
— hyperparathyroidism	96, 201
— odontogenic myxoma	110
— oral malignancy	136, 137
— osteopetrosis	211
— of Paget's disease	206
— in periosteal osteoclastoma	94
Radio-opaque calculi in salivary ducts	219
— materials, use of	19
Radiotherapy contra-indicated in ameloblastoma	103
— — giant-cell granuloma of jaws	92
— malignant disease (*Figs.* 22–26)	138, 139
— — — palliative	144
— — — preoperative	144
Ramus procedures in treatment of mandibular protrusion (*Fig.* 28)	163, 167, 168, 171
— surgical removal of needle medial to	262
Ranula (*Fig.* 11)	85
Reaction of degeneration	246
Re-animation procedures in facial paralysis	247
Rebound thrombosis	58
Receding chin, correction (*Fig.* 27)	149, 154, 155
Reconstruction after excision of cancer	145
Red cell appearances and abnormalities	14
— — sedimentation rate (E.S.R.)	15
Red-cell count	13
Regeneration of new bone	184
Rehabilitation of patient after cancer excision	147
Renal osteodystrophy	202
— rickets	202
Reparative granuloma, giant-cell	89, 93
Respiratory rate	13
Retention cyst, mucous	84
— — of submandibular duct	87
Reticuloses of oral cavity	129
Reticulum-cell sarcoma, diagnosis from malignant granuloma	119
Retrognathia, mandibular, extreme, correction (*Fig.* 27G)	157
Retrognathism, mandibular, correction (*Fig.* 27)	149, 153, 154, 155, 156
Retromandibular salivary duct, stricture	224
Rhabdomyoma, embryonal	68
Rheumatoid arthritis of temporomandibular joint	240
Rhinoliths	266
Rib grafts	191, 192

INDEX 279

	PAGE
Rickets, renal	202
Riedel's thyroiditis or struma	35
Road dirt in tissues	267
Rodent ulcer	10
Root(s) localization	19
— or tooth in soft tissues	263
Rubber base impression material	268
Rubella causing cervical node enlargement	26

SAGITTAL splitting operation for correction of mandibular deformity (*Figs.* 29G–31) 154, 163, 169
Salivary ducy calculi
 (*Figs.* 38–46) 218, 226
— — obstruction due to causes in wall 224
— — — — to compression . . 224
— — traumatic injuries to . . 224
— gland(s), actinomycosis of . . 255
— — adenocystic carcinoma of 141, 144
— — distension and infiltration, swelling due to . . . 225
— — infections, acute . . . 216
— — lesion causing mucocele . . 84
— — major . . (*Figs.* 38–42) 216–231
— — — neoplasms . (*Fig.* 42) 226, 227
— — mucoepidermoid carcinoma of 144
— — neoplasms of, biopsy . . 229
— — swellings, persistent . (*Fig.* 42) 226
— — — recurrent . . . 216
— — — — differential diagnosis . 226
— secretion, decreased, in Sjögren's syndrome 225
Salmon patch 71
Sarcoma, primary, of oral cavity . 129
— reticulum-cell, diagnosis from malignant granuloma . . 119
— treatment of 141
Scalp infection causing cervical lymphadenopathy . . . 26
Scars, inconspicuous, incisions leading to 36
Schönlein-Henoch syndrome . 53
Schwannoma 66
Second arch syndrome . . 232, 233
Sedimentation rate, red cell (E.S.R.) 15
Sela and Ulmansky, mucous retention cyst of 85
Serological tests 20
Serum calcium estimation . . 21
— — — in investigation of hyperparathyroidism . . 201
— inorganic phosphates estimation 21
Sexual precocity in fibrous dysplasia of bone 195
Sialo-adenitis, acute . . . 216
Sialo-angiectasis causing recurrent salivary gland swellings . 217
— secondary 218
Sialography 19
Sinus arrhythmia . . . 12
— exploration and fistulae . . 19
— multiple, in actinomycosis
 (*Fig.* 46) 255
Sinusitis, pain of 6, 7
Sjögren's syndrome . . . 224
Skeletal diseases . (*Figs.* 35, 36) 195–215

	PAGE
Skeletal signs and symptoms of hyperparathyroidism	200
Skin crease, incision in or parallel to	36
— edges, protection of, during operation	37
— incisions in oral surgery	36
— pigmentation in fibrous dysplasia of bone	195
Skin-graft with mandibular prosthesis in correction of receding chin	151
Skull in cleidocranial dysostosis	212
Sliding genioplasty (*Fig.* 27B) 151, 154, 155	
Sling operations in treatment of facial paralysis	247
Smoking, keratosis from	122
Socket, bleeding from extraction	44
— pack	44
Soft-tissue(s), actinomycosis of (*Fig.* 46) 255, 256	
— cysts, benign . (*Figs.* 9, 11) 81–88	
— non-pyogenic infections of	250
— radiographs	18
— repair after excision of cancer	146
— pack	
— tooth or root in	263
South American blastomycosis	259
' Speckled ' leucoplakia	123
Spider naevus . . . 71, 72, 73	
Squamous-cell carcinoma of antrum	132
— — keratinizing . (*Figs.* 18, 19) 123	
— — palliation of	145
— — of salivary gland	229
— — treatment of (*Figs.* 23, 26) 139, 141	
Stereoscopic radiographs	18
Sternomastoid tumour	32
Steroids, systemic, contra-indicated in rheumatoid arthritis of condyles	240
Still's disease affecting temporomandibular joint	240
Strawberry patch . . . 71, 73	
Stricture, salivary duct	224
Struma lymphomatosa	35
— Riedel's	35
Sturge-Weber syndrome	72
Subapical osteotomy	180
Sublingual calculi	218
— dermoid cyst	30
— gland, excision in treatment of ranula	86
Subluxation of temporomandibular joint	334
Submandibular calculi . 218, 219, 224	
— — removal of	219
— duct, retention cyst of	87
— gland excision . (*Figs.* 38, 39) 219	
— infection	216
— incisions	38
— lymph-nodes, enlarged . 25, 26	
— swelling due to dermoid cyst	83
Submental lymph-nodes, enlarged 25, 26	
— swelling due to dermoid cyst	81
Submucous fibrosis	126
— — limiting movement at temporomandibular joint	238
Subperiosteal giant-cell granuloma of jaws . . (*Fig.* 12) 91	
— osteotomy of Obwegeser	163
— resection of condyle	179

ORAL SURGERY PART II

Subsigmoid osteotomy, vertical (*Fig.* 28E) 168
'Sulphur granules' of actinomycosis 254
Supraclavicular lymph-nodes, left, carcinomatous deposits in . 33
Suprahyoid block, bilateral (*Fig.* 26) 143
Supranuclear facial paralysis . . 245
Surgical exploration of temporo-mandibular joint . . . 243
Surgicel in haemostasis . . . 41
Suturing skin incisions . . . 38
Swabs, haemostasis through pressure with 41
Sweating and flushing, gustatory . 247
Swellings of neck, differential diagnosis . . . (*Figs.* 1, 2) 24–35
— oral, with no apparent cause . 135
Symphysial alveolar osteotomy (*Fig.* 29 C) 175
Syphilis causing cervical node enlargement 28
— of soft tissues 250
— tests for 17
Syphilitic leucoplakia . . . 122
— lymphadenopathy . . . 28

Tar and road dirt in tissues . . 267
Telangiectasia, hereditary, haemorrhagic (H.H.T.) . 55, (*Fig.* 7) 71, 73
Telangiectasis 71
Temperature of patient . . . 12
Temporomandibulae joint, ankylosis of . . . . . . (*Fig.* 45) 235
— — arthritis and arthrosis of . . 239
— — causes of limited opening . 237
— — developmental disturbances . 232
— — causes of limited opening . 237
— — diseases . (*Figs.* 44, 45) 232–244
— — functional derangement . . 241
— — pain 7
— — radiography and radiology of . 243
— — surgical exploration . . . 243
— — traumatic injury to (*Figs.* 44, 45) 233
Terminal illness, management of . 145
Tetanus limiting openings of temporo-mandibular joint . . . 239
Thoma's oblique osteotomy of ramus (*Fig.* 28 G) 168
Thrombasthenia 53
Thrombocythaemia 53
Thrombocytopenia, conditions in which there is 52
— drugs, causing 53
— essential 52
Thrombocytopenic purpura, idiopathic 52
Thromboplastin 45
Thrombosis of cavernous haemangioma 73
— due to withdrawal of anticoagulant 58
Thrush, oral 257
Thyroglossal cyst 30
Thyroid gland, carcinoma of . . 25
— — enlargement(s), classification . 33
— — examination of patient . . 34
Thyroiditis, Riedel's 35
Tomography 18

Tongue, carcinoma of 10, (*Figs.* 18, 19) 123, 130, 139, 140
— dermoid cysts of . . . 81, 83
— leucoplakia of . (*Figs.* 18, 19) 123
— syphilitic lesions of . . . 250
— tuberculosis of 251
Tonsils, ectopic oral 87
Tooth (teeth) in cleidocranial dysostosis 212
— eruption, incomplete, in hemifacial microsomia 232
— extraction in haemophilia . . 49
— fragments in soft tissues following facial trauma 265
Tooth, resorption of roots, in giant-cell granuloma of jaw . . 91
— or root in soft tissues . . . 263
— sacrifice of, in ostectomy of body of mandible 162
— — in radiotherapy . . . 138
— socket, bleeding from . . . 44
Torus mandibularis 76
— palatinus 76
Toxic goitre 33, 34
Toxoplasmosis causing cervical node enlargement 27
Tracheostomy, elective . . . 193
Tranexamic acid in haemophilia . 50
Transosseous wires in immobilization of fragments 181
Tratman's odontome . . . 113
Traumatic arthritis of temporo-mandibular joint (*Figs.* 44, 45) 233
— haemangioma 74
Treacher-Collins syndrome . . 232
Trigeminal neuralgia, pain of . 6, 7
Trismus limiting opening of temporo-mandibular joint . . . 239
Tubercular swellings of neck (*Fig.* 1) 27
— ulcers 10, 11
Tuberculoma of tongue . . . 251
Tuberculosis, oral manifestations . 251
— primary oral lesion . . . 28
Tuberculous cervical lymphadenitis (*Fig.* 1) 27
— fissures of tongue 251
— papillomas of tongue . . . 251
— ulcer of tongue 251
Tuberosity, bilateral fibrous enlargement 64
Tularaemia causing cervical node enlargement 26

Ulcer (*see under specific sites*)
— examination of 10
— malignant . . . 10, 11, 135
Undercutting of wound edges . . 37
Uniform myoblastoma . . . 68
Urinary tract signs and symptoms in hyperparathyroidism . . . 201
Urine, examination of . . . 16

Vaginitis, candidal . . 257, 258
Vasoconstrictors, use of, to reduce haemorrhage 42
V.D.R.L. slide test 17
Venous engorgement following bilateral neck dissection . . 142
Verrucous carcinoma 123

INDEX

Vertical subsigmoid osteotomy in ascending ramus (*Fig.* 28E) 168
Vincent's acute ulcerative gingivitis . 44
Vitamin K and prothrombin deficiency 51, 52
Von Recklinghausen's neurofibromatosis 66
Von Willebrand's disease . . 53, 54

WARD condylotomy 242
Warthin's tumour 228
Wassermann reaction . . . 17
Wassmund's maxillary osteotomy (*Fig.* 29D) 176
— procedure to reduce prominent premaxilla . . (*Fig.* 27E) 155
Wegener's granulomatosis and malignant granuloma 118
Weight taking 13
White patches in mouth . . . 121
— — — treatment 125

White sponge naevus 121
White-cell count 14
Winstanley oblique osteotomy of ramus 169
Wiring of bone-ends in mandibular section 162, 165, 167, 168, 173, 174
— in immobilization of fragments after osteotomy . . 162, 180
Wood in soft tissues 267
Wound edges, undercutting of . . 37
Wound site, infection at, causing haemorrhage 43
Wry-neck due to sternomastoid tumour 32

Y-SHAPED osteotomy for mandibular protrusion . . (*Fig.* 29E, F) 165

ZYGOMATIC bone, fracture of, injuring infra-orbital nerve . . . 249
Zygomatico-frontal region, exposure 38